Public Mental Health

PUBLIC MENTAL HEALTH

EDITED BY WILLIAM W. EATON AND
THE FACULTY, STUDENTS, AND
FELLOWS OF THE DEPARTMENT OF MENTAL HEALTH,
BLOOMBERG SCHOOL OF PUBLIC HEALTH

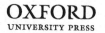

OXFORD
UNIVERSITY PRESS

OXFORD
UNIVERSITY PRESS

Oxford University Press is a department of the University of Oxford.
It furthers the University's objective of excellence in research, scholarship,
and education by publishing worldwide.

Oxford   New York
Auckland   Cape Town   Dar es Salaam   Hong Kong   Karachi
Kuala Lumpur   Madrid   Melbourne   Mexico City   Nairobi
New Delhi   Shanghai   Taipei   Toronto

With offices in
Argentina   Austria   Brazil   Chile   Czech Republic   France   Greece
Guatemala   Hungary   Italy   Japan   Poland   Portugal   Singapore
South Korea   Switzerland   Thailand   Turkey   Ukraine   Vietnam

Oxford is a registered trade mark of Oxford University Press
in the UK and certain other countries.

Published in the United States of America by
Oxford University Press
198 Madison Avenue, New York, NY 10016

© Oxford University Press 2012

First issued as an Oxford University Press paperback, 2014.

Library of Congress Cataloging-in-Publication Data
Public mental health / edited by William W. Eaton and the faculty, students,
and fellows of the Department of Mental Health,
Bloomberg School of Public Health.
p. ; cm.
Includes bibliographical references and index.
ISBN 978-0-19-539044-5 (hardcover : alk. paper); 978-0-19-021116-5 (paperback : alk. paper)
I. Eaton, William W.   II. Johns Hopkins Bloomberg
School of Public Health. Dept. of Mental Health.
[DNLM: 1.   Mental Disorders.   2.   Mental Health Services.
3.   Public Health Practice. WM 140]

616.89—dc23
2012003715

Contents

Preface

SOMETIME IN the first few years of the 20th century, Clifford Whittingham Beers, soon to be the founder of the mental hygiene movement in America, approached Adolph Meyer, the chief psychiatrist at the new Johns Hopkins University Hospital, asking for commentary on Beers's manuscript *A Mind That Found Itself*. Meyer provided the commentary and introduced Beers to William Henry Welch, the new dean of the Johns Hopkins University School of Hygiene and Public Health. The ensuing friendship and collaboration with Beers led Welch to spend more than a decade as president of the National Committee on Mental Hygiene, an organization that would later become the National Mental Health Association and eventually Mental Health America, now the nation's leading advocacy organization for mental health. The relationship with Beers also led Welch to include mental health as an integral component of the conceptual foundation of the Johns Hopkins University School of Hygiene and Public Health.

Meyer, an Austrian neurologist, had studied the brains of victims of pellagra, a form of psychosis caused by nutritional deficiency—a cause established through the epidemiologic investigations of Joseph Goldberger. When Meyer immigrated to America, he broadened his neurological approach to include a life course, psychobiological framework. This framework was carried into the School of Hygiene and Public Health in 1936 by Paul V. Lemkau, one of Meyer's last psychiatry residents. After completing classic studies in psychiatric epidemiology, Lemkau published a textbook in 1956, *Mental Hygiene and Public Health*, that expanded the targets of prevention services in public health to include both children's mental health clinics and school-based prevention services. As the only compendium of its kind on the topic, the book was read widely, was translated into 14 languages, and served as the program guide for public health departments around the world.

In 1961, Lemkau became the first chair of the Department of Mental Hygiene. In 2003, the department changed its name to the Department of Mental Health, the mission of which is "to advance understanding of mental and behavioral disorders, to develop, implement, and evaluate methods to prevent and control these disorders, and to promote mental health in the population." The Department of Mental Health is the only department-level unit in a school of public health dedicated to research and practice specifically on mental and behavioral outcomes. Now, as at its inception, the population-based life course psychobiological framework is still central to the work of the department. Fifty years after the founding of the department, 55 years after the publication of *Mental Hygiene and Public Health*, and a century after the beginning of the School of Hygiene and Public Health, this volume continues that unique historical tradition.

William W. Eaton, (Interim Chair, 2001–2004, Chair, 2004–2012)
Wallace Mandell (Interim Chair, 1993–1995)
Sheppard G. Kellam (Chair, 1982–1993)
Department of Mental Health
Bloomberg School of Public Health
Johns Hopkins University

Acknowledgments

THIS BOOK was made possible by an anonymous donation to establish the Center for Mental Health Initiatives in the Department of Mental Health, Bloomberg School of Public Health, Johns Hopkins University. The book's authors have profited enormously from the policy-writing and editorial expertise of Teddi Fine, for which the faculty are extremely grateful.

Contributors

Sharon Abramowitz, PhD
Postdoctoral Fellow, 2010–2011
Department of Mental Health
Johns Hopkins Bloomberg School of Public Health
Assistant Professor
Department of Anthropology & Center for African
    Studies
University of Florida

Deborah Agus, JD
Adjunct Assistant Professor
Department of Mental Health
Johns Hopkins Bloomberg School of Public Health
Director, Behavioral Health Leadership
    Institute, Inc.

Pierre Alexandre, PhD, MSc, MPH
Associate Professor
Department of Mental Health
Johns Hopkins Bloomberg School of Public Health

Melissa Azur, PhD
Doctoral student, 2002–2007
Department of Mental Health

Johns Hopkins Bloomberg School of Public Health
Researcher
Mathematica Policy Research

Judith K. Bass, PhD, MPH
Assistant Professor
Department of Mental Health
Johns Hopkins Bloomberg School of Public
    Health

O. Joseph Bienvenu, MD, PhD
Associate Professor (joint appointment)
Department of Mental Health
Johns Hopkins Bloomberg School of Public
    Health
Primary Appointment: Department of Psychiatry
    and Behavioral Sciences
School of Medicine
Johns Hopkins University

Catherine P. Bradshaw, PhD, MEd
Associate Professor
Department of Mental Health
Johns Hopkins Bloomberg School of Public Health

Michelle C. Carlson, PhD
Associate Professor
Department of Mental Health
Johns Hopkins Bloomberg School of Public Health

Sandy Chon, MHS
MHS student, 2008–2009
Senior Research Program Coordinator
Department of Mental Health
Johns Hopkins Bloomberg School of Public Health
Department of Medicine, School of Medicine
Johns Hopkins University

Yi-Fang Chuang, MD
Doctoral Student
Department of Mental Health
Johns Hopkins Bloomberg School
    of Public Health

Diana Clarke, MSc, PhD
Adjunct Assistant Professor
Department of Mental Health
Johns Hopkins Bloomberg School of Public Health
Research Statistician
Research Division
American Psychiatric Association

Lulu Dong, MHS
MHS student, 2008–2009
Department of Mental Health
Johns Hopkins Bloomberg School of Public Health
Graduate Student,
Department of Psychology
Emory University

William W. Eaton, PhD
Sylvia and Harold Halpert Professor and Chair
Department of Mental Health
Johns Hopkins Bloomberg School of Public Health

Dana Eldreth, PhD
Postdoctoral Fellow, 2008–2010
Department of Mental Health
Johns Hopkins Bloomberg School of Public Health
Research Neuroscientist
RTI International

Anita Everett, MD
Assistant Professor (joint appointment)
Department of Mental Health
Johns Hopkins Bloomberg School of Public Health
Primary Appointment: Department of Psychiatry
    and Behavioral Sciences
School of Medicine
Johns Hopkins Bayview Medical Center

Alden L. Gross, PhD
Doctoral Student, 2006–2011
Department of Mental Health
Johns Hopkins Bloomberg School of Public Health
Research Fellow
Hebrew SeniorLife

Ronald C. Kessler, PhD
Senior Associate
Department of Mental Health
Johns Hopkins Bloomberg School of Public Health
McNeil Family Professor of Health Care Policy
Harvard Medical School

Jean Ko, PhD
Doctoral Student, 2005–2010
Department of Mental Health
Johns Hopkins School of Public Health

S. Janet Kuramoto, PhD, MHS
Doctoral Student, 2007–2012
Department of Mental Health
Johns Hopkins Bloomberg School of Public Health
Senior Scientific Research Associate
American Psychiatric Institute for Research and
    Education/American Psychiatric Foundation

Sachiko Kuwabara, MA, PhD
Doctoral Student, 2007–2012
Department of Mental Health
Johns Hopkins Bloomberg School of Public Health

Lareina N. LaFlair, MPH
Doctoral Student
Department of Mental Health
Johns Hopkins Bloomberg School of Public Health

Phillip J. Leaf, PhD
Professor
Department of Mental Health
Johns Hopkins Bloomberg School of Public Health

Su Yeon Lee
Doctoral Student
Department of Mental Health
Johns Hopkins Bloomberg School of Public Health

Julie A. Leis, PhD
Doctoral Student, 2006–2011
Department of Mental Health
Johns Hopkins Bloomberg School of Public Health
Postdoctoral Fellow
Department of General Pediatrics and Adolescent
    Medicine
Johns Hopkins University School of Medicine

Jeannie-Marie S. Leoutsakos, PhD
Assistant Professor (joint appointment)
Department of Mental Health
Johns Hopkins Bloomberg School of Public Health
Primary Appointment: Department of Psychiatry
and Behavioral Sciences
Johns Hopkins School of Medicine
Bayview Medical Center

Brion Maher, PhD
Associate Professor
Department of Mental Health
Johns Hopkins Bloomberg School of Public Health

Wallace Mandell, PhD, MPH
Professor Emeritus
Department of Mental Health
Johns Hopkins Bloomberg School of Public Health

Ronald W. Manderscheid, PhD
Adjunct Professor
Department of Mental Health
Johns Hopkins Bloomberg School of Public Health
Executive Director
National Association of County Behavioral Health
and Developmental Disability Directors

Silvia S. Martins, MD, PhD
Associate Scientist
Department of Mental Health
Johns Hopkins Bloomberg School
of Public Health

Pallab K. Maulik, MBBS, MPH, PhD
Doctoral Student, 2005–2009
Department of Mental Health
Johns Hopkins Bloomberg School
of Public Health
Head, Research and Development
George Institute for Global Health

Paul McHugh, MD
Professor (joint appointment)
Department of Mental Health
Johns Hopkins Bloomberg School
of Public Health
Primary Appointment: Department of Psychiatry
and Behavioral Sciences
School of Medicine
Johns Hopkins University

Tamar Mendelson, PhD
Assistant Professor
Department of Mental Health
Johns Hopkins Bloomberg School
of Public Health

Ramin Mojtabai, MD, PhD, MPH
Associate Professor
Department of Mental Health
Johns Hopkins Bloomberg School
of Public Health

Preben Bo Mortensen, MD, DrMedSci
Adjunct Professor
Department of Mental Health
Johns Hopkins Bloomberg School
of Public Health
Director
National Center for Register Based Research
Aarhus University

Gerald Nestadt, MD, MPH
Professor (joint appointment)
Department of Mental Health
Johns Hopkins Bloomberg School
of Public Health
Primary Appointment: Department of Psychiatry
and Behavioral Sciences
School of Medicine
Johns Hopkins University

Atieh Novin, MHS
MHS Student, 2009–2010
Department of Mental Health
Student College of Medicine Drexel University
Johns Hopkins Bloomberg School
of Public Health

Laysha Ostrow
Doctoral Student
Department of Mental Health
Johns Hopkins Bloomberg School
of Public Health

Elise T. Pas, PhD
Assistant Scientist
Department of Mental Health
Johns Hopkins Bloomberg School
of Public Health

George W. Rebok, PhD
Professor
Department of Mental Health
Johns Hopkins Bloomberg School
of Public Health

Kimberly Roth, MHS
Research Associate
Department of Mental Health
Johns Hopkins Bloomberg School
of Public Health

Norman Sartorius, MD, PhD, MA
Senior Associate
Department of Mental Health
Johns Hopkins Bloomberg School of Public Health
President
Association for the Improvement of Health
    Programmes
Geneva, Switzerland

Shekhar Saxena, MD
Adjunct Professor
Department of Mental Health
Johns Hopkins Bloomberg School of Public Health
Director
Department of Mental Health and Substance
    Abuse
World Health Organization
Geneva, Switzerland

David L. Shern, PhD
Senior Associate
Department of Mental Health
Johns Hopkins Bloomberg School of Public Health
President and CEO
Mental Health America

Carla L. Storr, ScD, MPH
Adjunct Professor
Department of Mental Health
Johns Hopkins Bloomberg School of Public Health
Professor
Department of Family and Community Health
University of Maryland School of Nursing

Elizabeth A. Stuart, PhD
Associate Professor
Department of Mental Health
Johns Hopkins Bloomberg School of Public Health

Holly C. Wilcox, PhD
Assistant Professor (joint appointment)
Department of Mental Health
Johns Hopkins Bloomberg School of Public Health
Primary Appointment: Department of Psychiatry
    and Behavioral Sciences
School of Medicine
Johns Hopkins University

Benjamin Zablotsky
Doctoral Student
Department of Mental Health
Johns Hopkins Bloomberg School of Public Health

Peter P. Zandi, PhD, MPH, MHS
Associate Professor
Department of Mental Health
Johns Hopkins Bloomberg School of Public Health

Introduction

WILLIAM W. EATON

THERE IS an increasing awareness of the importance of mental and behavioral disorders in the field of public health. Recent years have seen the publication of two textbook-style collections of readings in psychiatric epidemiology (Susser, Schwartz, Morabia, & Bromet, 2006; Tsuang, Tohen, & Jones., 2011), a collection of readings in mental health services research (Levin, Hennessy, & Petrila, 2010), the proceedings of a conference on the public health approach to mental and behavioral disorders (Cottler, 2011), and a book on mental health of the population, focusing on policy (Cohen & Galea, 2011). This volume covers the breadth of the emerging field of public mental health more systematically than those others. An added advantage is that the authors and coauthors have a home in the Department of Mental Health of the Johns Hopkins Bloomberg School of Public Health. As faculty, postdoctoral fellows, and students, they are expressing both the orientation and

the curriculum of this unusual department, lending a degree of uniformity of conceptual framework and style that may not be found in other collections of readings.

The 18 chapters of this volume are divided into six sections. The first section, chapters 1–3, focuses on the nature of the target outcomes themselves. Chapter 1 introduces readers to the prevalence of mental and behavioral disorders and the burden of disability associated with them. The chapter focuses on 17 of the most important disorders, choosing them to represent the several hundred disorders whose precise descriptions are found in the *Diagnostic and Statistical Manual of Mental Disorders* (DSM) (American Psychiatric Association, 1994) and in chapter 5 of the International Classification of Diseases (World Health Organization, 1993) which focuses on mental disorders. The choices of outcomes in this chapter reflect the importance of the disorders as well as their ability to exemplify important aspects of mental and behavioral disorders in general. The chapter includes diagnostic criteria for 6 of the 15 disorders. Chapter 2 presents an antidote to the theoretical agnosticism of the DSM in a critique and commentary by Paul McHugh, whose widely read textbook *The Perspectives of Psychiatry* (McHugh & Slavney, 1998) is used in the introductory course in the Hopkins department of mental health. Chapter 3 presents yet another antidote to the shallow taxonomy of the DSM in exploring the relationship of culture to psychopathology, the possibility that unique mental syndromes exist in different cultures, and the problems inherent in public health research around the world if it is assumed that the DSM syndromes are universal and exhaustive.

The second section consists of two chapters that focus on methodologies for gathering and analyzing data necessary for understanding the public health approach to mental and behavioral disorders. Chapter 4 deals with the measurement of psychopathology, with an emphasis on population-based life course approaches. Assessment of mental and behavioral disorders is more difficult than measurement in many areas of medicine, because of the lack of simple and valid biological markers for the presence of mental and behavioral disorders. In effect, the measurement must always involve talking to individuals or observing their behaviors in ways that can be described to others and replicated by them if necessary, consistent with the scientific method. Chapter 5 addresses several unusual quantitative methodologies that have arisen in psychiatry and public health or are in use by researchers and practitioners in public mental health.

Section three consists of two chapters about the descriptive epidemiology of the mental and behavioral disorders. Chapter 6 estimates rates of incidence of specific disorders and charts them for each sex across the life span, consistent with the life course epidemiological approach, which is highly useful to psychiatric epidemiology. It also considers the natural history of the mental and behavioral disorders, including both the considerable degree of comorbidity they exhibit over the life course and their effects on mortality. Chapter 7 considers the relationship between the prevalences of mental and behavioral disorders and commonly used demographic descriptors of individuals such as education, marital status, race/ethnicity, and urbanicity of residence.

The fourth section of the book, chapters 8–11, explores mechanisms of risk; two chapters focus on so-called biological risk and two on social-psychological risk. Chapter 8 reviews the genetics of mental and behavioral disorders. Chapter 9 considers the relationship of disorders to brain function. Chapter 10 reviews the relationship of stresses throughout the life course in the general population to risk for episodes of disorder. Chapter 11 examines the special situation of traumatic stress and its effect on risk for disorders.

The volume's fifth section, five chapters in all, explores the behavioral health service system. Chapter 12 discusses mental and behavioral disorders in the context of the legal system. Chapter 13 presents an overview of the mental health service system in the United States. Chapter 14 discusses the existing systems of services provided in community behavioral care in the United States. Chapter 15 examines pathways to the service system and the effects of stigma on both access to and utilization of mental health services. Chapter 16 gives an overview of the wide range in capacity and availability of mental health services around the globe.

The concluding section begins with chapter 17, on prevention of mental and behavioral disorders, reviewing both the history of successful prevention strategies for mental and behavioral disorders and an array of techniques with proven efficacy that have not been adequately disseminated. Chapter 18 provides an overview of what can be done in the future to address the the prevention and control of mental and behavioral disorders.

Public Mental Health is intended as an introduction to population-based research on mental and behavioral disorders and a guide and reference for public health departments around the world. This work, with others, should reinforce the importance of mental and behavioral disorders in the public health framework.

References

American Psychiatric Association. (1994). *Diagnostic and Statistical Manual of Mental Disorders* (4th ed.) Washington, DC: Author.

Cohen, N., & Galea, S. (2011). *Population mental health: Evidence, policy and public health practice.* New York, NY: Routledge.

Cottler, L. (2011). *Mental health in public health.* New York, NY: Oxford University Press.

Levin, B. L., Hennessy, K. D., & Petrila, J. (2010). *Mental health services: A public health perspective.* New York, NY: Oxford University Press.

McHugh, P. R., & Slavney, P. R. (1998). *The perspectives of psychiatry* (2nd ed.). Baltimore, MD: Johns Hopkins University Press.

Susser, E., Schwartz, S., Morabia, A., & Bromet, E. J. (2006). *Psychiatric epidemiology.* New York, NY: Oxford University Press.

Tsuang, M., Tohen, M., & Jones, P. (2011). *Textbook in psychiatric epidemiology* (3rd ed.). New York, NY: John Wiley & Sons.

World Health Organization. (1993). *ICD-10 classification of mental and behavioral disorders—diagnostic criteria for research.* Geneva, Switzerland: Author.

Public Mental Health

SECTION I

The Nature of Mental and Behavioral Disorders

1

The Burden of Mental Disorders

WILLIAM W. EATON

PIERRE ALEXANDRE

O. JOSEPH BIENVENU

DIANA CLARKE

SILVIA S. MARTINS

GERALD NESTADT

BENJAMIN ZABLOTSKY

Key Points

- A systematic review shows the prevalences of 17 mental disorders

- Five disorders (simple phobia, major depressive disorder, alcohol abuse or dependence, personality disorders, and dementia) have prevalences of over 4% in the general population

- Estimates of severity of and impairment due to the 17 mental disorders display a range of individual burdens

- Six disorders (autism, major depressive disorder, personality disorders, schizophrenia, bipolar disorder, and dementia) have disability weights higher than 0.35

- New methods for estimating disease burden in the population reveal the importance of mental disorders

- Neuropsychiatric disorders produce more population disease burden in the developed world than any other category of disease, second only to the category of infectious and parasitic diseases in the world as a whole

INTRODUCTION

One of the first challenges when building epidemiologic knowledge about a disorder, disease, or condition is to establish its immediate, short-term, and long-term impact on life, health, and disability, a concept known as its health-related burden. Until the 1980s the epidemiology of mental disorders lagged far behind other areas of health care because of disagreements about diagnostic thresholds for specific mental disorders (Morris, 1975) and an overall dearth of reliable assessments (Helzer, Clayton, et al., 1977; Helzer, Robins, et al., 1977) and of measures of prevalence and incidence of disorders (President's Commission on Mental Health, 1978). Then, in 1980, the explicit diagnostic criteria in the third edition of the *Diagnostic and Statistical Manual of Mental Disorders* (DSM-III) (American Psychiatric Association [APA], 1980) provided the foundation for the population measurement of mental disorders—the so-called third generation of psychiatric epidemiology (Dohrenwend & Dohrenwend, 1982)— that began with the establishment of the NIMH Epidemiologic Catchment Area program (Eaton, Regier, Locke, & Taube, 1981; Regier et al., 1984; Robins & Regier, 1991) and continues to this day.

The slow growth of epidemiologic knowledge in behavioral health was amplified by the fact that population trends in acute diseases have been technically easier to describe than have trends in chronic or other nonfatal disorders such as mental illnesses. This picture of slow growth in the field was markedly altered with the Global Burden of Disease (GBD) study (Murray & Lopez, 1996). Whereas prior work had measured the burden of disease using traditional measures of mortality, the GBD study incorporated illness-related disability into an overall measure of disease burden with the concept of the disability-adjusted life year (DALY), described in more detail below. The ability to combine measures of burden from nonfatal, impairing conditions with those of conditions causing death disclosed the profound impact mental disorders have on the burden of illnesses worldwide.

The GBD study found that in 1990 mental disorders, as a broad category, were responsible for 21% of the total disease burden in the world; only infectious and parasitic diseases (41%) and cardiovascular diseases (26%) were more damaging. In the study's latest update (World Health Organization [WHO], 2008), infectious and parasitic diseases accounted for 19.8% of all the DALYs in the world, followed by neuropsychiatric disorders, which accounted for 13.1% (figure 1-1). There are several strictly neurologic conditions in the category of neuropsychiatric disorders, such as epilepsy (0.5% of all DALYs), of all DALYS multiple sclerosis (0.1%), and Parkinson's disease (0.1%), but the category is dominated by psychiatric conditions, notably unipolar depressive disorder (4.3%), alcohol use disorders (1.6%), self-inflicted injuries (1.3%), schizophrenia (1.1%), bipolar disorder (0.9%), Alzheimer's disease (0.7%), drug use disorders (0.5%), panic disorder (0.5%), obsessive-compulsive disorder (0.3%) and posttraumatic stress disorder (0.2%). Figure 1-2 shows the 24 most important specific causes of DALYs in the world, among which four are mental or behavioral disorders—only lower respiratory infections and diarrheal conditions are more important than unipolar depressive disorder. In high-income countries the category of neuropsychiatric conditions is the leading cause of DALYs, accounting for 18.3%, ahead of cardiovascular diseases (17.4%) and malignant neoplasms (17.3%).

This chapter briefly describes the features of 17 major mental disorders and summarizes current data on the burden of disease associated with each. Key diagnostic features of six selected disorders, presented in abbreviated form in text boxes throughout the chapter, are based on the fourth edition of the *Diagnostic and Statistical Manual of Mental Disorders* (DSM-IV) (APA, 1994). For details of the other disorders the reader is referred to the DSM-IV itself.

This review expands upon the range of mental disorders considered in the GBD study, updates the literature, and provides information on the range and depth of sources of information on burden. Because the available literature on burden of disease is insufficiently robust to sustain a formal meta-analysis (Fryers et al., 2004), this chapter presents summary measures associated

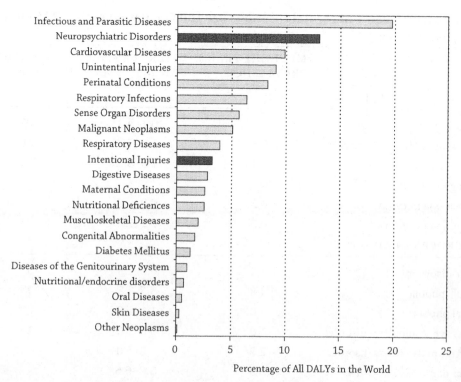

FIGURE 1-1 **Disability-Adjusted Life Years by Category in the World, 2004.**

Source: World Health Organization, 2008.

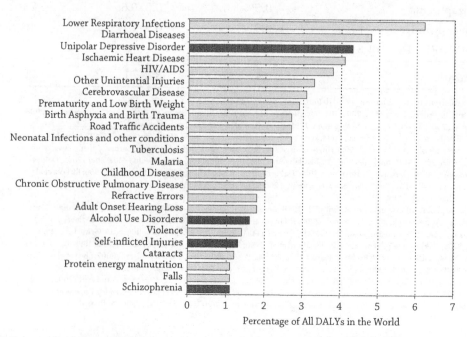

FIGURE 1-2 **Disability-Adjusted Life Years by Specific Cause in the World, 2004.**

Source: World Health Organization, 2008.

Table 1-1. Prevalence of Mental Disorders per 100 Population in the 12 Months Prior to Interview[a]

	MEDIAN 1-YEAR PREVALENCE	INTERQUARTILE RANGE	NO. OF STUDIES INCLUDED
DISORDERS IN CHILDREN			
Autistic disorder[a]	0.2	0.1–0.2	10
Attention deficit hyperactivity[a]	2.6	1.8–7.0	21
Conduct disorder[a]	2.1	1.5–3.3	18
Eating disorders[a]			
Anorexia nervosa	0.3	0.2–0.3	4
Bulimia nervosa	0.3	0.1–1.1	4
DISORDERS IN ADULTS			
Panic disorder	0.9	0.6–1.9	33
Simple phobia	4.8	3.5–7.3	25
Social phobia	2.8	1.1–5.8	30
Obsessive–compulsive disorder	1.0	0.6–2.0	19
Posttraumatic stress disorder	2.2	1.2–5.0	4
Major depressive disorder	5.3	3.6–6.5	42
Drug abuse/dependence	1.8	1.1–2.7	11
Alcohol abuse/dependence	5.9	5.2–8.1	14
Personality disorders	9.1	9.0–14.4	5
Schizophrenia	0.5	0.3–0.6	23
Bipolar disorder	0.6	0.3–1.1	16
DISORDERS IN THE ELDERLY			
Dementia	5.4	3.2–7.1	25

[a]Exceptions to the 12-month period definition are described in the text.

Panic disorder: Alonso et al., 2004; Bijl, Ravelli & van Zessen, 1998; Bland, Newman, & Orn, 1988; Bromet et al., 2008; Cho et al., 2007; Eaton, Dryman, & Weissman, 1991; Faravelli et al., 1997; Girolamo, Morosini, Gigantesco, & Kessler, 2008; Grant et al., 2006; Gureje et al., 2008; Haro et al., 2008; Huang et al., 2008; Hwu, Yeh, & Chang, 1989; Jacobi et al., 2004; Kessler et al., 1994, 2005; Kringlen, Torgersen, & Cramer, 2001, 2006; Levinson, Lerner, Zilber, Levav, & Polakiewicz, 2008; McConnell, Bebbington, McClelland, Gillespie, & Houghton, 2002; Medina-Mora et al., 2005; Oakley-Brown, Joyce, Wells, Bushnell, & Hornblow, 1989; Oakley-Brown, Wells, & Scott, 2008; Offord et al., 1996; Pirkola et al., 2005; Posada-Villa et al., 2008; Sanderson & Andrews, 2002; Shen et al., 2006; Vicente et al., 2006; Wells et al., 2006; D. R. Williams et al., 2008.

Social phobia: Alonso et al., 2004; Bijl et al., 1998; Bromet et al., 2008; Cho et al., 2007; Girolamo et al., 2008; Grant et al., 2005; Gureje et al., 2008; Haro et al., 2008; Huang et al., 2008; Jette, Patten, Williams, Becker, & Wiebe, 2008; Kawakami et al., 2005; Kessler et al., 1994, 2005; Kringlen et al., 2001, 2006; Lepine & Lellouch, 1995; Medina-Mora et al., 2005; Oakley-Browne et al., 1989, 2008; Offord et al., 1996; Pakriev, Vasar, Aluoja, Saarma, & Shlik, 1998; Pirkola et al., 2005; Posada-Villa et al., 2008; Rocha, Vorcaro, Uchoa, & Lima-Costa, 2005; Sanderson & Andrews, 2002; Shen et al., 2006; Stein, Walker, & Torgrud, 2000; Vicente et al., 2006; Wells et al., 2006; D. R. Williams et al., 2008.

Simple phobia: Alonso et al., 2004; Bijl et al., 1998; Cho et al., 2007; Faravelli et al., 1997; Kawakami et al., 2005; Kessler et al., 1994, 2005; Kringlen et al., 2001, 2006; McConnell et al., 2002; Medina-Mora et al., 2005; Oakley-Browne et al., 1989; Offord et al., 1996; Pakriev et al., 1998; Shen et al., 2006; Stinson et al., 2007; Vicente et al., 2006; Wells et al., 2006.

Table 1-1. (continued)

Sources cited below are those not included in the reviews cited in the text:

Autistic Disorder: Chakrabarti & Fombonne, 2001; Ellefson, Kampmann, Billstedt, Gillberg, & Gillber, Parner, Schendel, & Thorsen, 2008.

Attention Deficit Hyperactivity Disorder: Costello et al., 1996; Roberts, Roberts, & Xing, 1999; Srinath e Zwirs et al., 2007.

Conduct Disorder: Studies cited above for Attention Deficit Disorder, and Bird et al., 2001.

Eating Disorders: Morande, Celada, & Casas, 1999; Pelaez Fernandez, Labrador, & Raich, 2007; Rojo et al., 1

Major depressive disorder: Ahola et al., 2005; Amoran, Lawoyin, & Lasebikan, 2007; Andrews, Henderson, & 2001; Beals et al., 2005; Bijl et al., 1998; Bland, Newman, & Orn, 1988; Bourdon, Rae, Locke, Narrow, & Regier, 1992; Bromet et al., 2008; Compton, Conway, Stinson, & Grant, 2006; Faravelli, Guerrini, Aiazzi, Incerpi, & Pallanti, 1990; Girolamo et al., 2008; Gureje et al., 2008; Haro et al., 2008; Hasin, Goodwin, Stinson, & Grant, 2005; Huang et al., 2008; Hwang & Myers, 2007; Hwu et al., 1989; Karam et al., 2008; Kessler et al., 1994, 2003; S. Lee et al., 2007; Levinson et al., 2008; McConnell et al., 2002; Medina-Mora et al., 2005; Oakley-Browne et al., 1989, 2008; Offord et al., 1996; Ohayon & Hong, 2006; Posada-Villa et al., 2008; Shen et al., 2006; Slone et al., 2006; Szadoczky, Papp, Vitrai, Rihmer, & Furedi, 1998; Vicente et al., 2006; Vorcaro, Lima-Costa, Barreto, & Uchoa, 2001; Wang, 2004; D. R. Williams et al., 2007, 2008.

Obsessive–compulsive disorder: Andrade, Walters, Gentil, & Laurenti, 2002; Andrews et al., 2001; Bijl et al., 1998; Bland, Newman, & Orn, 1988; Canino et al., 1987; Chen et al., 1993; Cillicilli et al., 2004; Degonda, Wyss, & Angst, 1993; Faravelli et al., 1997; Ford et al., 2007; Grabe et al., 2000; Hwu et al., 1989; Jenkins et al., 1997; Kessler et al., 2005; C. K. Lee et al., 1990; Mohammadi et al., 2004; Stefansson, Lindal, Bjornsson, & Guomundsdottir, 1991; Weissman, Myers, & Harding, 1978.

Drug abuse/dependence: Andrews et al., 2001; Bijl et al., 1998; Bourdon et al., 1992; Grant, 1996; Grant, Stinson, et al., 2004; Jacobi et al., 2004; Kessler et al., 1994, 2005; Kringlen et al., 2001; Medina-Mora et al., 2006; Substance Abuse and Mental Health Services Administration, 2007.

Alcohol abuse/dependence: Andrews et al., 2001; Bijl et al., 1998; Bourdon et al., 1992; Bromet et al., 2005; Grant, 1996; Grant, Dawson, et al., 2004; Harford, Grant, Yi, & Chen, 2005; Jacobi et al., 2004; Kessler et al., 1994, 2005; Kringlen et al., 2001; Neumark, Lopez-Quintero, Grinshpoon, & Levinson, 2007; Ogborne & DeWit, 2001; Substance Abuse and Mental Health Services Administration, 2007.

Personality disorders: Coid, Yang, Tyrer, Roberts, & Ullrich, 2006; Grant, Hasin, et al., 2004; Lenzenweger, Lane, Loranger, & Kessler, 2007; Samuels et al., 2002; Torgersen, Kringlen, & Cramer, 2001.

Schizophrenia: McGrath et al., 2008.

Bipolar disorder: Bland, Newman, & Orn, 1988; Bourdon et al., 1992; Faravelli et al., 1990; Hwu et al., 1989; Kessler et al., 1994; Levinson et al., 2008; McConnell et al., 2002; Merikangas et al., 2007; Oakley-Browne et al., 1989, 2008; Offord et al., 1996; Pakriev et al., 1998; Bijl, Ravelli, & van Zessen, 1998; Szadoczky et al., 1998.

Dementia: Bachman et al., 1992; Ben-Arie, Swartz, Teggin, & Elk, 1983; Breitner et al., 1999; Chandra et al., 1998; deSilva, Gunatilake, & Smith, 2003; Ebly, Parhad, Hogan, & Fung, 1994; Farrag, Farwiz, Khedr, Mahfouz, & Omran, 1998; Fillenbaum et al., 1998; Graves et al., 1996; Hendrie et al., 1995; Herrera, Caramelli, Silveira, & Nitrini, 2002; Kim, Jeong, Chun, & Lee, 2003; Kiyohara et al., 1994; Kua, 1991; D. Y. Lee et al., 2002; Lobo et al., 2000; Ogura et al., 1995; Phanthumchindra, Jitapunkul, Sitthi-Amorn, Bunnag, & Ebrahim, 1991; Rajkumar, Kumar, & Thara, 1997; Senanarong et al., 2001; Shaji, Promodu, Abraham, Roy, & Verghese, 1996; Suh, Kim, & Cho, 2003; Vas et al., 2001; Woo et al., 1998.

with the individual disorders, including estimates of prevalence (table 1-1) and disabilities (table 1-2). To the extent possible, the chapter builds on existing reviews that most often focused on a single disorder. The examination of prevalence for each disorder presents essential summary data, including the number of studies conducted, the median prevalence or relative risk, and the interquartile range. Data on mortality, use of services, and costs are presented elsewhere in this volume.

METHODS

One-year prevalence is the most common form of prevalence reported in studies of the 17 mental disorders considered in this chapter (see table 1-1). One-year prevalence is a hybrid between lifetime prevalence and point prevalence, recording the history of a disorder within the 12-month period prior to the assessment (Eaton et al., 1985). It differs from lifetime prevalence by focusing solely on a single-year period; it differs from period prevalence because members of the study population who entered during the study period but died before assessment are not included in the numerator of the prevalence rate. Since the vast majority of these disorders typically endure for a year or more, 1-year prevalence is not too different from the point prevalence. While limiting this review to 1-year prevalence helps reduce variation due to differences in reporting period, it also results in the exclusion of many studies because they reported either lifetime or point prevalence rates. Point and lifetime prevalence rates were considered for some disorders in childhood, as described

2. Disability Associated with Mental Disorders

	GBD DISABILITY WEIGHT[a]	CPES PERCENT SEVERE SHEEHAN DISABILITY[b]
DISORDERS IN CHILDREN		
Autism	0.55[c]	NA
Attention deficit hyperactivity disorder	0.15[d]	NA
Conduct disorder	NA	NA
Eating disorders	0.28[c]	NA
DISORDERS IN ADULTS		
Panic disorder	0.17	47
Social phobia	NA	36
Simple phobia	NA	19
Obsessive–compulsive disorder	0.13	47
Posttraumatic stress disorder	0.11	NA
Major depression	0.35[e]	58
Drug abuse/dependence	0.25	39[f]
Alcohol abuse/dependence	0.16[e]	14[f]
Personality disorders	0.54[g]	NA
Schizophrenia	0.53[e]	NA
Bipolar disorder	0.40[e]	83
DISORDERS IN THE ELDERLY		
Dementia	0.7	NA

GBD = Global Burden of Disease study; CPES = Collaborative Psychiatric Epidemiologic Surveys; NA = not available.

[a]Except as indicated, disability weights are from Murray and Lopez, 1996, annex table 3, untreated form, age group 15–44.

[b]Percentage with marked or extremely severe impairment in Sheehan Disability Scale (SDS), as employed in the CPES. The SDS estimate for bipolar disorder was based on the most severe SDS rating for depression and mania. Bipolar disorder and its SDS estimate were present in the National Comorbidity Survey Replication and National Survey of American Life components of the CPES. Obsessive–compulsive disorder and simple phobia and their SDS estimates were present only in the National Comorbidity Survey Replication component of the CPES.

[c]Dutch weights from Vos and Mathers, 2000, table 3.

[d]Top of range of Dutch weights reported by Vos and Mathers, 2000, for mild and moderate impairment.

[e]Disability weights from Mathers, Lopez, and Murray, 2006; depression is moderate level.

[f]Dependence only.

[g]Locally derived weight for borderline personality disorder from Vos and Mathers, 2000.

below, for which there were few or no data on 1-year prevalence (see table 1-1). Only studies of the general population, rather than individuals in treatment settings, were included in the review of prevalence, since a large proportion of individuals with mental disorders never end up in treatment. Except where noted for individuals with schizophrenia and autism, studies of samples drawn from clinics or from the records of health maintenance organizations were excluded. To enhance the statistical stability of the findings, the studies' sample sizes needed to be larger than 500; to minimize response bias, studies with response rates of less than 60% were also excluded. Also excluded were studies that focused on specific demographic groups or populations (e.g., defined by narrow age ranges, gender, migrant status, or socioeconomic status) and studies of populations with a particular condition (e.g., only persons with a history of schizophrenia or with a history of stroke). In contrast, population-based studies of one ethnic group or one national group were included as long as they fit within the definition of general population. In studies reporting data from more than one ethnic group and from all groups combined, the rate for the combined group was reported or computed if possible; otherwise rates for specific ethnic groups were reported as if the data had been gathered in separate studies. When genders were reported separately along with sample numbers for each, the rate for the combined total was estimated and reported.

This review focuses solely on mental disorders that meet specific diagnostic criteria as assessed using structured or semistructured diagnostically oriented interviews, undertaken in person or by telephone. Chapter 4 describes the measurement characteristics of these methods. Reported study diagnoses had to match exactly the named diagnoses; thus in the case of major depressive disorder, for example, studies reporting groups of disorders such as depressive disorders or mood disorders were excluded. Two-stage studies were included when the second stage yielded a specific diagnosis. In studies reporting both a diagnosis according to the DSM-III, revised DSM-III (DSM-III-R), or DSM-IV (APA, 1980, 1987, 1994) and a diagnosis according to the 8th, 9th, or 10th revision of the International Classification of Disease (ICD) (WHO, 1967, 1977, 1993), the prevalence rate associated with the DSM diagnosis was used. These constraints resulted in the exclusion of a significant number of studies.

Measures of disability were based on estimates of the GBD study (Murray & Lopez, 1996), as well as estimates from both the Collaborative Psychiatric Epidemiology Surveys (CPES, described below) (Alegria, Jackson, Kessler, & Takeuchi, 2008) and the Canadian Community Health Survey (Statistics Canada, 2008). Disability is a general term for decline in functioning and is distinct from both impairment and handicap (WHO, 1980, 2001). An impairment is an abnormality of structure or function due to a disease or condition and is somewhat more difficult to define for mental disorders than physical conditions. For example, production of insulin is impaired in diabetes, cognitive ability is impaired while an individual is intoxicated,

but the precise impairment of structure or function is harder to specify for anxiety disorders such as panic disorder. In diabetes the impairment can produce ketoacidosis, bringing on a decline in functioning—that is, a disability—with fatigue, slurred speech, stupor, and even coma. This decline in function closely resembles alcoholic intoxication. Use of insulin by the diabetic can produce hypoglycemic episodes, not too different from panic attacks, with arousal, irritability, heart racing, sweating, and trembling. Although panic attacks and hypoglycemic episodes are distressing, a decline in functioning is less obvious, and individual variations in compensating factors may lead the same impairment to be more disabling in one person than in another. A handicap results from a disability when the society treats the individual differently and disadvantageously, as when diabetics and alcoholics are deprived of their right to drive an automobile. The focus of what follows is on disabilities associated with mental disorders.

The disability weights used in the GBD study were developed through a consensus process in which experts rates symptomatic and behavioral vignettes. The raters were asked to make choices comparing prevention programs that would extend life for a healthy person (e.g., a program that would extend life for a healthy person by one year) with prevention programs that would extend life for a person with a disabling health condition (say, for two years). Ratings ranged from 0.0 (no disability during a given single year) to 1.0 (death). Higher intermediary values indicated more disability and, consequently, a lower quality of life. A value of 0.5 indicates the individual would have the same quality of life for two years as a completely healthy individual with a value of 0.0 would experience in one year. These ratings enable comparison of population aspects of the burden of both fatal and nonfatal conditions. Thus, for example, for quadriplegia the severity rating is 0.90; for blindness, 0.62; for multiple sclerosis, 0.41; for deafness, 0.33; for rheumatoid arthritis, 0.21; and for watery diarrhea, 0.07 (Murray & Lopez, 1996). Ratings for adult psychiatric conditions reported in table 1-2 are from the GBD study or its later replication (Lopez, Mathers, Ezzati, Jamison, & Murray, 2006). For childhood conditions the ratings in table 1-2 are from a Dutch study that used similar methodology (Vos and Mathers, 2000).

The CPES (Alegria et al., 2008) data set combines three surveys, each with representative samples of adult populations in the United States: (1) the National Comorbidity Survey Replication, which includes the entire adult population (Kessler, Chiu, Demler, Merikangas, & Walters, 2005); (2) the National Survey of American Life, which focuses on the African American population (Jackson et al., 2004); and (3) the National Latino and Asian American Survey, which focuses on the Latino American and Asian American populations (Alegria et al., 2004).

The combined sample size for the CPES is 20,130; each of the component national surveys individually met this review's eligibility criteria. The CPES surveys used the Sheehan Disability Scale (SDS) (Sheehan, Harnett-Sheehan, & Raj, 1996) to assess disability resulting from many of the disorders addressed in this review (see table 1-2). The SDS is a brief, self-report measure that assesses functional impairments on a 10-point discretized analog scale (0 = no disability; 1–3 = mild disability; 4–6 = moderate disability, 7–9 = marked disability, and 10 = extreme disability). It was designed for clinical trials and has been used in hundreds of research studies and translated into 48 languages (Sheehan, 2008).

The SDS was used in the CPES's separate disorder-related sections, with separate questions relating to the extent to which each of four areas of functioning—work, household, relationship, and social roles—was impaired in the worst month of the past year for the problems associated with the given disorder (Kessler et al., 2003). In the current analysis, the threshold of disability was based on a rating of marked to extreme disability (i.e., an SDS value of 7 or higher) and reports the percentage of individuals meeting criteria for a given disorder and marked to extreme disability on one or more of the four SDS role domains. This reporting method makes it possible to multiply the percentage of individuals with this level of disability by the median prevalence to obtain an estimate of the prevalence in the population of people with the most severe disability. This advantage is important because there is typically a wide range of impairment and disability in the population of individuals with a given disorder.

The CPES did not include SDS data for alcohol or drug disorders; these measures of disability were available from the Canadian Community Health Survey. That survey's cycle 1.2, a probability sample of 36,984 community-dwelling respondents representative of the population of Canada over 15 years of age, had a special focus on mental health and well-being (Statistics Canada, 2008). Substance-related diagnoses in that survey were limited to alcohol or drug dependence, including cases with physiological dependence, with evidence of tolerance or withdrawal, or without physiological dependence (APA, 1994).

To the extent possible, tables 1-1 and 1–2 were based on prior systematic reviews identified using the PubMed bibliographic retrieval system. To cast the widest net possible, the search terms for each disorder varied, but they always included the terms *population* and *prevalence* and the specific disorder. For example, based on the foregoing search terms, the review of depressive disorder began with the article by Waraich, Goldner, Somers, and Hsu (2004), which reported on population-based studies of 1-year prevalence using standardized, diagnostically oriented assessments published from 1980 through 2000. Studies appearing after the reviews cited in the tables are included in the references to this chapter.

Important disorders of children include autistic disorder, attention deficit hyperactivity disorder (ADHD), conduct disorder, and eating disorders. There is some difficulty in collecting the prevalence rates for these disorders, because the age distributions of the studies included vary somewhat. Similarly, the prevalence period under consideration varies from study to study, from lifetime prevalence to various hybrids of period prevalence to point prevalence. Although the age range (children and adolescents) is more limited than the entire span of adulthood, these differences influence the rates presented in ways that are difficult to interpret. There were no strong prior reviews of these disorders.

ASSESSING THE BURDEN

Autistic Disorder

Autistic disorder is characterized by the presence of social deficits, language abnormalities, and stereotyped and repetitive behaviors prior to 3 years of age (APA, 1994). (See Diagnostic Criteria 1-1.) This review of autistic disorder adds three studies to the review by Fombonne (2003), while deeming 8 of the 32 studies included in the Fombonne review appropriate to our selection criteria. The current review also relied on the literature review of J. G. Williams, Higgins, and Brayne (2006), who noted 37 studies after searching MEDLINE from 1966 to 2001 for epidemiologic data on

---

Diagnostic Criteria 1-1. Diagnostic Criteria for 299.00 Autistic Disorder

A. A total of six (or more) items from (1), (2) and (3) with at least two from (1), and one each from (1), and one each from (2) and (3):
  (1) Qualitative impairment in social interaction, as manifested by at least two of the following:
    (a) Marked impairment in the use of multiple nonverbal behaviors such as eye-to-eye gaze, facial expression, body postures and gestures to regulate social interaction.
    (b) Failure to develop peer relationships appropriate to development level.
    (c) a lack of spontaneous seeking to share enjoyment, interests or achievements with other people (e.g., by a lack of showing, bringing, or pointing out objects of interest).
    (d) Lack of social or emotional reciprocity.
  (2) Qualitative impairments in communication as manifested by at least one of the following:
    (a) Delay in a total lack of, the development of spoken language(not accompanied by an attempt to compensate through alternative modes of communication such as gesture or mime)
    (b) In individuals with adequate speech, marked impairment in the ability to initiate or sustain a conversation with others
    (c) Stereotyped and repetitive use of language or idiosyncratic language
    (d) Lack of varied, spontaneous make believe play or social imitative play appropriate to developmental level
  (3) Restricted repetitive and stereotyped patterns of behavior, interests, and activities , as manifested by at least one of the Following:
    (a) Encompassing preoccupation with one or more stereotyped and restricted patterns of interest that is abnormal either in intensity or focus
    (b) Apparently inflexible adherence to specific, nonfunctional routines and rituals
    (c) Stereotyped and repetitive motor mannerisms (e.g., hand or finger flapping or twisting or complex whole–body movements)
    (d) Persistent preoccupation with parts of objects
B. Delays or abnormal functioning in at least one of the following areas, with onset prior to age 3 years: (1) social interaction (2) language as used in social communication, or (3) symbolic imaginative play.
C. The disturbance is not better accounted for by Rett's Disorder or Childhood Disintegrative Disorder.

Source: Reprinted with permission from the *Diagnostic and Statistical Manual of Mental Disorders, Fourth Edition, Text Revision*, (Copyright ©2000). American Psychiatric Association.

autism. Including the Williams review sources and the current review, there were 10 studies, from two continents, with prevalence estimates ranging from 4.5 cases per 10,000 in Norway in 1998 to 60 cases per 10,000 in Sweden the following year, with a median of 18.95 and an interquartile range of 12.20–22.00 cases per 10,000. Data have been converted to estimates per 100 population for presentation in table 1-1.

Autism is a severe disorder for which it is not possible to obtain a self-rating of disability using the SDS, even in the case of autistic adults. Since the clinical scales used to determine the disorder's presence were based on collecting lifetime history, generally from parents, prevalence rates were generally listed as lifetime. The GBD disability weight for autism is 0.55, comparable to that for schizophrenia and not too different from those for blindness and multiple sclerosis. This level of disability shows the considerable impact of autism on an individual's functioning and the need for a high level of care by parents and others. In the most recent edition of the DSM (APA, 1994), the diagnosis of Asperger's syndrome has been added—an illness of lesser impairment considered to be within the autism spectrum.

Attention Deficit Hyperactivity Disorder

Attention deficit hyperactivity disorder is characterized by a persistent pattern of inattentiveness, hyperactivity, or both in a child prior to the age of 7 years. Significant impairment is necessary in two or more settings to satisfy diagnostic criteria (APA, 1994). This review of ADHD builds on the work of Polanczyk and Jensen (2008), who presented 71 ADHD-related prevalence studies between 1997 and 2007, of which 17 were included in the review. Four additional studies were included, one from before the review and three from after the review. Together, the included studies contain estimates from all six populated continents. Because screening questions require a parent to evaluate a child's development over time, 3-month, 6-month, 1-year, and lifetime prevalence rates were accepted in the review presented here. Prevalence rates

ranged from 0.46 cases per 100 in the United Arab Emirates in 1998 to 11.2 cases per 100 in Australia in 2003, with a median of 2.60 and an interquartile range of 1.80–7.00 per 100 across all 21 studies in the review. Under the GBD system, the level of disability ranges widely, with a rating of 0.15 for moderate ADHD (see table 1-2).

Conduct Disorder

Conduct disorder is characterized by a repetitive and persistent pattern of behaviors that violate societal norms and display a disregard for the basic rights of others. Onset can be either in childhood or in adolescence. Typical behaviors include aggressive conduct, deceitfulness, theft, and serious violations of rules. There was no appropriate prior review, but 18 studies meeting the criteria of this review were located, of which only one (Bird et al., 2001) was independent from the studies identified for the review of ADHD discussed above. As with ADHD, prevalence rates accepted in the review presented here included 3-month, 6-month, 1-year, and lifetime rates. Prevalence rates ranged from 0.2 per 100 in India in 2005 to 5.8 per 100 in the United States and Puerto Rico, with a median of 2.1 and an interquartile range of 1.5–3.3. Although this disorder is important and not rare, neither the GBD nor the CPES provides measures of disability for conduct disorder.

Eating Disorders

Anorexia nervosa and bulimia nervosa constitute the two major eating disorders. Individuals with either disorder are preoccupied with body shape and weight. (See Diagnostic Criteria 1-2.) Typical symptoms of the former include a fear of gaining weight, a misperception about one's own body, and an unwillingness to attempt to maintain healthy body weight. Bulimia nervosa is characterized by binge eating and compensatory methods to subsequently prevent weight gain (e.g., purging). Only five epidemiologic studies meeting the methodological criteria were located, and therefore this review includes all prevalence periods. Studies were excluded if they did not differentiate between anorexia nervosa and bulimia nervosa. The

Diagnostic Criteria 1-2. Diagnostic Criteria for 307.1 Anorexia Nervosa

A. Refusal to maintain body weight at or above a minimally normal weight for age and height (e.g., weight loss leading to maintenance of body weight less than 85% of that expected; or failure to make expected weight gain during period of growth, leading to body weight less than 85% of that expected).
B. Intense fear of gaining weight or becoming fat, even though underweight.
C. Disturbance in the way in which one's body weight or shape is experienced, undue influence of body weight or shape on self-evaluation, or denial of the seriousness of the current low body weight.
D. In postmenarcheal females, amenorrhea, i..e., the absence of at least three consecutive menstrual cycles. (A woman is considered to have amenorrhea if her periods occur only following hormone, e.g., estrogen, administration.)

Specify type:
Restricting type: during the current episode of Anorexia Nervosa, the person has not regularly engaged in binge-eating or purging behavior (i.e. self-induced vomiting or the misuse of laxatives, diuretics, or enemas).
Binge-Eating/Purging Type: during the current episode of Anorexia Nervosa, the person has regularly engaged in binge-eating or purging behavior (i.e., self-induced vomiting or the misuse of laxatives, diuretics, or enemas).

Source: Reprinted with permission from the *Diagnostic and Statistical Manual of Mental Disorders, Fourth Edition, Text Revision,* (Copyright ©2000). American Psychiatric Association.

median prevalence rates were 0.28 cases per 100 for anorexia nervosa and 0.30 per 100 for bulimia nervosa. Eating disorders are moderately disabling, with a GBD weight of 0.28 (see table 1-2.)

Anxiety Disorders

The anxiety disorders are characterized by a combination of fearful thoughts, physiological activity, and behavioral avoidance. Diagnostic categories are based on the addition of temporal aspects to this so-called tripartite model. We present the relationship between these disorders and disability following a brief discussion of each of the major anxiety disorders, their symptoms, and their population prevalence.

PANIC DISORDER

In panic disorder, while fear, physiological activity, and temporal aspects are distinguishing features, the core symptom is the panic attack: a spell of fear accompanied by physiological symptoms over a period of a few minutes. Any 4 of a list of 13 possible symptoms, among them rapid heartbeat, chest pain, and a smothering sensation, must accompany the attack. Panic disorder may be diagnosed only if one or more panic attacks occur spontaneously (out of the blue and not associated with a particular stimulus or situation). The diagnosis also requires that attacks or extreme concern over their recurrence extend over at least 1 month. This review of panic disorder, along with those below for social phobia and simple phobia, builds on the review by Somers, Goldner, Waraich, and Hsu (2006) of 15 studies from 1980 through 2004. An additional 18, nonduplicated studies resulting from the current study's search were eligible for data abstraction. The population base for the review of panic disorder, social and simple phobia represents more than 200,000 sampled and assessed persons. The estimates of 1-year prevalence for panic disorder ranged from 0.1 per 100 in rural villages in Taiwan to 3.2 per 100 in Florence, Italy, with a median of 0.9 and an interquartile range of 0.6–1.9. All six East Asian studies had prevalence estimates in the lowest quartile. Of these three anxiety disorders, only panic was included in the GBD study, and its disability weight is relatively low (0.17 in table 1-2).

SIMPLE PHOBIA

Phobias primarily involve fearful cognition (thinking) and behavioral avoidance, with or without physical symptoms. Simple phobia is an unreasonable fear of a specific object or situation that is so strong that the individual endures the situation only with extreme distress or avoids it altogether, to the extent that the avoidance interferes with normal functioning. Common simple phobias include fear of heights, water, blood, snakes, bugs, and enclosed places. The range of possible objects or situations that give rise to phobias is so great that some refer to phobias as the "common cold of psychiatry." The current review yielded 1-year prevalence rate estimates of all simple phobias (without regard to the focus) that ranged from 0.2 per 100 in Derry, Northern Ireland, to 11.1 per 100 in Oslo, Norway. The median prevalence was 4.8; the interquartile range was 3.5–7.3.

SOCIAL PHOBIA

Social phobia resembles simple phobia but the feared situation is very specific: social interaction. The current review found that 1-year prevalence estimates for social phobia ranged from 0.2 per 100 in Korea and in Nigeria to 44.2 per 100 in Udmurtia, a Russian republic, with a median of 2.8 and interquartile range of 1.1–5.8. All three East Asian studies had prevalence rates of social phobia in the lowest quartile. The wide ranges found for both simple and social phobias across racial and ethnic groups suggest that these two disorders are culturally plastic.

OBSESSIVE-COMPULSIVE DISORDER

Obsessive–compulsive disorder is characterized by persistent thoughts and recurring behaviors that cause distress or impair functioning. Nineteen studies were identified that assessed the prevalence of obsessive–compulsive disorder. The search for relevant titles was aided by a relatively comprehensive, albeit nonsystematic, review (Fontenelle, Mendlowicz, &Versiani, 2006). Across all studies, the median 1-year prevalence of obsessive–compulsive disorder was 1.0 per 100, with interquartile range of 0.6–2.0.

POSTTRAUMATIC STRESS DISORDER

Posttraumatic stress disorder links the cognitive, physiological, and behavioral aspects of anxiety to a specific traumatic event. (See Diagnostic Criteria 1-3.) There are characteristic attempts to avoid thinking about the trauma or being reminded of it, which elicit physiological symptoms of anxiety. The current review identified four studies that met review criteria and included a 12-month prevalence rate; several studies reporting lifetime prevalence rates were not included. The median prevalence rate across the four studies included was 2.2 cases per 100. Prevalences reported here were drawn from general populations, not from populations that had experienced a recent collective trauma such as a weather-related disaster, war, or forced migration. In the latter populations, prevalence rates would vary widely based on the nature and extent of the collective trauma, making the data less generalizable to the general public.

The patterns of symptoms in all of these anxiety disorders occur commonly in the general population without always exacting much distress or impairment. Most often, symptoms never reach a diagnostic threshold, but even below the diagnostic threshold, they can be disabling. Panic disorder and obsessive–compulsive disorder incur moderately high disability according to the SDS methods, but according to the GBD method disability is low. The SDS measures contrast with the disability weights used in the GBD studies presumably because the latter are ratings by objective rates, whereas the SDS ratings are from the individual suffering from the disorder. For example, panic disorder and obsessive–compulsive disorder are distressing to the individual, with 47% of subjects reporting marked or extreme disability on the SDS for both, while the GBD rating for panic disorder is 0.17 and that for obsessive–compulsive disorder is 0.13—both less than the GBD rating of 0.21

Diagnostic Criteria 1-3. Diagnostic Criteria for 309.81 Posttraumatic Stress Disorder

A. The person has been exposed to a traumatic event in which both of the following was present:

   (1) the person experienced, witnessed, or was confronted with an event or events that involved actual or threatened death or serious injury, or a threat to the physical integrity of self or others.

   (2) the person 's response involved intense fear, helplessness, or horror. **Note**: In children, this may be expressed instead by disorganization or agitated behavior

B. the traumatic event is persistently reexperienced in one (or more) of the following ways:

   (1) recurrent and intrusive distressing recollections of the event, including images, thoughts, or perceptions **Note**: In young children , respective play may occur in which themes or aspects of the trauma are expressed .

   (2) recurrent distressing dreams of the event. **Note**: In children, there may be frightening dreams without recognizable content.

   (3) acting or feeling as if the traumatic event were recurring (included a sense of reliving the experience. illusions , hallucinations, and dissociative flashbacks episodes, including those that occur on awakening or when intoxicated). **Note**: in young children trauma –specific may occur.

   (4) intense psychological distress at exposure to internal or external cues that symbolize or resemble an aspect of the traumatic event.

   (5) physiological reactivity on exposure to internal or external cues that symbolize or resemble an aspect of the traumatic event.

C. persistent avoidance of stimuli associated with the trauma and numbing of general responsiveness (not present before the trauma). as indicated by three (or more) of the following:

   (1) efforts to avoid thoughts, feelings, or conversations associated with the trauma

   (2) efforts to avoid activities, places, or people that arouse recollections of the trauma

   (3) inability to recall an important aspect of the trauma

   (4) markedly diminished interest or participation in significant activities

   (5) feeling of detachment or estrangement from others

   (6) restricted range of affect (e.g. ., unable to have loving feelings)

   (7) sense of foreshortened future (e.g. does not expect to have a career, marriage, children, or a normal life span

D. Persistent systems of increased arousal (not present before the trauma), as indicated by two (or more) of the following:

   (1) difficulty falling and staying asleep

   (2) irritability or outbursts of anger

   (3) difficulty concentrating

   (4) hypervigilance

   (5) exaggerated startle response

E. Duration of disturbance (symptoms in Criteria B,C, and D) is more than 1 month.

Source: Reprinted with permission from the *Diagnostic and Statistical Manual of Mental Disorders, Fourth Edition, Text Revision,* (Copyright ©2000). American Psychiatric Association.

for rheumatoid arthritis. Persons experiencing panic attacks often suspect they are having a heart attack, even visiting emergency rooms with nontrivial frequency. However, once the attack has subsided, the residual impairment diminishes. Obsessive–compulsive disorder also has a relatively low GBD rating but a high SDS percentage, presumably because it is highly distressing to the individual but not quite as impairing and disruptive from the perspective of others in the social environment. One can surmise this rating difference might exist for social phobias, for which no GBD value is available but for which 36% of subjects report severe impairment on the SDS measure.

Affective Disorders

MAJOR DEPRESSIVE DISORDER

Major depressive disorder is a syndrome characterized by the cardinal symptoms of sadness or of loss of pleasure and interest, coupled with somatic symptoms such as problems with weight, fatigue, sleep, and concentration. (See Diagnostic Criteria 1–4.) The syndrome lasts for at least several weeks. The epidemiologic findings for major depressive disorder presented here build on the review by Waraich and colleagues (2004), who examined studies from 1980 through 2000 and found 13 that met their study criteria. For the current review, a PubMed search using the combined keywords *population prevalence* and *depressive disorder* yielded 3,935 titles, of which 2,477 were published in 2000 or later. While 59 of these appeared relevant, only 29 nonduplicated studies that met this review's criteria were added to the studies in Waraich's review (2004). The final 42 studies included in this review represent 290,471 persons. One-year prevalence rates ranged from 0.64 per 100 in Taipei, Taiwan, to 15.4 per 100 in the Russian republic of Udmurtia, with a median of 5.3 and interquartile range of 3.6–6.5. Six of the nine studies in the lowest quartile were in East Asia; otherwise, no obvious conclusions were evident regarding study location, method, or the period during which it was conducted.

Some persons meeting criteria for major depressive disorder can be so severely impaired

that they are led to commit suicide; others may be nearly stuporous or unable to carry out even the simplest of tasks. Still other individuals meeting the criteria for major depression may experience little impairment save for the distress produced by the syndrome (Kessler et al., 2003). Not surprisingly, major depressive disorder is one of the most disabling disorders, whether measured using the GBD (rating of 0.35 for the moderate form) or the SDS (58% reporting severe disability). Thus using the GBD schema, moderate forms of major depressive disorder compare roughly to multiple sclerosis (0.41) and deafness (0.33). However, the disability rating associated with the severe form of major depressive disorders is 0.62, matching that for blindness.

BIPOLAR DISORDER

Bipolar disorder generally consists of one or more episodes of mania usually followed or preceded by an episode of major depression. Mania refers to extreme elation and grandiosity that lasts at least 1 week (APA, 1994). Because manic episodes represent such a large deviation from normal behavior, they immediately generate problems for both the individual and those in his or her social environment.

This review of bipolar disorder expands on the review of studies from 1980 through 2000 by Waraich and colleagues (2004), who found 12 studies from that period that met their criteria. The current review adds 5 studies published later than 2000. Studies that did not present data specifically for bipolar I disorder (such as those focused on bipolar II diagnoses) were excluded from the current review. As with schizophrenia, bipolar disorder is often difficult to diagnose by anyone other than a medically trained clinician. But, since so few reports were based on register systems, the current review includes population-based survey studies as long as they used a standardized structured interviews. The median prevalence was 0.6 per 100 , with a relatively small interquartile range of 0.3–1.1. The GBD disability weight for this disorder (0.40) is slightly above that for major depressive disorder and nearly as high as for schizophrenia, and the percentage rating of severe disability on the Sheehan

Diagnostic Criteria 1-4. Criteria for Major Depressive Episode

A. Five (or more) of the following symptoms have been present during the same 2-week period and represent a change from previous functioning; at least one of the symptoms is either (1) depressed mood or (2) loss of interest or pleasure. **Note:** Do not include symptoms that are clearly due to a general medical condition, or mood- incongruent delusions or hallucinations.

(1) depressed mood most of the day, nearly every day indicated by either subjective report (e.g. feels sad and empty) or observation made by others (e.g. appears tearful). Note: in children and adolescents can be in irritable mood.

(2) markedly diminished interest or pleasure in all, or almost all, activities most of the day, nearly every day (as indicated by either subjective account or observation made by others).

(3) significant weight loss when not dieting or weight gain (e.g., a change of more than 5% of body in a month a increase in appetite nearly every day **Note**: In children, consider failure to make expected weight gains.

(4) insomnia or hypersomnia every day

(5) psychomotor agitation or retardation nearly every day (observable by others, not merely subjective feeling or being slowed down)

(6) fatigue or loss of energy nearly every day

(7) Feeling of worthlessness or excessive or in appropriate guilt (which may be delusional) nearly every day (not merely self-reproach or guilt about being sick)

(8) diminished ability to think or concentrate, or indecisiveness, nearly every day (ether by subjective account or as observed by others)

(9) recurrent thoughts of death (not just fear of dying), recurrent suicidal ideation without a specific plan, or a suicide attempt or specific plan for committing suicide

B. The symptoms do not meet criteria for a Mixed Episode (see p.33)

C. The symptoms cause clinically significant distress or impairment in social, occupational, or other important areas of functioning.

D. The symptoms are not due to direct physiological effects of a substance (e.g. a drug of abuse, a medication) or a general medical condition (e.g. Hypothyroidism).

E. The symptoms are not better accounted for by Bereavement. i.e., after the lost of a loved one, the symptoms persist for longer than 2 months or are characterized by marked functional impairment, morbid preoccupation with worthlessness, suicidal ideation, psychotic symptoms or psychomotor retardation.

Source: Reprinted with permission from the *Diagnostic and Statistical Manual of Mental Disorders, Fourth Edition, Text Revision*, (Copyright ©2000). American Psychiatric Association.

scale (83%) is higher than for any other disorder with an SDS rating.

Cognitive Disorders: Schizophrenia and Dementia

Because they both involve cognitive impairments, we present schizophrenia and dementia together.

SCHIZOPHRENIA

Schizophrenia (initially named "adolescent dementia" by Kraepelin, 1919), involves hallucinations (e.g., seeing things that aren't there, hearing voices when no one is speaking) or delusions (believing things that are not true and even patently absurd). The disorder also gives rise to chaotic speech or behavior. (See Diagnostic Criteria 1-5.) Bipolar disorder,

Diagnostic Criteria 1-5. Diagnostic Criteria for Schizophrenia

A. characteristic symptoms: Two (or more) of the following, each present for a significant portion of time during a 1- month period (or less if successfully treated):
   (1) delusions
   (2) hallucinations
   (3) disorganized speech (e.g., Frequent derailment or incoherence)
   (4) grossly disorganized or catatonic behavior
   (5) negative symptoms, i.e., affective flattening, alogia or avolition
   Note: only one Criterion A Symptom is required if delusions are bizarre or hallucinations consist of a voices conversing with each other.

B. Social/occupational dysfunction: for a significant portion of the time since the onset of the disturbance, one or more major areas of functioning such as work, interpersonal relations, or self care are markedly below the level achieved prior to the onset (or when the onset is in childhood or adolescence, failure to expected achieve level of interpersonal, academic, or occupational achievement).

C. Duration: continuous signs of the disturbance persist for at least 6 months. This 6-month period must include at least 1 month of symptoms (or less if successfully treated) that meet Criterion A (i.e., active phase symptoms) and may include periods of prodromal or residual symptoms. During these prodromal or residual periods, the signs of the disturbance may be manifested by only negative symptoms or two or more symptoms listed in the Criterion A present in an attenuated form (e.g., odd beliefs, unusual perceptual experiences).

D. Schizoaffective and Mood Disorder exclusions: Schizoaffective Disorder and Mood Disorder With Psychotic Features have been ruled out because either (1) no Major Depressive, Manic or Mixed Episodes have occurred concurrently with the active –phase symptoms; or (2) if the mood episodes have occurred during active,-phase symptoms, their total duration has been brief relative to the duration of the active and residual periods.

E. Substance/general medical condition exclusion: The disturbance is not due to the direct physiological effects of a substance (e.g., a drug of abuse, a medication) or a general medical condition.

F. Relationship to a Pervasive Development Disorder: If there is a history of Autistic Disorder or another Pervasive Development Disorder, the additional diagnosis of Schizophrenia is made only if prominent delusions or hallucinations are also present for at least a month (or less if successfully treated).

Classification of longitudinal course (can be applied only after at least 1 year has elapsed since the initial onset of active-phase symptoms):
Episodic with Interepisode Residual Symptoms (episodes are defined by the reemergence of prominent psychotic symptoms); also specify if: **With Prominent Negative Symptoms Episodic with No Interepisode Residual Symptoms Continuous** (prominent psychotic symptoms are present throughout the period of observation); also specify: **With prominent Negative symptoms**
Single Episodes in Partial Remission also specify: with Prominent Negative Symptoms Single Episode in Full Remission other or Unspecified Pattern

Source: Reprinted with permission from the *Diagnostic and Statistical Manual of Mental Disorders, Fourth Edition, Text Revision,* (Copyright ©2000). American Psychiatric Association.

discussed above, was formerly named manic–depressive insanity; these two disorders were considered the major psychoses—that is, disorders in which there is lack of understanding or contact with reality.

The current review of schizophrenia was taken directly, without updating, from the recent work of McGrath, Saha, Chant, and Welham (2008). Of all the disorders presented here, schizophrenia is the one for which prevalence is least likely to be underestimated by reliance on data from medical records and also the one for which the diagnosis by an interviewer without medical training is most suspect (Eaton & Chen, 2006).

Since diagnostic criteria for schizophrenia demand an element of chronicity (6 months), the studies in the current review include both point prevalence and 1-year prevalence. There were 23 relevant studies, and the median prevalence was 0.5 per 100. The interquartile range for schizophrenia prevalence is the smallest in table 1-1, from 0.3 to 0.6 per 100. According to the methodology of the GBD study, schizophrenia has the highest disability rating (0.53) of all mental illnesses among adults. It is difficult to imagine the results had the SDS methodology had been applied to persons meeting diagnostic criteria for schizophrenia, since they often lack insight into their condition.

DEMENTIA

With an onset that usually begins after age 65, dementia is a condition that results in gradual, global deterioration in cognitive functioning. This review of the prevalence of dementia builds on earlier work by Ferri and colleagues (2005) that includes further online data (http://www.alz.co.uk/research/consensus.html). Only studies including diagnoses based on an international, documented operational system (such as DSM or ICD) were included. Studies of dementia were required to focus on older adults, defined here as individuals 60 years of age or older, and to be included in the review the overall prevalence rates had to be reported for both sexes and all ages combined. Six studies focused on persons 60 or older; the balance focused on individuals 65 years of age or older. The studies varied in the number of stages of assessment (from one to three), with some studies including just an initial quick screen of cognitive impairment and other studies incorporating a consensus diagnosis of dementia by experts in a third stage of assessment. For this disorder, the definition of general population was expanded to include institutional populations, since in Japan, Europe, and the United States many older adults live in institutional retirement communities. The review by Ferri and colleagues included data from two other systematic reviews of 12 studies (Hoffman et al., 1991) and 11 studies (Lobo et al., 2000) in Europe. Because the studies summarized in those two reviews could not be identified separately, the results presented in table 1-1 potentially underestimate European studies and more generally underestimate the overall variation in studies. The current review found the median prevalence for dementia to be 5.4 per 100 of the population over the age of 60, with an interquartile range of 3.2–7.1.

Substance Use Disorders

Use of substances such as alcohol, illegal drugs, and prescription medications can have adverse effects on how an individual thinks, feels, and acts. Depending on the substance, associated disability, context, and pattern of use, an individual may meet criteria for psychiatric diagnosis (APA, 1994).

Substance abuse involves a pattern of use that is disabling. Since use of an illegal substance can lead to criminal arrest, its use alone is sufficient to yield a diagnosis of substance abuse. For legal substances such as prescription medications and alcohol, impairment may arise within the context of the legal, social, or psychological consequences of the use. In contrast, substance dependence involves a physiological craving in which the substance is required in increasing frequency or in greater and greater doses or in which the pattern of use comes to dominate the life of the individual. (See Diagnostic Criteria 1-6.) This review combines the categories of abuse and dependence, separating the disorders connected to illegal drugs from those linked to alcohol.

Diagnostic Criteria 1-6. Criteria for Substance Dependence

F. Maladaptive pattern of substance use, leading to clinically significant impairment or distress, as manifested by three (or more) of the following, occurring at any time in the same 12-month period.

    (1) Tolerance, as defined by either of the following:

        (f) a need for markedly increased amounts of substance to achieve intoxication or desired affect

        (g) markedly diminished effect with continued use of the same amount of the substance.

    (2) Withdrawal, as manifested by either of the following:

        (f) the characteristic withdrawal syndrome for substance (refer to Criteria A and B of the Criteria sets for Withdrawal from the specific substances)

        (g) markedly diminished effect with continued use of the same amount of the substance.

    (3) Withdrawal, as manifested by either of the following:

        (f) the characteristic withdrawal syndrome for substance (refer to Criteria A and B of criteria sets for Withdrawal from the specific substances)

        (g) the same (or closely related) substance is taken to relieve or avoid the withdrawal symptoms

    (4) the substance is often taken in larger amounts or over a longer period o than was intended.

    (5) there is a persistent desire or unsuccessful efforts to cut down or control substance use.

    (6) a great deal of time is spent in activities necessary to obtain the substance (e.g., visiting multiple doctors or driving long distances) use the substance (e.g., chain smoking) , or recover from side effects

    (7) important social, occupational, or recreational activities are give up or reduced because of substance use.

    (8) the substance use is continued despite knowledge of having persistent or recurrent physical or psychological problem that is likely to have caused or exacerbated by the substance (e.g., current cocaine use despite recognition than an ulcer was made worse by alcohol consumption)

Specify if

With Physiological Dependence: evidence of tolerance or withdrawal (i.e., either item 1 or 2 is present)

Without Physiological Dependence: no evidence of tolerance or withdrawal (i.e., neither Item 1 nor 2 is present)

Source: Reprinted with permission from the *Diagnostic and Statistical Manual of Mental Disorders, Fourth Edition, Text Revision,* (Copyright ©2000). American Psychiatric Association.

The current review's search for studies of drug use disorder yielded 1,417 titles. Of the 467 that were examined closely, only 11 met our criteria. The 1-year prevalence rates ranged from 0.4 per 100 in Mexico to 3.6 per 100 in the United States, and the median prevalence was 1.8. About half of the studies were conducted in the United States. All of the studies yielding 1-year prevalence rates in the lowest quartile were conducted outside the United States (specifically, in Mexico, Germany, and Norway). The prevalence in the single Australian study was in the highest quartile. The large range of prevalence rates is comparable to that found for the phobias and further suggests that a strong cultural basis underpins the prevalence of these disorders.

The current review's literature search for alcohol use disorder yielded 14 studies that met inclusion criteria. The range was from a low of 4.1 per 100 in Germany to a high of 10.6 per 100 in Norway. The median 1-year prevalence was 5.9 per 100, and the interquartile range was 5.2–8.1. No obvious relationships were detected with variables such as the place of the study, the method, or the calendar time during which the prevalence was estimated.

Drug abuse and dependence have significant consequences for both impairment and disability, including a GBD disability weight of 0.25. Thirty-nine percent of CPES respondents reported a severe disability according to the SDS scale (see table 1-2). When examining disabilityrelated to alcohol disorders, the SDS estimation procedure included only the more severe alcohol dependence. Even so, the associated disability was lower than for abuse or dependence on illicit drugs, with only 14% of subjects reporting severe impairment due to alcohol dependence on the SDS scale. The relatively low GBD disability weight for alcohol abuse or dependence (0.16) parallels the SDS percentage (see table 1-2), arguing against the notion that the SDS self-report measure reflects denial of impairment.

Personality Disorders

Personality disorders are unusual maladaptive patterns of behavior that both persist over time and occur in a wide range of situations. Whether these patterns should be considered disorders or whether they are nothing more than strong deviations from normal behavior remains the subject of some controversy (as discussed in chapter 2). Perhaps as a result, little epidemiologic research has focused on the personality disorders. The current review identified 629 studies of personality disorders, of which 168 were examined closely. Those focused on a single personality disorder were excluded. More than 20 studies report total prevalence of all personality disorders, but

a significant number were studies of clinical samples, had restricted age ranges, or used assessments not meeting the current review criteria. Ultimately only five studies met inclusion criteria, the fewest among all diagnostic categories in the current review. Relaxing the review criteria did not significantly alter the prevalence rates. Thus the current review includes only those five studies. (See table 1-1.) The median prevalence was 9.1 per 100, with an interquartile range of 9.0–14.4. No estimates have been obtained to suggest the level of impairment associated with personality disorders in general; however, the Dutch study (Vos and Mathers, 2000) reports severe disability (0.54) for one subtype, borderline personality disorder.

DISCUSSION

This review has shown that mental disorders have high prevalences in the general population compared with many other health conditions. Even schizophrenia and bipolar disorder, with the lowest prevalences among the disorders considered here (i.e., under 1.0 per 100), are more prevalent than many infectious diseases and chronic medical conditions. These two disorders with high levels of associated impairment may be considered the less common but more severe mental disorders. Three other disorders—panic disorder, obsessive–compulsive disorder, and drug abuse or dependence—might also be considered less common, with median prevalences under 2.0 per 100. Major depressive disorder, the phobias, and alcohol abuse or dependence are the common mental disorders, with median prevalence rates greater than 5.0 per 100.

In contrast to many diseases that rank as significant sources of disability in the developed nations, such as heart disease, most mental disorders have their onsets in childhood or young adulthood (as discussed in chapter 6). This relatively early onset contributes to their importance in the algebra of calculating DALYs (see figure 1-1). The chronicity of the mental disorders (also discussed in chapter 6) further contributes to their significance in the GBD estimates. Major depressive disorder stands apart from the other disorders because of its high prevalence, as well as its high associated impairment as measured by either GBD rating or the percentage of subjects with extreme disability on the Sheehan scale. This explains its place in the GBD study as the mental disorder claiming the highest percentage of DALYs. A surprise in these comparative results is the high median prevalence for personality disorder, at more than 9.0 per 100.

Almost all of the studies included in this review and summarized in tables 1-1 and 1-2 were conducted in the so-called third generation of psychiatric epidemiologic research, which was inaugurated with the NIMH Epidemiologic Catchment Area program (Eaton et al., 1981; Regier et al., 1984) and include a number of studies from around the world using similar methodologies (e.g., Bland, Orn, & Newman, 1988), a separate body of work following the National Comorbidity Survey (Kessler et al., 1994), and additional results of many recent national surveys from the World Mental Health 2000 study included in table 1-1 (Kessler, Haro, Heeringa, Pennell, & Ustun, 2006; Kessler & Ustun, 2008). This feature of the review results from the requirement for structured diagnostic interviews such as the Diagnostic Interview Schedule (Robins, Helzer, Croughan, & Ratcliff, 1981) and its descendants, including the Composite International Diagnostic Interview Schedule (Robins et al., 1988). These and other similar instruments are reliable but yield results that correspond only moderately well with the results of psychiatric interviews (Eaton, Hall, Macdonald, & McKibben, 2007; Wittchen 1994), as discussed further in chapter 4. However, they are the only alternatives for population-based studies in psychiatric epidemiology, where such a large percentage of cases do not seek or obtain treatment.

In 1996, Murray and Lopez reported, with respect to the GBD study, that "our understanding of the descriptive epidemiology of many, if not most, conditions is not advanced" (p. 41). Based on the findings presented here, is it possible now to say that the situation has been remedied, at least with respect to mental disorders? Can it be concluded that the third generation of research is complete, given the increasingly strong body of global research on the prevalence of mental disorders? The answer is mixed at best. The prevalence of mental disorders has been well studied in general, yet for some disorders even the prevalence estimates are based on merely a handful of studies. Further, while the burden of disability associated with mental disorders has been well described for clinical populations, the data are sparse for the general population, where the majority of cases of these disorders exist, undetected and untreated.

REFERENCES

Ahola, K., Honkonen, T., Isometsa, E., Kalimo, R., Nykyri, E., Aromaa, A., & Lönneqvist, J. (2005). The relationship between job-related burnout and depressive disorders: Results from the Finnish Health 2000 Study. *Journal of Affective Disorders, 88*(1), 55–62.

Alegria, M., Jackson, J. S., Kessler, R. C., & Takeuchi, D. (2008). *Collaborative Psychiatric Epidemiologic Surveys (CPES), 2001–2003 (United States).* Ann Arbor, MI: Inter-University Consortium for Political and Social Research.

Alegria, M., Takeuchi, D., Canino, G., Duan, N., Shrout, P., Meng, X. L., … Gong, F. (2004). Considering context, place and culture: the National Latino and Asian American Study. *International Journal of Methods in Psychiatric Research, 13*(4), 208–220.

Alonso, J., Angermeyer, M. C., Bernert, S., Bruffaerts, R., Brugha, T. S., Bryson, H., … Vollebergh, W. A. M. (2004). Prevalence of mental disorders in Europe: Results from the European Study of the Epidemiology of Mental Disorders (ESE-MeD) project. *Acta Psychiatrica Scandinavica, 420*(Suppl.), 21–27.

American Psychiatric Association. (1980). *Diagnostic and statistical manual of mental disorders* (3rd ed.). Washington, DC: Author.

American Psychiatric Association. (1987). *Diagnostic and statistical manual of mental disorders* (3rd ed., rev.). Washington, DC: Author.

American Psychiatric Association. (1994). *Diagnostic and statistical manual of mental disorders* (4th ed.). Washington, DC: Author.

Amoran, O., Lawoyin, T., & Lasebikan, V. (2007). Prevalence of depression among adults in Oyo State, Nigeria: A comparative study of rural and urban communities 3. *Australian Journal of Rural Health, 15*(3), 211–215.

Andrade, L., Walters, E. E., Gentil, V., & Laurenti, R. (2002). Prevalence of ICD-10 mental disorders in a catchment area in the city of Sao Paulo, Brazil. *Social Psychiatry and Psychiatric Epidemiology, 37*(7), 316–325.

Andrews, G., Henderson, S., & Hall, W. (2001). Prevalence, comorbidity, disability and service utilization: Overview of the Australian National Mental Health Survey. *British Journal of Psychiatry, 178,* 145–153.

Bachman, D. L., Wolf, P. A., Linn, R., Knoefel, J. E., Cobb, J., Belanger, A.,...White, L. R. (1992). Prevalence of dementia and probable senile dementia of the Alzheimer type in the Framingham study. *Neurology, 42*(1), 115–119.

Beals, J., Manson, S. M., Whitesell, N. R., Mitchell, C. M., Novins, D. K., Simpson, S.,...Manson, S. M. (2005). Prevalence of major depressive episode in two American Indian reservation populations: Unexpected findings with a structured interview. *American Journal of Psychiatry, 162*(9), 1713–1722.

Ben-Arie, O., Swartz, L., Teggin, A. F., & Elk, R. (1983). The coloured elderly in Cape Town: A psychosocial, psychiatric and medical community survey. Part II. Prevalence of psychiatric disorders. *South African Medical Journal, 64*(27), 1056–1061.

Bijl, R. V., Ravelli, A., & van Zessen, G. (1998). Prevalence of psychiatric disorder in the general population: Results of the Netherlands Mental Health Survey and Incidence Study (NEMESIS). *Social Psychiatry and Psychiatric Epidemiology, 33*(12), 587–595.

Bird, H. R., Canino, G. J., Davies, M., Zhang, H., Ramirez, R., & Lahey, B. B. (2001). Prevalence and correlates of antisocial behaviors among three ethnic groups. *Journal of Abnormal Child Psychology, 29*(6), 465–478.

Bland, R. C., Newman, S. C., & Orn, H. (1988). Period prevalence of psychiatric disorders in Edmonton. *Acta Psychiatrica Scandinavica, 338*(Suppl.), 33–42.

Bland, R. C., Orn, H., & Newman, S. C. (1988). Lifetime prevalence of psychiatric disorders in Edmonton. *Acta Psychiatrica Scandinavica, 338*(Suppl.), 24–32.

Bourdon, K. H., Rae, D. S., Locke, B. Z., Narrow, W. E., & Regier, D. A. (1992). Estimating the prevalence of mental disorders in U.S. adults from the Epidemiologic Catchment Area survey. *Public Health Reports, 107*(6), 663–668.

Breitner, J. C., Wyse, B. W., Anthony, J. C., Welsh-Bohmer, K. A., Steffens, D. C., Norton, M. C.,...Khachaturian, A. (1999). APOE-epsilon4 count predicts age when prevalence of AD increases, then declines: The Cache County study. *Neurology, 53*(2), 321–331.

Bromet, E. J., Gluzman, S. F., Paniotto, V. I., Webb, C. P., Tintle, N. L., Zakhozha, V.,...Schwartz, J. E. (2005). Epidemiology of psychiatric and alcohol disorders in Ukraine: Findings from the Ukraine world mental health survey. *Social Psychiatry and Psychiatric Epidemiology, 40*(9), 681–690.

Bromet, E. J., Gluzman, S. F., Tintle, N. L., Paniotto, V. I., Webb, C. P. M., Zakhozha, V.,...Schwartz, J. E. (2008). The state of mental health and alcoholism in Ukraine. In R. C. Kessler & T. B. Ustun (Eds.), *The WHO world mental health surveys: Global perspectives on the epidemiology of mental disorders* (pp. 431–445). New York, NY: Cambridge University Press.

Canino, G. J., Bird, H. R., Shrout, P. E., Rubio-Stipec, M., Bravo, M., Martinez, R.,...Guevarra, L. M. (1987). The prevalence of specific psychiatric disorders in Puerto Rico. *Archives of General Psychiatry, 44*(8), 727–735.

Chakrabarti, S., & Fombonne, E. (2001). Pervasive developmental disorders in preschool children. *Journal of the American Medical Association, 285*(24), 3093–3099.

Chandra, V., Ganguli, M., Pandav, R., Johnston, J., Belle, S., & DeKosky, S. T. (1998). Prevalence of Alzheimer's disease and other dementias in rural India: The Indo-US study. *Neurology, 51*(4), 1000–1008.

Chen, C. N., Wong, J., Lee, N., Chan-Ho, M. W., Lau, J. T., & Fung, M. (1993). The Shatin community mental health survey in Hong Kong. II. Major findings. *Archives of General Psychiatry, 50*(2), 125–133.

Cho, M. J., Kim, J. K., Jeon, H. J., Suh, T., Chung, I. W., Hong, J. P.,...Hahm, B. J. (2007). Lifetime and 12-month prevalence of DSM-IV psychiatric disorders among Korean adults. *Journal of Nervous and Mental Disease, 195*(3), 203–210.

Cillicilli, A. S., Telcioglu, M., Askin, R., Kaya, N., Bodur, S., & Kucur, R. (2004). Twelve-month prevalence of obsessive–compulsive disorder in Konya, Turkey. *Comprehensive Psychiatry, 45*(5), 367–374.

Coid, J., Yang, M., Tyrer, P., Roberts, A., & Ullrich, S. (2006). Prevalence and correlates of personality disorder in Great Britain. *British Journal of Psychiatry, 188,* 423–431.

Compton, W. M., Conway, K. P., Stinson, F. S., & Grant, B. F. (2006). Changes in the prevalence of major depression and comorbid substance use disorders in the United States between 1991–1992 and 2001–2002. *American Journal of Psychiatry, 163*(12), 2141–2147.

Costello, E. J., Angold, A., Burns, B. B., Stangl, D. K., Tweed, D. L., Erkanli, A., & Worthman, C. M.

(1996). The Great Smoky Mountains Study of Youth: Goals, design and prevalence of DSM-III-R disorders. *Archives of General Psychiatry, 53*(12), 1129–1131.

Degonda, M., Wyss, M., & Angst, J. (1993). The Zurich Study. XVIII. Obsessive–compulsive disorders and syndromes in the general population. *European Archives of Psychiatry and Clinical Neuroscience, 243*(1), 16–22.

deSilva, H. A., Gunatilake, S. B., & Smith, A. D. (2003). Prevalence of dementia in a semi-urban population in Sri Lanka: Report from a regional survey. *International Journal of Geriatric Psychiatry, 18*(8), 711–715.

Dohrenwend, B. P., & Dohrenwend, B. S. (1982). Perspectives on the past and future of psychiatric epidemiology: The 1981 Rema Lapouse Lecture. *American Journal of Public Health, 72*(11), 1271–1279.

Eaton, W. W., & Chen, C.-Y. (2006). Epidemiology. In J. A. Lieberman, T. S. Stroup, & D. O. Perkins (Eds.), *The American psychiatric publishing textbook of schizophrenia* (pp. 17–38). Washington, DC: American Psychiatric Press.

Eaton, W. W., Dryman, A., & Weissman, M. M. (1991). Panic and phobia. In L. N. Robins & D. A. Regier (Eds.), *Psychiatric disorders in America: The Epidemiologic Catchment Area study* (pp. 155–179). New York, NY: Free Press.

Eaton, W. W., Hall, A. L., Macdonald, R., & McKibben, J. (2007). Case identification in psychiatric epidemiology: A review. *International Review of Psychiatry, 19*(5), 497–507.

Eaton, W. W., Regier, D. A., Locke, B. Z., & Taube, C. A. (1981). The Epidemiologic Catchment Area program of the National Institute of Mental Health. *Public Health Reports, 96*(4), 319–325.

Eaton, W. W., Weissman, M. M., Anthony, J. C., Robins, L. N., Blazer, D. G., & Karno, M. (1985). Problems in the definition and measurement of prevalence and incidence of psychiatric disorders. In W. W. Eaton & L. G. Kessler (Eds.), *Epidemiologic field methods in psychiatry: The NIMH Epidemiologic Catchment Area program* (pp. 311–326). Orlando, FL: Academic Press.

Ebly, E. M., Parhad, I. M., Hogan, D. B., & Fung, T. S. (1994). Prevalence and types of dementia in the very old: Results from the Canadian Study of Health and Aging. *Neurology, 44*(9), 1593–1600.

Ellefsen, A., Kampmann, H., Billstedt, E., Gillberg, I. C., & Gillberg, C. (2007). Autism in the Faroe Islands: An epidemiological study. *Journal of Autism and Developmental Disorders, 37*(3), 437–444.

Faravelli, C., Guerrini, D. B., Aiazzi, L., Incerpi, G., & Pallanti, S. (1990). Epidemiology of mood disorders: A community survey in Florence. *Journal of Affective Disorders, 20*(2), 135–141.

Faravelli, C., Salvatori, S., Galassi, F., Aiazzi, L., Drei, C., & Cabras, P. (1997). Epidemiology of somatoform disorders: A community survey in Florence. *Social Psychiatry and Psychiatric Epidemiology, 32*(1), 24–29.

Farrag, A., Farwiz, H. M., Khedr, E. H., Mahfouz, R. M., & Omran, S. M. (1998). Prevalence of Alzheimer's disease and other dementing disorders: Assiut-Upper Egypt study. *Dementia and Geriatric Cognitive Disorders, 9*(6), 323–328.

Ferri, C. P., Prince, M., Brayne, C., Brodaty, H., Fratiglioni, L., Ganguli, M.,…Scufca, M. (2005). Global prevalence of dementia: A Delphi consensus study. *Lancet, 366*(9503), 2112–2117.

Fillenbaum, G. G., Heyman, A., Huber, M. S., Woodbury, M. A., Leiss, J., Schmader, K. E.,…Trapp-Moen, B. (1998). The prevalence and 3-year incidence of dementia in older Black and White community residents. *Journal of Clinical Epidemiology, 51*(7), 587–595.

Fombonne, E. (2003). The prevalence of autism. *Journal of the American Medical Association, 289*(1), 87–89.

Fontenelle, L. F., Mendlowicz, M. V., & Versiani, M. (2006). The descriptive epidemiology of obsessive–compulsive disorder. *Progress in Neuropsychopharmacology and Biological Psychiatry, 30*(3), 327–337.

Ford, B. C., Bullard, K. M., Taylor, R. J., Toler, A. K., Neighbors, H. W., & Jackson, J. S. (2007). Lifetime and 12-month prevalence of *Diagnostic and Statistical Manual of Mental Disorders,* fourth edition disorders among older African Americans: Findings from the National Survey of American Life. *American Journal of Geriatric Psychiatry, 15*(8), 652–659.

Fryers, T., Brugha, T., Morgan, Z., Smith, J., Hill, T., Carta, M.,…Lehtinen, V. (2004). Prevalence of psychiatric disorder in Europe: The potential and reality of meta-analysis. *Social Psychiatry and Psychiatric Epidemiology, 39*(11), 899–905.

Girolamo, G. D., Morosini, P., Gigantesco, S. D., & Kessler, R. C. (2008). The prevalence of mental disorders and service use in Italy: Results from the National Health Survey 2001–2003. In R. C. Kessler & T. B. Ustun (Eds.), *The WHO world mental health surveys: Global perspectives on the epidemiology of mental disorders* (pp. 364–387). New York, NY: Cambridge University Press.

Grabe, H. J., Meyer, C., Hapke, U., Rumpf, H. J., Freyberger, H. J., Dilling, H., & John, U. (2000).

Prevalence, quality of life and psychosocial function in obsessive–compulsive disorder and subclinical obsessive–compulsive disorder in northern Germany. *European Archives of Psychiatry and Clinical Neuroscience, 250*(5), 262–268.

Grant, B. F. (1996). DSM-IV, DSM-III-R, and ICD-10 alcohol and drug abuse/harmful use and dependence, United States, 1992: A nosological comparison. *Alcoholism: Clinical and Experimental Research, 20*(8), 1481–1488.

Grant, B. F., Dawson, D. A., Stinson, F. S., Chou, S. P., Dufour, M. C., & Pickering, R. P. (2004). The 12-month prevalence and trends in DSM-IV alcohol abuse and dependence: United States, 1991–1992 and 2001–2002. *Drug and Alcohol Dependence, 74*(3), 223–234.

Grant, B. F., Hasin, D. S., Blanco, C., Stinson, F. S., Chou, S. P., Goldstein, R. B.,...Huang, B. (2005). The epidemiology of social anxiety disorder in the United States: Results from the National Epidemiologic Survey on Alcohol and Related Conditions. *Journal of Clinical Psychiatry, 66*(11), 1351–1361.

Grant, B. F., Hasin, D. S., Stinson, F. S., Dawson, D. A., Chou, S. P., Ruan, W. J., & Pickering, R. P. (2004). Prevalence, correlates, and disability of personality disorders in the United States: Results from the National Epidemiologic Survey on Alcohol and Related Conditions. *Journal of Clinical Psychiatry, 65*(7), 948–958.

Grant, B. F., Hasin, D. S., Stinson, F. S., Dawson, D. A., Goldstein, R. B., Smith, S.,...Saha, T. D. (2006). The epidemiology of DSM-IV panic disorder and agoraphobia in the United States: Results from the National Epidemiologic Survey on Alcohol and Related Conditions. *Journal of Clinical Psychiatry, 67*(3), 363–374.

Grant, B. F., Stinson, F. S., Dawson, D. A., Chou, S. P., Dufour, M. C., Compton, W.,...Kaplan, K. (2004). Prevalence and co-occurrence of substance use disorders and independent mood and anxiety disorders: Results from the National Epidemiologic Survey on Alcohol and Related Conditions. *Archives of General Psychiatry, 61*(8), 807–816.

Graves, A. B., Larson, E. B., Edland, S. D., Bowen, J. D., McCormick, W. C., McCurry, S. M.,...Uomoto, J. M. (1996). Prevalence of dementia and its subtypes in the Japanese American population of King County, Washington State: The Kame project. *American Journal of Epidemiology, 144*(8), 760–771.

Gureje, O., Adeyemi, O., Enyidah, N., Ekpo, M., Udofia, O., Uwakwe, R., & Wakil, A. (2008). Mental disorders among adult Nigerians: Risks, prevalence, and treatment. In R. C. Kessler &

T. B. Ustun (Eds.), *The WHO world mental health surveys: Global perspectives on the epidemiology of mental disorders* (pp. 211–237). New York, NY: Cambridge University Press.

Harford, T. C., Grant, B. F., Yi, H. Y., & Chen, C. M. (2005). Patterns of DSM-IV alcohol abuse and dependence criteria among adolescents and adults: Results from the 2001 National Household Survey on Drug Abuse. *Alcoholism: Clinical and Experimental Research, 29*(5), 810–828.

Haro, J. M., Alonso, J., Pinto-meza, A., Vilagut, G., Fernandez, A., Codony, M.,...Autonell, J. (2008). The epidemiology of mental disorders in the general population of Spain. In R. C. Kessler & T. B. Ustun (Eds.), *The WHO world mental health surveys: Global perspectives on the epidemiology of mental disorders* (pp. 406–430). New York, NY: Cambridge University Press.

Hasin, D. S., Goodwin, R. D., Stinson, F. S., & Grant, B. F. (2005). Epidemiology of major depressive disorder: Results from the National Epidemiologic Survey on Alcoholism and Related Conditions. *Archives of General Psychiatry, 62*(10), 1097–1106.

Helzer, J., Clayton, P., Pambakian, L., Reich, T., Woodruff, R., & Reveley, M. (1977). Reliability of psychiatric diagnosis: II. The test/retest reliability of diagnostic classification. *Archives of General Psychiatry, 34*(2), 136–141.

Helzer, J., Robins, L., Taibleson, M., Woodruff, R., Reich, T., & Wise, E. (1977). Reliability of psychiatric diagnosis: A methodological review. *Archives of General Psychiatry, 34*(2), 129–133.

Hendrie, H. C., Osuntokun, B. O., Hall, K. S., Ogunniyi, A. O., Hui, S. L., Unverzagt, F. W.,...Musick, B. S. (1995). Prevalence of Alzheimer's disease and dementia in two communities: Nigerian Africans and African Americans. *American Journal of Psychiatry, 152*(10), 1485–1492.

Herrera, E., Jr., Caramelli, P., Silveira, A. S., & Nitrini, R. (2002). Epidemiologic survey of dementia in a community-dwelling Brazilian population. *Alzheimer Disease and Associated Disorders, 16*(2), 103–108.

Hoffman, A., Rocca, W. A., Brayne, C., Breteler, M. M., Clarke, M., Cooper, B,...Amaducci, L. (1991). The prevalence of dementia in Europe: A collaborative study of 1980–1990 findings. Eurodem Prevalence Research Group. *International Journal of Epidemiology, 20*(3), 736–748.

Huang, Y., Liu, Z., Zhang, M., Shen, Y., Tsang, A., He, Y., & Lee, S. (2008). Mental disorders and service use in China. In R. C. Kessler & T. B. Ustun (Eds.), *The WHO world mental health surveys: Global perspectives on the epidemiology of mental disorders* (pp. 447–473). New York, NY: Cambridge University Press.

Hwang, W. C., & Myers, H. F. (2007). Major depression in Chinese Americans: The roles of stress, vulnerability, and acculturation. *Social Psychiatry and Psychiatric Epidemiology, 42*(3), 189–197.

Hwu, H. G., Yeh, E. K., & Chang, L. Y. (1989). Prevalence of psychiatric disorders in Taiwan defined by the Chinese Diagnostic Interview Schedule. *Acta Psychiatrica Scandinavica, 79*(2), 136–147.

Jackson, J. S., Torres, M., Caldwell, C. H., Neighbors, H. W., Nesse, R. M., Taylor, R. J., . . . Williams, D. R. (2004). The National Survey of American Life: A study of racial, ethnic and cultural influences on mental disorders and mental health. *International Journal of Methods in Psychiatric Research, 13*(4), 196–207.

Jacobi, F., Wittchen, H. U., Holting, C., Hofler, M., Pfister, H., Muller, N., & Lieb, R. (2004). Prevalence, co-morbidity and correlates of mental disorders in the general population: Results from the German Health Interview and Examination Survey (GHS). *Psychological Medicine, 34*(4), 597–611.

Jenkins, R., Lewis, G., Bebbington, P., Brugha, T., Farrell, M., Gill, B., & Melzer, H. (1997). The National Psychiatric Morbidity surveys of Great Britain: Initial findings from the household survey. *Psychological Medicine, 27*(4), 775–789.

Jette, N., Patten, S., Williams, J., Becker, W., & Wiebe, S. (2008). Comorbidity of migraine and psychiatric disorders: A national population-based study. *Headache, 48*(4), 501–516.

Karam, E. G., Mneimneh, Z. N., Karam, A. N., Fayyad, J. A., Nasser, S. C., Dimassi, H., & Salamoun, M. M. (2008). Mental disorders and war in Lebanon. In R. C. Kessler & T. B. Ustun (Eds.), *The WHO world mental health surveys: Global perspectives on the epidemiology of mental disorders* (pp. 265–278). New York, NY: Cambridge University Press.

Kawakami, N., Takeshima, T., Ono, Y., Uda, H., Hata, Y., Nakane, Y., . . . Kikkawa, T. (2005). Twelve-month prevalence, severity, and treatment of common mental disorders in communities in Japan: Preliminary findings from the World Mental Health Japan Survey 2002–2003. *Psychiatry and Clinical Neuroscience, 59*(4), 441–452.

Kessler, R. C., Berglund, P., Demler, O., Jin, R., Koretz, D., Merikangas, K. R., . . . Wang, P. S. (2003). The epidemiology of major depressive disorder: Results from the National Comorbidity Survey Replication (NCS-R). *Journal of the American Medical Association, 289*(23), 3095–3105.

Kessler, R. C., Chiu, W. T., Demler, O., Merikangas, K. R., & Walters, E. E. (2005). Prevalence, severity, and comorbidity of 12-month DSM-IV disorders in the National Comorbidity Survey Replication. *Archives of General Psychiatry, 62*(6), 617–627.

Kessler, R. C., Haro, J. M., Heeringa, S. G., Pennell, B. E., & Ustun, T. B. (2006). The World Health Organization world mental health survey initiative. *Social Psychiatry and Psychiatric Epidemiology, 15*(3), 161–166.

Kessler, R. C., McGonagle, K. A., Zhao, S., Nelson, C. B., Hughes, M., Eshleman, S., . . . Kendler, K. S. (1994). Lifetime and 12-month prevalence of DSM-III-R psychiatric disorders in the United States: Results from the National Comorbidity Survey. *Archives of General Psychiatry, 51*(1), 8–19.

Kessler, R. C., & Ustun, T. B. (Eds). (2008). *The WHO world mental health surveys: Global perspectives on the epidemiology of mental disorders.* New York, NY: Cambridge University Press.

Kim, J., Jeong, I., Chun, J. H., & Lee, S. (2003). The prevalence of dementia in a metropolitan city of South Korea. *International Journal of Geriatric Psychiatry, 18*(7), 617–622.

Kiyohara, Y., Yoshitake, T., Kato, I., Ohmura, T., Kawano, H., Ueda, K., & Fujishima, M. (1994). Changing patterns in the prevalence of dementia in a Japanese community: The Hisayama study. *Gerontology, 40*(Suppl. 2), 29–35.

Kraepelin, E. (1919). *Dementia praecox and paraphrenia.* Edinburgh, UK: Livingstone.

Kringlen, E., Torgersen, S., & Cramer, V. (2001). A Norwegian psychiatric epidemiological study. *American Journal of Psychiatry, 158*(7), 1091–1098.

Kringlen, E., Torgersen, S., & Cramer, V. (2006). Mental illness in a rural area: A Norwegian psychiatric epidemiological study. *Social Psychiatry and Psychiatric Epidemiology, 41*(9), 713–719.

Kua, E. H. (1991). The prevalence of dementia in elderly Chinese. *Acta Psychiatrica Scandinavica, 83*(5), 350–352.

Lee, C. K., Kwak, Y. S., Yamamoto, J., Rhee, H., Kim, Y. S., Han, J. H., . . . Lee, Y. H. (1990). Psychiatric epidemiology in Korea. Part II: Urban and rural differences. *Journal of Nervous and Mental Disease, 178*(4), 247–252.

Lee, D. Y., Lee, J. H., Ju, Y. S., Lee, K. U., Kim, K. W., Jhoo, J. H., . . . Woo, J. I. (2002). The prevalence of dementia in older people in an urban population of Korea: The Seoul study. *Journal of the American Geriatric Society, 50*(7), 1233–1239.

Lee, S., Tsang, A., Zhang, M. Y., Huang, Y. Q., He, Y. L., Liu, Z. R., . . . Kessler, R. C. (2007). Lifetime prevalence and inter-cohort variation in DSM-IV disorders in metropolitan China. *Psychological Medicine, 37*(1), 61–71.

Lenzenweger, M. F., Lane, M. C., Loranger, A. W., & Kessler, R. C. (2007). DSM-IV personality disorders in the National Comorbidity Survey Replication. *Biological Psychiatry, 62*(6), 553–564.

Lepine, J. P., & Lellouch, J. (1995). Classification and epidemiology of social phobia. *European Archives of Psychiatry and Clinical Neuroscience, 244*(6), 290–296.

Levinson, D., Lerner, Y., Zilber, N., Levav, I., & Polakiewicz, J. (2008). The prevalence of mental disorders and service use in Israel: Results from the National Health Survey, 2003–2004. In R. C. Kessler & T. B. Ustun (Eds.), *The WHO world mental health surveys: Global perspectives on the epidemiology of mental disorders* (pp. 346–363). New York, NY: Cambridge University Press.

Lobo, A., Launer, L. J., Fratiglioni, L., Andersen, K., Di, C. A., Breteler, M. M.,...Hofman, A. (2000). Prevalence of dementia and major subtypes in Europe: A collaborative study of population-based cohorts. *Neurology, 54*(11, Suppl. 5), s4–s9.

Lopez, A., Mathers, C. D., Ezzati, M., Jamison, D. T., & Murray, C. J. L. (Eds.) (2006). *Global burden of disease and risk factors*. New York, NY: Oxford University Press.

Mathers, C., Lopez, A. D., & Murray, C. (2006). The burden of disease and mortality by condition: Data, methods, and results for 2001. In A. D. Lopez, C. D. Mathers, M. Ezzati, D. T. Jamison, & C. J. L. Murray (Eds.), *Global burden of disease and risk factors* (pp. 45–240). New York, NY: Oxford University Press.

McConnell, P., Bebbington, P., McClelland, R., Gillespie, K., & Houghton, S. (2002). Prevalence of psychiatric disorder and the need for psychiatric care in Northern Ireland: Population study in the district of Derry. *British Journal of Psychiatry, 181*, 214–219.

McGrath, J., Saha, S., Chant, D., & Welham, J. (2008). The epidemiology of schizophrenia: A concise overview of incidence, prevalence and mortality. *Epidemiologic Reviews, 30*, 67–76.

Medina-Mora, M. E., Borges, G., Fleiz, C., Benjet, C., Rojas, E., Zambrano, J.,...Aguillar-Gaxiola, S. (2006). Prevalence and correlates of drug use disorders in Mexico. *Revista Panamericana de Salud Pública, 19*(4), 265–276.

Medina-Mora, M. E., Borges, G., Lara, C., Benjet, C., Blanco, J., Fleiz, C.,...Zambrano, J. (2005). Prevalence, service use, and demographic correlates of 12-month DSM-IV psychiatric disorders in Mexico: Results from the Mexican National

Comorbidity Survey. *Psychological Medicine, 35*(12), 1773–1783.

Merikangas, K. R., Akiskal, H. S., Angst, J., Greenberg, P. E., Hirschfeld, R. M., Petukhova, M., & Kessler, R. C. (2007). Lifetime and 12-month prevalence of bipolar spectrum disorder in the National Comorbidity Survey Replication, 11. *Archives of General Psychiatry, 64*(5), 543–552.

Mohammadi, M. R., Ghanizadeh, A., Rahgozar, M., Noorbala, A. A., Davidian, H., Afzali, H. M.,...Teranidoost, M. (2004). Prevalence of obsessive–compulsive disorder in Iran. *BMC Psychiatry, 4*, 2.

Morande, G., Celada, J., & Casas, J. J. (1999). Prevalence of eating disorders in a Spanish school-age population. *Journal of Adolescent Health, 24*(3), 212–219.

Morris, J. N. (1975). *Uses of epidemiology* (3rd ed.). Edinburgh, UK: Churchill Livingstone.

Murray, C. J. L., & Lopez, A. D. (1996). *The global burden of disease*. Boston, MA: Harvard University Press.

Neumark, Y. D., Lopez-Quintero, C., Grinshpoon, A., & Levinson, D. (2007). Alcohol drinking patterns and prevalence of alcohol-abuse and dependence in the Israel National Health Survey. *Israel Journal of Psychiatry and Related Science, 44*(2), 126–135.

Oakley-Browne, M. A., Joyce, P. R., Wells, J. E., Bushnell, J. A., & Hornblow, A. R. (1989). Christchurch Psychiatric Epidemiology Study, Part II: Six month and other period prevalences of specific psychiatric disorders 2. *Australian and New Zealand Journal of Psychiatry, 23*(3), 327–340.

Oakley-Browne, M. A., Wells, J. E., & Scott, K. M. (2008). Te Rau Hinengaro: The New Zealand Mental Health Survey. In R. C. Kessler & T. B. Ustun (Eds.), *The WHO world mental health surveys: Global perspectives on the epidemiology of mental disorders* (pp. 486–508). New York, NY: Cambridge University Press.

Offord, D. R., Boyle, M. H., Campbell, D., Goering, P., Lin, E., Wong, M., & Racine, Y. A. (1996). One-year prevalence of psychiatric disorder in Ontarians 15 to 64 years of age. *Canadian Journal of Psychiatry, 41*(9), 559–563.

Ogborne, A. C., & DeWit, D. (2001). Alcohol use, alcohol disorders, and the use of health services: Results from a population survey. *American Journal of Drug and Alcohol Abuse, 27*(4), 759–774.

Ogura, C., Nakamoto, H., Uema, T., Yamamoto, K., Yonemori, T., & Yoshimura, T. (1995). Prevalence of senile dementia in Okinawa, Japan. *International Journal of Epidemiology, 24*(2), 373–380.

Ohayon, M. M., & Hong, S. C. (2006). Prevalence of major depressive disorder in the general population of South Korea. *Journal of Psychiatric Research, 40*(1), 30–36.

Pakriev, S., Vasar, V., Aluoja, A., Saarma, M., & Shlik, J. (1998). Prevalence of mood disorders in the rural population of Udmurtia. *Acta Psychiatrica Scandinavica, 97*(3), 169–174.

Parner, E. T., Schendel, D. E., & Thorsen, P. (2008). Autism prevalence trends over time in Denmark: Changes in prevalence and age at diagnosis. *Archives of Pediatrics and Adolescent Medicine, 162*(12), 1150–1156.

Pelaez Fernandez, M. A., Labrador, F. J., & Raich, R. M. (2007). Prevalence of eating disorders among adolescent and young adult scholastic population in the region of Madrid (Spain). *Journal of Psychosomatic Research, 62*(6), 681–690.

Phanthumchindra, K., Jitapunkul, S., Sitthi-Amorn, C., Bunnag, S. C., & Ebrahim, S. (1991). Prevalence of dementia in an urban slum population in Thailand: Validity of screening methods. *International Journal of Geriatric Psychiatry, 6*, 639–646.

Pirkola, S. P., Isometsä, E., Suvisaari, J., Aro, H. J. M., Poikolainen, K., Koskinen, S.,...Lönnqvist, J. K. (2005). DSM-IV mood-, anxiety- and alcohol use disorders and their comorbidity in the Finnish general population: Results from the Health 2000 Study. *Social Psychiatry and Psychiatric Epidemiology, 40*(1), 1–10.

Polanczyk, G., & Jensen, P. (2008). Epidemiologic considerations in attention deficit hyperactivity disorder: A review and update. *Child and Adolescent Psychiatric Clinics of North America, 17*(2), 245–260, vii.

Posada-Villa, J., Rodriguez, M., Duque, P., Garzon, A., Aguilar-Gaxiola, S., & Breslau, J. (2008). Mental disorders in Colombia: Results from the World Mental Health Survey. In R.C. Kessler & T. B. Ustun (Eds.), *The WHO world mental health surveys: Global perspectives on the epidemiology of mental disorders* (pp. 131–143). New York, NY: Cambridge University Press.

President's Commission on Mental Health. (1978). *Report to the President from the President's commission on mental health* (Vol. 1). Washington, DC: US Government Printing Office.

Rajkumar, S., Kumar, S., & Thara, R. (1997). Prevalence of dementia in a rural setting: A report from India 1. *International Journal of Geriatric Psychiatry, 12*(7), 702–707.

Regier, D. A., Myers, J. K., Kramer, M., Robins, L. N., Blazer, D. G., Hough, R. L.,...Locke, B. Z. (1984). The NIMH Epidemiologic Catchment Area (ECA) program: Historical context, major objectives, and study population characteristics. *Archives of General Psychiatry, 41*(10), 934–941.

Roberts, R. E., Roberts, C. R., & Xing, Y. (1999). Rates of DSM-IV psychiatric disorders among adolescents in a large metropolitan area. *Journal of Psychiatric Research, 41*(11), 959–967.

Robins, L. N., Helzer, J. E., Croughan, J., & Ratcliff, K. S. (1981). National Institute of Mental Health Diagnostic Interview Schedule: Its history, characteristics, and validity. *Archives of General Psychiatry, 38*(4), 381–389.

Robins, L. N., & Regier, D. A. (1991). *Psychiatric disorders in America—the Epidemiologic Catchment Area study.* New York, NY: Free Press.

Robins, L., Wing, J. K., Wittchen, H. U., Helzer, J. E., Babor, T. F., Burke, J.,...Towle, J. H. (1988). The Composite International Diagnostic Interview: An epidemiologic instrument suitable for use in conjunction with different diagnostic systems and in different cultures. *Archives of General Psychiatry, 45*(12), 1069–1077.

Rocha, F. L., Vorcaro, C. M., Uchoa, E., & Lima-Costa, M. F. (2005). Comparing the prevalence rates of social phobia in a community according to ICD-10 and DSM-III-R. *Revista Brasiliera Psiquiatria, 27*(3), 222–224.

Rojo, L., Livianos, L., Conesa, L., Garcia, A., Dominguez, A., Rodrigo, G.,...Vila, M. (2003). Epidemiology and risk factors of eating disorders: A two-stage epidemiologic study in a Spanish population aged 12–18 years. *International Journal of Eating Disorders, 34*(3), 281–291.

Samuels, J., Eaton, W. W., Bienvenu, O. J., III, Brown, C. H., Costa, P. T., Jr., & Nestadt, G. (2002). Prevalence and correlates of personality disorders in a community sample. *British Journal of Psychiatry, 180*, 536–542.

Sanderson, K., & Andrews, G. (2002). Prevalence and severity of mental health–related disability and relationship to diagnosis. *Psychiatric Services, 53*(1), 80–86.

Senanarong, V., Poungvarin, N., Sukhatunga, K., Prayoonwiwat, N., Chaisewikul, R., Petchurai, R.,...Viriyavejakul, A. (2001). Cognitive status in the community dwelling Thai elderly. *Journal of the Medical Association of Thailand, 84*(3), 408–416.

Shaji, S., Promodu, K., Abraham, T., Roy, K. J., & Verghese, A. (1996). An epidemiological study of dementia in a rural community in Kerala, India. *British Journal of Psychiatry, 168*, 745–749.

Sheehan, D. V. (2008). Sheehan Disability Scale. In A. J. Rush, M. B. First, & D. Blacker (Eds.), *Handbook of psychiatric measures* (2nd ed., pp. 100–102). Washington, DC: American Psychiatric Press.

Sheehan, D. V., Harnett-Sheehan, K., & Raj, B. A. (1996). The measurement of disability. *International Clinical Psychopharmacology, 11*(Suppl. 3), 89–95.

Shen, Y. C., Zhang, M. Y., Huang, Y. Q., He, Y. L., Liu, Z. R., Cheng, H.,...Kessler, R. C. (2006). Twelve-month prevalence, severity, and unmet need for treatment of mental disorders in metropolitan China. *Psychological Medicine, 36*(2), 257–267.

Slone, L. B., Norris, F. H., Murphy, A. D., Baker, C. K., Perilla, J. L., Diaz, D.,...Gutiérrez Rodriguez Jde, J. (2006). Epidemiology of major depression in four cities in Mexico. *Depression and Anxiety, 23*(3), 158–167.

Somers, J. M., Goldner, E. M., Waraich, P., & Hsu, L. (2006). Prevalence and incidence studies of anxiety disorders: A systematic review of the literature. *Canadian Journal of Psychiatry, 51*(2), 100–113.

Srinath, S., Girimaji, S. C., Gururaj, G., Seshadri, S., Subbakrishna, D. K., Bhola, P., & Kumar, N. (2005). Epidemiological study of child and adolescent psychiatric disorders in urban and rural areas of Bangalore, India. *Indian Journal of Medical Research, 122*(1), 67–79.

Statistics Canada. (2008). *Canadian Community Health Survey (CCHS): Mental Health and Wellbeing—Cycle 1.2.* Retrieved May 2, 2011, from http://www.statcan.gc.ca/dli-ild/data-donnees/ftp/cchs-escc-eng.htm

Stefansson, J. G., Lindal, E., Bjornsson, J. K., & Guomundsdottir, A. (1991). Lifetime prevalence of specific mental disorders among people born in Iceland in 1931. *Acta Psychiatrica Scandinavica, 84*(2), 142–149.

Stein, M. B., Walker, J. R., & Torgrud, L. J. (2000). Social phobia symptoms, subtypes, and severity: Findings from a community survey. *Archives of General Psychiatry, 57*(11), 1046–1052.

Stinson, F. S., Dawson, D. A., Patricia Chou, S., Smith, S., Goldstein, R. B., June Ruan, W., & Grant, B. E. (2007). The epidemiology of DSM-IV specific phobia in the USA: Results from the National Epidemiologic Survey on Alcohol and Related Conditions. *Psychological Medicine, 37*(7), 1047–1059.

Substance Abuse and Mental Health Services Administration. (2007). *Results from the 2006 National Survey on Drug Use and Health: National findings.* Rockville, MD: Substance Abuse and Mental Health Services Administration, US Department of Health and Human Services.

Suh, G. H., Kim, J. K., & Cho, M. J. (2003). Community study of dementia in the older Korean rural population. *Australian and New Zealand Journal of Psychiatry, 37*(5), 606–612.

Szadoczky, E., Papp, Z., Vitrai, J., Rihmer, Z., & Furedi, J. (1998). The prevalence of major depressive and bipolar disorders in Hungary: Results from a national epidemiologic survey. *Journal of Affective Disorders, 50*(2–3), 153–162.

Torgersen, S., Kringlen, E., & Cramer, V. (2001). The prevalence of personality disorders in a community sample. *Archives of General Psychiatry, 58*(6), 590–596.

Vas, C. J., Pinto, C., Panikker, D., Noronha, S., Deshpande, N., Kulkarni, L., & Sachdeva, S. (2001). Prevalence of dementia in an urban Indian population. *International Psychogeriatrics, 13*(4), 439–450.

Verhulst, F.C., van der Ende, J., Ferdinand, R.F., & Kasius, M.C. (1997). The prevalence of DSM-III-R diagnoses in a national sample of dutch adolescents. *Archives of General Psychiatry, 54*(4), 329–336.

Vicente, B., Kohn, R., Rioseco, P., Saldivia, S., Levav, I., & Torres, S. (2006). Lifetime and 12-month prevalence of DSM-III-R disorders in the Chile psychiatric prevalence study. *American Journal of Psychiatry, 163*(8), 1362–1370.

Vorcaro, C. M., Lima-Costa, M. F., Barreto, S. M., & Uchoa, E. (2001). Unexpected high prevalence of 1-month depression in a small Brazilian community: The Bambui study. *Acta Psychiatrica Scandinavica, 104*(4), 257–263.

Vos, T., & Mathers, C. D. (2000). The burden of mental disorders: A comparison of methods between the Australian burden of disease studies and the Global Burden of Disease study, *Bulletin of the World Health Organization, 78*(4), 427–438.

Wang, J. L. (2004). Rural–urban differences in the prevalence of major depression and associated impairment. *Social Psychiatry and Psychiatric Epidemiology, 39*(1), 19–25.

Waraich, P., Goldner, E. M., Somers, J. M., & Hsu, L. (2004). Prevalence and incidence studies of mood disorders: A systematic review of the literature. *Canadian Journal of Psychiatry, 49*(2), 124–138.

Weissman, M. M., Myers, J. K., & Harding, P. S. (1978). Psychiatric disorders in a U.S. urban community: 1975–1976. *American Journal of Psychiatry, 135*(4), 459–462.

Wells, J. E., Browne, M. A., Scott, K. M., McGee, M. A., Baxter, J., & Kokaua, J. (2006). Prevalence, interference with life and severity of 12 month DSM-IV disorders in Te Rau Hinengaro: The

New Zealand Mental Health Survey. *Australian and New Zealand Journal of Psychiatry, 40*(10), 845–854.

Williams, D. R., Gonzalez, H. M., Neighbors, H., Nesse, R., Abelson, J. M., Sweetman, J., & Jackson, J. S. (2007). Prevalence and distribution of major depressive disorder in African Americans, Caribbean Blacks, and non-Hispanic Whites: Results from the National Survey of American Life. *Archives of General Psychiatry, 64*(3), 305–315.

Williams, D. R., Herman, A., Stein, D. J., Heeringa, S. G., Jackson, P. B., Moomal, H., & Kessler, R. C. (2008). Twelve-month mental disorders in South Africa: Prevalence, service use and demographic correlates in the population-based South African Stress and Health Study. *Psychological Medicine, 38*(2), 211–220.

Williams, J. G., Higgins, J. P., & Brayne, C. E. (2006). Systematic review of prevalence studies of autism spectrum disorders. *Archives of Disease in Childhood, 91*(1), 8–15.

Wittchen, H. U. (1994). Reliability and validity studies of the WHO—Composite International Diagnostic Interview (CIDI): A critical review. *Journal of Psychiatric Research, 28*(1), 57–84.

Woo, J. I., Lee, J. H., Yoo, K. Y., Kim, C. Y., Kim, Y. I., & Shin, Y.S. (1998). Prevalence estimation of dementia in a rural area of Korea. *Journal of the American Geriatric Society, 46*(8), 983–987.

World Health Organization. (1967). *Manual of the International Statistical Classification of Diseases, Injuries, and Causes of Death (ICD-8).* Geneva, Switzerland: Author.

World Health Organization. (1977). *International Classification of Diseases, 9th revision (ICD-9).* Geneva, Switzerland: Author.

World Health Organization. (1980). *International Classification of Impairments, Disabilities, and Handicaps (ICIDH).* Geneva, Switzerland: Author.

World Health Organization. (1993). *ICD-10 classification of mental and behavioral disorders: Diagnostic criteria for research.* Geneva, Switzerland: Author.

World Health Organization. (2001). *International Classification of Functioning, Disability, and Health.* Geneva, Switzerland: Author.

World Health Organization. (2008). *The global burden of disease: 2004 update.* Geneva, Switzerland: Author.

Zwirs, B. W. C., Burger, H., Schulpen, T. W. J., Wiznitzer, M., Fedder, H., & Buitelaar, J. K. (2007). Prevalence of psychiatric disorders among children of different ethnic origin. *Journal of Abnormal Child Psychology, 35*, 556–566.

2

The Perspectives of Psychiatry:
The Public Health Approach

PAUL R. MCHUGH

Key Points

- The *Diagnostic and Statistical Manual of Mental Disorders* (DSM) functions as a field guide in which psychiatric diagnoses are made based on the clinical presentations rather than on any aspects of the generative nature of the disorders

- A field guide brings consistency to nomenclature and identification but being heuristically barren it offers no help to understanding and in clinical matters no direction to preventive or treatment interventions

- Reordering DSM listings would encourage conceptualization of mental disorders according to perspectives of generation and would enhance its public health value

- Four important perspectives that relate mental disorders to their sources are disease, dimension, behavior, and life story

- Certain perspectives tend to illuminate certain disorders, and other perspectives other disorders, but together they comprise a comprehensive approach to patient services and care

---

INTRODUCTION:
THE PROBLEM

Today, all who aim to improve the mental and behavioral well-being of the public confront an awkward but conspicuous problem. Although contemporary psychiatric epidemiologic research indicates that some kind of mental disorder afflicts more than 50% of the American people at some time in their lives (Kessler et al., 2005; Wang et al., 2005), it fails to suggest any pathways for either preventing or remedying these matters.

The reason why is not hard to discern. The current standard method to identify mental disorders that is codified in the official *Diagnostic and Statistical Manual of Mental*

Disorders (DSM) (American Psychiatric Association [APA], 1980, 1987, 1994) functions as a field guide. It identifies cases based on expressed symptoms (the counterparts of field marks in naturalists' guide books); symptom criteria act as the clinic-based equivalent of a plumed crest or colored breast used by bird-watchers to identify a bird on the wing.

Specifically, DSM's nosology operates without considering the nature, cause, or mechanism behind a mental or behavioral disorder. Although this approach does bring consistency to public health efforts to name and enumerate mental disorders (a justification for the DSM itself), it offers nothing to advance either prevention or remediation of disorders, as such efforts are dependent on knowledge of causes or mechanisms.

How can one mount significant population-based efforts to prevent or treat chronic or recurrent disorders when their grounds are not well understood or even a matter of interest? Thus the so-called atheoretical (and actually a-conceptual) nature of the nosology of the fourth edition of the DSM (DSM-IV) (APA, 1994) and its immediate predecessors has led to an impasse in the conduct of a public health mission. The situation is ripe for change.

The goal of this chapter is to demonstrate how the field of clinical psychiatry is ready to effect that change. A scientific foundation has been laid by basic, clinical, epidemiologic, and services research on mental disorders that provides an intelligible, comprehensive picture of much that is fundamental to their etiology and their nature. By combining identification with research-based understanding of the nature of mental disorders, public health psychiatry can find ways to advance rational public mental health policies. Reciprocally, such policies can advance clinical psychiatry in much the same way as public health enterprises have so often advanced general medical care (Morris, 1975).

Although all physicians have the same basic education, a fundamental difference appears to exist between the ways in which those who specialize in mental disorders and those who specialize in physical disorders approach clinical diagnosis and therapeutic decision making. Internists and neurologists, who concentrate on body and brain, depend on their knowledge of the physical functioning of bodily parts to identify the disorders they diagnose and treat. They address and answer questions such as "Where in the patient's body is the proposed disruption localized?" and "What process of nature does this disruption represent?" In contrast, psychiatrists, who concentrate on mental life and behavior and depend on the DSM to identify disorders by symptomatic criteria, make every diagnostic exercise a question of confidence, asking, "Am I sure I'm diagnosing this patient in a reliable fashion?"

These basic distinctions in approach explain why physical medicine and psychological medicine have diverged. The former—answering "where" and "what" questions such as the localization of a disorder (in the heart, lung, kidney, etc.) and its nature as a pathologic process (infectious, vascular, neoplastic, nutritional, etc.)—appears far more aligned with the natural sciences than does the latter. Ultimately, this alignment of physical medicine with science led to answers to even more fundamental questions such as "how" a disorder progresses and "why" it affects certain persons and not others. The process of answering these questions led to diagnostic intelligibility, to rational, individual treatment, and to coherent public health measures.

The Clinical Descriptions and Diagnostic Guidelines of the 10th revision of the International Classification of Diseases (ICD-10) (World Health Organization, 1992) present a clear example of this approach in the form of a systematic heuristic taxonomy of disorders based on organ structures and functional mechanisms affected by etiopathologic processes. In the ICD-10, most clinical signs and symptoms of a particular disease process (the "what?") are explained through the localization of its pathology to a definite organ or organ part (the "where?").

Ernst Mayr (1997) observed, "Any classification which takes causation into account is subject to severe constraints that prevent it from becoming a purely artificial system" (p. 137). In fact, the causal presumptions driving a classification often can prompt research that challenges and refines those very presumptions. For example, challenges to the notion in an earlier iteration of the ICD that peptic ulcer results from an inflammatory process affecting the mucosal lining of the stomach and duodenum led to a demonstration that in reality the underlying culprit is an intraintestinal *Helicobacter* infection that is readily susceptible to antibiotic treatment (Forbes et al., 1994; Marshall et al., 1988; Marshall & Warren, 1984).

Unfortunately, with psychiatry dominated by the symptom-focused DSM, nothing of this hypothesis-challenging, progress-inducing heuristic approach can occur. There simply is no concept of etiopathology to challenge. Rather, the "powers that be"—the creators of the DSM—define what mental disorders exist; rank-and-file clinicians, working by rote, decide which patients meet the predetermined diagnostic criteria; and no one wonders what is real.

APPROACHING A SOLUTION

To quote another authority, the evolutionary theorist Stephen Jay Gould (1989) observed that "Classifications [should be] theories about the basis of natural order, not dull catalogues compiled only to avoid chaos" (p. 98). Applying this concept to the practice of psychiatry, either in general or in public health, calls for the definition of its own natural order.

Psychiatrists are physicians who identify, study, and treat disorders of human conscious mental life. This definition pinpoints the problem of building a systematic taxonomy on the concepts of localization and process ("where?" and "what?") given the mental, subjective domain of life represented by consciousness. Consciousness is a biological domain characterized by unique features such as an internal, subjective nature, expressed functionally in terms of a first-person experience ("I" think, feel, know, need, etc.), and carrying inherent powers for both choice and response. None of these features have the tangible, corporeal characteristics customarily studied by a sensate culture of science and medicine, and from which such concepts as localization and process emerge naturally.

We can resolve this dilemma by clarifying the relationship between the tangible brain and the intangible mind. The conscious mind is not a product of the brain in the way bile is a product of the liver or urine is the product of the kidneys. Rather, mind is an emergent property, engendered by and dependent on an unknown (perhaps unknowable [McGinn, 1999]) aspect of how neuronal systems in the brain are organized and function. As an emergent property, the features of mind should not be studied simply for their content, as if mind were a product such as urine or bile. Rather, the features of mind should be considered in the context of how they affect and are affected by the life of their subject. On this idea, after all, rests the justification of the science of psychology.

Although human consciousness is subjective, it is not without form. Rather, the conscious mind has a composite nature structured around several functional, interactive, operative modes or modalities. These are identified by psychologists as the intrinsic modalities, the self-differentiating modalities, the teleologic modalities, and the extrinsic/experiential modalities (see figure 2-1).

The first, most obvious and fundamental attributes of mind are those that make up the intrinsic modalities and encompass the wakeful aspect of consciousness and such cerebral faculties such as memory, perception, language, and affect. The attributes of mind that constitute the self-differentiating modalities include several psychological features that, in their individuating variation, characterize each person and encompass intelligence, affective temperament, and maturational stage. The attributes of mind that constitute the teleologic modalities include fluctuating appetites or drives, such as hunger and thirst, that give rise to inclinations and behavioral choices when the individual seeks satisfaction. The attributes of mind that constitute the extrinsic/experiential modalities include the emotional and cognitive responses to life events, both transient and persistent, through which responses the family, social networks, education, occupation, and culture exert their influence on psychosocial development, individuation, and character formation.

Normal, healthy mental or emotional life arises from the dynamic interaction of these four modalities of mind, both with each other

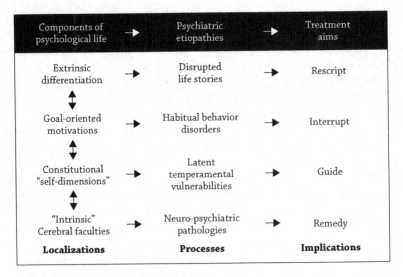

Components of psychological life	→	Psychiatric etiopathies	→	Treatment aims
Extrinsic differentiation	→	Disrupted life stories	→	Rescript
↕				
Goal-oriented motivations	→	Habitual behavior disorders	→	Interrupt
↕				
Constitutional "self-dimensions"	→	Latent temperamental vulnerabilities	→	Guide
↕				
"Intrinsic" Cerebral faculties	→	Neuro-psychiatric pathologies	→	Remedy
Localizations		**Processes**		**Implications**

Figure 2-1 **Comprehensive Representation of Hierarchical "Proximate" Causes in Psychiatry: Biopsychiatric components, processes, and treatments.**

and with the environment within which the individual develops and responds. The modalities are, as well, the psychological sites at which the etiopathic processes that generate mental unrest and disorder can be localized and from which the symptomatic effects of these processes are comprehended.

THE PERSPECTIVES OF PSYCHIATRY

To make sense of mental disorders, the perspectives of psychiatry take advantage of this composite nature of the conscious mind with its distinct modalities. We (McHugh and Slavney 1998) refer to the explanatory concepts as the perspectives of psychiatry to emphasize, by metaphor, that each is a way of looking at mental or behavioral unrest through which one can discern the modality locus and etiopathic process that may explain both the nature and cause of the unrest. As the metaphoric use of the term *perspectives* implies, for any patient presenting with a mental disorder, each perspective illuminates certain aspects of the causal nature of the problem but must be combined with other perspectives that further illuminate the particular example.

Like the modalities of the conscious mind, the distinct perspectives of psychiatry are

systematically interrelated and complementary. Because each perspective has particular methodological characteristics, any one stands in some theoretical tension with the others. However, in practice, they join together to illuminate every diagnostic formulation. To make these features clear, what follows (1) describes the method of reasoning tied to each perspective, (2) shows how, by identifying etiopathic processes disrupting, disturbing, or acting through the modalities of consciousness, the perspectives render clinical presentations more causally intelligible; and (3) explains how thinking about mental disorders in these ways illuminates a role for public health psychiatry in the treatment and prevention of those disorders. (see figure 2-2). Figure 2-3 displays a simple acronym (HIDE) we have found useful in capturing and transmitting the meanings of each perspective.

The Disease Perspective and the Intrinsic Modalities of Consciousness

Some mental disorders are the direct, conscious expression of a disease process that damages or disrupts the neuronal integrity of the brain, hence their identification by the

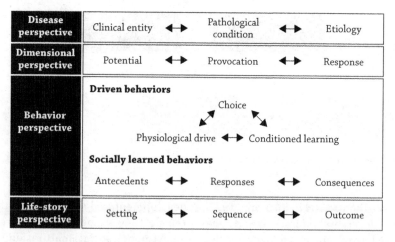

Disease perspective	Clinical entity	↔	Pathological condition	↔	Etiology
Dimensional perspective	Potential	↔	Provocation	↔	Response

Behavior perspective

Driven behaviors

Choice

Physiological drive ↔ Conditioned learning

Socially learned behaviors

Antecedents	↔	Responses	↔	Consequences

Life-story perspective	Setting	↔	Sequence	↔	Outcome

Figure 2-2   **The Perspectives of Psychiatry.**

Adapted from McHugh & Slavney, 1998.

perspective of disease (see figure 2-4). As a bodily organ like any other, the brain is subject to the same pathologies (vascular, infectious, neoplastic, etc.) that affect other body parts. The brain also is affected by unique pathologic processes (irritative, degenerative, neurotoxic, etc.). Any of these neuropathologic conditions can disrupt mechanisms sustaining the intrinsic modalities of mind, resulting in demonstrable signs and symptoms indicative of that disruption.

Thus the disease perspective encompasses those mental disorders that represent the disruption of such intrinsic features as wakefulness (delirium), cognition (dementia), affect (bipolar disorder), and the like. Disorders that fall within this perspective ultimately can be attributed to a specific "broken" part of the brain, a pathologic entity that, by disrupting the natural integrative mechanisms of neural circuitry, gives rise to the psychological signs and symptoms. And such a "broken part" within the brain can be the result of abnormal genes, toxins, infections, or other forms of etiopathy. Complete knowledge about a mental disorder resulting from a brain disease emerges when it is possible to identify an etiology underlying the brain pathology—that is, to discern a pathogenesis for the "broken part"—and then to link the broken part to the expressed symptoms of the disorder—that is, discern the pathophysiology of the diagnostic syndrome.

In this way, psychiatrists who adopt the disease perspective see clinical presentations in which a disruption of a basic cerebral faculty such as memory or consciousness is evident as neuropathologic. As a result, they seek to employ treatments either to alter the pathophysiologic mechanisms , thereby relieving the symptoms, or to cure the provocative or sustaining pathogenetic process, thus preventing the pathology.

In the history of psychiatric public health, this perspective is best exemplified by examples such as the treatment and prevention of brain disruptions caused by niacin deficiency in pellagra dementia (Goldberger, Wheeler, & Syden, 1920), the risk for psychosis among individuals infected with syphilis (Dattner,

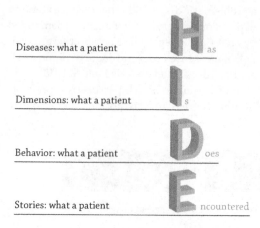

Diseases: what a patient _____ as

Dimensions: what a patient _____ s

Behavior: what a patient _____ oes

Stories: what a patient _____ ncountered

Figure 2-3   **Simplifying Sources and Process.**

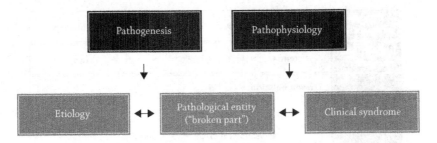

Figure 2-4   **The Disease Perspective Process.**

Kaufman, & Thomas,1947; Martin, 1972), and the risk for cerebral infarctions and aphasia associated with untreated hypertension (Kurtzke, 1983). We expect and await opportunities to view bipolar disorder and schizophrenia as disorders best illuminated by the perspective of disease.

The Dimensional Perspective and the Self-Differentiating Modalities of Consciousness

Many psychiatric problems arise not from a disease of brain but from aspects of the self-differentiating modalities (individuating characteristics of intelligence, temperament, and maturation) that render an individual vulnerable to emotional distress under certain provocative and challenging life circumstances. These latent, constitutional features are graded ("dimensional") psychological characteristics of humankind. Individuals at some extreme along the continuum of features, such as those with low intelligence, high extraversion, and high "neuroticism" (a term used in early psychiatry to suggest constitutional emotional instability), carry a vulnerability to emotional distress and excessive emotional responses in situations others handle successfully.

Just as the self-differentiating modalities influence the trajectory of personal development and educational attainment, so too do they shape and influence emotional adjustment, social maturation, and interpersonal relationships. It is also clear that within these modalities there also exist protective factors against disorders, represented by features of psychological resilience and strength (Rutter, 2000).

The dimensional perspective identifies a class of disorders best viewed as the product of an individual's affective or cognitive potential and some confrontation with provocative life circumstances that elicits excessive, disruptive emotional or behavioral responses (see figure 2-5). Suboptimal cognitive capacity (e.g., IQ less than 85) and affective features of high neuroticism, low conscientiousness, or immaturity represent particular problematic dispositional potentials.

The dimensional perspective grapples with the disorders listed on Axis II of DSM-IV (APA, 1994). However, the perspectives approach, by emphasizing the gradation in these human psychological features, helps discern effects of a problematic disposition that do not extend to expressions satisfying all the criteria demanded by an Axis II category. The perspective also can help make sense of several depressive and anxiety disorders listed on Axis I in DSM-IV.

From a public health perspective, preventing the distress and disruptions these aspects

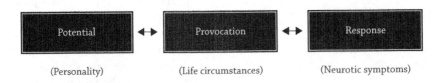

Figure 2-5   **The Dimensional Perspective Process.**

of human mental life bring about turns on finding a "goodness of fit" in the life circumstances of these individuals (Chess & Thomas, 1996). In particular, among youth, this means encouraging such efforts as responding to the educational needs of the cognitively subnormal with remediation and apt pacing of subject matter, and also rendering a school environment less emotionally challenging or threatening to children who are either excessively shy or excessively aggressive. Recognition by public health psychiatrists of the need to encourage families and schools to find ways to better support, strengthen, and guide such dimensionally at-risk children early in their development has proven of great value to their later life success and emotional contentment.

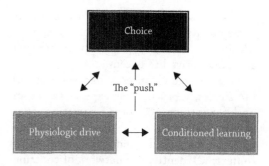

Figure 2-6 **The Behavioral Perspective Process.**

The Behavior Perspective and the Teleologic Modalities of Consciousness

The regular, quasirhythmic alterations in attention and perception produced by drives such as hunger, thirst, sleep, and sexual interest and by their satisfaction are the prime expressions in consciousness of the teleologic modalities. In his one enduring achievement in psychology, Sigmund Freud was the first to draw attention to these psychic states and how they affect conscious mental life. He noted the way in which these hungers wax and wane, affecting an individual's "attitude" toward his or her setting and impelling such complex, goal-directed, motor-sensory activities as eating, sleeping, and sexual activity. Both the behaviors and their provocative, affective attitudes are shaped by their psychosocial consequences and are sustained by conditioned learning over time. See figure 2-6.

For psychiatrists, the behavior perspective identifies the disruptions of choice and self-control manifest in such conditions as anorexia nervosa and bulimia nervosa, sexual paraphilias, and drug abuse and dependency. Exposure to drugs with high abuse potential (e.g., alcohol, cocaine, and heroin) can alter brain transmitter systems, producing and sustaining drug cravings, drug seeking, and drug consumption.

Public health psychiatry explores the role of supply and demand in these drug-related

behaviors and strives to understand the social contexts and characteristics of individuals who become substance dependent. The goal is to identify and promote social environments in which individuals can overcome their destructive habits. For substance abusers, three approaches to the contingencies of those behaviors that have met with success in interrupting drug dependence are methadone programs that offer drive reduction, voucher and monitoring programs that provide direct rewards and punishments, and programs analogous to Alcoholics Anonymous that support and sustain abstinence through peer-group engagement (Higgins, Silverman, & Heil, 2008)

The implication of this work for public health psychiatry is that addicts—whatever the focus of the addiction—neither suffer from a "disease" nor have an obsessive–compulsive disorder. Rather, such individuals have a behavioral disorder that, beginning with their choice to use substances of abuse, leads to a sustained need to continue the use because of the features of reward tied to ingesting these drugs—in other words, dependence. Forms of treatment and assistance that reframe both the context and contingencies promoting the behavioral choices ultimately can help them stop (Heyman, 2009).

The Life Story Perspective and the Extrinsic/Experiential Modality of Consciousness

The life story perspective—resting on the expressions in consciousness of the extrinsic/experiential modality—can enable psychiatrists to make sense of certain distressful disruptions of mental life by identifying them as responses within that modality to particular personal and provocative life encounters or socioenvironmental circumstances. When working with life stories, a psychiatrist expects to accomplish three things: (1) forge a narrative of setting and sequence that makes the distressful outcome meaningful and appropriate to its context; (2) identify the network of contributions from personal events, life circumstances, and social demands that play mediating roles in this outcome; and (3) identify instances in which a better understanding of situation and response would relieve or prevent the disruptive state of mind (see figure 2-7).

In the simplest terms, psychiatrists turn to the life story perspective to explain grief from losses, shame from humiliations, homesickness from difficulties in acculturation, jealousy from threats to valued personal relationships, and anxieties from fears about one's physical or social integrity. In addition, the life story perspective can explain how an individual's worldview, thought habits, assumptions, and expectations have been shaped through experiences and reflections on them. From this personal framework emerge disorders such as hysteria, adult gender identity disorder, false memory syndrome, and disordered expressions such as are found in religious scrupulosity and sociopolitical fanaticisms. With life story reasoning, psychiatrists can identify patients who need help to reframe their thinking and planning—a process at the very heart of psychotherapy.

Perhaps the most frequent contemporary considerations employing life story reasoning in public health psychiatry relate to posttraumatic stress disorder—a condition provoked by a variety of traumatic events and of particular concern during war and military campaigns.

The almost century-long history of recognizing such states of mind in combat soldiers and other traumatized individuals, as well as the various ways of understanding, treating, and preventing such conditions, represents a most significant contribution of public health psychiatry (McHugh & Treisman, 2007; McNally, 2003; Rosen & Lilienfeld, 2008; Shephard, 2000).

COMBINATIONS OF PERSPECTIVES FOR SPECIFIC SERVICES

Pure examples of the four perspectives provide only a partial demonstration of the value they have as approaches to differentiating among classes of mental disorders and as guides to psychiatric treatment and prevention. Disorders of human mental life are more complex than implied by single examples of what in fact are interrelated perspectives. The vast majority of patients demonstrate the interactions of several perspectives at once in their mental afflictions. For example, the disease perspective can be applied to schizophrenia, but the course of schizophrenia and even its risk may be exacerbated by the challenge of complex social tasks and life planning, which is illuminated by the life story perspective (Eaton & Harrison, 2001). Disorders best connected to the dimensional perspective are strongly affected by physical as well as emotional provocations; prognosis may depend on the life narrative selected by the individual as an explanation for the provocative issue. Although the social environment is tightly related to disorders understood through the behavioral perspective, in that exposure to drugs or constraints on life choices differ among natural groups and classes, neuronal effects and heritable factors certainly also influence drug and alcohol use, suggesting that the disease and dimensional

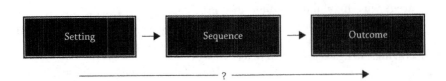

Figure 2-7 **The Life Story Perspective Process.**

Table 2-1 Some Examples of DSM Diagnoses Clustered by Causal "Perspectives"

DISEASES	DIMENSIONS	BEHAVIORS	ENCOUNTERS
Delirium	Mental retardation	Anorexia nervosa	Adjustment disorder
Schizophrenia	Anti-social personality	Sexual paraphilia	Bereavement
Bipolar disorder	Obsessive compulsive personality	Alcohol dependence	Posttraumatic stress disorder

perspectives can offer extra illumination of these matters.

Thus the clinician will find all four perspectives valuable in treating the whole patient, looking in effect for clues to etiology or mechanism that may help both in diagnosis and in treatment planning. Moreover, the perspectives are of help to the public health researcher and practitioner first as signposts to guide epidemiologic research in the search for clues to etiology (Morris, 1975) and then to suggest population-based interventions.

CONCLUSION

The four perspectives described in this chapter represent together an heuristic approach those at the Johns Hopkins School of Public Health have suggested as a response to the current psychiatric nosology. Table 2.1 exemplifies with some common diagnoses of DSM-IV how conditions can be encompassed within the perspectives classification structure, allowing psychiatrists and public health investigators to retain the advantages of diagnostic consistency but distinguish mental disorders by their likely generation.

American psychiatry has had more than 30 years of experience with the field guide method of diagnosis imposed on it by the DSM (APA, 1980, 1987, 1994). That manual's original goals of reducing doctrinal chaos and bringing diagnostic reliability to the field have been achieved. The time has arrived for psychiatry to follow the rest of medicine by differentiating disorders according to their likely underlying natures expressed through causes and mechanisms and so discern the most suitable ways for their coherent scientific study. The perspectives of psychiatry represent our way at the Johns Hopkins School of Public Health of moving in that direction.

REFERENCES

American Psychiatric Association. (1980). *Diagnostic and statistical manual of mental disorders* (3rd ed.). Washington, DC: Author.

American Psychiatric Association. (1987). *Diagnostic and statistical manual of mental disorders* (3rd ed., rev.). Washington, DC: Author.

American Psychiatric Association. (1994). *Diagnostic and statistical manual of mental disorders* (4th ed.). Washington, DC: Author.

Chess, S., & Thomas, A. (1996). *Temperament: Theory and practice*. New York, NY: Brunner/Mazel.

Dattner, B., Kaufman, S. S., & Thomas, E. W. (1947). Penicillin in treatment of neurosyphilis. *Archives of Neurology and Psychiatry, 58*(4), 426–435.

Eaton, W. W., & Harrison, G. (2001). Life chances, life planning, and schizophrenia: A review and interpretation of research on social deprivation. *International Journal of Mental Health, 30*, 58–81.

Forbes, G. M., Glaser, M. E., Cullen, D. J., Warren, J. R., Christiansen, K. J., Marshall, B. J., & Collins, B. J. (1994). Duodenal ulcer treated with *Helicobacter pylori* eradication: Seven-year follow-up. *Lancet, 343*(8892), 258–260.

Goldberger, J., Wheeler, G. A., & Syden, E. (1920). A study of the relation of family income and other economic factors to pellagra incidence in seven cotton-mill villages of South Carolina in 1916. *Public Health Reports, 355*(46), 2673–2714.

Gould, S. J. (1989). *Wonderful life: The Burgess Shale and the nature of history*. New York, NY: W. W. Norton.

.Heyman, G. M. (2009) *Addiction: A disorder of choice*. Cambridge, MA: Harvard University Press.

Higgins, S. T., Silverman K., & Heil, S. H. (2008). *Contingency management in substance abuse treatment*. New York, NY: Guilford.

Kessler, R. C., Berglund, P., Demler, O., Jin, R., Merikangas, K. R., & Walters, E. E. (2005). Lifetime prevalence and age-of-onset distributions of DSM-IV disorders in the National Comorbidity Survey Replication. *Archives of General Psychiatry, 62*(6), 593–602.

Kurtzke, J. F. (1983). Epidemiology and risk factors in thrombotic brain infarction. In M. J.

G. Harrison & M. L. Dyken (Eds.), *Cerebral vascular disease* (pp. 27–45). London, UK: Butterworths.

Marshall, B. J., Goodwin, C. S., Warren, J. R., Murray, R., Blincow, E. D., Blackbourn, S. J., . . . Sanderson, C. R. (1988). Prospective double-blind trial of duodenal ulcer relapse after eradication of *Campylobacter pylori*. *Lancet, 2*, 1437–1442.

Marshall, B. J., & Warren, J. R. (1984). Unidentified curved bacilli in the stomach of patients with gastritis and peptic ulceration. *Lancet, 1*, 1311–1315.

Martin, J. P. (1972). Conquest of general paralysis. *British Medical Journal, 3*, 159–160.

Mayr, E. (1997). *This is biology: The science of the living world*. Cambridge, MA: Harvard University Press.

McGinn, C. (1999). *The mysterious flame: Conscious minds in a material world*. New York, NY: Basic Books.

McHugh, P. R., & Slavney, P. R. (1998). *The perspectives of psychiatry* (2nd ed.). Baltimore, MD: Johns Hopkins University Press.

McHugh, P. R., & Treisman, G. (2007). PTSD: A problematic diagnostic category. *Journal of Anxiety Disorders, 21*(2), 211–222.

McNally, R. J. (2003). *Remembering trauma*. Cambridge, MA: Belknap Press/Harvard University Press.

Morris, J. N. (1975). *Uses of epidemiology* (3rd ed.). Edinburgh, UK: Churchill Livingstone.

Rosen, G. M., & Lilienfeld, S. O. (2008). Posttraumatic stress disorder: An empirical analysis of core assumptions. *Clinical Psychology Review, 28*(5), 837–868.

Rutter, M. (2000). Resilience reconsidered: Conceptual considerations, empirical findings, and policy implications. In J. P. Shonkoff & S. J. Meisels (Eds.), *Handbook of early childhood intervention* (2nd ed., pp. 651–682). New York, NY: Cambridge University Press.

Shephard, B. (2000). *A war of nerves: Soldiers and psychiatrists, 1914–1994*. London, UK: Jonathan Cape.

Wang, P. S., Lane, M., Olfson, M., Pincus, H. A., Wells, K. B., & Kessler, R. C. (2005). Twelve-month use of mental health services in the United States: Results from the National Comorbidity Survey Replication. *Archives of General Psychiatry 62*(6), 629–640.

World Health Organization. (1992). *International statistical classification of diseases and related health problems* (10th ed.). Geneva, Switzerland: Author.

3

Global Mental Health Issues: Culture and Psychopathology

JUDITH K. BASS

WILLIAM W. EATON

SHARON ABRAMOWITZ

NORMAN SARTORIUS

Key Points

- Most research on mental health has been conducted in the limited cultural framework of high-resource countries

- The cultural and contextual influences on the presentation and prevalence of mental health problems in low- and middle-income countries are only now beginning to be understood

- Both local ("emic") and universal ("etic") approaches are useful in understanding the impact of culture and context on mental health

- In different cultures mental illness may be seen as a psychological, medical, or social condition (or some combination)

- In different cultures differing aspects of risk and resiliency affect rates, courses, and outcomes of disorders

- Culture is related to how a population understands the etiology of a mental disorder and is therefore related to what are seen as appropriate treatments and judicious interventions

INTRODUCTION

Little is known about mental health–related problems in countries with cultures and resources different from those of highly resourced European and North American nations. Most research on mental health and mental illnesses has been conducted in high-resource contexts, resulting in a wealth of information within a limited cultural framework. The reasons that less epidemiologic research has been conducted in countries with moderate to low resources include a lack of researchers and resources for scientific inquiry and the cultural, social, political, and economic variations throughout the world (Lund et al., 2010; Rahman & Prince, 2009).

This gap in public mental health knowledge persists despite the well-publicized Global Burden of Disease reports that have posited that mental health problems are likely to represent an increasingly significant part of the direct and indirect disease burden in both industrialized and developing countries over the coming decades (Prince et al., 2007). In their most recent publication, Lopez and colleagues (Mathers, Lopez, & Murray, 2006) estimated that in 2001, unipolar depressive disorders were the third leading cause of disability in high-income countries (see chapter 1) and the seventh leading cause in low- and middle-income ones. Populations of low-resource countries are particularly vulnerable to the disabling effects of mental disorders, including effects on both economic and social development (Patel & Kleinman, 2003). Because the mental well-being and cognitive capacity of an entire population are intrinsically linked to economic and social prosperity (Beddington et al., 2008, Lund et al., 2010), mental health must be considered a key component for economic development.

This chapter begins with a definition of culture that will be useful in exploring the issue of global mental health, followed by a delineation of approaches to clarify the interrelationship of culture and mental health. The next section examines current knowledge of mental disorders in low-resource contexts using approaches from anthropology (the culture-bound approach) and epidemiology (the cross-cultural or transnational approach). It is followed by discussion of both social behaviors and functionality, issues associated with mental health that are affected by the culture in which a person lives. What follows is an exploration of risk and resiliency factors, including an examination of the difficulty inherent in differentiating between culture-specific vulnerabilities and vulnerabilities associated more generally with the effects of poverty in a low-resource environment. Finally, the chapter delineates how culture and context can influence the selection and adaptation of behavioral interventions and treatments.

DEFINING CULTURE AND ITS IMPACT ON MENTAL HEALTH

Culture can be understood as the collection of norms, beliefs, values, and attitudes shared by a collection of people within an institution, organization, or group. For the purposes of this chapter, culture is defined as relating to shared language, values, and perceptions of the world, which inform how people within a culture experience life emotionally and how they behave in relation to other people, supernatural forces or gods, and the environment (Helman, 1994). Under this definition, culture can be thought of as a construct that both shapes experiences and provides a framework for understandings and beliefs. Thus one might infer that culture could affect psychopathology by providing content for its expression, yielding different forms of expression in different cultures even for the same mental disorders (Good, 1997). Cultural differences also affect risk and resiliency factors that themselves affect the etiology of mental disorders, thereby influencing prevalence and incidence rates across cultures. Further, culture has an impact on the interpretation of the illness by care providers and on the selection and adaptation of appropriate prevention and intervention strategies (Good & Del Vecchio Good, 1986; Jenkins, 1988; Kleinman, 1986).

One way to investigate mental disorders from a global perspective is to begin with the "etic/emic" approach popularized by linguistic anthropologists. The original methodological distinction in linguistic anthropology was between phon*emics,* the linguistic designation of phonemes as units of meaning, and phon*etics,* the study of universal units of sound that the linguist can represent no matter in which culture they occur or how they are represented in language (Pike, 1967). Thus the emic approach treats matters as culture bound, while the etic approach is transcultural. In its purest form, the emic approach assumes that each culture is unique and therefore that the expression of disorder is culturally specific. In contrast, a strict etic approach assumes that cultural variation is more an outcome of idiosyncratic variation than substantive difference. The culture-bound, emic approach assumes insider or grounded knowledge and gives preeminence to local cultural paradigms of meaning, forms of knowledge, and forms of social practice. The transcultural, etic approach takes an outsider perspective and seeks to find universal patterns (and diagnoses) across cultures. Often, researchers with an etic orientation seek to build knowledge paradigms that generalize across the human condition in an effort to identify commonalities, explain local quirks and variations, and find underlying common truths (Goodenough, 1970; Harris, 1976).

The legitimacy of any attempt to examine mental health through the lens of culture rests on researchers' and practitioners' recognition that language is constitutive of how people understand, interpret, and find their way through the world. Language is the structural foundation on which people create categories, build systems of meaning, define who is an insider or an outsider, and describe both normal and abnormal behavior. While initially these meaning and language distinctions may seem abstruse, both lie at the core of understanding mental illness in a cultural perspective. When a case of psychosis or neurasthenia is observed in China, is it defined as psychosis or neurasthenia, consistent with Western psychiatric classification. Or is it defined according to local definitions of spirit attack, religious persecution, or social suffering (Kleinman, 1986)? How one defines a problem has significant implications for how one recognizes symptoms of mental illness,

understands mental illness among populations, builds treatment paradigms and interventions, and interprets the disorder's social and health effects.

CURRENT KNOWLEDGE OF MENTAL DISORDERS

Different approaches to the study of culture and mental health represent methodological distinctions rather than a debate about the nature of "truth" in global mental health. Locally based, culture-bound descriptions of symptoms, definitions, and social impacts help explain the ways in which populations assign meaning to mental illness and disorders. In contrast, transcultural studies help explain how disorders occur, vary, and respond to intervention across populations. Some disorders, such as depression, may lend themselves particularly well to cultural interpretation and variation; other disorders, such as schizophrenia, may have biological substrates that override cultural variations and present more similarities than differences from a transcultural perspective.

The Culture-Bound Approach

At the heart of the culture-bound approach lies the question of the nature and meaning of symptoms of a mental disorder (Biehl & Moran-Thomas, 2009). An assumption of the culture bound approach is that manifestations of mental illnesses are defined by the cultures in which they occur, as reflected in the complaints and symptoms reported by individuals and in the behaviors and signs observed by the clinician and researcher. Mental illnesses are commonly identified and patterned syndromes of symptoms that can reliably be found across cases and, presumably, across populations. However, symptoms are highly mediated by the cultural environments in which they occur. For example, a vast literature has emerged demonstrating that among persons with schizophrenia, the content of auditory delusions (hearing voices) and other symptoms are often linked to the cultural and social conditions of their production—from traditional cultural tropes to new, culturally relevant artifacts (e.g., radios, loudspeakers, or, in the United States, space aliens or the Central Intelligence Agency) to culturally specific pattern formations of selfhood and subjectivity (Estroff, 1989).

The changing description of syndromes has been recognized throughout the history of medicine. In the 18th century, the German novel *Die Leiden des Jungen Werther* described the way in which a character with major depressive disorder expressed sadness using metaphors and idioms of such strong impact that the book was banned (Phillips, 1974). Later, in the early annals of psychoanalysis, Freud (1957) noted that because each patient's symptom report was so uniquely manipulated within the patient's own interpretive framing of the disorder, often little relationship existed between the reported symptom and the "etic"-ally observed symptom noted by the doctor. Symptoms not only form the basis of observation and diagnosis of an illness but also are used by patients to make social claims to certain kinds of recognition of a particular illness status. Symptoms are what patients and healing professionals use together to create a distinction between what is normal and abnormal. They are the conceptual bases on which to determine who is experiencing mental illness and who, while experiencing symptoms, might otherwise be fully functional in social, physical, and emotional capacities.

The manifestation of depressive illnesses varies by culture. For example, in many countries, somatic complaints such as headache and fatigue are often the common presenting symptoms of depression. Kleinman's (1982) early work on neurasthenia in China found a "bioculturally patterned illness experience (a special form of somatization) related to either depression and other diseases or to culturally sanctioned idioms of distress and psychosocial coping" (p. 117). In later reflections on his China work, Kleinman noted that while he once observed considerable commonalities across cultures, he now sees greater, more significant cultural variations (Kleinman, 2004). Another widely known example in the crosscultural psychiatric literature comes from Nigeria. Among Nigerian students, a once widely experienced phenomenon—"brain fag"—included symptoms related to the head,

ranging from sensations of heat, heaviness, and emptiness to a sensation of skin crawling (Prince, 1968). To investigate the relationship between these locally defined, somatic symptoms and the emotional and cognitive symptoms of depression, Okulate and Jones (2002) adapted a standard measure (the Patient Health Questionnaire) to include these symptoms. They found that the somatic symptoms did not co-occur with the depression symptoms, indicating that in this population these expressions of brain fag did not appear to be manifestations of depression. However, Okulate and Jones did find a grouping of cognitive symptoms, similar to those found by Prince (1985) and Morakinyo (1985), that may reflect a culture-specific syndrome associated with concentration and other cognitive issues. Even these findings, however, are not without controversy. In a critique of the research literature on culture and somatization, Kirmayer and Young (1998) questioned the extent to which the brain fag syndrome was a function of local cultural idioms or of other structural experiences common among the affected students, such as high-stakes school examinations, class background, and school social conditions.

Yet another example of cultural differences can be seen in the variations of presenting symptoms and definitions of a panic attack. In the United States, panic attacks often are characterized by heart palpitations and shortness of breath—two signs that suggest panic to the sufferer and to others. A study of Khmer refugees, however, found that the most prominent symptoms included dizziness and neck tension (Hinton, Um, & Ba, 2001). In Nigeria, the feeling of "extreme heat" in the is was a common description of a panic attack head (Ebigbo, 1986; Hinton & Hinton, 2002), while in some Latin American cultures, trembling limbs or a feeling of "nerves" is most common (Lewis-Fernandez et al., 2002). This is not to suggest that heart palpitations, dizziness, and nervous feelings do not occur in all of these individuals. Rather, individuals of different cultures may describe the same presenting symptoms in very different ways, an important issue when considering how to talk about these problems, how to advertise services or treatments, and how to design assessment tools for epidemiologic and treatment research.

In addition to cultural variations in individual symptoms, significant cultural variations in syndromes (frequently recurring groupings of psychiatric and somatic complaints, symptoms, behaviors, and signs) have been analyzed over the last several decades. In some situations, the expression of signs and symptoms is so unusual that no match appears to exist in the Western diagnostic system, leading to the designation of a culture-bound syndrome—that is, a disorder with a regularly observed collection of psychiatric and somatic symptoms that occurs only in a single culture. Culture-bound syndromes have such local specificity that they cannot be validly applied to other cultural contexts, nor can they be validly included within a predefined diagnosis.

A major challenge for global mental health research is the sheer dearth of information to help clarify which disorders are universal in cause and manifestation, and thus amenable to research using transcultural approaches, and which disorders require a more localized, specific approach to their investigation. Researchers have used both methodologies to extend public health knowledge of mental disorders around the world.

Many syndromes regarded as culture-bound can often be similar to well-known syndromes and disorders in a range of other cultures. Thus, both "oro" and "mal de ojo" can be defined as anxiety disorders. Even for syndromes with no obvious connection to Western diagnoses (e.g., according to the *Diagnostic and Statistical Manual of Mental Disorders* (DSM-IV) [American Psychiatric Association, (1994] or the ICD-10 Classification of Mental and Behavioral Disorders (1992), it is usually possible to detect similar syndromes that go by different names in other cultures: for example, the startle-match behavior in "latah," in Malaysia resembles "jumping loggers" in French Canada and "mali-mali" in the Philippines (Simon, 1996). One complex example from studies of depression among the Hopi has found five distinct indigenous syndromes that align none too perfectly with conventional classifications of that disorder: worry sickness, unhappiness, heartbrokenness, drunken-like craziness, and

disappointment. Each of these syndromes differs in symptoms, duration, and patterns of comorbidity with alcoholism (a major public health problem among this population), but only one, unhappiness, shares parameters with Western-defined depressive disorder (Manson, Shore, & Bloom, 1985).

Culture-bound syndromes have been investigated widely over the last three decades and received specific mention in a glossary addition to the fourth edition of the DSM-IV (American Psychiatric Association [APA], 1994; Mezzich et al., 1999). While there is increasing agreement in the global mental health literature about the legitimacy of culture-bound syndromes, some debate has emerged regarding the requisite for cultural specificity. If syndromes such as spirit possession or haunting can be identified in multiple cultural contexts, should they be defined as culture bound simply because they are not included in Western psychiatric diagnostic frameworks? Or should such syndromes still be classified as non–culture bound even if they cannot be found universally? Not all scientists and clinicians concur with the concept of culture-bound syndromes. In fact, a large number of psychiatrists argue that all mental disorders can be classified within preexisting psychiatric nosology. This ongoing debate perhaps indicates the most extreme—and least constructive—manifestation of the epistemological divide that can separate emic and etic analysts of culture in the realm of global mental health.

The Transcultural Approach

The assumption of the transcultural approach to global public mental health research is that universal symptom patterns define disorders across cultures. The patterns, as currently defined in the DSM and the International Classification of Disease manuals, have been investigated and clarified through scientific inquiry conducted for the most part in North American and European samples. In a collaborative effort led by the World Health Organization's (WHO) Mental Health Division, the International Pilot Study of Schizophrenia (IPSS) sought to demonstrate the universality of this particular mental disorder (Jablensky et al., 1992; WHO, 1975, 1979). Despite early reports suggesting that schizophrenia did not exist in certain non-Western cultures (Fortes & Mayer, 1966), most Western-educated psychiatrists at the time of the WHO study believed that schizophrenia was universal. The IPSS explored 10 different cultures, using similar study designs and diagnostic methods to identify possible cases and assess them in an equivalent fashion for the presence of schizophrenia. Figure 3-1 presents some of the findings. The horizontal axis shows 20 groups of signs and symptoms related to psychosis in general and to schizophrenia in particular (selected from 27 available in the IPSS). The vertical axis represents the percentage of individuals presenting with each of the 20 signs and symptoms who met diagnostic criteria for schizophrenia. For clarity, the figure shows findings from 5 of the 10 cultures studied: Aarhus (Denmark) and London (England) representing "Western" cultures, and Ibadan (Nigeria), Agra (India), and Cali (Colombia) representing "non-Western" cultures. The investigators interpreted the similar patterns to mean that the symptom picture of schizophrenia was similar across all the cultures in

which it had been identified. They thus concluded that the transcultural approach was appropriate for schizophrenia. Even so, long-term follow-up of the IPSS cases showed large differences in outcome for developing versus developed countries (Hopper et al, 2007).

The IPSS opened the way for transcultural studies of other disorders based on the assumption of universality. One of those transcultural prevalence studies of mental illness was conducted by the Cross-National Collaborative Group (CNCG) in the 1980s in 10 countries and territories (United States, Puerto Rico, Canada, France, West Germany, Italy, Lebanon, Taiwan, Korea, and New Zealand) (Weissman et al., 1996). Using the Diagnostic Interview Schedule on a total sample of more than 38,000 community subjects, the researchers were able to generate lifetime rates for several disorders in the third edition of the DSM (DSM-III) (APA, 1980). Wide variations were found across countries for different disorders, with Taiwan generally showing the lowest lifetime prevalence rates among adults: 1.5 cases per 100 for major depressive disorder; 0.3 per 100 for bipolar disorder; 0.4 for panic disorder; and 0.4 for obsessive–compulsive disorder (Weissman et al., 1996). Lebanon

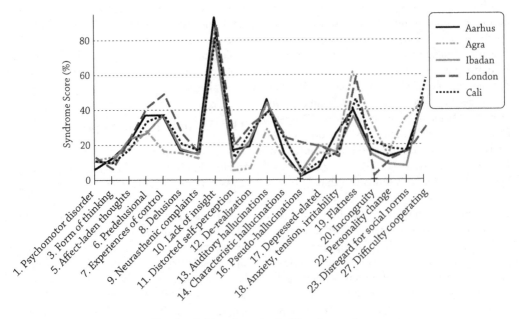

Figure 3-1   **Syndrome Profiles for Schizophrenics in Five Countries.**

Source: Based on data from table 9, World Health Organization, 1979.

had the highest lifetime prevalence rates for major depressive disorder, with 19.0 cases per 100 adults. New Zealand had the highest rates of bipolar disorder, with 1.5 cases per 100 adults. Paradoxically, Lebanon had the lowest rate of suicide attempts among adults (0.7 per 100), while Puerto Rico had the highest (5.9 per 100).

Following the CNCG studies, the WHO conducted the International Consortium of Psychiatric Epidemiology surveys in 10 countries (Canada, United States, Brazil, Chile, Mexico, Czech Republic, Germany, Netherlands, Turkey, and Japan) (Andrade et al., 2003). More than 37,000 adults were surveyed using the Composite International Diagnostic Interview (CIDI), which generated diagnoses according to both the revised DSM-III (APA, 1987) and DSM-IV. Results from this set of surveys include lifetime prevalence rates of major depressive disorder of 3 per 100 individuals in Japan, 6–9 per 100 individuals in Turkey, the Czech Republic, Mexico, Canada, and Chile, and 11–17 per 100 individuals in Germany, Brazil, the Netherlands, and the United States. Rates of any lifetime mental disorder ranged from greater than 40 per 100 individuals in the United States and the Netherlands to 20 per 100 individuals in Mexico and 12 per 100 individuals in Turkey. Significant variation in age ranges and sampling strategies across the sites limits the ability to draw inferences about these differences. Some sites included participants as young as 15 years, some included adults through age 54, and others included participants over age 70. Four sites used national samples, five collected data in a single major city, and one (Chile) surveyed four provinces.

With their focus on lifetime disorder, these initial cross-national surveys yielded no information on either 12-month or current (time of interview) disorder prevalence, nor did they amass data on the severity and treatment of mental illnesses. Thus the WHO established its World Mental Health (WMH) Survey Consortium to address these limitations. In conducting the new surveys, the WMH chose to expand the assessment tool (the CIDI) to include detailed questions about disorder severity, impairment, and treatment before implementing coordinated surveys in 28 countries around the world, including less developed countries in each region (Kessler & Ustun, 2004). Initially, six of the countries included in this round of surveys were classified as developing countries (China, Colombia, Lebanon, Mexico, Nigeria, and Ukraine); ongoing WMH surveys have added data from other countries. (For more information, consult the website http://www.hcp.med.harvard.edu/wmh/.)

Using DSM-IV diagnostic criteria (APA, 1994), the WMH survey found the 12-month prevalence of mood disorder to be lowest in Nigeria, at 0.8 cases per 100 individuals sampled (with a range from 0.5 to 1.0) and highest in the United States, at 9.6 (with a range from 5.9 to 7.8) (Demyttenaere et al., 2004). However, major depressive disorder accounted for 84% of all mental illness in Nigeria, compared with 72% in the United States. The proportion of respondents with some mental illness who received mental health care during the 12 months before being interviewed varied widely across surveys, from a low of 8.0% in Nigeria to a high of 15.3% in the United States; among serious cases, only 49.7–64.5% in developed countries and 14.6–23.7% in less developed countries received any treatment at all (Demyttenaere et al., 2004). Critically, these study findings may be limited by the performance of the survey in parts of the world where local concepts and phrases used to describe syndromes of mental illness are less consonant with the concepts defined in the survey instrument.

Combined Approaches

Clearly, untangling the relationship between cultural manifestations of mental illness and symptoms of illness themselves is a complicated endeavor, sensitive to a broad array of confounding factors. To try to uncover the nuances in how cultures experience and describe mental disorders, some researchers have employed qualitative methods to identify symptoms relevant to local populations but not included in standard DSM case definitions of specific psychiatric disorders. A finding of Wilk and Bolton's (2002) Uganda investigation into mental problems among adults affected by the human immunodeficiency virus (HIV) epidemic was that although many local symptoms matched DSM-IV criteria for major depressive disorder, additional symptoms—"hating the world," "bad, criminal or reckless behavior," and "unappreciative of assistance"—were relevant manifestations of locally defined depression that warranted incorporation into the disorder criteria. By creating a framework that enables locally identified symptoms to be coanalyzed with preexisting diagnostic frameworks, this approach manages to integrate both emic and etic interpretations. While focusing on linguistic relevance and local meaning, the approach also includes the capacity to generalize to and compare with other populations, albeit with the addition of specific linguistic adaptations.

An alternative approach to examining local experiences of mental illness involves ethnographic investigation of local illness experiences and the transposition of those ethnographic findings to standardized data collection measures. Both Sheper-Hughes, who studied schizophrenia in Northern Ireland (2001) and maternal attachment in impoverished favelas (slums) in northeastern Brazil (1993), and Lock (1995), who studied the interpretation of menopause in Japanese and American women, conducted studies exemplifying this emic-driven approach. Scheper-Hughes's powerful critique in *Death Without Weeping* (1993) demonstrated that the absence of affect shown by mothers toward their newborn infants was not symptomatic of a mental disorder such as postpartum depression. Rather, the response was a highly practical, local, population-wide product of a shockingly high infant mortality rate. Similarly, Lock showed that contrary to conventional medical wisdom, many of the psychological and somatic symptoms assumed to be a part of the universal medical phenomenon of menopause were in fact highly culturally idiosyncratic. Japanese women reported neither the mood swings nor the hot flashes so commonly reported among women in the United States; when asked specifically about those symptoms, Japanese women thought they were odd occurrences.

The virtue of the foregoing approach lies in its tendency to yield a great deal of culturally valid information about illness experiences. The disadvantage of the approach, however, is that the findings are not readily generalizable to broader populations, in part because of the specificity of local social and structural conditions and also the usually small convenience samples involved in ethnographic research.

SOCIAL BEHAVIORS AND FUNCTIONALITY

Social functioning is a subtle element of global mental health that often goes unconsidered in the anthropological and public health literature. Social functioning is deeply intertwined with and rooted in the conditions of culture and the norms of social behavior in which it is observed. For example, visualize a picture of two uniformed men holding hands and hugging in a mess hall on a Marine Corps base in North Carolina in the 1990s. In that cultural environment, such behaviors might well be identified as aberrant, with potential legal, professional, or therapeutic implications for the men. In contrast, consider two men engaging in the same behaviors while telling stories and drinking tea among a group of male peers in Morocco or Guinea. In these contexts, the behaviors would be recognized and accepted as normative. The same intense sensitivity to context applies when considering culture and psychopathology. Even without the ability to identify with precision the standardized symptoms from the DSM-IV or WHO frameworks, when confronted with an individual with a mental illness in their midst, family, friends, and neighbors often know at an intuitive level that the person is not well. Mental illnesses often straddle the imperceptible social line between normal and abnormal, making mental illness both a psychological or psychiatric condition and a social condition.

At times an individual's social functioning in a non-Western cultural context may define in part an experience of mental illness that would not be recognized if measured by universal diagnostic scales. For example, in a study of mental problems among new mothers in the Democratic Republic of Congo, researchers identified a local syndrome that, while manifesting in ways similar to depression,

Table 3-1 Operationalizing Culture in Global Mental Health Research

DEFINITION OF "CULTURE"	OPERATIONALIZATION OF "CULTURE"
Shared language	Comprehensive linguistic analysis of symptoms and syndromes
Local experience	Phenomenological description
Local meaning	Ethnographic description of local classification of illness and description of local healing approaches, with a hermeneutic analysis
Peer analysis	Interviews with family or significant others regarding subjects' functioning, experiences, and interpretations of behavior
Social functioning	Ability to carry out "normal" behaviors on a daily basis
Social networks	Links and nodes signifying density of social networks
Social support	Number and types of social resources available to subject
Structural conditions	Conditions of health supports, wealth, exposure, risk, violence, discrimination, physical protection, and stability available to subject
Psychiatric evaluation	Often considers personal history and illness history of subject, but discounts culture as a salient factor in presentation of symptoms

This table contributed by Sharon Abramowitz.

also included symptoms specific to the local population that are not part of the DSM diagnostic model, among them feeling tormented, a lack of peace, anger, self-pity, and baseless argumentativeness (Bass, Ryder, Lammers, Mukaba, & Bolton, 2008). While these symptoms are not unique to the population (i.e., not culture bound), they generally are not included in standard screens or assessment tools used to identify cases of depression. In addition to uncovering a type of real and widespread treatable psychological distress, the study discovered that some of the items in a standard, globally used measure of postpartum depression (the Edinburgh Postpartum Depression Scale) were not valid for the local population. For example, one of the scale questions asks how often the subject has "looked forward to the future with enjoyment." When this question was piloted with the local women, many said they did not think about the future; their focus was on the here and now, with a particular emphasis on daily efforts to survive and provide for their family. This finding emphasizes the importance both of understanding local expressions for case definition and of recognizing the role cultural variations in symptoms play in making valid cross-cultural comparisons.

These findings and those of Wilk and Bolton (2002) regarding locally defined expressions of depression direct attention to the issue of social functioning. In the Western DSM framework, social functioning is considered an Axis V diagnostic category, a recommended but not required axis on which to base a psychiatric diagnosis. However, in non-Western settings, impairments in social functioning constitute a key factor that distinguishes a person with mental illness from "normal" members of the community. Across the globe, much informal diagnostic work related to mental disorders—whether by families, neighbors, or clinicians—revolves around poorly defined, highly perceived local categories of social functioning. Many community members may be unable to classify a person as mentally ill according to a symptom-based diagnostic framework, but most can identify those who are functionally impaired based on their failure to observe social conventions. In her work on trauma in Liberia, Abramowitz (2009) demonstrated that community members with mental illnesses were often known to their communities by common attributes: failing to wash or dress appropriately (e.g., hair becoming nappy, not buttoning shirts, or not wearing belts); speaking excessively, loudly, or without coherence in social gatherings; aggressive, violent, criminal, or reckless behavior; or hoarding behaviors such as gathering and pocketing trash from the street. In an environment in which both formal employment and school enrollment were exceedingly rare, these behaviors functioned as more locally relevant, legitimate proxies for shortcomings in social functioning than did conventional Western social functioning indexes.

Research in global mental health thus often demands that researchers subordinate their expectations about what mental illness looks like and reconsider mental health and mental illness within local frameworks of what is normal or abnormal. At the same time, researchers must retain sufficient independence from local contexts to identify treatable disorders that the community may take for granted as normal in everyday life. To do so, a few researchers have designed and sought to implement ways to "operationalize" culture in the study of global mental health. (See table 3-1 for a list of some of these approaches.) However, most research in global mental health largely has overlooked culture as a salient determinant of mental illness.

RISK AND RESILIENCY FACTORS

Discussion of risk and resiliency factors in global mental health research begins by reconsidering the IPSS. While IPSS investigators concluded that rates of schizophrenia were not widely divergent across cultures, subsequent studies from around the world have found significant variation in aspects of mental illness such as recurrence of psychotic episodes, chronicity, long-term disability, and social and community integration of the affected individual (see discussions in Hopper, 1991, and Jenkins & Jenkins, 2004). Why might this be so?

Considerable qualitative research has demonstrated that social factors play an important role in promoting the resilience of persons with mental disorders or in exacerbating the illnesses and their courses and outcomes. A familiar case—the course of schizophrenia among persons in the United States—is illustrative. Such individuals often experience recurring

psychotic episodes, have a poor prognosis for avoiding disease chronicity, and are socially marginalized (Bromet et al., 2011; Bromet, Naz, Fochtmann, Carlson, & Tanenberg-Karant, 2005). In contrast, in Italy, social policies provide strong support to families of people with schizophrenia and enable the individual with the disorder to be integrated into local labor structures, community functions, and local, nonspecialized health care systems (Donnelly, 1992; Leff, 1998). Research from India has found that social pressure promoting marriage acts as a protective factor against divorce or abandonment by their families for people with serious mental illnesses (Leff et al., 1987; Srivastava, Stitt, Thakar, Shah, & Chinnasamy, 2009). Finally, in Africa, Patel (1998) has found that communities surrounding people with schizophrenia often explain the illnesses using local explanatory models that integrate religious or spiritual motifs and that may have a protective or at least a socially integrative effect on the affected individual. (See the next section for a further discussion of explanatory models.) Social and cultural factors such as these can exert a long-term effect on the overall severity of schizophrenia, so much so that they may appear to alter the expected course of illness itself.

In global mental health research, culture and context can influence both the mechanisms by which risk and resiliency factors affect the rates, courses, and outcomes of disorders and the ways in which a culture can create conditions that promote mental health. Considerations of culture need to take into account multiple aspects of mental illness, ranging from culturally normative attitudes and practices to locally associated sets of symptoms and social attitudes towards mentally ill persons. Efforts to integrate culture into the study of mental illness also need to take into account large-scale structural paradigms, including local, state, and national treatment paradigms; available systems of intervention; the politics of health; and the ways in which mental health trends intersect with demographic trends.

Context and culture can directly affect the experience of mental illness through their interaction with demographic factors such as gender, age, poverty, and marital status. Gender, in particular, has repeatedly been shown to be important in investigating mental health issues. Women have been found to experience higher rates of mood and anxiety disorders than men (Hopcroft & Bradley, 2007; Kessler, McGonagle, Swarz, Blazer, & Nelson, 1993; Van de Velde, Bracke, & Levecque, 2010), whereas men show higher rates of substance use (e.g., Gureje et al., 2007; Kessler, et al., 1994). Women's greater vulnerability to mood and anxiety disorders may be associated with a range of factors, including not only biological differences but also social roles (e.g., childbearing and child rearing, running the home, caring for the sick, and ways of earning income), social expectations (e.g., relating to reproduction, gender preferences for children, issues of infertility, and stigma or blame for infertility), gender inequality in power and status, and vulnerability to domestic violence. Similarly, while men's greater vulnerability to substance use disorders may be associated with biological factors, it also may be related to cultural expectations regarding such issues as employment and unemployment; the ability to achieve life course expectations such as marriage, childbearing, and land or home ownership; and socially tolerated modes of coping.

Age, like gender, is an important predictor across cultures of variations in mental illness. There is considerable local specificity in the types of mental illness that arise at different points in the life cycle. For example, in poor, urban non-Western settings, youth often report increased depression and aggressive behavior to be due to their real or perceived dearth of life opportunities resulting from poverty and unemployment. In contrast, middle-class US youth are increasingly diagnosed with depression, attention deficit hyperactivity disorder, and drug dependency for an entirely different, often not entirely clear set of reasons, including possibly the cultural acceptability of these diagnoses in the United States.

The role of culture in understanding the influence of both age, particularly in the younger years, and the developmental process is also important. Culture can exert an influence not only on expectations about children developmental trajectory but also on the roles and responsibilities of children and youth and on the rights afforded to children. For example, the age of female maturation can affect expected roles and expectations (e.g., the age of marriage and the taking on of "adult" roles in child care and household duties).

Culture also may influence the prevalence and recognition of disorder, as in the example of postpartum depression. Rates of postpartum depression are high also in low-resource countries. In India and Pakistan, for example, two studies estimated the prevalences at 23 per 100 individuals (Patel, Rodrigues, & Desouza, 2002) and 28 per 100 individuals (Rahman, Iqbal, & Harrington, 2003), respectively. A review of studies from around the world found variation in rates of postpartum depression but its existence in all sites (Halbreich & Karkun, 2006). In addition, the aforementioned studies found that causes varied across cultures. For example, the India study found that beyond the issues of poor marital relations and economic difficulties that are commonly seen globally, the stress of child gender preference was a particular risk factor for the local population (Patel et al., 2002).

Culturally normative attitudes and behaviors—often with long histories—can have a direct influence on the prevalence of certain disorders. However, while these attitudes and behaviors can have powerful explanatory effects, researchers must be wary of crossing the line from recognizing culture as one of many explanations to using culture as a means of prediction. Consider, for example, alcohol use and abuse in Russia. Since the 10th century, alcohol has been referenced as a central component of Russian life. While consumption of alcohol, particularly as part of a meal, is common across many populations, in Russia the majority of alcohol traditionally consumed is spirit based (e.g., vodka), and drinking often takes the form of bingeing (McKee, 1999). Drinking is an important part of the traditional Russian culture, with particular celebrations involving alcohol and specific toasts. Even the definition of what constitutes excessive drinking differs when one compares many of the former Soviet republics with the United States or other Western nations.

Eating disorders provide another example in which cultural attitudes can influence prevalence rates. Research has found that a variety of sociocultural factors are associated with the development of eating disorders and that rates of the disorders vary across cultural and economic groups in the West. Historically, eating disorders have been less common in non-Western countries, so much so that they have been considered by some to be culture-bound syndromes of Western cultures (Lee, 1996; Prince, 1985). Some researchers explain these differences as due to variations in ideals of beauty. For example, rising rates of both bulimia nervosa and anorexia in the West (Eagles, Johnston, Hunter, Lobban, & Millar, 1995; Lucas, Beard, O'Fallon, & Kurland, 1991; Willi, Giacometti, & Limacher, 1990) have been associated with the recent emphasis on thinness exemplified in the Miss America competitions and choices of Playmate models (Garfinkel & Garner, 1982; Rubinstein & Caballero, 2000; Wiseman, Gray, Mosimann, & Ahrens, 1992). Other researchers have shown that cultures in which the social roles of women are restricted have lower rates of eating disorders (Bemporad, 1997).

In addition to variations in culture, differences in the prevalence and incidence of disorders in low-income countries also can be attributed to factors that are not culture specific. Although social and environmental stressors commonly associated with mental illnesses (e.g., violence, low socioeconomic status, trauma, and illness) exist globally, many of these stressors are greatly exacerbated in the developing world by the presence of diseases like HIV, high rates of poverty, war, and the simple lack of a health infrastructure.

While a considerable body of research documents the high burden of psychiatric disorders in a range of HIV-infected populations in the United States (Chander, Himelhock, & Moore, 2006; Lyketsos, Hanson, Fishman, McHugh, & Treisman, 1994; Orlando et al., 2002) and other industrialized countries (Gordillo, del Amo, Soriano, & González-Lahoz, 1999; Skydsbjerg, Lunn, & Hutchings, 2001), the developing world contains the majority (90%) of cases of global HIV infection (UNAIDS: http://www.unaids.org/en/media/unaids/contentassets/dataimport/pub/factsheet/2009/20091124_fs_global_en.pdf). Part of the burden of HIV-related mental illness is associated with the disease itself, including HIV-related dementias and psychotic disorders. However, the social rejection, stigma, lack of access to treatment, and problem of orphans in low-resource areas amplify the burden and increase the risk for distress and disorder. Of particular concern is the impact of parental HIV infection on children. Children face many challenges when living with an HIV-infected caregiver (Rotheram-Borus, Stein, & Lester, 2006). Despite their own developmental needs, many adolescent children assume responsibility for household tasks, care for younger siblings, and provide emotional support for other family members.

In their review, Patel and Kleinman (2003) identified 11 studies that explored the relationship between poverty and mental illness in low- or moderate-income countries (defined by World Bank standards). They identified a number of factors related to increased risk of mental illness: poor living conditions (including quality of housing), polluted water and air, increased risks of violence and accidents, hopelessness and humiliation (including the stigma of poverty, lack of hope for self or family, and humiliation associated with handouts or begging), lack of access to education (including costs of uniforms, books, and school fees), and general health problems (including greater susceptibility to illness and malnutrition).

CULTURAL INFLUENCES ON THE SELECTION AND ADAPTATION OF INTERVENTIONS

Because non-Western explanatory models of caring for common mental health problems such as depression, anxiety, and posttraumatic and somatoform disorders often do not match the Western biomedical model, care needs to be taken when selecting and adapting intervention strategies for these cultures. Individuals from cultures that, for example, explain mental problems as spiritual in nature or as products of relationships with other people may be less likely to accept pharmacologic treatment for their problems than individuals in cultures that have a more biomedical approach to the disorders. With few randomized controlled trials for mental disorders having been conducted in non-Western countries, conclusions regarding the efficacy and effectiveness of different intervention programs are limited. Existing evidence focuses on the common syndromes of depression, anxiety, and somatoform disorders.

A randomized controlled trial of cognitive behavioral therapy for medically unexplained symptoms (i.e., somatoform disorder) conducted in Sri Lanka found that intervention participants had significantly reduced scale scores compared with treatment-as-usual controls, indicating the intervention's efficacy (Sumathipala et al., 2008). A randomized controlled trial in Goa, India, compared the effectiveness of a general psychological treatment, antidepressants, and a placebo in the treatment of common mental disorders (Patel et al., 2003). Outcome improvements for those receiving antidepressants were found after only two months of treatment; however, the effect was not maintained at 12-month follow-up. Another randomized controlled trial, comparing a multifaceted, stepped care approach with treatment as usual for women with major depressive disorder in three primary care settings in Santiago, Chile, found an overall positive intervention effect (Araya et al., 2003). The investigators also demonstrated that the program successfully used nonmedical workers and was well received by study participants, as evidenced by participation rates greater than 85%. Randomized controlled trials of group interpersonal psychotherapy (IPT) showed the modality to be an effective option for the treatment of depression among Ugandan adults affected by HIV (Bass et al., 2006; Bolton et al., 2003) and among Ugandan adolescents affected by war and trauma (Bolton et al., 2007).

These last two studies in Uganda were implemented using a culturally adapted version of IPT, developed specifically for use by counselors with minimal previous mental health training. Verdeli and colleagues (2003) describe the adaptation as the result of consultation with trainee group leaders to ensure that modifications fit with the local cultural worldview. For example, the researchers were challenged by a cultural norm that prohibits any negative mention of the dead. Yet the IPT process, when working to manage depressive symptoms following the death of a loved one, includes recognizing both the strengths and weaknesses of the person who died, Thus the therapy was modified to both reflect and respect this cultural attitude while maintaining the essence of the therapeutic process.

CONCLUSION

Understanding the impact of culture on mental health requires recognizing that while much more remains to be learned, knowledge is growing with each new study that seeks to understand how mental problems are understood, expressed, and treated in cultures different from our own. While some disorders, particularly severe ones such as schizophrenia, tend to present similarly around the world, the experience of these disorders may differ by community, culture, and resources available. Other disorders, such as depression and anxiety, not only may be understood and treated differently in different cultures but also may manifest with different core and presenting complaints.

Variations in culture and resource availability also affect the selection and implementation of prevention and intervention services. While historically, mental health services have not been high on the health care priority list in low-resource countries, the recognition that mental health is a human right and that there is "no health without mental health" (Patel, Saraceno, & Kleinman, 2006) is changing that picture.

Given the growing evidence for the importance and treatability of mental disorders globally, the Movement for Global Mental Health (http://www.globalmentalhealth.org) was established to call on advocates, researchers, and service providers to use the best available scientific evidence in planning services and to do so based on the principles of human rights.

REFERENCES

Abramowitz, S. (2009). *Psychosocial Liberia: Managing suffering in post-conflict life* (Doctoral dissertation). Available from ProQuest Dissertations and Theses database. (UMI No. 3365067)

American Psychiatric Association. (1980). *Diagnostic and statistical manual of mental disorders* (3rd ed.). Washington, DC: Author.

American Psychiatric Association. (1987). *Diagnostic and statistical manual of mental disorders* (3rd ed., rev.). Washington, DC: Author.

American Psychiatric Association. (1994). *Diagnostic and statistical manual of mental disorders* (4th ed.). Washington, DC: Author.

Andrade, L., Caraveo-Anduaga, J. J., Berglund, P., Bijl, R. V., De Graaf, R., Vollenbergh, W., ... Wittchen, H. U. (2003). The epidemiology of major depressive episodes: Results from the International Consortium of Psychiatric Epidemiology (ICPE) surveys. *International Journal of Methods in Psychiatric Research, 12*(1), 3–21.

Araya, R., Rojas, G., Fritsch, R., Gaete, J., Rojas, M., Simon, G., & Peters, T. J. (2003). Treating depression in primary care in low-income women in Santiago, Chile: A randomized controlled trial. *Lancet, 361*(9362), 995–1000.

Bass, J., Neugebauer, R., Clougherty, K. F., Verdeli, H., Wickramaratne, P., Ndogoni, L., ... Bolton, P. (2006). Group interpersonal psychotherapy for depression in rural Uganda: Six-month follow-up of a randomized controlled trial. *British Journal of Psychiatry, 288,* 567–573.

Bass, J. K., Ryder, R. W., Lammers, M. C., Mukaba, T. N., & Bolton, P. A. (2008). Postpartum depression in Kinshasa, Democratic Republic of Congo: Validation of a concept using a mixed-methods cross-cultural approach. *Tropical Medicine and International Health, 13,* 1534–1542.

Beddington, J., Cooper, C. L., Field, J., Goswami, U., Huppert, F. A., Jenkins, R., ... Thomas, S. M. (2008). The mental wealth of nations. *Nature, 455*(7216), 1057–1060.

Bemporad, J. R. (1997). Cultural and historical aspects of eating disorders. *Theoretical Medicine, 18*(4), 401–420.

Biehl, J. & Moran-Thomas, A. (2009). Symptoms: Subjectivities, social ills, technologies. *Annual Review of Anthropology, 38,* 267–288.

Bolton, P., Bass, J., Betancourt, T., Speelman, L., Onyango, G., Clougherty, K., ... Verdeli, H. (2007). Interventions for depression symptoms among adolescent survivors of war and displacement in Northern Uganda: A randomized controlled trial. *Journal of the American Medical Association. 298*(5), 519–527.

Bolton, P., Bass, J., Neugebauer, R., Clougherty, K. F., Verdeli, H., Wickramaratne, P., ... Weissman, M. (2003). A clinical trial of group interpersonal psychotherapy for depression in rural Uganda. *Journal of the American Medical Association, 289*(23), 3117–3124.

Bromet, E. J., Kotov, R., Fochtmann, L. J., Carlson, G. A., Tanenberg-Karant, M., Ruggero, C., &

Chang, S. W. (2011). Diagnostic shifts during the decade following first admission for psychosis. *American Journal of Psychiatry, 168*(11): 1186–1194.

Bromet, E. J., Naz, B., Fochtmann, L. J., Carlson, G. A., & Tanenberg-Karant, M. (2005). Long-term diagnostic stability and outcome in recent first-episode cohort studies of schizophrenia. *Schizophrenia Bulletin, 31,* 639–649.

Chander, G., Himelhoch, S., & Moore, R. D. (2006). Substance abuse and psychiatric disorders in HIV-positive patients: Epidemiology and impact on antiretroviral therapy. *Drugs, 66*(6): 769–789.

Demyttenaere, K., Bruffaerts, R., Posada-Villa, J., Gasquet, I., Kovess, V., Lepine, J.-P., ... Ustun, T. B. (2004). Prevalence, severity and unmet need for treatment of mental disorders in the World Health Organization World Mental Health (WMH) Surveys. *Journal of the American Medical Association, 291,* 2581–2590.

Donnelly, M. (1992). *The politics of mental health in Italy.* London, UK: Routledge.

Eagles, J. M., Johnston, M. I., Hunter, D., Lobban, M., & Millar, H. R. (1995). Increasing incidence of anorexia nervosa in the female population of northeast Scotland. *American Journal of Psychiatry, 152,* 1266–1271.

Ebigbo, P. (1986). A cross-sectional study of somatic complaints of Nigerian females using the Enugu Somatization Scale. *Culture, Medicine, and Psychiatry, 10,* 167–186.

Estroff, S. E. (1989). Self, identity, and subjective experiences of schizophrenia: In search of the subject. *Schizophrenia Bulletin, 15,* 189–196.

Fortes, M., & Mayer, D. (1966). Psychosis and social change among the Tallensi of Northern Ghana. *Cahiers d'Études Africains, 6*(21), 5–40.

Freud, S. (1957). The sense of symptoms. In J. Strachey (Ed.), *The standard edition of the complete psychological works of Sigmund Freud* (Vol. 16, pp. 257–272). London, UK: Hogarth.

Garfinkel, P. E., & Garner, D. M. (1982). *Anorexia nervosa: A multidimensional perspective.* New York, NY: Brunner Mazel.

Good, B. (1997). Studying mental illness in context: Local, global, or universal? *Ethos, 25*(2), 230–248.

Good, B., & Del Vecchio Good, M. J. (1986). The cultural context of diagnosis and therapy: A view from medical anthropology. In A. H. Tuma & J. D. Maser (Eds.), *Anxiety and the anxiety disorders* (pp. 297–323). Hillsdale, NJ: Lawrence Erlbaum.

Goodenough, W. H. (1970). *Description and comparison in cultural anthropology* (pp. 104–119). Cambridge, MA: Cambridge University Press.

Gordillo, V., del Amo, J., Soriano, V., & González-Lahoz, J. (1999). Sociodemographic and psychological variables influencing adherence to antiretroviral therapy. *AIDS, 13*(13), 1763–1769.

Gureje, O., Degenhardt, L., Olley, B., Uwakwe, R., Udofia, O., Wakil, A., . . . Anthony, J. C. (2007). A descriptive epidemiology of substance use and substance use disorders in Nigeria during the early 21st century. *Drug and Alcohol Dependence, 91*(1), 1–9.

Halbreich, U., & Karkun, S. (2006). Cross-cultural and social diversity of prevalence of postpartum depression and depressive symptoms. *Journal of Affective Disorders, 91*(2–3), 97–111.

Harris, M. (1976). History and significance of the emic/etic distinction. *Annual Review of Anthropology, 5*, 329–350.

Helman, C. G. (1994). *Cultura, saúde e doença* [Culture, health and disease]. Porto Alegre, Brazil: Artes Médicas.

Hinton, D., & Hinton S. (2002). Panic disorder, somatization, and the new cross-cultural psychiatry: The seven bodies of a medical anthropology of panic. *Culture, Medicine, and Psychiatry, 26*, 155–178.

Hinton, D., Um, K., & Ba, P. (2001). A unique panic-disorder presentation among Khmer refugees: The sore-neck syndrome. *Culture, Medicine, and Psychiatry, 25*, 297–316.

Hopcroft, R. L., & Bradley, D. B. (2007). The sex difference in depression across 29 countries. *Social Forces, 85*(4), 1483–1507.

Hopper, K. (1991). Some old questions for the new cross-cultural psychiatry. *Medical Anthropology Quarterly, 5*(4), 299–330.

Hopper, K., Harrison, G., Janca, A., & Sartorius, N. (2007) *Recovery from Schizophrenia: an International Perspective.* New York, Oxford University Press.

Jablensky, A., Sartorius, N., Ernberg, G., Anker, M., Korten, A., Cooper, J. E., . . . Bertelsen, A. (1992). Schizophrenia: Manifestations, incidence and course in different cultures. A World Health Organization ten-country study. *Psychological Medicine, 20*(Suppl.), 1–97.

Jenkins, J. (1988). Ethnopsychiatric interpretations of schizophrenic illness: The problem of *nervios* within Mexican-American families. *Culture, Medicine, and Psychiatry, 12*, 301–329.

Jenkins, J. D., & Jenkins, J. H. (2004). *Schizophrenia, culture, and subjectivity: The edge of experience.* Cambridge, UK: Cambridge University Press.

Kessler, R. C., McGonagle, K. A., Swartz, M., Blazer, D. G., & Nelson, C. B. (1993). Sex and depression in the National Comorbidity Survey I: Lifetime prevalence, chronicity and recurrence. *Journal of Affective Disorders, 29*(2–3), 85–96.

Kessler, R. C., & Ustun, T. B. (2004). The World Mental Health (WMH) Survey Initiative version of the World Health Organization (WHO) Composite International Diagnostic Interview (CIDI). *International Journal of Methods in Psychiatric Research, 13*(2), 93–121.

Kirmayer, L. J., & Young, A. (1998). Culture and somatization: Clinical, epidemiological, and ethnographic perspectives. *Psychosomatic Medicine, 60*(4), 420–430.

Kleinman, A. (1982). Neurasthenia and depression: A study of somatization and culture in China. *Culture, Medicine, and Psychiatry, 6*(2), 117–190.

Kleinman, A. (1986). *Social origins of distress and disease: Depression, neurasthenia, and pain in modern China.* New Haven, CT: Yale University Press.

Kleinman, A. (2004). Culture and depression. *New England Journal of Medicine, 35*, 951–953.

Lee, S. (1996). Reconsidering the status of anorexia nervosa as a Western culture-bound syndrome. *Social Science & Medicine, 42*, 21–34.

Leff, J. (1998). *Care in the community: Illusion or reality?* West Sussex, UK: John Wiley & Sons.

Leff, J., Wig, N. N., Ghosh, A., Bedi, H., Menon, D. K., Kuipers, L., . . . Sartorius, N. (1987). Expressed emotion and schizophrenia in north India. III. Influence of relatives' expressed emotion on the course of schizophrenia in Chandigarh. *British Journal of Psychiatry, 151*, 166–173.

Lewis-Fernandez, R., Guarnaccia, P. J., Martinez, I. E., Salmán, E., Schmidt, A., & Liebowitz, M. (2002). Comparative phenomenology of *ataques de nervios*, panic attacks, and panic disorder. *Culture, Medicine, and Psychiatry, 26*, 199–223.

Lock, M. (1995). *Encounters with aging: Mythologies of menopause in Japan.* Berkeley, CA: University of California Press.

Lopez, A. D., Mathers, C. D., Ezzati, M., Jamison, D. T., & Murray, C. J. L. (Eds.). (2006). *Global burden of disease and risk factors.* Washington, DC: World Bank.

Lucas, A. R., Beard, C. M., O'Fallon, W. M., & Kurland, L. T. (1991). 50-year trends in the incidence of anorexia nervosa in Rochester, MN: A population-based study. *American Journal of Psychiatry, 148*, 917–922.

Lund, C., Breen, A., Flisher, A. J., Kakuma, R., Corrigall, J., Joska, J. A., . . . Patel, V. (2010). Poverty and common mental disorders in low and middle income countries: A systematic review. *Social Science and Medicine, 71*, 517–528.

Lyketsos, C. G., Hanson, A., Fishman, M., McHugh, P. R., & Treisman, G. J. (1994). Screening for psychiatric morbidity in a medical outpatient clinic for HIV infection: The need for a psychiatric presence. *International Journal of Psychiatric Medicine, 24*(2), 103–113.

Manson, S. M., Shore, J. H., & Bloom, J. D. (1985). The depressive experience in American Indian communities: A challenge for psychiatric theory and diagnosis. In A. Kleinman & B. Good (Eds.), *Culture and depression: Studies in the anthropology and cross-cultural psychiatry of affect and disorder.* Los Angeles, CA: University of California Press.

Mathers, C.D., Lopez, A.D. & Jurray, C.J.L. (2006). The Burden of Disease and Mortality by Condition: Data, Methods, and Results for 2001. Chapter 3, pages 45–240 in Lopez, A.D., Mathers, C.D., Ezzati, M., Jamison, D.T., & Murray, C.J.L., Global Burden of Disease nd Risk Factors, New York, Oxford University Press.

McKee, M. (1999). Alcohol in Russia. *Alcohol, 34*(6), 824–829.

Mezzich, J., Kirmayer, L., Kleinman, A., Fabrega, H., Parron, D., Good, B.,…Manson, S. (1999). The place of culture in DSM-IV. *Journal of Nervous and Mental Disease, 187*(8), 457–464.

Morakinyo, O. (1985). The brain-fag syndrome in Nigeria: Cognitive deficits in an illness associated with study. *British Journal of Psychiatry, 146,* 209–210.

Okulate, G. T., & Jones, O. B. (2002). Two depression rating instruments in Nigerian patients. *Nigerian Postgraduate Medical Journal, 9*(2), 74–78.

Orlando, M., Burnam, M. A., Beckman, R., Morton, S. C., London, A. S., Bing, E. G., & Fleishman, J. A. (2002). Re-estimating the prevalence of psychiatric disorders in a nationally representative sample of persons receiving care for HIV: Results from the HIV Cost and Service Utilization study. *International Journal of Methods in Psychiatric Research, 11*(2), 75–82.

Patel, V. (1998). *Culture and common mental disorders in Sub-Saharan Africa.* East Sussex, UK: Psychology Press.

Patel, V., Chisholm, D., Rabe-Hesketh, S., Dias-Saxena, F., Andrew, G., & Mann, A. (2003). Efficacy and cost-effectiveness of drug and psychological treatments for common mental disorders in general health care in Goa, India: A randomised, controlled trial. *Lancet, 361*(9351), 33–39.

Patel, V., & Kleinman, A. (2003). Poverty and common mental disorders in developing countries. *Bulletin of the World Health Organization, 81,* 609–615.

Patel, V., Rodrigues, M., & Desouza, N. (2002). Gender, poverty, and postnatal depression: A study of mothers in Goa, India. *American Journal of Psychiatry, 159,* 43–47.

Patel, V., Saraceno, B., & Kleinman, A. (2006). Beyond evidence: The moral case for international mental health. *American Journal of Psychiatry, 163,* 1312–1315.

Phillips, D. P. (1974). The influence of suggestion on suicide: Substantive and theoretical implications of the Werther effect. *American Sociological Review, 39,* 340–354.

Pike, K. L. (1967). *Language in relation to a unified theory of structure of human behavior* (2nd ed.). The Hague, Netherlands: Mouton.

Prince, M., Patel, V., Saxena, S., Maj, M., Maselko, J., Phillips, M. R., & Rahman, A. (2007). No health without mental health. *Lancet, 370,* 859–877,

Prince, R. (1968). Psychotherapy without insight: An example from the Yoruba of Nigeria. *American Journal of Psychiatry, 124*(9), 1171–1176.

Prince, R. (1985). The concept of culture-bound syndromes: Anorexia nervosa and brain-fag. *Social Science and Medicine, 21*(2), 197–203.

Rahman, A., Iqbal, Z., & Harrington, R. (2003). Life events, social support, depression and childbirth: Perspectives from a rural population in a developing country. *Psychological Medicine, 33,* 1161–1167.

Rahman, A., & Prince, M. (2009). Mental health in the tropics. *Annals of Tropical Medicine and Parasitology, 103*(2), 95–110.

Rotheram-Borus, M. J., Stein, J. A., & Lester, P. (2006) Adolescent adjustment over six years in HIV-affected families. *Journal of Adolescent Health, 39*(2), 174–182.

Rubinstein, S., & Caballero, B. (2000). Is Miss America an undernourished role model? *Journal of the American Medical Association, 283,* 1569.

Scheper-Hughes, N. (1993). *Death without weeping: The violence of everyday life in Brazil.* Berkeley, CA: University of California Press.

Scheper-Hughes, N. (2001). *Saints, scholars, and schizophrenics: Mental illness in rural Ireland* (20th anniversary ed.). Berkeley, CA: University of California Press.

Simon, R. C. (1996). *Boo! culture, experience, and the startle reflex,* New York, Oxford University Press.

Skydsbjerg, M., Lunn, S., & Hutchings, B. (2001). Psychosocial aspects of human immunodeficiency virus (HIV) infection in a pre-HAART sample. *Scandinavian Journal of Psychology, 42*(4), 327–333.

Srivastava, A. K., Stitt, L., Thakar, M., Shah, N., & Chinnasamy, G. (2009). The abilities of improved schizophrenia patients to work and live independently in the community: A 10-year, long-term outcome study from Mumbai, India. *Annals of General Psychiatry, 13*(8), 24.

Sumathipala, A., Siribaddana, S., Abeysingha, M. R., De Silva, P., Dewey, M., Prince, M., & Mann, A. H. (2008). Cognitive-behavioural therapy versus structured care for medically unexplained symptoms: Randomised controlled trial. *British Journal of Psychiatry, 193*(1), 51–59.

Van de Velde, S., Bracke, P., & Levecque, K. (2010). Gender difference in depression in 23 European countries: Cross-national variation in the gender gap in depression. *Social Science and Medicine, 71*(2), 305–313.

Verdeli, H., Clougherty, K., Bolton, P., Speelman, L., Ndogoni, L., Bass, J., . . . Weissman M. (2003). Adapting group interpersonal psychotherapy for a developing country: Experience in rural Uganda. *World Psychiatry, 2*(2), 114–120.

Weissman, M., Bland, R. C., Canino, G. J., Faravelli, C., Greenwald, S., Hwu, H., . . . Yeh, E.-K. (1996). Cross-national epidemiology of major depression and bipolar disorder. *Journal of the American Medical Association, 276*(4), 293–299.

Wilk, C., & Bolton, P. (2002). Local perceptions of the mental health effects of the Uganda Acquired Immunodeficiency Syndrome epidemic. *Journal of Nervous and Mental Disease, 190*(6), 394–397.

Willi, J., Giacometti, G., & Limacher, B. (1990). Update on the epidemiology of anorexia nervosa in a defined region of Switzerland. *American Journal of Psychiatry, 147*, 1514–1517.

Wiseman, C. V., Gray, J. J., Mosimann, J. E., & Ahrens, A. H. (1992). Cultural expectations of thinness in women: An update. *International Journal of Eating Disorders, 11*, 85–89.

World Health Organization. (1975). *Schizophrenia: A multinational study*. Geneva, Switzerland: Author.

World Health Organization. (1979). *Schizophrenia: An international follow-up study*. New York, NY: John Wiley & Sons.

World Health Organization. (1992). *ICD-10: The ICD-10 Classification of Mental and Behavioral Disorders; Clinical descriptions and diagnostic guidelines*, Geneva, World Health Organization

SECTION II

Methods

4

Assessment of Distress, Disorder, Impairment, and Need in the Population

WILLIAM W. EATON

RAMIN MOJTABAI

ELIZABETH A. STUART

JEANNIE-MARIE S. LEOUTSAKOS

S. JANET KURAMOTO

Key Points

- Evolution of methods of assessment of mental disorders helps demarcate three generations in the history of psychiatric epidemiology

- A range of quantitative methods for judging success in assessment (reliability and validity) is available

- Modalities of assessment include short questions on distress, brief screening scales oriented toward a syndrome, structured diagnostic interviews, and structured and semistructured psychiatric examinations

- Agreement between modalities of assessment is only moderate

- Population-based surveys of mental disorders involve large numbers of assessments, and quality control is important

- Extrapolation of survey results to areas not surveyed (indirect estimation) is possible

INTRODUCTION

A public health approach to health and illness involves exploration of both the presence and absence of diseases and disorders. Because the emphasis is on populations, not individuals, the assessment instruments employed must be appropriate for use not only across large groups but also for replication in work by other researchers and clinicians. This chapter introduces the reader to current approaches to public health assessment and to common assessment tools now in use for assessing large numbers of people.

Mental disorders and mental health provide unusual opportunities for understanding assessment in populations, because measurement is often more complex than in other fields of medicine and health. For example, no simple indicators can attest to the presence or absence of disease; assessment data are derived primarily from talking with or observing the behavior of each individual in the study group. Symptoms of many mental disorders resemble those of transient disturbances in cognition, emotion, or behavior that occur across the lifetime of the population in general. Many of these short-term disturbances are subclinical, involving rapid recovery and little, if any, change in functioning. As a result, they fail to meet the requirement of the fourth revision of the *Diagnostic and Statistical Manual of Mental Disorders* (DSM) (American Psychiatric Association [APA], 1994) that the disorder be clinically significant, involving distress or impairment and manifesting the specific signs and symptoms of the putative disorder. Therefore this chapter discusses the assessment and measurement not only of distress and impairment but also of specific mental disorders themselves.

Population-based studies have many purposes, among them, developing clues to disease etiology (Morris, 1975) that may link to laboratory and clinical findings and, ultimately, may guide prevention efforts. This analytic interest is served by population-based studies of the prevalence and incidence of mental disorders. A second important end product of assessment in medicine and public health is to determine the need for treatment. At the level of the individual, diagnosis and assessment of need guide treatment decisions. From the population point of view, diagnosis and assessment of need in large numbers of individuals provides the numerator for various forms of rates, the essential tool of the epidemiologist. Assessment of need at the level of the population is part of the community diagnosis mentioned by Morris (1975) in his volume *Uses of Epidemiology*. Population-based needs assessment should be the basis of health service planning. This chapter integrates the assessment of mental disorders, distress, and impairment with the field of needs assessment.

HISTORICAL BACKGROUND

Psychiatric epidemiology—the population approach to mental disorders—has existed since at least the middle of the 19th century, that is, before or concomitantly with the beginning of epidemiologic study as a whole. The history of psychiatric epidemiology was characterized in the 1981 Rema Lapouse Award lecture by Bruce and Barbara Dohrenwend (Dohrenwend & Dohrenwend, 1982) as spanning three historical epochs or generations.

First Generation

The first generation of psychiatric epidemiology, roughly from the end of 19th century until around 1955, consisted primarily of surveys of mental hospitals and other institutions in which persons with mental disorders resided. Classic first-generation studies include the Chicago study of urbanization and mental illness (Faris & Dunham, 1939), studies of inmates of institutions in New York State by Malzberg (1952a, 1952b, 1953), the New Haven study of social class and mental illness (Hollingshead and Redlich, 1958), and the Model Reporting Areas, in which states and communities reported the characteristics of state hospital populations to the National Institute of Mental Health (M. Kramer, 1969). In these studies, medical records provided information about specific psychiatric diagnoses.

In the 19th century, the prevalence of mental disorders in the community was estimated by taking censuses of the residents of asylums, poorhouses, and other institutions in which people with mental illnesses were housed (Humphreys, 1890; Tuke, 1892/1976). Data resulting from such exercises often were referred to as statistics of insanity, although the term included sociodemographic correlates of mental disorders as well. In the latter part of the 19th century, interest in these data grew, concomitantly with growing concern about the rising prevalence of mental disorders; these data provided one of the few ways in which one could investigate whether prevalence in fact was increasing (Humphreys, 1890). Historical research continues to explore past trends in the prevalence of mental disorders (Torrey & Miller, 2001).

This method of estimating the burden of mental illness in a population had a number of benefits. First, relying on regularly collected administrative data incurred little extra cost. Second, an institutional census likely captured the majority of people with the most serious mental illnesses, since in the era before the introduction of antipsychotic medications many people with mental disorders entered and remained for long periods in psychiatric hospitals. Finally, because the vast majority of patients in asylums allegedly suffered from the most serious mental disorders, the clinical significance of these cases was rarely in doubt.

The method's major limitation was that it equated need for treatment with treatment itself. Neither these statistics of insanity nor their modern counterparts—psychiatric registries—capture the majority of individuals with less severe mental disorders that go untreated. This important limitation was clear even to early observers of trends in mental health and illness. As one early observer (Humphreys, 1890) noted, "Insanity being...a relative term, there are a large number of persons who are on the borderline, who are or are not lunatics according to the convenience or affluence of their friends" (p. 248). It also was soon recognized that other factors, including social class and even such factors as geographical distance, could affect whether an individual was placed in a mental facility (Humphreys, 1890; Jarvis, 1866).

Recognizing the limitations of data on utilization of treatment facilities, investigators, as early as the 19th century, sought other methods to estimate the prevalence of mental disorders. In Massachusetts in 1855, Edward Jarvis conducted what remains one of the most extensive and impressive surveys of mental disorders undertaken anywhere in the world (Commission on Lunacy, 1855/1971). Jarvis attempted to count both treated and untreated cases of mental disorders across the state. The definition of mental illness in Jarvis's survey and, indeed, in the view of mid-19th-century psychiatry was limited to very severe cases that required custodial care. He approached physicians, clergymen, and other knowledgeable individuals in every locality, asking each to report on known cases of mental illness and mental retardation (then respectively termed "lunacy" and "idiocy"). Information on institutionalized patients was obtained from facility administrators.

Jarvis estimated the prevalence of severe cases of mental illness to be less than one-fourth of one percent. While only about half of the identified cases were found in institutions, all of those with severe mental illness, in Jarvis's judgment, actually needed institutional care. Based on his findings, Jarvis argued for an increased number of psychiatric beds in Massachusetts. Despite these findings and a growing body of epidemiologic studies over the following century that continued to show that as many as 75% of individuals with significant psychiatric problems never sought treatment (Link & Dohrenwend, 1980), the problem of untreated mental illness received little public attention until the second half of the 20th century.

Analysis of utilization data to estimate both the burden of mental illness and, indirectly, the need for treatment has continued to this day, providing policymakers with vital information on demand for psychiatric services at the local, state, and national levels (Baldwin & Evans, 1971; de Salvia, Barbato, Salvo, & Zadro, 1993; Goodman, Rahav, Popper, Ginath, & Pearl, 1984; Hall, Robertson, Dorricott, Olley, & Millar, 1973; M. Kramer, 1969; Munk-Jorgensen, Kastrup, & Mortensen, 1993; O'Hare, 1987; Pedersen,

Gotzsche, Moller, & Mortensen, 2006; Rahav, 1981; Selten & Sijben, 1994; ten Horn, Geil, Gulbinat, & Henderson, 1986; Thornicroft, Johnson, Leese, & Slade, 2000; J. K. Wing, 1989; J. Wing & Fryers, 1976; L. Wing et al., 1967). In their modern incarnation as local and national registries, these data also provide valuable information on the broad range of risk factors for the development of mental disorders.

Second Generation

The second generation of psychiatric epidemiology benefited from the development of surveys of persons residing in households in the general population, a practice that began during and just after World War II. At that time, diagnosis and treatment of mental disorders was dominated by the psychoanalytic model; population-based studies focused more on the broad rubric of mental disorders than on specific disorders or diagnoses. Thus, these early household interview surveys were designed to estimate the probability that an individual would be diagnosed by a psychiatrist as meeting criteria for any mental disorder. Findings from these studies led to a renewed recognition of and concern about the fact that many individuals in need of care for mental disorders were not receiving it, the very issues Jarvis (1866) had highlighted 100 years earlier. This awareness resulted in part from the discovery of a high prevalence of psychiatric morbidity among military personnel serving in World War II (Brill & Beebe, 1956). Almost one-fifth of some 26 million men between ages 18 and 37 were identified as suffering from some type of mental disorder. Replicated in a number of postwar general population surveys (Dohrenwend, 1980; Leighton, Harding, Macklin, Macmillan, & Leighton, 1963; Srole, Langner, Michael, Kirkpatrick, & Rennie, 1962), these findings made clear that estimating the prevalence of mental disorders based on service utilization data alone captures only the tip of the iceberg of mental illness in the community (Link & Dohrenwend, 1980). Classic studies during this second generation include the Midtown Manhattan study (Srole et al., 1962), among the first to explore the

role of stress in the etiology of mental disorders, and the Stirling County study in Atlantic Canada (Leighton et al., 1963), which emphasized the impact of social integration on the development of mental disorders.

Third Generation

The third generation began around 1980, the time of the neo-Kraepelinian revolution in diagnosis embodied in the third revision of the DSM (DSM-III) (APA, 1980). The neo-Kraepelinian model of mental disorders assumes that much like physical disorders, mental disorders are discrete, biologically based disease entities with relatively clear boundaries. The emphasis on specific disorders was picked up in a cartoon in *The New Yorker* (figure 4-1). Concomitant with the new nosology, many investigators felt the need for more reliable, standardized methods to assess the

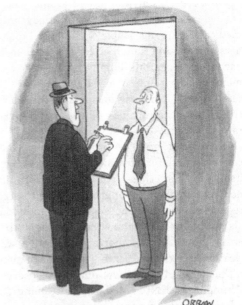

"You have been chosen in a random selection to take part in a nationwide survey. Question Number One: 'What kind of a nut would you say you are?'"

Figure 4-1 **Specificity of Mental Disorders.**

prevalence of these disorders in population surveys. The incorporation of DSM-III criteria into the Epidemiologic Catchment Area (ECA) study's structured interview schedule—called the Diagnostic Interview Schedule (DIS)—addressed this need (Eaton, Regier, Locke, & Taube, 1981; Klerman, 1986, 1990; Regier et al., 1984).

The ECA spawned a new generation of population surveys of mental disorders that continues to this day and has served as a model for studies in the US and abroad. Compared with earlier general population surveys, the ECA's most important innovation was its focus on specific mental disorders, a methodological approach now widely used in general population surveys worldwide (Demyttenaere et al., 2004). Important US examples of such studies (described in greater detail in chapter 7) include both the National Comorbidity Survey (NCS) of the 1990s (Kessler, 1994) and the National Comorbidity Survey—Replication (NCS-R) a decade later (Kessler & Merikangas, 2004). In addition, several other nationally representative surveys on substance use in the US, such as the National Survey of Drug Use and Health (Substance Abuse and Mental Health Services Administration, 2010) and the National Epidemiologic Survey on Alcohol and Related Conditions (Grant et al., 1994), included measures of a range of mental disorders as well as substance use disorders.

METHODS FOR JUDGING SUCCESS IN ASSESSMENT

A large number of assessment technologies developed to obtain information on individuals also can help estimate the population prevalence of specific mental disorders or groups of them. Before we briefly describe a selection of these measures, two key issues—reliability and validity—warrant exploration. Reliability addresses whether a measure yields consistent results, and validity addresses whether we are measuring what we think we're measuring. When building assessment tools, the goal is to yield instruments that are both highly reliable and valid. It is difficult to overstate the negative consequences of unreliable or invalid measurement. Unreliable measurement attenuates any

true association between two measures, clouding the ability to study etiologic clues. Invalid measurement biases estimates of the prevalence of a disorder and of the disorder's relationship to risk factors and outcomes, which in turn compromises estimates of need for treatment as well as the study of etiology.

Reliability

Reliability is the consistency of a measurement. For a measurement to be useful, it must be reliable. For example, a perfectly reliable yardstick or tape measure would yield the same height (e.g., 1.6 meters) each time a particular person was measured. In contrast, an unreliable tool (e.g., estimates of height by observers at a distance) would yield highly variable measurements. For this reason, mental health research employs several types of research designs which focus on the consistency of measurement, among them:

- test–retest reliability, which refers to the correlation between consecutive measurements on the same individuals (Bohrnstedt, 2010)
- inter-rater reliability, which refers to consistency among measurements conducted by different raters (Shrout & Fleiss, 1979)
- internal consistency reliability, which refers to consistency of responses to similar items (Bohrnstedt, 2010).

The third type of reliability measure—internal consistency—was developed for variables such as cognitive abilities and emotions that lack an easy-to-access physical indicator (like height), for which assessment sometimes takes the form of many not-quite-equivalent forms of measurement, such as questions on personality tests. These forms of inquiry are not identical, in order to prevent practice effects (when people perform better on subsequent tests because they get used to the particular test) and reactivity effects (when the very act of asking about a feeling or thought causes people to change their response). Internal consistency reliability can be assessed under such circumstances by quantifying the consistency of answers across items. For more detail on the development of reliable measurements, see DeVellis (1991).

Quantitative estimates of reliability—reliability coefficients—take different forms, depending on which of the three research designs is used and the level of measurement of the variable whose reliability is being assessed (see table 4-1). For dichotomous variables, such as the presence or absence of a disorder, the kappa coefficient (κ) is used when the design is of the test–retest or inter-rater form (Fleiss, Gurland, & Cooper, 1971). For continuous variables in these two situations, the correlation coefficient (r) is used. In the situation of multiple items, Cronbach's alpha coefficient (α) is used for continuous and dichotomous variables, though in the latter case it is called the Kuder-Richardson 20 coefficient (KR-20). The intraclass correlation coefficient (ICC) can be used in all six situations (Shrout & Fleiss, 1979). An important common feature of all these reliability coefficients is that perfect reliability yields a value of 1.0. When a reliability coefficient is less than around .40, research results are severely threatened. In general, a reliability coefficient value of .60 is considered moderately good; a coefficient value of .80 or higher is considered good or excellent (Altman, 1991; Landis & Koch, 1991).

Reliability was an important motivation for the APA to undertake its 1980 comprehensive revision of the DSM. Reviews of the diagnostic reliability of assessments based on the previous two editions found reliability not only to be well below a level acceptable to most researchers but also to be so low as to support popular arguments of the myth of mental illness. Thus in six projects reviewed by Spitzer and Fleiss (1974), the average kappa value for a diagnosis of neurotic depression was .26, for anxiety neurosis the average was .45, and for schizophrenia the average was .57 (Helzer et al., 1977; Spitzer & Fleiss, 1974). In comparison, in DSM-III field trials (Spitzer, Forman, & Nee, 1979), the value of kappa in the test–retest design for major affective disorder was .77, for anxiety disorder .43, and for schizophrenia .82. Later studies of revisions to both the DSM-III and the International Classification of Diseases (World Health Organization, 1992, 1993), which included increasingly precise operational criteria for diagnosis, revealed kappa values that were higher still (see table 1.1 in Eaton, 2001).

Validity

A measure's validity is the degree to which it measures what it is purported to measure. That is, validity refers to the strength of the relationship between the measurement and the concept or construct represented by the name of the variable (e.g., major depressive disorder or distress). A measure can have very high reliability but low validity if it gets consistent results but in fact is not measuring what it is supposed to be measuring. Classic descriptions of validity include Cronbach and Meehl (1955) and Messick (1995). For discussions of validity specifically related to psychiatric diagnoses, see E. Robins and Guze (1970) and Spitzer (1983). Chapter 3 of this volume discusses issues of reliability and validity associated with cross-cultural work. There are several types of validity as discussed below. *Criterion validity* is assessed by comparison

Table 4-1. Coefficients for Reliability

	MEASURES			
DESIGN	CONTINUOUS		CATEGORICAL	
Test–retest	r	ICC	κ	ICC
Inter-rater	r	ICC	κ	ICC
Multiple item	α	ICC	KR-20	ICC

r = Pearson or Spearman correlation coefficient; ICC = intraclass correlation coefficient; κ = kappa coefficient; α = Cronbach's alpha; KR-20 = Kuder-Richardson coefficient.

with some standard measure in which there is complete confidence that it measures what it purports to measure—sometimes called the gold standard. When measuring height, a gold standard might be the yardstick or tape measure; one might compare this measure with assessments by observers at a distance, noting any discrepancy between the two. With few exceptions, instruments that measure mental health or mental illness lack such a gold standard; no directly observable variables, such as blood tests, indicate the presence or absence of a mental disorder or the level of a trait (Tsuang & Tohen, 2002). Instead, all possible data are gathered from existing interview, examination, and medical records, from as many points in time as possible, and from many observers; the data then are analyzed with expert assistance. This is referred to as the L-E-A-D (Longitudinal, Expert, All Data) standard, the closest to a gold standard as exists in the field of psychiatry. *Content validity* is the degree to which the many indicators represent the defined domain of content. This type of validity became much easier to determine after DSM-III delineated operational diagnostic criteria for specific mental disorders. For example, a scale to measure depressive disorder can be constructed readily to ensure good content validity, thanks to careful description of the nine symptom groups in DSM-III's operational criteria for diagnosis (APA, 1980). *Construct validity* refers to the degree to which measurement results demonstrate the predicted association with antecedents and outcomes. Again, in the case of depression, individuals' depression scores would be expected to have an inverse relationship to scores on scales of self-esteem, a closely related construct. Depression scores also would be consistent with known risk factors for depression, such as age and sex (Burvill, 1995), and with outcomes for which depression itself is a risk factor, such as myocardial infarction (Glassman, 2008).

The study of validity in behavioral health is more complex than in physical health and epidemiology generally, where the emphasis is on criterion validity and gold standards, such as biological measures, which are less often in doubt. In physical health and epidemiology, criterion validity often is quantified with reference to the indicators of sensitivity and specificity. *Sensitivity* is the proportion of cases identified by the gold standard measure that are similarly identified as positive in the population by the test measure. *Specificity* is the proportion of persons identified by the gold standard as not having the disorder that are correctly identified by the test measure as not having the disorder (Gordis, 2004). These two indicators apply specifically to dichotomous variables, such as the presence or absence of a disease. In psychiatric epidemiology, sensitivity and specificity indicators have been found to have utility for assessing specific diagnoses only since DSM-III was adopted (APA, 1980). However, their usefulness suffers from the lack of a gold standard in psychiatric diagnosis.

METHODS OF ASSESSMENT FOR LARGE NUMBERS OF INDIVIDUALS

As discussed earlier, one of the challenges in public mental health is to obtain reliable, valid, population-based information about mental disorders. Three broad types of assessment methods are available to help estimate the prevalence of mental disorders in a large number of individuals:

1. Structured or unstructured psychiatric examinations, in which psychiatrists assess DSM-diagnosed mental disorders—;
2. Structured diagnostic interviews, based on DSM criteria, conducted by interviewers without clinical training (the method that forms the bulk of psychiatric epidemiologic efforts to date);
3. Short scales that screen for potential cases of both diagnosable mental disorders as well as for subclinical distress, disability, and impairment.

We discuss each of these assessment tools in turn.

Psychiatric Examination

Examination by a well-trained psychiatrist in the context of a research study is the closest approximation to a gold standard in public mental health. The term *examination* implies that the examiner determines the presence or absence of the relevant sought-for sign, symptom, or diagnosis. In contrast to the structured psychiatric interview, in which an interviewer records the answers of the respondent, the psychiatric interview provides broad discretion and variation in how the examiner—the psychiatrist—obtains the information needed to make a diagnosis. As a result, the assessments made, even in research settings, can have low reliability. As described earlier in this chapter and in chapter 2, the delineation of diagnosis-specific operational criteria in DSM-III helped reduce the risk of poor inter-rater reliability. Yet despite the greater diagnostic precision, concern remained that variation in the conduct of the psychiatric examination or in the interpretation of that information would leave too much room for error. In response, both structured and semistructured examinations were designed to standardize the process.

Among the most important of these structured psychiatric examination tools are the Schedules for Clinical Assessment in Neuropsychiatry (SCAN) (J. K. Wing et al., 1990) and the Structured Clinical Interview for DSM (SCID) (Spitzer, Williams, Gibbon, & First, 1992; Williams et al., 1992). Both instruments involve recording information obtained in a face-to-face interview followed by application of a precise algorithm to the results to reach a diagnosis. The instruments differ in two key ways, however. The slightly more conversational SCAN examination amasses information on a wide range of signs and symptoms that are generally organized by syndrome—for example, starting with questions about physical health, then about worrying and tension, followed by obsessional symptoms, and so forth. This approach is sometimes referred to as a "bottom-up" approach, since information about a broad array of signs and symptoms is gathered without the benefit of an antecedent, presumptive presenting problem or hypothesis about diagnosis. The SCAN includes suggested interview questions, an example of which is shown in figure 4-2.

The SCAN glossary of symptoms and syndromes (J. K. Wing et al., 1990) requires clinicians to determine if the pattern of responses from the individual being examined meets minimum criteria for a particular disorder. For example, section 4 of the 236-page SCAN glossary (titled "Panics, Anxiety, and Phobias") includes the following entry:

> 4.020 Panic attacks
> Panic attacks are discrete episodes of marked autonomic anxiety, with a sudden onset, building rapidly (within minutes) to a crescendo and a maximum point. They may occur against a general background of autonomic anxiety or emerge with no symptomatic precursors. An attack may last up to an hour but dissipate gradually. Both free-floating and phobic forms of anxiety may be characterized by panic attacks (see item 4.055) and multiple ratings are then required. (p. 49)

Now I should like to ask you about feelings of anxiety or attacks of panic. When people get anxious or panicky they often feel very fearful. They may feel their heart beating fast, or maybe they start shaking or sweating, or feel they can't get their breath. Have you had feelings like that?

Response:

    0   Anxiety and panic attacks absent

    1   Anxiety and/or panic attacks present

Figure 4-2 **SCAN Question on Panic Attack.**

Item 4.055, referred to in the final sentence, occurs in the SCAN itself (J. K. Wing et al., 1990):

"Did the panics you mentioned always occur with one of these phobias, or did you also have them without any warning?"

The multiple ratings consist of four response values: 0—No phobias; 1—Only phobias; 2—Phobias with panic; and 3—panic rarely or never with phobias. (p. 66)

In contrast to the SCAN, the SCID instrument (Spitzer et al., 1992) often is referred to as a "top-down" approach, since each question has a specific relationship to a diagnostic algorithm. Instead of a symptom glossary, diagnostic criteria are placed next to the question. (See figure 4-3 for the SCID instrument's section on panic disorder.) Another significant difference between the two instruments is that the SCAN requires more clinical judgment and training than the SCID and also takes longer to administer.

These assessment tools have been used only in a limited number of epidemiologic studies, primarily because of the expense of training and employing clinicians to undertake the assessments (Eaton, Neufeld, Chen, & Cai, 2000; Phillips et al., 2009). These instruments most often are used to validate the results of less expensive assessment techniques such as those described below.

Structured Diagnostic Interviews

The DIS, designed to be administered by interviewers without clinical training, was developed in part to provide a reliable, valid assessment tool for use in conducting the NIMH ECA program survey (Robins et al, 1981; 1989). Different from semistructured examinations like the SCAN, which suggests questions to guide the clinically trained examiner, the DIS is a verbatim interview. The interviewer reads each question exactly as written, obviating the need for clinical training. Because the DIS was crafted concurrently with the creation of the DSM-III, the designers of the DIS (Robins, Helzer, and colleagues) and the creators of the DSM-III (Spitzer and colleagues), worked closely to keep the DIS aligned with DSM-III criteria, some of which were still being refined. As a result, for example, DIS questions on the durations of symptoms of depressive disorder used at the first ECA site (New Haven, Connecticut), asked whether symptoms had lasted a week or more, carrying forward the tradition of a research predecessor of the DSM, the Research Diagnostic Criteria (Spitzer, Endicott, & Robins, 1978). However, the second version of the DIS, employed at all but the first ECA site in New Haven, changed the duration to two weeks or more, consistent with DSM-III. Thus the DIS adhered to highly specific operational criteria in the new DSM-III, with questions that reflected those criteria so closely that slight changes in the criteria make it difficult to analyze together data from the several sites.

F. Anxiety Disorders Panic Disorder *Have you ever had a panic attack, when you suddenly felt frightened, anxious, or extremely uncomfortable?*	Panic Disorder Criteria A. At some time during the disturbance, one or more panic attacks (discrete periods of intense fear or discomfort) have occurred that were (1) unexpected, i.e., did not occur immediately before or on exposure to a situation that almost always causes anxiety, and (2) not triggered by situations in which the person was the focus of others' attention.

Figure 4-3   **SCID Instrument Section on Panic Disorder.**

Source: Adapted from Spitzer et al., 1992.

The content of the questions posed became critical; they needed to be both inference and affect free, with clear and identical meaning for the individuals being interviewed. Careful pilot testing was of assistance in the process. For example, version II of the DIS, used at the New Haven ECA site, included the question "Did you ever have problems with belly pain?" in the section on somatization disorder. In response, 36% of sampled adults ages 18–64 in New Haven answered positively. Following further pilot testing and discussion after the survey began, concern arose that as written, the question might be too broad; anyone might well respond positively, regardless of psychological status, making the question uninformative. Thus in the subsequent version, used at the Baltimore and subsequent sites, the language was altered to read, "Did you ever have a lot of problems with belly pain?" In Baltimore, 27% of sampled adults responded positively to the question, suggesting that even a small wording change (e.g., adding "a lot of...")could affect the apparent prevalence of a disorder. This example illustrates not only how the measuring instrument can affect validity but also just how difficult it is to establish a gold standard for the symptom of abdominal pain in the diagnosis of somatization disorder. Clearly, in psychiatric epidemiology, as in other areas of mental health care where most information is garnered through discussion, word choice is very important.

The questions asked by the DIS to generate a DSM-III diagnosis of panic disorder are shown in figure 4-4. As the figure shows, the set of questions fits on a single sheet of paper. The close relationship with DSM-III diagnostic criteria is apparent when one compares the questions with the diagnostic criteria for panic disorder found in the diagnostic manual.

A verbatim interview has the distinct advantage that it can be administered by persons without clinical training, facilitating its use in large, population-based studies without incurring prohibitive costs. However, some problems do arise in the conduct of a structured diagnostic interview. For example, rather than reflecting the presence of a psychiatric disorder, a positive response to a question on symptoms might reflect a trivial or transitory occurrence of the symptom. Or a positive response might be the result of a physical illness or injury or ingestion of drugs, alcohol, or other substances. For most psychiatric disorders, a symptom caused by ingestion of drugs or alcohol would not be considered as an indication of the disorder (the exception to this exclusionary rule is the alcohol and drug disorders themselves). Unfortunately, a lay interviewer does not have the clinical knowledge to make this important distinction. However, the DIS includes a way to manage this potential problem through the DIS Probe Flow Chart (see figure 4-5). The Probe Flow Chart is designed to mimic the questions a psychiatrist asks about the occurrence of symptoms and is potentially applicable to every symptom-related question on the DIS. It yields specific code values:

1. Response to the question is negative; symptom never occurred
2. Response to the question is positive, but the symptom was not severe enough to lead the respondent to tell a doctor or other health professional about [it], to take medication for it more than once, or to respond that it "interfered with [their] life a lot"
3. Response to the question is positive; and the symptom was severe, but, each time it occurred, it was caused by a medication, drug, or alcohol
4. Response to the question is positive and the symptom was severe, but, each time it occurred, it was caused by an illness or injury, or by a medication, drug, or alcohol
5. Response to the question is positive; the symptom was severe, and, at least once, it was not caused by illness, injury, medication, drug, or alcohol—making it a plausible psychiatric symptom.

It would appear from the Probe Flow Chart that each symptom-related question can receive a response value of 1 through 5. However, in the case of some symptoms and disorders, the presence of a symptom is considered inherently severe. For example, questions on somatic aspects of depression lack a code value of 2; other depression-related symptoms, such as a suicide gesture or attempt, are classified as not having potential substance or illness causes and so no 2, 3, or 4 code is

62. Have you ever had a spell or attack when all of a sudden you felt frightened, DECK 02
○ anxious or very uneasy in situations when most people would not be afraid?

  ① ② ③ ④ ⑤

  MD: _____ SELF: _____ 48/

┌───┐
│ **INTERVIEWER:** DID R TELL MD (CAUSE WRITTEN ON MD LINE IN Q. 62)?   │
│   NO... ①   │
│   C   YES .... ⑤ 49/ │
│   │
│ **INTERVIEWER:** If Q. 62 IS CODED "1," SKIP TO Q. 68.   │
│   **ALL** OTHERS, ASK Qs. 63-67.   │
└───┘

63. During one of your worst spells of suddenly feeling frightened or anxious or uneasy, did you ever notice
○ that you had any of the following problems? During this spell: (READ EACH SYMPTOM AND CODE
   "YES" OR "NO" FOR EACH. **REPEAT** THE PHRASE "DURING THIS SPELL" FOR EACH.)

		NO	YES	
A.	were you short of breath—having trouble catching your breath?	①	⑤	50/
B.	did your heart pound?	①	⑤	51/
C.	were you dizzy or light-headed?	①	⑤	52/
D.	did your fingers or feet tingle?	①	⑤	53/
E.	did you have tightness or pain in your chest?	①	⑤	54/
F.	did you feel like you were choking or smothering?	①	⑤	55/
G.	did you feel faint?	①	⑤	56/
H.	did you sweat?	①	⑤	57/
I.	did you tremble or shake?	①	⑤	58/
J.	did you feel hot or cold flashes?	①	⑤	59/
K.	did things around you seem unreal?	①	⑤	60/
L.	were you afraid either that you might die or that you might act in a crazy way?	①	⑤	61/

63. How old were you the **first** time you had one of these sudden spells of feeling frightened or anxious?
○ (IF R SAYS "WHOLE LIFE": **CODE 02**)

   ENTER AGE & [ ][ ] ⓪ ① ② ③ ④ ⑤ ⑥ ⑦ ⑧ ⑨
   GO TO Q. 65.   ⓪ ① ② ③ ④ ⑤ ⑥ ⑦ ⑧ ⑨   62/

┌───┐
│ **INTERVIEWER:** IF "DK" AND R IS **UNDER** 40: **CODE 01**   │
│   IF "DK" AND R IS 40 OR MORE: ASK A   │
└───┘

   A. Would you say it was before or after you were 40?

              Before 40 ...... (RECORD 01)
              After 40   .... (RECORD 95)
              Still DK   .... (RECORD 98)   64/

65. Have you ever had 3 spells like this close together—say within a 3-week period?
○

              No .... ①
              Yes .... ⑤   65/

66. Have spells like this occurred during at least 6 **different** weeks of your life?
○

              No .... ①
              Yes .... ⑤   66/

Figure 4-4   **Diagnostic Interview Schedule, Panic Disorder Section.**

Source: National Opinion Research Center, University of Chicago and Washington University, St. Louis, Missouri, DIS, Diagnostic Interview Schedule, Version III, 1981.

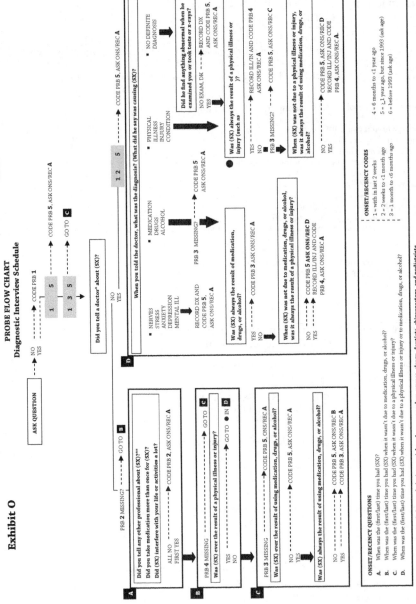

Figure 4-5 Diagnostic Interview Schedule Probe Flow Chart.

indicated. Until recently, because of these idiosyncrasies, interviewers were required to memorize the Probe Flow Chart and follow the structure of questions indicated by the pattern of response codes.

Over time, the DIS has evolved consistent with changes in the DSM; today, the DIS produces DSM-IV (APA, 1994) diagnoses. Interviewer training in the use of the DIS now requires about a week. Print and electronic copies of the DIS, its training schedule, and the computer-assisted DIS are available from Washington University and online at http://epi.wustl.edu/did/dishome.htm.

The Composite International Diagnostic Interview (CIDI) is a collective creation of the authors of the DIS and researchers from other countries who wanted an instrument that reflected both the nosologic categories of the International Classification of Diseases World Health Organization, 1992, 1993) and those of the DSM (Kessler & Ustun, 2004; L. Robins et al., 1988). The DIS is organized so that all or nearly all questions in a given diagnostic area occur together and are asked sequentially. In contrast, the CIDI is austerely diagnostic; the diagnostic algorithm is applied by the computer at each point in the interview. Thus when it is clear that, without regard to subsequent responses, a respondent will not meet diagnostic criteria, the corresponding follow-on questions are not scheduled to be asked. For example, dysphoria or anhedonia is required for a diagnosis of major depressive disorder (see chapter 1 for abbreviated diagnostic criteria for this disorder). Questions about these two symptoms are asked early in the interview; if the responses are negative, questions on the somatic aspects of depressive disorder are excluded altogether from the interview. While use of such skip patterns may shorten the interview, it also limits the ability to study subclinical syndromes, since not every diagnostic question is asked of each respondent. However, the space and time saved by using skip patterns made it possible to include additional questions relevant to the International Classification of Diseases and other diagnoses in the DSM. The CIDI, in a variety of forms, was used to gather data for the NCS (Kessler, 1994) and both its follow up (NCS-F) and

replication (NCS-R) about a decade later (Kessler & Merikangas, 2004), as well as in the World Mental Health 2000 surveys (Demyttenaere et al., 2004; Kessler & Ustun, 2004).

The validity of findings about the prevalence of disorders disclosed through structured interviews such as the DIS and its successor, the CIDI, has been a topic of ongoing discussion and debate (Anthony et al, 1985; Eaton, Hall, Macdonald, & McKibben, 2007; Henderson, 2000). Investigators evaluating the validity of structured interviews typically assess the concordance between the measures obtained in such interviews and diagnoses made by clinicians, usually using a semistructured interview instrument. Figure 4-6 presents data on the sensitivity and specificity of structured interviews compared with clinician diagnoses for seven mental disorders. Table 4-2 displays results of one of the 29 studies of criterion validity for major depressive disorder and serves as an example of concordance assessment. As

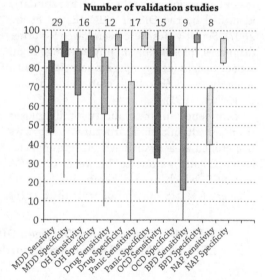

Number of validation studies

Sensitivity and specificity total and interquartile ranges

Figure 4-6 **Concordance Between Lay Interviewers and Psychiatrist Diagnosis.**
MDD = major depressive disorder; OH = alcohol disorder; OCD = obsessive–compulsive disorder; BPD = bipolar disorder; NAP = non affective psychosis.

Source: Reprinted with permission from Eaton et al., 2007.

the table shows, 349 subjects in the Baltimore ECA follow-up were interviewed with the DIS and then examined by psychiatrists using the SCAN. The psychiatrists did not know the results of the DIS interviews. According to the SCAN, 78 individuals were found to have a lifetime diagnosis of major depressive disorder (prevalence of 22%); the DIS found only 34 with the same lifetime diagnosis (prevalence of 10%). Twenty-three cases were identified with major depressive disorder by both instruments. If the SCAN is considered the gold standard in this study, sensitivity of the DIS is 23/78, or 29%. When it comes to specificity, according to the SCAN, 271 participants were recorded as negative for major depressive disorder; 260 were similarly identified as negative by the DIS, for a specificity of 96%.

In Figure 4-6. one quarter of the studies of depression (indicated by the bottom of the bar displaying the interquartile range) reported sensitivities of the structured interview below 46%. In other words, fewer than 46% of individuals whom a clinician would diagnose with major depression using the SCAN are similarly identified by the DIS or CIDI (Eaton et al., 2007). Sensitivities were even lower for other diagnoses, presumably highly contingent on lack of insight into symptoms associated with some disorders (Eaton, Romanoski, Anthony, & Nestadt, 1991).

Confidence in the validity of diagnoses from lay-administered structured interviews has eroded as a result both of discrepancies in prevalence estimates between the ECA and NCS, which used different instruments (Regier et al., 1998), and of wide differences

within and across countries in prevalence estimates found using different translations of the CIDI (Demyttenaere et al., 2004). Based on these findings, it probably is fair to say that the validity of case ascertainment in psychiatric epidemiology remains in question (Eaton et al., 2007). The measurement weaknesses appear most evident when one compares prevalence rates found in different studies. In such cases, seemingly small departures of sensitivity or specificity from 100% can easily generate large differences in the numbers above and below a stated threshold, with corresponding large differences in prevalence. For studies of the association of antecedent and consequent variables with the presence of a disorder, the errors due to unreliability tend to cancel out, weakening the degree of association but not resulting in a high or low bias. Fortunately, methods using sensitivity and specificity can help correct estimates of prevalence (Rogan & Gladen, 1978).

The ECA findings and later population surveys modeled after it met with disbelief among some clinicians and investigators. For example, when asked to comment on the results of the NCS-R survey on lifetime prevalence of mental disorder, Paul McHugh, MD, of the Johns Hopkins University famously said, "Fifty percent of Americans mentally impaired—are you kidding me?" (Carey, 2005). Typically, criticism of the findings has focused on:

- the growing number of psychiatric disorders included in the successive editions of the DSM
- the uncertain validity of these diagnoses, especially when evaluated using lay-administered structured interviews (despite

Table 4-2. Concordance Between DIS and SCAN Lifetime Diagnoses of DSM-III-R Major Depressive Disorder, Baltimore ECA Follow-up

RESULTS ACCORDING TO DIS	RESULTS ACCORDING TO SCAN		TOTAL
	ABSENT	PRESENT	
Absent	260	55	315
Present	11	23	34
Total	271	78	349

the generally low sensitivity of the measures compared with psychiatrist examinations, discussed above)

- the uncertain association of psychiatric diagnosis with need for treatment (as discussed in chapter 15).

The 1980 revision of the DSM is now considered a watershed event in the history of psychiatry (Shorter, 1997). With 265 distinct disorders, DSM-III included 85 more disorders than were found in the DSM-II (APA, 1980). The number has continued to grow, with 292 disorders listed in the DSM-III-R (APA, 1987) and 297 in the DSM-IV (APA, 1994). At this point, many researchers and clinicians doubt that a compendium of this number of distinct disorders provides a useful means through which to categorize abnormal human behavior (Carey, 2005; Praag, 1993). These doubts are compounded by speculations about the role special interest groups and pharmaceutical companies may have played in promoting an expanded set of diagnostic categories (Carey, 2008; Kirk & Kutchins, 1992). Third-party payers typically reimburse only for the treatment of disorders listed in the DSM, and development and government approval of patents for new psychotherapeutic medications hinge on their capacity for effective treatment of DSM-listed disorders.

Screening Scales for Disorder, Distress, and Impairment

The instruments reviewed above—SCAN, SCID, DIS, CIDI—were designed to make diagnoses in large populations specifically to explore the epidemiology of mental disorders. Each instrument requires an hour or more to administer and an interviewer (whether a clinician or a trained layperson) to engage in a face-to-face encounter with each respondent. In contrast, screening scales, sometimes computer-based or self-administered questionnaires, are designed to be administered in just a few minutes and not necessarily in a face-to-face encounter. Such modalities may fit best within a primary care setting, since these scales are intended to identify individuals who

may need a more detailed follow-up interview or perhaps a little bit more attention from a primary care provider.

Many scales have been designed to screen for and measure stress, distress, or demoralization: conditions reflecting an individual's averse emotional state arising from the perception that the demands of the environment may exceed his or her capacity to respond (Cohen, Kamarck, & Mermelstein, 1983; Cohen, Kessler, & Underwood Gordon, 1995; Goldberg, 1972, 1978; Goldberg & Hillier, 1979; Link & Dohrenwend, 1980). Distress is the most common concomitant of many mental disorders; scales for distress therefore also screen for mental disorders, particularly common mood and anxiety disorders. Scales of distress were created during World War II to help identify individuals at risk for combat reaction (now known as posttraumatic stress disorder). These same instruments were revised and used in studies during the second generation of psychiatric epidemiology, such as the Midtown Manhattan and Stirling County studies (Leighton et al., 1963; Srole et al., 1962). Since then, many new scales have been developed and calibrated to optimize their capacity to screen for a general set of specific diagnoses.

The K-6, for example, is a six-item scale initially developed to screen for general distress (Kessler et al., 2002) and later applied to screen for serious mental illnesses (Kessler, Barker, et al., 2003). It has been used in a number of general population surveys, among them, the US National Health Interview Survey (CDC, 2011) and the Australian National Survey of Mental Health and Well-Being (Furukawa, Kessler, Slade, & Andrews, 2003). The K-6 asks: "During the past 30 days, how often did you feel...so sad that nothing could cheer you up?...nervous?...restless or fidgety?...hopeless?...that everything was an effort?...worthless?"

Scales of distress such as this can be used, as they were during the second generation of psychiatric epidemiologic inquiry, to assess the likelihood that a particular individual in the survey population represents a case of mental disorder. When combined with structured diagnostic interviews, distress scales can help quantify the level of distress associated with a particular disorder and the overall need for care in the population.

Some screening scales are oriented toward a specific diagnosis or group of disorders. Thus, the State–Trait Anxiety Inventory uses 20 questions to screen for anxiety disorders in general (Spielberger, 1983). The CAGE scale screens for alcohol disorders with four questions (Aertgeerts, Buntinx, & Kester, 2004). The revision of the Center for Epidemiologic Studies Depression Scale (CESD-R) has 20 questions that precisely target DSM-IV operational criteria for major depressive disorder (Eaton, Muntaner, Smith, & Tien, 2004). The CESD-R includes two questions for each of nine criteria and one additional question each for the criteria of dysphoria and problems with sleep. The CESD-R can be printed readily on the front and back of a single sheet of paper and completed in a few minutes, either in a face-to-face interview or over the telephone. An online version (see http://cesd-r.com) both generates ordinal categories of the probability that the individual meets criteria for major depressive disorder and includes recommendations based on the screen that can be e-mailed to the respondent or to a treating clinician. The Primary Health Questionnaire-9 is another scale designed specifically to screen for depression (Beck, Steer, Ball, & Ranieri, 1996; Kroenke, Spitzer, & Williams, 2001). The title of the scale suggests its efficiency; it includes but a single question for each of nine DSM symptom groups.

As with physical illnesses, mental disorders differ widely in the degree of impairment and disability they produce. Screening measures of impairment and disability have been developed to capture these differences with precision and specificity. The Sheehan Disability Scales (Sheehan, 2008; Sheehan, Harnett-Sheehan, & Raj, 1996) use a visual analog scale to assess impairment in work, family, and social life that may result from a specific disorder. The respondent is asked to:

Think about the month or longer when your...(specific disorder)...was most severe. Using the 0–10 on the scale where 0 means no interference and 10 means very severe interference, what number describes how much your (disorder) interfered with each of the following activities during that time.

- Your home management like cleaning, shopping, and taking care of the house/apartment?
- Your ability to work?
- Your ability to form and maintain close relationships with other people?
- Your social life?

A number of other measures of impairment and disability are in wide use. The US Department of Labor surveys include a single question on work disability: "During the last three months, were there any times when you were kept from your work, school or usual activities for at least one whole day because of an injury or because you weren't feeling well? How many days?" The Baltimore ECA site (Kouzis & Eaton, 1995) added the question "Were you kept from your usual activities because of an emotional problem or trouble with your nerves?" The results of each generate an integer-level response value, expressed as a number of days.

As with distress, disability and impairment are not inevitable consequences of mental disorders. Table 4-3 shows the distribution of responses on the Sheehan Disability Scales and days out of work for 622 individuals meeting the criteria for major depressive disorder in the NCS-R. (See also Table 1-2 which compares the SDS to the Global Burden of Disease DALYs measures.) While many individuals with depressive disorders are severely impaired, a substantial minority who meet criteria for depressive disorder have little or no resulting impairment. Whether people who meet criteria for a mental disorder such as depression but who are not impaired should be considered to be above or below the diagnostic threshold remains a matter of some controversy. (Kessler, Merikangas, et al., 2003). The debate pits those who wish to understand the etiology of a disorder, without regard to any associated impairment, against those

Table 4-3. Distribution of Severity in 622 Persons Meeting Criteria for Major Depressive Disorder, National Comorbidity Study—Replication

	NONE	MILD	MODERATE	SEVERE	VERY SEVERE
	PERCENTAGES				
Home	9	22	35	27	7
Work	20	26	26	18	10
Relationship	15	22	29	27	7
Social	12	17	28	31	12
Highest severity for any of above domains	3	10	28	40	19
	DAYS PER YEAR				
Annual days out of role	0	3	11	33	96

Source: Adapted from Kessler et al., 2003.

who want to focus resources on individuals in greatest need of treatment, as described in greater detail below.

ADMINISTRATION OF ASSESSMENTS TO LARGE POPULATIONS

Recruiting and Training Interviewers

The quality of information gleaned from population-level studies of mental disorders depends not only on the content of the questions asked but also on the person asking the questions and on how those questions are asked. This section describes general methods by which to administer surveys related to public mental health. A discussion of how to define a target population and select a sample, both relevant to this topic, is found in chapter 5.

Interviewers to conduct structured diagnostic interviews such as the DIS and CIDI can be recruited through many means: newspaper advertisements, bulletin boards, employment agencies, and survey research firms. The part-time, flexible nature of interviewing is attractive to some people; interviewing does not demand high educational attainment, though many who respond to advertisements will have taken college courses at one time or another. Without regard to education, interviewers must be able to read interview questions aloud with good diction and precisely as written and to remember details of the interview to guide the process. They should be both patient and persistent with respondents, without being overtly assertive. In the conduct of psychiatric interviews, they must be willing and able to talk about and to elicit responses on subjects many people consider private or sensitive.

Training of interviewers typically takes from a few days to a few weeks. The process often results in considerable attrition; many interviewer recruits prove unsuitable. They forget aspects of the training, cannot read questions in a conversational tone, are too instructive or assertive, cannot be trained to stick to the verbatim script, or are too embarrassed by the interview content. Training sessions typically begin with group instruction (lectures, videos, and demonstrations), followed by role-playing exercises in groups of two, and then supervised or videotaped individual interviews with test subjects.

Laptop computers that assist in the interview process markedly simplify interviewer training. Questions are presented on the computer screen and read by the interviewer; responses are entered directly into the laptop database instead of being marked on paper copy. Further, the computer program accepts only responses within the legitimate range of the question, providing the kind of editing that otherwise often occurs during data entry. The program includes an algorithm that leads the interviewer to the next appropriate question based on the pattern of previous responses, relieving the interviewer of making that determination. If the subject agrees, portions of the interview may be recorded directly by the computer, capturing a wider range of meaning than is possible with short or yes/no responses. The savings realized from the use of computer-assisted interviews typically are much greater than the cost of purchasing laptop computers for interviewers. Several commercial computer programs are available that help program questionnaires into the computers. Some of these programs use the features of the World Wide Web to enable data to be sent directly to a distant database without being stored on the laptop computer. (A comparison of 10 proprietary systems is available at: http://sprc.washington.edu/services/docs/ACASISoftwareAssessment.pdf.) In this case, all that is needed to conduct the interview is a subscription to the service and access to the Internet at the time of the interview. Laptop questionnaires can be particularly effective when the interview includes questions about potentially stigmatizing or sensitive topics, such as illegal behaviors, because the sensitive portion can be set up for self-administration by the respondent.

The skill of interviewing includes locating and scheduling an interview with a previously selected subject. When conducting a household survey, this process typically takes more time than the interview itself. Because a two-hour interview may require 5 to 10 separate attempts to locate the individual and to schedule the interview, many surveys expect a full-time interviewer to complete only one interview each day. Scheduling flexibility is important, since many interviews are conducted outside normal work hours.

Particularly in the early stages of fieldwork, interviewers should be closely supervised, during which time supervisors may discuss individual interviews in some detail with interviewers. Interviewers should feel free to ask questions of supervisors about judgments made during the interviews. In some cases, portions of an interview may be discussed after

each interview, depending on the response to a given question. For example, the ECA interviews required respondents to judge whether a given potentially psychiatric symptom was caused by a physical disorder or injury. Interviewers frequently questioned ambiguous responses, and in some cases the question was referred to the researchers, including the principal investigators, for input. Further, mistakes may be uncovered as data are edited and keyed for analysis, leading to interviewer retraining and in some situations to sending the interviewer back to the respondent for clarification of an important question.

It sometimes happens that a small minority of interviewers submit completed interview forms without actually having conducted the interviews—a practice called "curbstoning." To detect this practice, researchers often select a set percentage of interviews for validation by a telephone call or follow-up interview that asks a small proportion of the survey questions to ensure that the interview took place and was completed as expected. If the interview is assisted by computer, another form of interview validation can be provided by turning on the computer's recording capacity randomly, if the subject agrees. Curbstoning interviewers must be fired; their previously completed interviews must be conducted again.

Pay rates and structure can affect the quality of the data collected. Interviewers paid by the piece are apt to rush an interview, not giving respondents sufficient time to process the sometimes complex requests for information. Hence an hourly pay rate may be more appropriate. The process of locating and recruiting participants becomes more difficult as a survey progresses. Available and agreeable respondents are interviewed first, leaving a residue of designated subjects who are more difficult to locate, recruit, and schedule. Study directors may want to consider introducing a pay incentive at various stages of the survey to keep interviewers from becoming discouraged with the slower pace of obtaining interviews. Toward the end of the fieldwork, the accretion of subjects who are hard to recruit and interview leads many surveys to be conducted in a series of independent sample replicates released in stages, so that final completion rates can be estimated before the survey is finished. If a survey turns out to be more difficult than anticipated and funds run short, one or more replicates may be omitted in an effort to optimize the completion rate, even if the final sample size is smaller and has fewer replicates than anticipated.

Committees for the protection of human subjects (also called institutional review boards, or IRBs) are likely to require that field survey subjects agree in advance to participate and that they know, with some degree of precision, how long the interview will take, what it will contain, and whether any risks are involved. Psychiatric survey questions generally are considered sensitive; IRBs may be surprisingly cautious about the risks for subjects involved. IRBs generally require that an interview proceed only after a subject freely provides documented, written, informed consent. For example, it is not atypical for an IRB to consider whether the interview might prompt an emotional response or even an attempt at suicide by a sample subject. The potential of suicide risk among subjects in mental health surveys means that interviewers should be trained to recognize a serious suicide plan— one with an identified method and a precise time—and to respond to it. (For example, the interviewer might alert a spouse or relative, dial 911, or escort the respondent to an emergency room, much as would occur if the respondent had another type of health emergency, such as a sudden heart attack.) In general, however, respondents find interviews with emotional or psychiatric content interesting or even refreshing. Thus interviewers find it relatively simple to convince them that their answers are important and that no one else can answer for them. The number of mid-interview terminations by respondents during the 20,000-plus ECA interviews was trivially small; those terminations usually had to do with scheduling, such as the need to leave for work, the arrival at home of a family member during the interview, or the beginning of a TV show.

Hiring a Survey Contractor

Professional survey firms conduct many population-based, mental health–oriented surveys. These firms can convert an investigator's questionnaire into a field survey with great efficiency and often can design and execute a sampling strategy as well. The end product will be a clean data set ready for analysis. The economy of scale of employing a professional survey firm is such that the cost may be lower than if the survey were led by the research investigators themselves.

Engaging a survey firm requires a detailed description of the scope of work to be performed, including such details as questionnaire length, sensitivity of the questions, level of required training for interviewers, and the role of the researchers in that training. The scope of work should specify:

- the sample size and structure
- the number of callbacks to be undertaken in pursuit of any one designated respondent
- the interviewer pay rate (per hour, piece, or day)
- the percentage of interviews to be independently validated and the nature of such validation
- the supervisor-to-interviewer ratio
- the identification of who determines when sample replicates are released to the field
- the precise structure of the data file to be produced.

With these details in hand, a survey firm can estimate the cost of the survey and generate a predicted schedule for completion.

ASSESSMENT OF NEED IN INDIVIDUALS AND IN THE POPULATION

Population Need Assessed through Structured Diagnostic Surveys

The mental health estimates derived from these large-scale, population-based assessments can contribute to decisions about the need for treatment and the allocation of resources to meet those needs. Clinicians make decisions about recommended treatments for individual patients based, in part, on the individual's need for care. Mental health policy makers and service administrators often are challenged to decide how to most efficiently allocate limited resources. Their decisions should be based on the level of need of the populations being served. Unfortunately, need is difficult to conceptualize at both the individual and population levels. This final section focuses specifically on assessing need, building on previously discussed issues and concepts, such as diagnosis, distress, and impairment.

The concept of need is inherently ambiguous. As noted by J. K. Wing, Brewin, and Thornicroft (1992):

> Need can be defined either in terms of the type of impairment or other factor causing social disablement or of the model of treatment or other intervention required to meet it, for example hip replacement, insulin regime for diabetes, medication for auditory hallucinations. (p. 5)

In mental health, impairment and disability traditionally have been defined by psychiatric diagnosis itself. Some serious, disabling mental illnesses such as schizophrenia, bipolar disorder, and dementia most often are clearly associated with serious impairment. However, ambiguity remains when defining a need for care for individuals with other, less severe or disabling mental disorders, in part because of the kinds of measurement difficulties discussed in this chapter and in chapters 2 and 3. For example, Horwitz and Wakefield (2007) have argued that many cases of major depression are more likely normal reactions to stressful life conditions than biological disorders. Further, many well-defined mental disorders are self-limiting either in duration or extent of impairment, such as major depressive episodes that last only a few weeks or specific common phobias, some of which entail only trivial impairment. As noted earlier, absent a biological gold standard to distinguish bona fide cases of mental illness from normal variations in behavior, it is difficult to distinguish individuals in need of treatment from others whose symptoms are likely to resolve spontaneously or with general support from family and friends. Even with such a gold standard, however, resource allocation based on current conditions may be shortsighted. Kessler (2000) posits that defining need solely in the context of current illness and impairment essentially excludes preventive interventions from the range of needed services that should be funded by third-party payers.

The definition of need set forth by J. K. Wing and colleagues (1992) also requires a demonstration of benefit: responsiveness of the disorder to the application of the needed intervention. For many interventions, however, the benefits in any individual case may be uncertain. Thus, for example, a patient's psychotic symptoms may not respond to treatment with antipsychotic medications. This raises the question of whether the patient needed antipsychotic medication treatment in the first place (Priebe, Huxley, & Burns, 1999). This ambiguity about need is not unique to the mental health field; patients with common physical illnesses also have variable responses to treatments.

Distinguishing between need, on one hand, and demand for and use of services, on the other hand, is a common challenge when conceptualizing need for mental health care (Mechanic, 2003). Many individuals with mild or, on occasion, no psychopathology make use of mental health resources, including both psychotropic medications and psychotherapy. Some researchers and clinicians believe these interventions improve or enhance functioning among people otherwise physically and emotionally healthy (Elliott, 2003). Psychiatrist Peter Kramer (1993) famously has advocated the use of the antidepressant Prozac for conditions ranging from shyness to low self-esteem. Further, a growing movement advocates the use of cognition-enhancing medications, including stimulants, by healthy individuals to improve functioning at work and school (Greely et al., 2008). Long before these developments, psychoanalysts in the tradition of Freud and Jung advocated long-term talking therapy as a means of self-discovery and improved well-being. How are we, as a society, to decide if these demands represent legitimate needs? Who is to make this decision?

The relationship between need and demand is unsettling from yet another perspective. In the face of a significant health problem, such as a severe and persistent mental illness, a multiplicity of demands arise from different quarters: the patient, family, and health care providers. They must be juggled or balanced in some way. Norman Sartorius (2000) has suggested that needs for health care be defined as "the agglomerate of those demands of people having a health problem, their families and their communities" (p. 7). Unfortunately, to date, no one has shed light on how best to achieve a compromise among those competing demands.

The amount, duration, and scope of needed care are almost as important as the fact of the need itself. Today's mental health care system is complex; treatment options range from pharmacologic treatments of various kinds to a broad array of psychosocial treatments. Where care is provided even the medium through which it is provided can vary, from conventional psychiatric hospital and outpatient general medical settings to self-help groups and computer-administered therapies. To state solely that an individual needs mental health care provides little information about the content, intensity, duration, or setting of that needed treatment.

Based on these difficulties in conceptualizing the need for mental health care, some have proposed forgoing the term, at least as applied to population needs, and have suggested instead that the focus be on identifying problems and specifying intervention goals (Priebe et al., 1999). Nevertheless, the concept of need and its use in the literature remain popular in public health and health policy discussions. The term does continue to provide both a convenient summary measure of disability resulting from various disorders for which mental health care is indicated, in one form or another, and a terminology consistent with that employed elsewhere in health care where the need for treatment is arguably more clearly defined and more readily measured.

At the population level, decisions about the allocation of scarce resources often are based on factors other than need. From a public health perspective, the magnitude of the need for mental health care in a community often is inferred from the burden of disease in that community, measured by the prevalence of cases with serious mental disorders requiring some form of intervention. When defined objectively, this definition of mental health care need permits comparison across populations. Matched with corresponding estimates of mental health service utilization, measurements of need should allow policy makers to estimate the prevalence of met and unmet need for mental health care in different settings (Demyttenaere et al., 2004).

Estimates of population need for specific subgroups or small geographical regions are not always readily available. Because states and local authorities often use estimates of need to request or justify funding for services, however, researchers often are called upon to provide workable estimates of the need for care of such populations or regions. Such estimates usually are derived from data from censuses or surveys in which individuals in the general population are approached and assessed. Chapter 5 describes these indirect or synthetic estimates in more detail.

A fundamental innovation of the ECA was the systematic collection of survey data on the use of services to meet a particular mental health need. This aspect connects the tradition of the 19th and early 20th century of measuring need by counting the number of persons in treatment with the more recent tradition of estimating need based on survey data on prevalence. The ECA sought to determine why people used or did not use treatment services, what led to unmet need for care, and why some social groups were underserved (Eaton et al., 1981). To assess unmet need in specific population groups, the ECA strategy was to estimate the proportion seeking treatment among all individuals with mental disorders. Thus ECA researchers implicitly accepted a DIS-generated diagnosis as an indicator of need for treatment. Regions in which many people met the criteria for diagnosis but were not in treatment most likely lacked adequate mental health resources. This approach continues today as a method to identify unmet need for treatment in epidemiologic studies (Kessler et al., 1994).

Publication of prevalence rates of mental disorders from the ECA, NCS, and other population surveys raised questions about the ability of the health care system to meet the need for mental health care. Investigators involved in these studies were well aware of these concerns. Regier and colleagues (1998) wrote, "In the current U.S. climate of determining the medical necessity for care in managed health care plans, it is doubtful that 28% or 29% of the population would be judged to need mental health treatment in a year" (p. 113). These authors posited that in the same way that variations in blood pressure, pulse rate, or body temperature can affect diagnosis of physical disease, some cases found to meet diagnostic criteria for specific mental disorders during structured interviews might reflect milder disease states or "transient homeostatic responses to internal or external stimuli that do not represent true psychopathologic disorders" rather than serious mental disturbances (Regier et al., 1998, p. 114). Spitzer (1998) drew an analogy between mental and skin disorders: "Dermatology has skin cancer and warts. So, too, some mental disorders are devastating in their associated impairment (e.g., schizophrenia), whereas others (e.g., some animal phobias) are distressing but rarely cause serious impairment" (p. 12).

Often ignored in these discussions is the equally disturbing low sensitivity found in many lay-administered structured interviews, suggestive of high rates of false negatives (i.e., individuals with disorders not detected as cases by the structured interview) (Figure 4-6). Thus structured interviews based on subject self-reports can both overestimate and underestimate the proportion of cases in which a psychiatrist would diagnose a mental disorder.

In part as a result of these concerns, a consensus appears to be forming that diagnoses drawn from population surveys alone cannot stand as surrogate measures for need for treatment; additional criteria related to severity and impairment should be used to more accurately define treatment need (Mechanic, 2003; Regier et al., 1998). Indeed, researchers have sought to identify subgroups of individuals with more severe or persistent mental disorders within general epidemiologic samples such as the NCS and NCS-R (Kessler et al., 2005; Wang, Demler, & Kessler, 2002). This return to the use of measures of distress and impairment is reminiscent of pre-DSM-III population surveys that relied solely on those very measures to identify cases of mental illness (Leighton et al., 1963; Srole et al., 1962). Establishing standardized, valid measures of severity and functional impairment and ascertaining the levels at which those measures give rise to a need for treatment remain critical tasks for psychiatric epidemiology in the coming years.

Direct Clinician Assessment of Need

Most of the methods of assessing need for treatment discussed earlier use the identification of psychopathology as a proxy for need. An alternative approach might base determinations of need for treatment on direct clinical assessment. In the words of one commentator (Mechanic, 2003), "the most appropriate decisionmakers are clinicians with psychiatric expertise, guided by current knowledge of the evidence and best practice and appreciation of the costs and benefits of alternative treatment approaches" (pp. 18–19).

A small body of research has used these direct assessments to estimate community need for mental health care (Bebbington, Brewin, Marsden, & Lesage, 1996; Bebbington, Marsden, & Brewin, 1997; Messias, Eaton, Nestadt, Bienvenu, & Samuels, 2007). In the study reported by Messias and colleagues (2007), psychiatrists estimated need for mental health care for a subgroup of participants in the Baltimore ECA follow-up study. The psychiatrists rated both need for various forms of treatment and receipt of those treatments among individuals meeting diagnostic criteria for specific disorders. The authors estimated that almost 29% (nearly one-third) of the general population were in need of some form of treatment for a mental disorder. As those authors note, despite the different assessment method, this estimate of need does not differ markedly from the overall prevalence of mental disorders. They also found that over two-thirds of mental health treatment needs of participants identified by psychiatrists remained unmet (see figure 4-7).

Direct assessment by mental health professionals of mental health care needs has

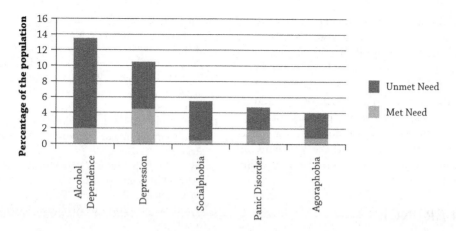

Figure 4-7   **Clinician-assessed need for and Utilization of Treatment, Baltimore ECA Follow-up Study.**

several advantages over methods that rely on proxy measures of need, such as diagnosis or impairment in role functioning based on structured self-report interviews. As noted earlier, because diagnosing and treating mental disorders is a routine part of their daily work, clinicians are positioned ideally to make decisions regarding mental health care needs. Also, needs estimates made by direct clinical assessments have more widespread credibility among policy makers and other stakeholders.

As with other methods discussed earlier, however, direct clinical assessment has limitations. Studies using clinician assessments are far more expensive than are studies relying on lay interviewers. In addition, clinicians' decisions might not be as valid for subjects residing in the community and not under care as the decisions they make in their conduct of clinical work, since the characteristics of individuals with psychiatric problems in community settings might not be routinely captured by available clinical assessment tools. Moreover, clinical decision making is a complex phenomenon, influenced by a clinician's training, experience, and subjective norms. Decisions made by individual clinicians may vary based on their theoretical orientations as well as where they were trained and have worked.

Despite these limitations, direct assessment of treatment needs by clinicians offers a new, potentially important approach to estimating the needs for mental health care in general population settings. Use of this approach

in future epidemiologic surveys could add to a small but growing literature bearing on both its reliability and validity. In the meantime, assessments of need for treatment will continue to be based on the prevalence of disorders disclosed through structured interviews and measures of distress and impairment from epidemiologic surveys.

CONCLUSION

Over the years, psychiatric epidemiology has made much progress, moving through three distinct periods in its history. Yet despite the progress, population-based assessment of mental disorders remains an ongoing challenge. With the advent of the third generation of psychiatric epidemiology—structured diagnostic interviews—the field has gained the capacity to make increasingly credible estimates of prevalence of a number of specific common disorders such as the mood and anxiety disorders and substance disorders. Consistent variation in prevalence rates across important social categories and population groups lend further credibility to the estimates (see chapter 7). The variation between groups permit prediction of prevalence estimates by geographic area using so-called indirect estimation techniques (see chapter 5). The structured diagnostic techniques described in this chapter can be repeated on individuals at different times, allowing estimation of the incidence of disorders and the study of the life course of the force of morbidity, as presented in chapter 6. Incidence data facilitate study of risk factors in a prospective fashion. However, disparities in prevalence estimates across studies and cultural settings are sufficiently large to raise questions about the validity of today's assessment techniques. The field has yet to resolve the problem of how best to conceptualize, let alone estimate, need for treatment. Many of these problems are inherent in the nature of mental disorders and mental health care.

REFERENCES

Aertgeerts, B., Buntinx, F., & Kester, A. (2004). The value of the CAGE in screening for alcohol abuse and alcohol dependence in general clinical populations: A diagnostic meta-analysis. *Journal of Clinical Epidemiology, 57*(1), 30–39.

Altman, D. G. (1991). *Practical statistics for medical research*. London, UK: Chapman & Hall.

American Psychiatric Association. (1980). *Diagnostic and statistical manual of mental disorders* (3rd ed.). Washington, DC: Author.

American Psychiatric Association. (1987). *Diagnostic and statistical manual of mental disorders* (3rd ed., rev.). Washington, DC: Author.

American Psychiatric Association. (1994). *Diagnostic and statistical manual of mental disorders* (4th ed.). Washington, DC: Author.

Anthony, J. C., Folstein, M. F., Romanoski, A.,...Gruenberg, E. M., (1985). Comparison of the lay Diagnostic Interview Schedule and a standardized psychiatric diagnosis: Experience in Eastern Baltimore. *Archives of General Psychiatry, 42*, 667–675.

Baldwin, J., & Evans, J. H. (1971). The psychiatric case register. *International Psychiatry Clinics, 8*(3), 17–38.

Bebbington, P., Brewin, C. R., Marsden, L., & Lesage, A. (1996). Measuring the need for psychiatric treatment in the general population: The community version of the MRC Needs for Care Assessment. *Psychological Medicine, 26*(2), 229–236.

Bebbington, P. E., Marsden, L., & Brewin, C. R. (1997). The need for psychiatric treatment in the general population: The Camberwell Needs for Care survey. *Psychological Medicine, 27*(4), 821–834.

Beck, A. T., Steer, R. A., Ball, R., & Ranieri, W. (1996). Comparison of Beck Depression Inventories-IA and -II in psychiatric outpatients. *Journal of Personality Assessment, 67*(3), 588–597.

Bohrnstedt, G. (2010). Measurement models for survey research. In P. V. Marsden & J. D. Wright (Eds.), *Handbook of survey research* (2nd ed., pp. 347–404). Bingley, UK: Emerald Group.

Brill, N. Q. & Beebe, G. W. (1956). *A follow-up study of war neuroses*. Washington, DC: Government Printing Office.

Burvill, P. W. (1995). Recent progress in the epidemiology of major depression. *Epidemiologic Reviews, 17*(1), 21–31.

Carey, G. (2005, June 7). Most will be mentally ill at some point, study says. *The New York Times*. Retrieved from http://www.nytimes.com/2005/06/07/health/07mental.html?_r=1

Carey, G. (2008, December 18). Psychiatrists revise the book of human troubles. *The New York Times*. Retrieved from http://www.nytimes.com/2008/12/18/health/18psych.html

Centers for Disease Control and Prevention. (2012). National Health Interview Survey, retrieved from http://www.cdc.gov/nchs/nhis.htm

Cohen, S. T., Kamarck, R., & Mermelstein, R. (1983). A global measure of perceived stress. *Journal of Health and Social Behavior, 24*(4), 385–396.

Cohen, S., Kessler, R. C., & Underwood Gordon, L. (1995). *Measuring stress: A guide for health and social scientists*. New York, NY: Oxford University Press.

Commission on Lunacy, 1. (1971). *Report on insanity and idiocy in Massachusetts*. Boston, MA: Harvard University Press. (Original work published 1855)

Cronbach, L. J., & Meehl, P. E. (1955). Construct validity in psychological tests. *Psychological Bulletin, 52*(4), 281–302.

Demyttenaere, K., Bruffaerts, R., Posada-Villa, J., Gasquet, I., Kovess, V., Lepine, J. P.,...Chatterji, S. (2004). Prevalence, severity, and unmet need for treatment of mental disorders in the World Health Organization World Mental Health Surveys. *Journal of the American Medical Association, 291*(21), 2581–2590.

de Salvia, D., Barbato, A., Salvo, P., & Zadro, F. (1993). Prevalence and incidence of schizophrenic disorders in Portogruaro: An Italian case register study. *Journal of Nervous and Mental Disease, 181*(5), 275–282.

DeVellis, R. F. (1991). *Scale development: Theory and applications*. Newbury Park, CA: Safe Publications.

Dohrenwend, B. P. (1980). *Mental illness in the United States: Epidemiological estimates*. New York, NY: Praeger.

Dohrenwend, B. P., & Dohrenwend, B. S. (1982). Perspectives on the past and future of psychiatric epidemiology: The 1981 Rema Lapouse Lecture. *American Journal of Public Health, 72*(11), 1271–1279.

Eaton, W. W. (2001). *The sociology of mental disorders* (3rd ed.). Westport, CT: Praeger.

Eaton, W. W., Hall, A. L., Macdonald, R., & McKibben, J. (2007). Case identification in psychiatric epidemiology: A review. *International Review of Psychiatry, 19*(5), 497–507.

Eaton, W. W., Muntaner, C., Smith, C. B., & Tien, A. Y. (2004). Revision of the Center for Epidemiologic Studies Depression (CESD) Scale. In M. Maruish (Ed.), *The use of psychological testing for treatment planning and outcomes assessment* (pp. 363–377). Mahwah, NJ: Lawrence Erlbaum.

Eaton, W. W., Neufeld, K., Chen L., & Cai, G. (2000). A comparison of self-report and clinical diagnostic interviews for depression: DIS and SCAN in the Baltimore ECA Followup. *Archives of General Psychiatry, 57*(3), 217–222.

Eaton, W. W., Regier, D. A., Locke, B. Z., & Taube, C. A. (1981). The Epidemiologic Catchment Area program of the National Institute of Mental Health. *Public Health Reports, 96*(4), 319–325.

Eaton, W. W., Romanoski, A., Anthony, J. C., & Nestadt, G. (1991). Screening for psychosis in the general population with a self-report interview. *Journal of Nervous and Mental Disease, 179*(11), 689–693.

Elliott, C. (2003). *Better than well: American medicine meets the American dream.* New York, NY: Norton.

Faris, R. E., & Dunham, W. (1939). *Mental disorders in urban areas.* Chicago, IL: University of Chicago Press.

Fleiss, J. L., Gurland, B. J., & Cooper, J. E. (1971). Some contributions to the measurement of psychopathology. *British Journal of Psychiatry, 119*(553), 647–656.

Furukawa, T. A., Kessler, R. C., Slade, T., & Andrews, G. (2003). The performance of the K6 and K10 screening scales for psychological distress in the Australian National Survey of Mental Health and Well-Being. *Psychological Medicine, 33*(2), 357–362.

Glassman, A. (2008). Depression and cardiovascular disease. *Pharmacopsychiatry, 41*(6), 221–225.

Goldberg, D. (1972). *The detection of psychiatric illness by questionnaire.* London, UK: Oxford University Press.

Goldberg, D. (1978). *Manual of the General Health Questionnaire.* Windsor, UK: National Federation for Educational Research.

Goldberg, D. P., & Hillier, V. F. (1979). A scaled version of the General Health Questionnaire. *Psychological Medicine, 9*(1), 139–145.

Goodman, A. B., Rahav, M., Popper, M., Ginath, Y., & Pearl, E. (1984). The reliability of psychiatric diagnosis in Israel's psychiatric case register. *Acta Psychiatrica Scandinavica, 69*(5), 391–397.

Gordis, L. (2004). *Epidemiology* (3rd ed.). Philadelphia, PA: Elsevier.

Grant, B., Harford, T., Dawson, D., Chou, P., Dufour, M., & Pickering, R. (1994) Prevalence of DSM-IV alcohol abuse and dependence: United States, 1992. *Alcohol Health and Research World, 18,* 243–248.

Greely, H., Sahakian, B., Harris, J., Kessler, R. C., Gazzaniga, M., Campbell, P., & Farah, M. J. (2008). Towards responsible use of cognitive-enhancing drugs by the healthy. *Nature, 456*(7223), 702–705.

Hall, D., Robertson, N. C., Dorricott, N., Olley, P. C., & Millar, W. M. (1973). The north-east Scottish psychiatric case register: The second phase. *Journal of Chronic Diseases, 26*(6), 375–382.

Helzer, J., Clayton, P., Pambakian, L., Reich, T., Woodruff, R., & Reveley, M. (1977). Reliability of psychiatric diagnosis: II. The test/retest reliability of diagnostic classification. *Archives of General Psychiatry, 34*(2), 136–141.

Henderson, S. (2000). The central issues. In G. Andrews & S. Henderson (Eds.), *Unmet need in psychiatry* (pp. 422–428). Cambridge, MA: Cambridge University Press.

Hollingshead, A. B., & Redlich, F. C. (1958). *Social class and mental illness.* New York, NY: John Wiley & Sons.

Horwitz, A. V., & Wakefield, J. C. (2007). *The loss of sadness: How psychiatry transformed normal sorrow into depressive disorder.* New York, NY: Oxford University Press.

Humphreys, N. A. (1890). Statistics of insanity in England with special reference to its increasing prevalence. *Journal of the Royal Statistical Society, 53,* 201–252.

Jarvis, E. (1866). Influence of distance from and nearness to an insane hospital on its use by the people. *American Journal of Psychiatry, 22,* 361–406.

Kessler, R. (1994). The National Comorbidity Survey of the United States. *International Review of Psychiatry, 6,* 365–376.

Kessler, R. C. (2000). Some considerations in making resource allocation decisions for the treatment of psychiatric disorders. In G. Andrews & S. Henderson (Eds.), *Unmet need in psychiatry* (pp. 59–84). Cambridge, MA: Cambridge University Press.

Kessler, R. C., Andrews, G., Colpe, L. J., Hiripi, E., Mroczek, D. K., Normand, S. L., ... Zaslavsky,

A. M. (2002). Short screening scales to monitor population prevalences and trends in nonspecific psychological distress. *Psychological Medicine, 32*(6), 959–976.

Kessler, R. C., Barker, P. R., Colpe, L. J., Epstein, J. F., Gfroerer, J. C., Hiripi, E.,...Zaslavsky, A. M. (2003). Screening for serious mental illness in the general population. *Archives of General Psychiatry, 60*(2), 184–189.

Kessler, R. C., Demler, O., Frank, R. G., Olfson, M., Pincus, H. A., Walters, E. E.,...Zaslavsky, A. M. (2005). Prevalence and treatment of mental disorders, 1990 to 2003. *New England Journal of Medicine, 352*(24), 2515–2523.

Kessler, R. C., McGonagle, K. A., Zhao, S., Nelson, C. B., Hughes, M., Eshleman, S.,...Kendler, K. S. (1994). Lifetime and 12-month prevalence of DSM-III-R psychiatric disorders in the United States. Results from the National Comorbidity Survey. *Archives of General Psychiatry, 51*(1), 8–19.

Kessler, R. C., & Merikangas, K. R. (2004). The National Comorbidity Survey Replication (NCS-R): Background and aims. *International Journal of Methods in Psychiatric Research, 13*(2), 60–68.

Kessler, R., Merikangas, K., Berglund, P., Eaton, W., Koretz, D., & Walters, E. (2003). Mild disorder should not be eliminated from the DSM-V. *Archives of General Psychiatry, 60*(11), 1117–1122.

Kessler, R. C., & Ustun, T. B. (2004). The World Mental Health (WMH) Survey Initiative version of the World Health Organization (WHO) Composite International Diagnostic Interview (CIDI). *International Journal of Methods in Psychiatric Research, 13*(2), 93–121.

Kirk, S. A., & Kutchins, H. (1992). *The selling of DSM.* New York, NY: Aldine DeGruyter.

Klerman, G. L. (1986). The National Institute of Mental Health–Epidemiologic Catchment Area (NIMH-ECA) program. Background, preliminary findings and implications. *Social Psychiatry, 21*(4), 159–166.

Klerman, G. L. (1990). Paradigm shifts in USA psychiatric epidemiology since World War II. *Social Psychiatry and Psychiatric Epidemiology, 25*(1), 27–32.

Kouzis, A. C., & Eaton, W. W. (1995). Emotional disability days: Prevalence and predictors. *American Journal of Public Health, 84*(8), 1304–1307.

Kramer, M. (1969). *Applications of mental health statistics: Uses in mental health programmes of statistics derived from psychiatric services and selected vital and morbidity records.* Geneva, Switzerland: World Health Organization.

Kramer, P. (1993). *Listening to Prozac.* New York, NY: Viking.

Kroenke, K., Spitzer, R. L., & Williams, J. B. W. (2001). The PHQ-9: Validity of a brief depression severity measure. *Journal of General Internal Medicine, 16*(9), 606–613.

Landis, J. R., & Koch, G. G. (1991). An application of hierarchical kappa-type statistics in the assessment of majority agreement among multiple observers. *Biometrics, 33*(2), 363–374.

Leighton, D. C., Harding, J. S., Macklin, D. B., Macmillan, A. M., & Leighton, A. H. (1963). *The character of danger: Psychiatric symptoms in selected communities.* New York, NY: Basic Books.

Link, B., & Dohrenwend, B. P. (1980). Formulation of hypotheses about the true prevalence of demoralization in the United States. In B. S. Dohrenwend, M. S. Gould, B. Link, R. Neugebauer, & R. Wunsch-Hitzig (Eds.), *Mental illness in the United States: Epidemiological estimates* (pp. 114–132). New York, NY: Praeger.

Malzburg, B. (1952a). Rates of discharge and rates of mortality among first admissions to the New York civil state hospitals. *Mental Hygiene, 36*(1), 104–120.

Malzburg, B. (1952b). Rates of discharge and rates of mortality among first admissions to the New York civil state hospitals. II. *Mental Hygiene, 36*(4), 618–638.

Malzburg, B. (1953). Rates of discharge and rates of mortality among first admissions to the New York civil state hospitals. III. *Mental Hygiene, 37*(4), 619–654.

Mechanic, D. (2003). Is the prevalence of mental disorders a good measure of the need for services? *Health Affairs, 22*(5), 8–20.

Messias, E., Eaton, W., Nestadt, G., Bienvenu, O. J., & Samuels, J. (2007). Psychiatrists' ascertained treatment needs for mental disorders in a population-based sample. *Psychiatric Services, 58*(3), 373–377.

Messick, S. (1995). Validity of psychological assessment: Validation of inferences from persons' responses and performances as scientific inquiry into score meaning. *American Psychologist, 50*(9), 741–749.

Morris, J. N. (1975). *Uses of epidemiology* (3rd ed.). Edinburgh, UK: Churchill Livingstone.

Munk-Jorgensen, P., Kastrup, M., & Mortensen, P. B. (1993). The Danish psychiatric register as a tool in epidemiology. *Acta Psychiatrica Scandinavica, 370*(Suppl.), 27–32.

O'Hare, A. (1987). *Three county and St. Loman's psychiatric case registers.* Dublin, UK: Cahill.

Pedersen, C. B., Gotzsche, H., Moller, J. O., & Mortensen, P. B. (2006). The Danish civil registration system: A cohort of eight million persons. *Danish Medical Bulletin, 53*(4), 441–449.

Phillips, M. R., Zhang, J., Shi, Q., Song, Z., Ding, Z., Pang, S.,...Wang, Z. (2009). Prevalence, treatment, and associated disability of mental disorders in four provinces in China during 2001–05: An epidemiological survey. *Lancet, 373*(9680), 2041–2053.

Praag, H. M. (1993). *"Make-believes" in psychiatry, or, the perils of progress.* New York, NY: Brunner/ Mazel.

Priebe, S., Huxley, P., & Burns, T. (1999). Who needs needs? *European Psychiatry, 14*(4), 186–188.

Rahav, M. (1981). The psychiatric case register of Israel: Initial results. *Israel Journal of Psychiatry and Related Sciences, 18*(4), 251–267.

Regier, D. A., Kaelber, C. T., Rae, D. S., Farmer, M. E., Knauper, B., Kessler, R. C., & Norquist, G. S. (1998). Limitations of diagnostic criteria and assessment instruments for mental disorders: Implications for research and policy. *Archives of General Psychiatry, 55*(2),109–115.

Regier, D. A., Myers, J. K., Kramer, M., Robins, L. N., Blazer, D. G., Hough, R. L.,...Locke, B. Z. (1984). The NIMH Epidemiologic Catchment Area (ECA) program: Historical context, major objectives, and study population characteristics. *Archives of General Psychiatry, 41*(10), 934–941.

Robins, E., & Guze, S. B. (1970). Establishment of diagnostic validity in psychiatric illness: Its application to schizophrenia. *American Journal of Psychiatry, 127*(7), 983–987.

Robins, L. N., Helzer, J. E., Croughan, J., & Ratcliff, K. (1981) National Institute of Mental Health Diagnostic Interview Schedule: Its history, characteristics, and validity, *Archives of General Psychiatry, 38*, 381–389.

Robins, L., Helzer, J., Cottler, L., & Goldring, E. (1989). *NIMH Diagnostic Interview Schedule Version III Revised,* Department of Psychiatry, Washington University-St. Louis.

Robins, L., Wing, J. K., Wittchen, H. U., Helzer, J. E., Babor, T. F., Burke, J.,...Towle, L. H. (1988). The Composite International Diagnostic Interview: An epidemiologic instrument suitable for use in conjunction with different diagnostic systems and in different cultures. *Archives of General Psychiatry, 45*(12), 1069–1077.

Rogan, W. J., & Gladen, B. (1978). Estimating prevalence from the results of a screening test. *American Journal of Epidemiology, 107*(1), 71–76.

Sartorius, N. (2000). Assessing needs for psychiatric services. In G. Andrews & S. Henderson (Eds.), *Unmet need in psychiatry* (pp. 3–7). Cambridge, UK: Cambridge University Press.

Selten, J. P., & Sijben, N. (1994). First admission rates for schizophrenia in immigrants to the Netherlands: The Dutch national register. *Social Psychiatry and Psychiatric Epidemiology, 29*(2), 71–77.

Sheehan, D. V. (2008). Sheehan Disability Scale. In A. J. Rush, M. B. First, & D. Blacker (Eds.), *Handbook of psychiatric measures* (2nd ed., pp. 100–102). Washington, DC: American Psychiatric Press.

Sheehan, D. V., Harnett-Sheehan, K., & Raj, B. A. (1996). The measurement of disability. *International Clinical Psychopharmacology, 11*(Suppl. 3), 89–95.

Shorter, E. (1997). *A history of psychiatry: From the era of the asylum to the age of Prozac.* New York, NY: John Wiley & Sons.

Shrout, P. E., & Fleiss, J. L. (1979). Intraclass correlations: Uses in assessing rater reliability. *Psychological Bulletin, 86*(2), 420–428.

Spielberger, C. D. (1983). *Manual for the State–Trait Anxiety Inventory (STAI: Form Y).* Palo Alto, CA: Consulting Psychologists Press.

Spitzer, R. L. (1983). Psychiatric diagnosis: Are clinicians still necessary? *Comprehensive Psychiatry, 24*(5), 399–411.

Spitzer, R. L. (1998). Diagnosis and need for treatment are not the same. *Archives of General Psychiatry, 55*(2), 120.

Spitzer, R. L., Endicott, J., & Robins, E. (1978). Research diagnostic criteria: Rationale and reliability. *Archives of General Psychiatry, 35*(6), 773–782.

Spitzer, R. L., & Fleiss, J. L. (1974). A reanalysis of the reliability of psychiatric diagnosis. *British Journal of Psychiatry, 125*, 341–347.

Spitzer, R. L., Forman, J. B. W., & Nee, J. (1979). DSM-III field trials I: Initial inter-rater diagnostic reliability. *American Journal of Psychiatry, 136*(6), 815–817.

Spitzer, R. L., Williams, J. B., Gibbon, M., & First, M. B. (1992). The Structured Clinical Interview for DSM-III-R (SCID). I: History, rationale and description. *Archives of General Psychiatry, 49*(8), 624–629.

Srole, L., Langner, T. S., Michael, S. T., Kirkpatrick, P., & Rennie, T. A. C. (1962). *Mental health in the metropolis: The Midtown Manhattan study.* New York, NY: McGraw Hill.

Substance Abuse and Mental Health Services Administration. (2010). *Results from the 2009 National Survey on Drug Use and Health: Volume I. Summary of national findings.* Rockville, MD: Substance Abuse and Mental Health Services

Administration, US Department of Health and Human Services.

ten Horn, C. H., Geil, R., Gulbinat, W. H., & Henderson, J. H. (1986). *Psychiatric case registers in public health: A worldwide inventory, 1960–1985.* Amsterdam, Netherlands: Elsevier Science.

Thornicroft, G., Johnson, S., Leese, M., & Slade, M. (2000). The unmet needs of people suffering from schizophrenia. In G. Andrews & S. Henderson (Eds.), *Unmet need in psychiatry* (pp. 197–217). Cambridge, UK: Cambridge University Press.

Torrey, E. F., & Miller, J. (2001). *The invisible plague: The rise of mental illness from 1750 to the present.* New Brunswick, NJ: Rutgers University Press.

Tsuang, M. T., & Tohen, M. (2002). *Textbook in psychiatric epidemiology.* Hoboken, NJ: John Wiley & Sons.

Tuke, D. H. (1976). *A dictionary of psychological medicine* (Vol. II). New York, NY: Arno Press. (Originally published 1892)

Wang, P. S., Demler, O., & Kessler, R. C. (2002). Adequacy of treatment for serious mental illness in the United States. *American Journal of Public Health, 92*(1), 92–98.

Williams, J. B. W., Gibbon, M., First, M. B., Spitzer, R. L., Davies, M., Borus, J.,…Wittchen, H. U. (1992). The Structured Clinical Interview for DSM-III-R (SCID) II: Multisite test–retest reliability. *Archives of General Psychiatry, 49*(8), 630–636.

Wing, J. K. (1989). *Health services planning and research: Contributions from psychiatric case registers.* London, UK: Gaskell.

Wing, J. K., Babor, T., Brugha, T., Burke, J., Cooper J. E., Giel, R.,…Sartorius, N. (1990). SCAN: Schedules for Clinical Assessment in Neuropsychiatry. *Archives of General Psychiatry, 47*(6), 589–593.

Wing, J. K., Brewin, C. R., & Thornicroft, G. (1992). Defining mental health needs. In G. Thornicroft, C. R. Brewin, & J. K. Wing (Eds.), *Measuring mental health needs* (pp. 1–17). London, UK: Royal College of Psychiatrists.

Wing, J., & Fryers, T. (1976). *Statistics from the Camberwell and Salford psychiatric registers, 1964–1974.* London, UK: MRC Psychiatry Unit, Institute of Psychiatry.

Wing, L., Wing, J. K., Hailey, A., Bahn, A. K., Smith, H. E., & Baldwin, J. A. (1967). The use of psychiatric services in three urban areas: An international case register study. *Social Psychiatry, 2,* 158–167.

World Health Organization (1992). *International statistical classification of diseases and related health problems* (10th rev.). Geneva, Switzerland: World Health Organization.

World Health Organization (1993). *ICD-10 classification of mental and behavioral disorders: Diagnostic criteria for research.* Geneva, Switzerland: World Health Organization.

5

An Introduction to Quantitative Methods Especially Relevant for Public Mental Health

ELIZABETH A. STUART

JEANNIE-MARIE S. LEOUTSAKOS

ALDEN L. GROSS

S. JANET KURAMOTO

WILLIAM W. EATON

Key Points

- Study designs include randomized experiments and nonexperimental studies, which include cross-sectional studies, cohort studies, and case–control studies
- Randomized experiments offer the best way to learn about causal effects of treatments, risk factors, or interventions
- Nonexperimental methods such as instrumental variables and propensity scores can also give insight into effects of treatments, risk factors, or interventions
- Methods for generalizing results from a sample to a carefully defined target population are available for both nonexperimental and experimental contexts
- Multilevel models are useful for investigating factors that operate at multiple levels, such as individuals nested within schools, which are in turn nested within communities
- Latent constructs that cannot be directly observed, such as depression, intelligence, or personality, can be modeled using latent variable methods
- Indirect estimation approaches can help in making inferences about relatively small geographic areas
- A variety of data sources for public mental health research are publically available

INTRODUCTION

What study designs and methods do researchers use to answer questions such as "What is the prevalence of depression in the population?" or "What interventions can help slow cognitive decline?" This chapter provides a brief introduction to some of the epidemiologic and statistical methods for and challenges to gathering and analyzing the data that underlie the research presented in this volume and in the field of public mental health as a whole. Not intended as a general introduction to epidemiologic and statistical methods, the chapter focuses more specifically on some of the data and methodological complexities particularly common in public mental health research. Readers interested in obtaining a more general overview of statistical methods should refer to books such as Rosner (2006) or van Belle, Fisher, Heagerty, and Lumley (2004). Readers interested in a more thorough treatment of some of the issues raised here should refer to Tsuang and Tohen (2002), particularly chapters 1, 4, and 5.

We explore three fundamental types of questions relevant to public mental health:

- estimating rates of disorders in a population across people, place, and time
- examining risk and protective factors associated with particular disorders
- exploring interventions to prevent disorders or to treat them once they emerge.

The ability to measure disorders and survey the population is necessary to address the first type of question. Both the first and second types of question fit within the common descriptive and analytic forms of epidemiology (e.g., Lilienfeld & Stolley, 1994; Mausner & Kramer, 1985). The second and third types of question also involve investigation of the impact of behaviors or interventions on individuals or populations over time. Thus, for example, explorations may seek to discern childhood experiences that act as risk factors for later problems or to understand the relative effectiveness of school-based interventions to prevent problem behavior.

While other chapters in this volume (including chapters 14 and 15) describe important interventions in public mental health, and chapter 4 describes field methods and ways of collecting vast amounts of data on populations, the current chapter addresses some of the most salient statistical issues encountered in analyzing data amassed when studying such interventions and in collecting such data.

The Ideal

Ideally, answers to these kinds of epidemiologic inquiries are gleaned from extensive, detailed information on each person in a large sample of individuals representative of the population of interest. In estimating prevalence, the population of interest most often is the general population itself. Thus the national prevalence of major depressive disorder is best estimated from a nationally representative sample of individuals to whom a clinical diagnostic interview is administered. In contrast, in exploring the impact of an intervention, the population of interest consists of individuals who have received (or could receive) the intervention. Ideally, in this context, individuals are assigned randomly to treatment and control groups and assessed both before and after the intervention. In this way, outcome differences between the two groups can be attributed specifically to the intervention rather than to any preexisting differences between individuals in the two groups. In some cases, longitudinal data on individuals are gathered by following them over time, either to examine development of behaviors, attitudes, or mental disorders or to identify any long-term intervention effects.

The Reality

Unfortunately, the ideal is often unattainable in reality. Individuals in a study rarely are representative of the target population. It often is hard to measure the disorders and correlates of interest, particularly when conducting a short survey. Researchers do not always get all of the information desired, whether because it is not available, because it is too expensive to obtain, or because some respondents simply do not provide it. Longitudinal data on individuals that span more than 5 to 10 years are rarely available, and even when these data are available, some study subjects drop out before the study period ends. Moreover, when examining the effects of public mental health interventions, researchers often cannot randomly assign individuals to treatment and control groups. Instead, researchers simply observe that some individuals received the treatment and others did not.

This chapter discusses specific epidemiologic and statistical methods that can help address these and other complexities inherent in public mental health inquiry. It begins with an exploration of study design, followed by a discussion of data analysis. Each section explores a few specific challenges and the methodological solutions used to surmount them. A final section discusses some of the primary data sources available for investigating public mental health in the United States. Throughout the chapter it is important to keep perspective and remember the ultimate interest, which is to answer important questions in public health, as illustrated in figure 5-1.

STUDY DESIGN

This section provides a brief overview of challenges encountered in planning, designing, and administering studies to explore issues affecting public mental health. For more information on measurement, assessment, and survey design, including both design challenges and ways of overcoming them, the reader is encouraged to review chapter 4.

Study Design Overview

Study designs can be either experimental or nonexperimental. Experimental studies seek to estimate the effect of exposure to a stimulus, activity, or behavior, such as a treatment or intervention. Fleming and Hsieh (2002) provide more extensive discussion and examples

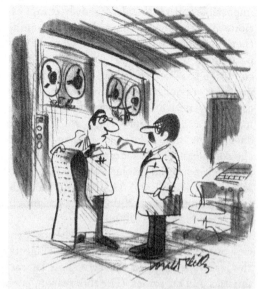

"Early on, Ed, I learned never to forget that these numbers are honest-to-God flesh-and-blood human beings."

Figure 5-1   Reminder of the Ultimate Interest in Using Data to Answer Important Questions in Public Health.

Source: Republished with permission of *The New Yorker*. ©*The New Yorker*.

of experimental and nonexperimental designs. In an experimental study, a researcher assigns some individuals (or groups, such as communities) randomly to treatment conditions (e.g., one or more conditions, within each of which subjects receive either an active treatment or are untreated). All of the individuals or groups are then followed over time to measure outcomes. In sufficiently large samples, randomization ensures that outcome differences are attributable to the intervention and not to preexisting differences between the treated and control groups. As a result, randomized designs can yield unbiased estimates of treatment effects.

However, randomized designs cannot answer all of the questions of interest in public mental health inquiry. For example, in studying risk factors for a particular mental disorder, randomizing individuals to adverse conditions (such as low socioeconomic status, homelessness, or unemployment) is both impossible and unethical. Moreover, complications can arise in randomized studies, among them noncompliance (subjects who do not participate in the intervention or treatment condition to which they were assigned), missing data, or poor intervention fidelity. In such cases alternative, nonexperimental designs may be a more appropriate study design choice. For more detailed information on the complexities of randomized experiments and their potential resolutions, see Frangakis and Rubin (2002); Jo, Asparouhov, Muthén, Ialongo, and Brown (2008); and McConnell, Stuart, and Devaney (2008).

In nonexperimental studies, with no control over the experiences of study subjects, the researcher instead observes their characteristics and outcomes. (For this reason, such studies sometimes are called naturalistic or observational studies.) Nonexperimental designs include cross-sectional studies, cohort studies, and case–control studies.

Cross-sectional studies are carried out at a particular point in time; data are collected on a sample of a population of interest, typically through respondent surveys, which may include objective measures of physical or cognitive function. Cross-sectional studies can be particularly useful for estimating a mental disorder's point prevalence or lifetime prevalence.

In contrast, cohort studies follow a sample population over time. A prospective cohort study establishes and follows a cohort of outcome-free (e.g., disease-free) individuals to assess who develops one or more disorders and when the disorders arise. Because they follow individuals over time, cohort studies are particularly useful for studying disorder incidence rates. One of the most well-known prospective cohort studies in the mental health field is the Epidemiologic Catchment Area (ECA) study (Eaton, Regier, Locke, & Taube, 1981). To conduct and interpret results from prospective cohort studies, it must be possible to follow up and ascertain disease status over a potentially long time interval and to accommodate any loss to follow-up that may occur over time.

In case–control studies, the third broad class of nonexperimental designs, a sample is selected based on the presence or absence of disorder (the cases and controls, respectively),

and current and past characteristics, risk factors, and exposures of the two populations are compared. While particularly effective for studying rare disorders, case–control designs are less useful for studying rare exposures and also are subject to the possibility of significant bias. Further, because subjects are selected based on their outcome status, the case–control design cannot be used to estimate prevalence or incidence rates in the population of interest. Data generated from the design can only generate estimated relative risks between exposed and unexposed individuals through odds ratios.

Design Challenge 1: Making Results Relevant to the Population of Interest

The individuals participating in a study may or may not represent the population of interest (the target population). Of course, the first step in any study is to specify the target population carefully and in advance. For example, voter surveys often refer to likely voters or registered voters as the target population; as such, findings might not generalize to nonvoters. Many other surveys focus on the household-residing population as a target, ignoring individuals who do not reside in households. Usually, the target population is related to a particular geographic location (e.g., Maryland or the continental United States). Whatever the target population designation, however, descriptive precision is key (e.g., the population of unionized carpenters, persons holding a license to drive an automobile, residents of correctional institutions, or persons with Spanish as their native language).

Some subtleties about the populations of interest need to be considered in working to define a target population. Defining the target population as all individuals residing in households in a given area—a typical definition for many public opinion and health surveys—may lead to undercounting of persons with mental disorders relative to a target population of all individuals living in that area, since some persons with mental disorders reside in general or mental hospitals, in nursing homes, in correctional facilities, or on the street with no fixed residence. The methodological shift from a focus on institutions in psychiatric epidemiology's first-generation epidemiologic surveys (described in chapter 4) to a focus on households in the second generation itself represents a redefinition of the target population. For example, interest in the prevalence of mental illness in a broader population than individuals residing in households led ECA study researchers to define the target population as the "normal residents" of a geographic area, such as Baltimore, Maryland (Leaf et al., 1985). Normal residents were identified as those persons who, while perhaps not residing in a household at the time of the survey, were attached in one way or another to the geographic area in question. Thus persons temporarily away from their customary households or residing in college dormitories, military barracks, general hospitals, or jails in the geographic area were to be included in the sample. Persons living permanently in institutions (e.g., prisons and mental hospitals) would be included in the population of the area in which the institution was located. To avoid prevalence variations based solely on higher rates of mental disorders in areas that include a prison or mental hospital, for example, researchers might choose to use a subject's address at entry to the institution, even if the relationship to the survey date was tenuous (as in the case of an individual whose address at admission to a mental hospital 20 years prior to the survey was inside a designated survey area). A well-conducted field survey will specify explicit methods to identify members of the target population and follow them for interview either at a distant location or on return to the geographic target area.

The prevalence of disorders differs greatly across residential settings, as shown in table 5-1. For example, in Baltimore in 1981, 50% of individuals in correctional institutions and 36% of those in mental hospitals had a history of a drug use disorder; the prevalence of schizophrenia was markedly higher among those living in mental hospitals than among those in other settings; and the prevalence of cognitive impairment was much higher among nursing home residents than in other residences. These findings effectively combine the approach taken in the first generation of psychiatric epidemiology (record-based searches of treatment facilities) with that taken in the third generation (diagnostic surveys). Although prevalence varies widely across settings, the effect of including or excluding the nonhousehold sector of the population is small, since such residents represent only a small proportion of the overall

Table 5-1. Proportion of Respondents Meeting Criteria for Six Categories of Mental Disorder in Their Lifetimes, by Residential Setting (N = 4,034)

	HOUSE HOLD	NURSING HOME	PRISON OR JAIL	MENTAL HOSPITAL
PERCENTAGES				
Drug disorder	5	2	50	36
Alcohol disorder	13	12	36	28
Major depression	4	2	8	24
Schizophrenia	2	2	2	23
Cognitive impairment	2	37	1	19
Any disorder	39	59	77	83
NUMBERS				
Total sample[a]	3,481	350	155	48

[a]Number of missing cases varies by diagnosis, from 7% to 13%.
Source: 1981 Baltimore Epidemiologic Catchment Area data.

population. For this reason, coupled with the additional challenges associated with gaining access to hospitals and correctional facilities, most national surveys do not include such residents in their samples.

When all individuals in a target population specified by a research design cannot be enumerated (counted and listed), researchers may rely on a sample of individuals thought to be representative of but not necessarily a subset of the target population. Such a sample, however, may differ from the target population with respect to relevant characteristics, place, or time, limiting the ability to apply study findings to the original target population and limiting generalizability. For example, questions about need for treatment for all individuals with major depressive disorders cannot be answered by a study that relies solely on Medicaid claims data. Not everyone who seeks treatment for a depressive disorder does so through Medicaid. Moreover, individuals who seek treatment for a depressive disorder or another mental illness represent a limited portion of all individuals affected by the disorder (Kessler et al., 2005; Mojtabai, 2009). A similar problem arises from so-called convenience samples, in which data are collected from a haphazard set of individuals, such as may be identified through Internet surveys or newspaper or magazine advertisements (Groves et al., 2009).

GENERALIZABILITY IN NONEXPERIMENTAL SETTINGS

Generalizability takes one of two forms: logical and statistical. A researcher makes a logical generalization by concluding that the variation and causal processes found in the study sample are identical to those in the target population. To achieve this type of generalizability, the study sample and the data collected on that sample are defined to include the same important sources of variation that exist in the target population, such as age, sex, race and ethnicity, socioeconomic position, and marital status. Although logical generalization occurs with little precision and often with minimal justification, it occurs routinely and for this reason is important. For example, indirect

estimation procedures described later in this chapter, particularly the so-called synthetic estimation of prevalence rates, involve logical generalization with the addition of some statistical procedures. Logical generalization can be made with respect to prevalence data as well as to the associations between mental disorders and other antecedent and concurrent factors.

In statistical generalization, quantitative procedures that can be described and replicated link the sample to the target population and specify any constraints on the ability to generalize from the sample. Statistical generalizations are based on population (or epidemiologic) samples: individuals who are probabilistically selected as representative of the specified target population. In mental health, the ECA study is one of the first nationwide exemplars of such generalization (Eaton & Kessler, 1985; L. N. Robins et al., 1984). The ECA study initially collected data from a representative sample of individuals aged 18 and above across five sites in the United States. Individuals at the Baltimore site have since been followed longitudinally for 25 years, providing information on trends and associations over time. Other examples of nationally representative epidemiologic studies in public mental health include many large national data sets, such as the National Comorbidity Survey (NCS) (Kessler & Walters, 2002) and others described later in this chapter. These studies have shown, for example, that most individuals meeting diagnostic criteria for common mental disorders—such as mood and anxiety disorders and alcohol and drug use disorders—are not receiving treatment (Kessler et al., 1999; Regier et al., 1993; Shapiro et al., 1984; Wang et al., 2005), severely compromising the generalizability of analyses of these disorders that are based on administrative records on individuals in treatment.

This inability to generalize from cases in treatment to the larger population of cases is referred to as Berkson's bias. Berkson (1946) argued that use of hospital inpatients as controls in studies of smoking and lung cancer induces a bias since smokers are more likely than nonsmokers to be admitted to the hospital. Thus Berkson's bias would suggest both a bias in samples from clinics, as opposed to those from general household-residing populations, and a possibility that clinic populations are more likely to have health conditions than populations not selected in this way. In contrast, general population studies in high-resource countries, including investigations with more intensive assessment than is undertaken in ECA- or NCS-style surveys, show that the majority of individuals with serious mental disorders such as schizophrenia do come into the treatment system (Eaton, 1985, 1991). Thus the relative value of survey-based data compared with administrative records often is dependent on both the place and the disorder being studied.

Population-based study samples usually are obtained from sampling frames, essentially lists of every individual in the target population (Kish, 1965). Simple random sampling, in which the desired number of study participants is randomly selected from the larger sampling frame, is the most straightforward sampling method. However, since enumerating a complete target population often is difficult (e.g., obtaining a list of the population of the entire United States), multistage methods, discussed below, often are used. For example, a random sample of US counties first would be selected; individuals within the selected counties then would be selected as the sample invited to take a survey. In this case, enumeration of the population is necessary only for the selected counties. On occasion, the population may be stratified as well, to ensure that the sample includes diverse subpopulations (e.g., different racial or ethnic groups, degrees of educational attainment, or income levels).

Household surveys are crucial to studies of the epidemiology of mental disorders and mental health. The following discussion of the process of household surveys is intended to help researchers and clinicians better understand the procedures involved in this type of survey design and to aid in subsequent data analysis. Many good texts are available for additional information on this topic, among them Groves et al. (2009), Lohr (2009), and Sudman (1976).

The basic principle of sampling is that each individual in the target population is recruited for the survey with a known probability (called the selection probability) greater than zero. In other words, everyone in the population had some probability of being selected. Generalization to the entire population is accomplished by weighting analytic results by the inverse of the selection probability, called the sample weight. The sample weight indicates the number of individuals in the population represented by each sample respondent.

In some sample surveys of relatively small, delineable populations—for example, all persons living in a defined neighborhood or all members of the United Mineworkers Union—the entire population can be listed, with unique consecutive numbers linked to each individual name. It then becomes a small job to select a random sample based on either a random number list or a random number generator (typically available in statistical software packages). On rare occasion, lists of large populations of households may be available, such as those from utility companies. More commonly, such a listing of an entire population is not available.

Thus in most large household samples, the population of study subjects is listed theoretically, that is, to the point that estimation of the probability of selection is possible. The most prominent form of such theoretical sampling occurs when listings are made by physical areas, in what is called area probability sampling. Typically, the listing includes geographic clusters, such as county or city blocks, the total populations of which are known from another source, such as a national census. Each cluster is selected in proportion to its known size (probability proportionate to size, or PPS). Then within each chosen cluster, and again using the PPS method, a smaller subcluster (e.g., one specific street) is selected. This process is repeated until the process reaches the household level. Through this multistage approach, the probabilities of selection at each level can be multiplied to generate a final probability of selection for each household, yet specific household listings are required only for the ultimate subclusters (e.g., streets) selected.

Once the sampled households for study participation are identified, they are approached to participate. Members of the household are enumerated by a field-worker, and a random selection from eligible household members is made. Some confounds must be avoided. For example, selecting a single respondent from each household implies that the probability of being selected from a single-person household is greater than the probability of selection from a multiple-person household. Similarly, a field-worker charged with identifying respondents might recognize and immediately interview a willing, available respondent rather than interview another household resident selected from the subsequent random pick. To prevent such departures from the rules, field procedures sometimes specify that household or respondent designation be performed by different personnel and under a separate set of procedures from the interview itself—a procedure termed independent listing.

In sample-based surveys, the probability of selection for each person in the sample must be known before undertaking data analysis (Horvitz & Thompson, 1952). If the probability of selection is estimable at each stage of sampling, the sample weights at each stage can be multiplied to generate a final sample weight. Thus in a multistage sample, in which counties are first selected and then individuals are selected from within the selected counties, the final sample weight for an individual is the product of the inverse of the probability of the individual's county being selected and the inverse of the probability of the individual being selected within the county.

The distinction between being selected to participate in a survey and actually participating is an important consideration in conducting and analyzing field surveys. Many individuals selected for a survey may not participate, either because they decline to do so or because they cannot be located. The proportion of individuals selected who participate in the study is called the survey completion rate. Analysis is complicated because while the probability of selection into the survey sample is known, the probability of actually participating (responding) is not known. Survey analysis methods, including nonresponse weighting adjustments

(Groves et al., 2009), compensate for this difficulty.

GENERALIZABILITY IN EXPERIMENTAL SETTINGS

Representativeness (or lack thereof) is also an important problem in randomized trials that seek to estimate the effect of a treatment or intervention. Frequently, randomized trials are conducted in samples of individuals whose demographic characteristics or disease severity are far different from those of most people (Rothwell, 2005). Many of the same challenges to generalizability found in nonexperimental designs are also present in experimental settings. In either case, it remains critical to identify an appropriate source population or sampling frame from which inferences can be made about the target.

In randomized trials, however, the key issue is whether differences between the participants in a trial and the target population are related specifically to the associations between exposure (treatment) and outcome. For example, Zimmerman and colleagues (2005) found that patients excluded from a depression treatment trial were more chronically ill than those included in the trial. Such a situation could limit generalizability, since conclusions regarding the treatment's effectiveness were established only for those with acute, not chronic, depression. Similarly, many medication trials eliminate persons with comorbid disorders from consideration, even though comorbidity is more often the rule than the exception and may affect treatment efficacy.

Another high-profile example related to the generalizability of study findings comes from studies of hormone replacement therapy. Differences in women's ages and the point at which they began hormone replacement therapy provide one explanation for discrepancies in findings about the effects of hormone replacement therapy on postmenopausal women between the Women's Health Initiative randomized trial and the Nurse's Health Study nonexperimental study (Grodstein, Clarkson, & Manson, 2003). Similar discrepancies may arise when individuals enter a randomized trial at different points in the disease process, as in studies on the use of nonsteroidal anti-inflammatory drugs, such as aspirin or ibuprofen, to prevent Alzheimer's disease, an illness in which there may be important differences in the phases of preclinical illness of study participants (Hayden et al., 2007). Further, quite simply, individuals who agree to participate in a clinical trial of a medication may be different from those who do not want the type of treatment they receive to be decided by a random flip of a coin (US General Accounting Office, 1994).

Nonetheless, randomized trials do have the previously mentioned benefits that the probability of pretreatment differences between groups is estimable with a known probability and that the treatment effect in the study sample, similarly, is estimable. The treatment effect in this context is referred to as the efficacy of the treatment; the ability to obtain an accurate estimate of this effect for individuals in the study sample is termed internal validity. In contrast, external validity is the degree to which the effects estimated in the randomized trial are generalizable to the broader population. Finally, the corresponding effect of treatment in the general population, carried out under real-life conditions, is termed effectiveness rather than efficacy (Flay et al., 2005; Imai, King, & Stuart, 2008; Shadish, Cook, & Campbell, 2002).

External validity is a critical concept, because few means exist to account for potential differences between a randomized trial sample and a target population. The recent emphasis on effectiveness trials marks one effort to help improve external validity. Traditionally, efficacy trials in behavioral health often involved a small set of volunteer subjects and were conducted in laboratory rather than real-world settings (Pasamanick, Scarpitti, & Dinitz 1967; Stein & Test, 1980). In contrast, effectiveness trials aim to enroll a broad set of patients and are conducted in real-world settings (Flay, 1986). For example, both Ialongo and colleagues (1999) and Bradshaw, Koth, Thornton, and Leaf (2009) describe studies of school-based interventions carried out in school districts. Olds and colleagues (2007) describe an effectiveness trial carried out in a public obstetric and pediatric care system in which nurses visit the homes of families with new infants. The challenges encountered in providing these interventions in real-world settings mean that the results found in these effectiveness trials may be quite different from results seen in more controlled settings (e.g., a lab or clinical setting).

Practical clinical trials represent a further step to advance external validity. These large-scale effectiveness trials aim to enroll a large, representative sample so that detected effects will readily be generalizable to a broad population (Insel, 2006; March et al., 2005). Among the practical clinical trials funded by the National Institute of Mental Health are the Sequenced Treatment Alternatives to Relieve Depression trial, known as STAR*D, comparing treatments for adults with depression (Rush et al., 2004), and the Clinical Antipsychotic Trials of Intervention Effectiveness (CATIE) trial, comparing antipsychotic treatments for psychosis and Alzheimer's disease (Stroup et al., 2003). The primary drawback of practical clinical trials such as these is their high cost, driven by large samples and longitudinal follow-up. Practical clinical trials often cost in the tens of millions of dollars; some cost as much as $30,000 per participant (Tunis, Stryer, & Clancy, 2003). In addition, despite their cost, even these large, well-designed, well-implemented studies are not without complications. For example, in long-term trials like the CATIE study, researchers need to account for individuals who, during the course of the study, may have had several treatments of varying duration, discontinued treatments for a variety of reasons, or never took their assigned treatments at all.

The balance between internal and external validity has prompted some researchers to supplement randomized trials with observational studies, since observational data are often available on larger, more representative samples of individuals (Imai et al., 2008). The use of large administrative data sets, such as Medicare claims or health insurance records, while posing some challenges to generalizability, do allow study among a broad array of individuals rather than among a convenience sample. The next section explores some of the challenges inherent in the use of nonrandomized studies to estimate causal effects.

Design Challenge 2: Estimating Causal Effects Using Nonexperimental Studies

Many research questions in public mental health are descriptive, such as estimating the percentage of individuals in the population with a disorder or comparing disorder rates among races. However, some questions ask about causality. For example, some studies seek to estimate the impact of a deliberate intervention on a desired outcome, such as determining how well a prevention or treatment program works for a specific population (e.g., Kellam et al., 2008; Olds et al., 2007). Another area of interest is the extent to which particular exposures (e.g., the experience of trauma, poverty, a drug culture, or physical illness) affect various populations. In public mental health research, many research questions involve identifying factors (e.g., trauma, drug abuse, or poverty) that may predispose individuals to or act as risk factors for mental disorders. For example, studies have explored such potential relationships as the effect of truancy on the onset of drug use (Henry & Huizinga, 2007), the role of depression in cancer etiology (Gross, Gallo, & Eaton, 2010), and the effect of heavy adolescent drug use on employment status in adulthood (Stuart & Green, 2008).

Random assignment of individuals to treatment and control conditions is an ideal way to estimate the causal effect of an exposure or intervention. As mentioned previously, random assignment ensures that differences in background characteristics between treatment and control groups are strictly random. Because the only difference between the two groups is the treatment or exposure, any difference in outcomes must be attributable to the exposure in question. In statistical terms, randomized experiments of this kind yield internally valid, unbiased estimates of the effects of treatments or exposures.

In contrast, nonexperimental studies are not automatically guaranteed to be internally valid. Individuals in the treatment and comparison groups are likely to differ in ways beyond the study-specific treatment or exposure they received. For example, studies have found that compared with youth who do not use marijuana, adolescents with marijuana use problems are also more likely to smoke tobacco and to abuse or be dependent on alcohol (Harder, Stuart, & Anthony, 2008). The difficulty inherent in separating the effects of marijuana use problems from other differences between the groups means that bias would arise in a simple comparison of adolescents with and without marijuana use problems. This issue is formally known as confounding, a difference between treatment and comparison groups (or exposed and unexposed groups) on a pretreatment variable that also is related to the outcome (Altman et al., 2001).

Traditionally, statistical adjustment using regression analysis is used to alleviate confounding by observed variables and to estimate causal effects in nonrandomized studies. Potential confounders are included as predictors in the statistical model, and if the effect of the putative cause persists in the adjusted model, the causal inference is strengthened. However, such adjustment cannot mitigate all of the inherent weaknesses of nonrandomized studies. For example, sometimes the adjustment cannot include all potential confounders, either because of limited sample size or because the confounders were not measured in the first place. Further, it may not be possible to tease apart the outcome's explanatory variance common to the putative causal variable and the potential confounder and allocate it to one variable or the other. Finally, effect estimates from the regression adjustment can be biased if the regression model itself is not correctly specified, particularly if the distribution of potential confounders is quite different in the treatment and comparison groups (J. Robins & Greenland, 1986; Rubin, 1973).

A variety of nonexperimental study designs are employed to address the limitations in the use of traditional regression adjustment to control for confounding. Shadish and colleagues (2002) and West and colleagues (2008) present overviews of ways to estimate causal effects in nonexperimental settings, among them instrumental variables, interrupted time series, regression discontinuity designs, and propensity score matching methods.

INSTRUMENTAL VARIABLE METHODS

Instrumental variable methods are used when a randomly assigned (or thought to be randomly assigned) instrument influences receipt of the treatment of interest but does not directly affect the outcomes of interest (Angrist, Imbens, & Rubin, 1996). A public mental health study by Foster (2000) estimating the effect of added outpatient visits on outcomes of children and adolescents is illustrative. Foster used data from an evaluation of the Fort Bragg demonstration (Bickman et al., 1995), a study of a continuum-of-care model of mental health care for children that collected data from children at three military bases (three sites). Since the number of outpatient visits could not be randomized and is likely related to other characteristics of the children, Foster identified two instruments that probably affected the number of mental health visits by a child but did not have a direct effect on outcomes: date of entry into the evaluation, since the high cost of the demonstration constrained access to services later in the evaluation, and conduct of the demonstration in only one of the three sites, since the demonstration may have increased access to services. Exploring the validity of the underlying assumptions, Foster found that higher numbers of visits were associated with improved functioning.

INTERRUPTED TIME SERIES

Interrupted time series, a commonly used non-experimental design with a complex before/after design (Shadish et al., 2002), is used when an intervention is implemented at a particular time. Outcomes observed following the intervention are compared with outcomes that would have been expected in the absence of the intervention based on trends observed during the preintervention period. This method works best when many observations are made in advance of the intervention, so that patterns and trends over time are readily discernible. Biglan, Ary, and Wagenaar (2000) discuss the benefits of interrupted time series designs for estimating the effects of community-level interventions. They also address the underlying assumptions and possible threats to validity of such designs. Gibbons and colleagues (2007) employed this kind of design to examine the impact of government "black box" warnings about adolescent use of selective serotonin reuptake inhibitor (SSRI) antidepressants on both antidepressant prescription use and suicide rates. They found that the regulatory warnings were associated with decreased use of SSRIs by children and adolescents and that in turn the reduced use of SSRIs was associated with higher suicide rates among children and adolescents.

REGRESSION DISCONTINUITY

Related to interrupted time series, a third method, regression discontinuity (Cook, 2008) can be used when assignment to an intervention is determined by the score on an observed measure. Individuals on one side of the score receive the intervention; those on the other side do not. Regression discontinuity is used often in education research, in which program eligibility, such as for a remedial reading program, may depend on an achievement test score. Ludwig and Miller (2007) were able to estimate the effects of the federal Head Start program on education and health outcomes using a discontinuity in the initial funding of Head Start projects under which the 300 poorest counties in the country received grant-writing assistance from the federal government to help with their Head Start applications.

PROPENSITY SCORE MATCHING

A fourth approach to estimating causal effects in nonexperimental studies is propensity score matching (Stuart, 2010). Propensity scores, developed by Rosenbaum and Rubin (1983), represent the probability of receiving a treatment given observed characteristics. By creating treatment and comparison groups that are as similar as possible to one another, this method attempts to mimic a randomized experiment, at least with respect to the observed characteristics. The propensity score summarizes each individual's observed characteristics into a single variable. The propensity scores are then used to match, weight, or subclassify exposure groups in ways that make the observed covariate distributions as similar as possible across the two groups. Harder and colleagues (2008), for example, estimated the effects of heavy adolescent marijuana use on subsequent adult depression using previously available longitudinal data on a cohort of individuals followed from age 6 through their 20s (Kellam et al., 2008) and propensity score weighting to make observed background characteristics comparable between adolescent users and nonusers. In other research, Haviland, Nagin, and Rosenbaum (2007) combined propensity score matching and longitudinal methods to estimate the effect of joining a gang on later violent delinquency. Haviland's group matched young males who joined a gang at age 14 with nonjoiners who nonetheless had characteristics and trajectories of violence before age 14 similar to those of the gang joiners.

Unfortunately, the propensity score can control only for observed characteristics; unobserved differences, known as unmeasured confounding, may remain between the treatment and comparison groups. Sensitivity analyses can assess the extent to which the results may be the product of an unobserved confounder associated with both the treatment received and the outcome. (For an example, see Haviland et al., 2007.)

Design Challenge 3: Multilevel Influences and Effects

A variety of factors at many levels influence mental health and mental illness, from individual and family factors to community and broader geographic factors to time. Moreover, many mental health interventions, such as system-wide changes in service networks or community-wide preventive interventions, are carried out at the group level. As a consequence, both nonexperimental and experimental studies alike may need to measure effects of an exposure or intervention at one or more of the levels at which effects may be apparent. For example, many universal preventive interventions designed to reduce problem behavior in children are undertaken in schools or classrooms, among them the classroom-based Good Behavior Game (Dolan et al., 1993) and the school-wide Positive Behavioral Interventions and Supports (PBIS) program (Sugai, Horner, & Gresham, 2001). Similarly, there is growing interest in how neighborhood characteristics affect mental health (e.g., Furr-Holden et al., 2008).

Particular challenges arise in trying to evaluate interventions carried out at a group level. Random assignment of individuals to treatment or control groups often is not appropriate or even possible when interventions are administered at the group level. In that case, groups are randomized together in what is called a group randomized trial (Murray, 1998; Raudenbush & Bryk, 2002). A randomized evaluation (Bradshaw et al., 2009) of the PBIS program provides an example of this type of trial. Since it generally is not possible to randomly assign children to schools, 37 Maryland schools themselves were randomly assigned to receive or not to receive PBIS training. Other group randomized trials in public mental health include a study of a collaborative care model for treating adults with Alzheimer's disease in which physicians were the unit of randomization (Callahan et al., 2006) and an evaluation of the Guided Care program, designed to enhance the quality of care for older adults with multiple chronic conditions, in which randomization occurred at the level of primary care practices (Boult et al., 2008).

In group randomized trials, individual outcomes may be correlated more within a group than with individuals in other groups. For example, test scores among students at the same school are more likely to be similar to each other than are test scores of students from different schools. This correlation of measures is quantified by the intraclass correlation coefficient (ICC), the proportion of variance in a variable that is due to between-cluster variation.

This correlation has two key implications. First, if the ICC is considerable, a relatively large number of groups is needed to detect effects with sufficient statistical power, even with many individuals in each group. In fact, even with hundreds of individuals in each group, it is rare to have sufficient power to detect intervention effects with fewer than 8 to 10 groups in each treatment condition (Murray, 1998). The design effect quantifies this as the factor by which a study sample size with individual randomization would need to be multiplied to obtain the same statistical power as a study that uses group randomization (Donner & Klar, 2000; Eldridge, Ashby, & Kerry, 2006). Second, analyses must account for the group structure; analysis of individual-level outcomes that ignores the group structure is insufficient. Appropriate analysis techniques include either aggregating data across individuals and analyzing it at the group level or implementing multilevel models, such as random effects models, that explicitly model the group structure (Raudenbush & Bryk, 2002; Varnell, Murray, Janega, & Blitstein, 2004). When there are large numbers of groups—often over 40—it may be possible to use generalized estimating equations for analyses (Varnell et al., 2004).

Design Challenge 4: The Need for Long-Term Follow-up

The etiologically relevant period—the time between the first potential causal factor and the full expression of a disorder—is longer for most mental disorders than it is for other diseases and illnesses, as noted in previous chapters. Moreover, the physical and behavioral trajectory of many mental disorders extends over decades, often with periods of remission and exacerbation, as discussed in chapter 6. Thus even when a well-designed, randomized trial is conducted to assess intervention effects, many years, even decades, may pass before effects are seen, particularly with regard to preventive interventions designed to prevent substance abuse, delinquent behavior, or mental illness. In ideal settings, study participants are followed for many years, as in the Johns Hopkins Prevention and Intervention Research Center (PIRC) trials, which followed children from first grade into their early 30s

(Ialongo, Poduska, Werthamer, & Kellam, 2001; Kellam & Anthony, 1998). However, such long-term follow-up is expensive and resource intensive; consequently, it also is rare.

One means of overcoming the challenges related to long-term study population follow-up is the use of surrogate outcomes: measurable, short-term, proximal outcomes that are correlated with the more distal outcomes of interest. This approach is common in longitudinal medical studies in which the ultimate outcome is a participant's death. In such studies, surrogate outcomes such as blood pressure or cholesterol levels often are used to estimate intervention effects in a shorter time frame. Similarly, in long-term prevention studies of childhood interventions designed to affect subsequent adult behaviors (e.g., drug use or smoking), shorter-term, mediating adolescent behaviors may be examined instead of waiting for an extended period. A sizable literature on mediation analysis (Jo, 2008; MacKinnon, 2008) provides considerable guidance on ways to consider mediated effects and how effects can best be estimated.

The use of nonexperimental data to investigate causal effects provides another avenue through which to examine a normally long prodromal period. Data sets such as those from the PIRC or Woodlawn studies (Ensminger, Anthony, & McCord, 1997) include follow-ups, from age 6 to adulthood, of cohorts in well-delimited neighborhoods. These data sets can be used to investigate relationships between early-life exposures and much later outcomes. Using propensity score methods, Stuart and Green (2008) used the child-to-adult Woodlawn data to explore the effects of heavy adolescent drug use on employment, marital status, and drug use in the individuals' 30s and 40s. Employing publicly available data sets and the regression discontinuity design described earlier, Ludwig and Miller (2007) ascertained the long-term effects of childhood participation in Head Start. While Head Start appeared to have minimal effects on short-term educational outcomes such as test scores, it had a greater impact on longer term educational outcomes such as high school graduation and total years of completed education. Ongoing research continues to identify the best designs and analyses for ascertaining long-term effects of interventions in the absence of long-term data. Methods described by Stuart and Ialongo (2010) suggest ways to target resources by limiting long-term follow-up to a subset of study participants.

The availability of longitudinal data also makes it possible to examine disorders whose course varies over time, such as many mental illnesses characterized by exacerbations and remissions. It is not enough to observe multiple individuals in a cross-sectional manner at various stages of life; these analyses require repeated observations of the same set of individuals. Given the fluctuating nature of many mental disorders, repeated observation is critical to ensure that the feature of interest is not missed altogether. Longitudinal data also may be used to examine the onset of mental disorders, for example, by using survival analysis methods to examine the predictors and risk factors for the illness as well as the timing of onset.

While longitudinal data provide valuable information about change over time, repeated observations for each subject also can pose analytic complications. The use of analytic methods such as generalized estimating equations (Liang & Zeger, 1986), hierarchical linear models (Raudenbush & Bryk, 2002), and growth curve models (Goldstein, 1995; Singer & Willett, 2003) can account for the correlations of observations on the same individual over time.

Design Challenge 5: Rare Outcomes

Nonexperimental studies in general and studies of risk factors for later disorders in particular require long-term follow-up across the study population. Such a longitudinal approach is particularly relevant for studies of life course epidemiology investigating the link between early life experiences and disease risk later in life (Cannon, Huttunen, & Murray, 2002; Kuh & Ben-Shlomo, 1997). Many of these types of questions can be examined through long-term cohort studies. However, additional problems arise when the disorder in question is relatively rare (e.g., schizophrenia or autism), demanding a proportionately

large sample size to generate sufficient numbers of cases for analysis.

Two strategies are available to overcome this potential problem. The first is to select a high-risk sample—a specific cohort in which a larger-than-expected number of cases are expected to be found. Such a sample might include, for example, individuals at high genetic risk for schizophrenia (Watt & Saiz, 1991) or, to study longitudinal predictors of autism spectrum disorders, siblings of children with autism (Landa & Garrett-Mayer, 2006). The second strategy is to use existing cohorts for whom many years of data are available and, as in a case–control design, to evaluate the data retrospectively. Use of this method, however, results in less control over both the quality and availability of early measures, as compared to a planned, prospective data collection for a specific purpose (Cannon et al., 2002).

DATA ANALYSIS

Unfortunately, even when the study design is as strong as possible, data analysis difficulties sometimes arise after the study design is completed. This section discusses some of these challenges, among them missing data and the need to model latent constructs.

Analysis Challenge 1: Missing Data

While a strong study design can help limit the occurrence of missing data, almost inevitably data gaps do occur. For example, some individuals selected for study participation fail to respond, either because they become unavailable or because they refuse to participate after being designated as subjects. This is known as unit nonresponse. Among the individuals who do participate, not all will respond to all questions, a gap known as item nonresponse. These twin sources of data loss are particularly important to recognize in studies of mental disorders, since nonresponse may be a product of the stigma and shame attached to the disorders or may be related to active symptomatology. Analyses that exclude individuals for whom complete data are not available may yield severely biased results, particularly if subjects who respond to an item are different from those who do not respond. In the 1-year follow-up of the ECA sample, for example, interview completion rates for older white women and younger black males were lower than those for other sample participants (Eaton, Anthony, Tepper, & Dryman, 1992).

Fortunately, methods are readily available to manage certain types of missing data, using methods such as maximum likelihood, multiple imputation, or weighting approaches. Excellent introductions to methods to manage missing data are found in Graham (2009) and Schafer and Graham (2002). The immediate focus here, however, is on what are referred to as nonignorable missing data, data that are not missing at random (Rubin, 1976)—in other words, data for which the "missingness" depends on unobserved factors. In other words, individuals with and without missing data are different from one another even after accounting for differences in observed variables. A few examples are illustrative. Survey subjects with very high or very low incomes may be more likely to refuse to provide information about their incomes. Similarly, individuals with depression may be less likely to respond to a survey. Thus even among individuals with the same observed characteristics, the distribution of variables with missing values (e.g., rates of depression, income levels) may be different for those not providing data than for those for whom data are available.

When nonignorable missing data such as these are a concern, researchers must guess why or when values are missing based on a model of the missing-data process using substantive or external information. Siddique and Belin (2008) have developed a method that uses a nonignorable-missing-data model to impute (fill in) missing data on subjects' levels of depression. Creation of the model was motivated by missing data in the WECare study of depression treatment for low-income minority women (Miranda et al., 2003). Subjects were randomly assigned to one of three interventions: medication, cognitive behavioral therapy, or usual care. Depression levels in the women were measured monthly or every other month over a 12-month period. Unfortunately, at each time point the follow-up interviews were missing for 24–38% of the women. Siddique and Belin used a procedure that imputes a prediction for each missing depression level by finding an individual with similar previously observed values and substituting that person's response for the missing response. They then modified the procedure slightly, using an approximate Bayesian bootstrap (ABB) imputation that enables the researcher to specify further the type of subjects to be selected in the imputation, such as those with higher outcome depression scores, if it is believed that such subjects are more likely to be missing. The ABB model enables the imputation process to incorporate a priori beliefs about the missing-data process. Researchers also may combine models or undertake analyses that use several possible models to examine the sensitivity of results to particular assumptions about the nonignorable missing data. Siddique and Belin recommend using procedures that allow for flexible relationships between the missing-data process and the outcomes themselves, since using an incorrect model for the nonignorable-missing-data process may be worse than simply using a method that assumes data are missing at random (Graham, 2009).

Pattern-mixture models, which apply different outcome models to individuals with different patterns of missing data, are another approach for handling nonignorable missing data. This approach was employed in a psychiatric trial of antipsychotic medications for the treatment of schizophrenia (Demirtas, 2005). Based on measures obtained early in the study, individuals who dropped out of the study's control condition appeared to be more severely ill than those who stayed in the study. In contrast, individuals who dropped out of the medication group appeared to be less severely ill than those who completed the study. Demirtas (2005) used a Bayesian pattern-mixture model that permitted disease status outcome to affect study completion and allowed this relationship to vary across treatment groups, thus accounting for the missing data. Like Siddique and Belin (2008), he stressed the need for flexible models that do not make strong assumptions about the missing-data process.

Analysis Challenge 2: Measuring and Modeling Mental Disorders as Latent Constructs

In mental health research, many of the concepts or variables of interest are not directly observable; these are often referred to as latent constructs or latent variables (Bollen, 2002). Such constructs encompass disorders such as schizophrenia and depression, as well as variables such as intelligence, socioeconomic status, and personality. Latent variables stand in contrast to observable, directly measurable variables such as height or weight. This section examines how latent variables are used and modeled in mental health.

LATENT VARIABLE MEASUREMENT MODELS

The measurement model for a latent construct includes both the latent variable itself and its indicators—observed variables that provide information on the latent construct. For example, the latent construct of depression might be measured by relevant observed signs and symptoms, such as sleep difficulties, weight change, and feelings of sadness as measured by a valid, reliable scale such as the Beck Depression Inventory (Beck, Steer, & Brown, 1996). Common to all measurement models are the assumptions that the indicator variables are caused by the latent variable and that correlations between indicator variables (such as the items on the Beck Depression Inventory in the depression example) can be explained by the presence of the latent variable. A more detailed discussion of the nature of latent variables can be found in Bollen (2002).

Typically, latent variable models are classified by whether the latent construct and its indicators are categorical or continuous variables (Bartholomew & Knott, 1999). Table 5-2 presents different latent variable models, classified into four types: factor analysis, latent trait analysis, latent profile analysis, and latent class analysis.

Factor analysis models, in which both latent variables (constructs) and indicators are continuous, can be either exploratory or confirmatory, depending on a researcher's goal (Kim & Mueller, 1978). The five-factor model of personality is a classic example (Eysenck, 1992; McCrae & Costa, 1992). In that example, the challenge of distilling all possible English-language descriptions of behavioral disposition into a few basic personality dimensions was accomplished using exploratory factor analysis and confirmatory factor analyses of factor structures from prior studies. In addition to providing insight into the structure of human personality, this factor analysis has facilitated inquiry into both risk factors for and outcomes of different personality constructs. In another example, Samuels and colleagues (2004) examined histories of arrest among individuals in the ECA study who had completed the 300-item Revised Neuroticism-Extroversion-Openness Personality Inventory (NEO PI-R) questionnaire (McCrae, 1991), which measures the domains of neuroticism, extroversion, openness, agreeableness, and conscientiousness. They found statistically significant lower scores on agreeableness and conscientiousness and higher scores on neuroticism among those who had been arrested.

Continuous latent variables with categorical indicators are modeled using dichotomous factor analysis or latent trait analysis.

Table 5-2. Forms of Latent Variable Analyses

		CONSTRUCTS	
		CONTINUOUS	CATEGORICAL
INDICATORS	CONTINUOUS	Factor analysis	Profile analysis
	CATEGORICAL	Dichotomous factor analysis; Latent trait analysis	Latent class analysis

Source: Adapted from Bartholomew & Knott, 1999.

(See table 5-2.) Latent trait analysis is associated closely with what is known as item response theory and is commonly used in the development of computer adaptive tests (Bock, 1997; Rost & Langeheine, 1997; van der Linden & Glas, 2000). The analysis of age differences in the symptomatology of depression by Gallo, Anthony, and Muthén (1994) offers one application of latent trait analysis in public mental health inquiry. Their work found that elderly individuals with depression were less likely to report dysphoria or anhedonia than their younger counterparts. Latent trait analysis facilitated modeling the relationship between the construct of depression and the indicators used to measure it, which were dichotomous diagnostic criteria for depression in the revision of the third edition of the *Diagnostic and Statistical Manual of Mental Disorders* (DSM-III-R) (American Psychiatric Association [APA], 1987).

Latent profile analysis models are used with categorical latent variables with continuous indicators. In contrast, latent class analysis models employ categorical, typically binary indicators (Bartholomew & Knott, 1999). (See table 5-2.) Perhaps because of the nature of the data typically available, latent class analysis models are the more commonly used of the two. Both models are useful when the observed data are thought to represent a mixture of groups of individuals and when group membership is not directly observed; they are thus sometimes called mixture models (B. Muthén, 2001). One of the earliest uses of a latent class model was in the analysis of symptoms of depression in the ECA study (Eaton, Dryman, Sorenson, & McCutcheon, 1989). Using dichotomous indicators based on DSM-III-R criteria (APA, 1987), three latent classes were identified. One of these was characterized by qualities comparable to those of major depression in DSM-III-R, providing empirical support for the utility of the diagnostic category in summarizing population variation.

Latent variable modeling has two key benefits. It can summarize a large number of items into a meaningful scale, reducing statistical and interpretation problems that arise when managing each item separately. For example,

had Samuels and colleagues (2004) analyzed arrest rates against each of the 300 questionnaire items for each individual, the results would have been difficult to interpret and summarize. Moreover, with a 0.05 type I error rate, 15 of the 300 items would have shown differences between the two groups at a statistically significant level solely by chance, thereby complicating interpretation. While this multiple-comparison issue can be dealt with using methods that adjust the *p*-values of hypothesis tests, such as the Bonferroni correction, or more sophisticated methods such as those proposed by Benjamini and Hochberg (1995), latent variable models can also help manage the problem by summarizing a large number of individual items with a smaller set of latent constructs, thereby reducing the number of dimensions to be analyzed. Further, since the reliability of a construct is higher than that of any one of the individual items, latent variable models can reduce measurement error, leading to increased analytic precision.

LATENT VARIABLE STRUCTURAL MODELS

In addition to modeling a latent construct and its indicators in a measurement model, there is value in simultaneously modeling the relationships among different latent constructs or regressing latent constructs on observed variables other than the latent variable indicators. This part of the model is referred as the structural model (see figure 5-2). In particular, the structural model includes the components of a latent variable model that reflect relationships among latent constructs or between latent constructs and other observed variables. A wide variety of latent variable models are available; see B. Muthén (2008) for a useful taxonomy.

In one public mental health example, Menard, Bandeen-Roche, and Chilcoat (2004) explored the natural clustering of childhood stressors using a latent class (measurement) model. They then regressed the latent classes on sociodemographic variables to determine if sex or other observable characteristics affected the probability of membership in each of the latent classes relative to a reference

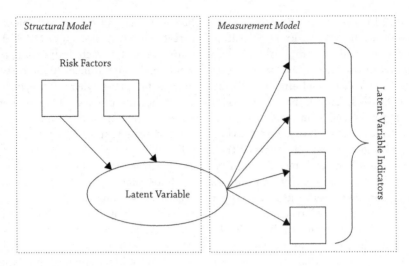

Figure 5-2 **Latent Variable Model.**

class (structural model). Before doing so, however, they needed to assess potential gender differences in the latent construct itself (in this case, the class structure of stressors). This issue of possible differences in the latent construct itself across groups (such as gender), referred to as measurement invariance or nondifferential measurement (Bandeen-Roche, Miglioretti, Zeger, & Rathouz, 1997), is crucial to the interpretation of such models. An example is illustrative. Begin with the assumption that the latent classes are ice cream flavors A and B. The determination that being male is associated with doubled odds of choosing flavor A would be meaningless if later it was determined that for boys flavor A was vanilla but for girls it was chocolate. This kind of issue also arises in longitudinal studies, in which measurement invariance over time is crucial.

Increasingly, as public mental health researchers are exploring processes, change, and development, the benefit of the flexibility of latent variable models for testing such hypotheses is becoming all the more apparent. For example, a mediated causal chain (A causes B, which in turn causes C) is difficult to model using standard regression (Kraemer, Stice, Kazdin, Offord, & Kupfer, 2001). The same analysis is more readily handled with a latent variable model, which can simultaneously estimate both relationships (A → B and B → C) (Netemeyer et al., 2001). Longitudinal factor

models (Corballis & Traub, 1970) and latent trait models (Dunson, 2003) permit modeling of change in the underlying continuous latent variable over time. In contrast, latent transition models (Collins & Wugalter, 1992) allow for the modeling of probabilities of individuals' switching between latent classes at different points in time.

Latent growth curve models can help in the identification of classes of developmental trajectories, a topic of recent growing interest. Predictors of these trajectories, as well as trajectory class–specific treatment effects, also can be modeled (B. Muthén & Muthén, 2000; B. Muthén et al., 2002). Latent growth curve models are particularly suited to public mental health research on how individuals develop over time and whether there are groups distinguished by different patterns of development. For more detail on these latent growth models, see Curran and Hussong (2003) and McArdle (2009).

The large sample sizes required are a significant obstacle to the use of latent variable models, especially in the analysis of clinical data (L. K. Muthén & Muthén, 2002). Moreover, while the models frequently are quite useful, their complexity may be a drawback. Although the past decade has been marked by exciting advances in the flexibility and availability of software for latent variable modeling, this flexibility may have had the adverse effects both of encouraging the creation of unnecessarily large, complex models and of increasing inattention to violations of model assumptions (Tomarken & Waller, 2005). Even more fundamental, the use of latent constructs precludes certainty about the validity of their measurements; lack of validity limits the strength of any inferences drawn from such models. Perhaps in the future, use of these models will prompt the discovery of biomarkers that in turn can refine the latent construct in a process of iterative validation. Similarly, by refining the estimation of latent variable measurement models, it may be possible to incorporate additional scientific information (Leoutsakos, Bandeen-Roche, Garrett-Mayer & Zandi, 2011).

Analysis Challenge 3: The Need for Prevalence Estimates in Small Areas

The desire to estimate prevalence or need in groups or geographic areas for which there is not sufficient observed information poses a particular challenge in public mental health research. For example, to help determine the need for services, a county may want to know the number of individuals in the county with dementia. However, it is unlikely that a single county has sufficient data to estimate this prevalence. The county might turn instead to methods for indirect estimation. These statistical techniques are able to generate estimates for particular groups or areas using national survey data by borrowing strength from other groups or geographic areas. Indirect estimation has been used to assess prevalence of such phenomena as unemployment (Schaible, 1996), insurance coverage (Yu, Meng, Mendez-Luck, Jhawar, & Wallace, 2007), substance use and abuse (Larson, 2003; Maxwell, 2000), smoking (Twigg & Moon, 2002), obesity (Malec, Sedransk, Moriarity, & LeClere, 1997), and mental disorders (Holzer, Jackson, & Tweed, 1981; Kessler et al., 1998; Messer, Liu, Hoge, Cowan, & Engel, 2004).

Two types of indirect estimation are most frequently used in public mental health inquiry: (1) extrapolating a disorder rate to a population not included in a survey sample (horizontal estimation), and (2) estimating need for a small geographic area that is part of a large-scale survey (vertical estimation or small-area estimation). The latter uses a larger survey to obtain estimates for smaller domains within the survey (e.g., making estimates for a small county using data from a large national survey in which the particular county had few respondents). In contrast, horizontal estimation extrapolates population estimates from a survey of one population to another population of interest (e.g., using a survey in one state to extrapolate to another state), taking advantage of known variations in prevalence based on population categories (Holzer et al., 1981).

Both vertical (Kessler et al., 1998) and horizontal (Holzer et al., 1981; Messer et al., 2004) estimation are used in epidemiologic studies of mental disorders. A number of epidemiologic estimates related to mental and substance use disorders are available on the World Wide Web. For example, state-level estimates for a range of mental health outcomes from the World Health Organization Composite International Diagnostic Interview (described in chapter 4) in the Collaborative Psychiatric Epidemiology surveys are available online at http://66.140.7.153/estimation/estimation.htm. County-level estimates also are available from that site with permission. State and regional estimates of the number of individuals using drugs, all from 2004–2006 iterations of the annual National Survey on Drug Use and Health (NSDUH) of the Substance Abuse and Mental Health Administration, are available online at http://oas.samhsa.gov/substate2k8/toc.cfm. The estimates were conducted using horizontal synthetic procedures and hierarchical Bayesian procedures, respectively, which are described further below.

Three basic approaches to indirect estimation are most commonly used: synthetic estimation, small-area estimation, and composite estimation.

SYNTHETIC ESTIMATION

Using estimates of the association between sociodemographic characteristics and mental disorders from another area, synthetic estimation predicts the rate of disorders in an area with known sociodemographic characteristics but unknown data on mental disorders (Schaible, 1996). A more complex estimator, called a regression estimator, can be used to improve predictions of the proportion of a population with a mental disorder by including categorical characteristics or continuous characteristics (Manton et al., 1985). One type of regression estimator, the regression synthetic estimation approach proposed by Holzer and colleagues (1981), employs logistic regression to do the predictions. This method is particularly helpful for estimating rates for rare, low-prevalence disorders, since subgroups with few or no cases can result in unstable crude rates. However, determining the precision of a synthetic estimate is not always straightforward; methods used to calculate such an estimate's variance include a Taylor series approximation (Yu et al., 2007) and the bootstrap (Knutson, Zhang, & Tabnak, 2008).

In both traditional and regression-based synthetic estimators, the characteristics used to predict mental disorders in the direct survey are assumed similarly to predict mental disorders in the target population (Goldsmith, Lin, Jackson, Manderscheid, & Bell, 1988). For example, if in one area males have higher rates of mental illness than females, it is assumed that males in the areas for which predictions are being made will similarly have higher rates of mental illness than females. Likewise, in vertical estimation, an estimated national-level relationship is assumed to be applicable at the local level (Twigg, Moon, & Jones, 2000). When this assumption does not hold, the resulting estimates are more likely to be inaccurate.

Indirect estimation of mental disorders is most appropriate under a number of specific situations. For example, indirect estimation using the regression synthetic estimator performs best if the predictors in the model are strongly related to mental disorders (Gonzales, Placek, & Scott, 1996; Kessler et al., 1998). However, the choice of predictors usually is driven by their availability in both direct and indirect surveys. Model diagnostics are also crucial. Kessler and colleagues (1998) describe a method using chi-square tests to examine model fit; standard model diagnostics, such as residual analysis and outlier influences, also may be used (Rao, 2003a, 2003b). In addition, an indirect estimate may be improved still further by including contextual effects in addition to demographic characteristics. Twigg and colleagues (2000), for example, used such multilevel modeling (Diez-Roux, 1998) to incorporate both contextual (e.g., community) and individual characteristics in predicting smoking and alcohol consumption in wards in the United Kingdom. Similarly, Kessler and colleagues (1998) used a combined model including individual, aggregate tract-level, and county-level predictors to estimate the proportion of individuals with mental illness within states.

SMALL-AREA ESTIMATION: METHODS THAT BORROW STRENGTH

Another common indirect estimation strategy is to use one geographic area to help learn about another, known as borrowing strength. Two small-area models that can increase the accuracy of an estimate through this strategy (Ghosh & Rao, 1994; Pfeffermann, 2002) are the nested error unit-level regression model (Battese, Harter, & Fuller, 1988) and the area-level random effects model (Fay & Herriot, 1979). The latter uses individual-level characteristics to estimate rates of mental disorders; the former uses group-level characteristics (Pfeffermann, 2002). The nested error regression model arguably is the most popular method of indirect estimation (Singh, Stukel, & Pfeffermann, 1998). This model reduces to a synthetic regression estimator under certain conditions (Malec et al., 1997).

Three other methods have been employed to estimate small-area models: the empirical best linear unbiased predictor (EBLUP), the empirical Bayes method (EB), and the hierarchical Bayes method (HB). EBLUP is best suited for normally distributed outcomes; both EB and HB can be applied to nonnormally distributed outcomes. Bayesian estimation, whether EB or HB, is increasingly popular in the conduct of indirect estimation, particularly vertical estimation, because of its ability to borrow strength (Ghosh & Rao, 1994; Malec et al., 1997). These Bayesian methods typically use additional (prior) information about the parameters of interest in the modeling process. For example, a model might incorporate a prior belief that rates of schizophrenia are unlikely to be greater than 20%. In the EB approach, prior knowledge such as this is driven, at least in part, by the data; in the HB approach, prior knowledge is not data driven (Ghosh & Rao, 1994; Manton et al., 1985). The survey-weighted HB method employed in NSDUH to produce state-level estimates for drug use and serious psychological distress is a classic example of the HB approach (Folsom, Shah, & Vaish, 1999; Wright, Sathe, & Spagnola, 2007; You & Rao, 2003). Several textbooks provide statistical details on how to use these small-area models (Longford, 2005; Rao, 2003a). For a more comprehensive review of small-area estimation techniques, see Longford (2005), Pfeffermann (2002), or Rao (2003a).

COMPOSITE ESTIMATORS

In some cases, both a direct estimate and an indirect estimate are available. For example, an imprecise direct estimate and an indirect estimate obtained using one of the approaches discussed above may be available for a small geographic area. In this case, a composite estimator, created by combining and weighting the values of the two estimates, may be employed (Manton et al., 1985). Alternative composite estimators are distinguished by the choice of weight (Ghosh & Rao, 1994; Singh et al., 1998). For example, in horizontal estimation (what might be thought of as extreme composite estimation), the weight given to the direct estimate is 0, since a direct survey does not exist. As a result, the estimate is dependent strictly on the synthetic estimator. However, more often, the direct and indirect estimates are weighted by their inverse variances to reflect the precision with which each is measured, with greater weight to the more precise one. In the case of composite estimators that incorporate small-area models, both direct and indirect estimates can be weighted instead by the size of the area-level variance relative to the total variance, giving added weight to the direct estimator if the areas are heterogeneous (Ghosh & Rao, 1994; Pfeffermann, 2002).

Composite estimators also can be estimated within a Bayesian framework, as seen in the work of Manton and colleagues (1985), who used EB methods to estimate the prevalence of mental disorders. Use of a Bayesian approach has two major advantages. First, the approach yields an estimate of the posterior variance, a measure that indicates the estimate's precision (Malec et al., 1997). Second, Bayesian approaches generally rely less on the main assumption of horizontal synthetic estimation, namely, that the direct survey's estimated relationships between predictors and mental disorders hold for the target population. However useful, Bayesian estimation also can be complicated and computationally intensive compared with the traditional synthetic estimator (Ghosh & Rao, 1994; Rao, 2003a).

OTHER APPROACHES

Other indirect estimation procedures used in mental health epidemiologic study include demographic profile models (Manton et al., 1985), the National Institute of Mental Health's rank by race, Grosser's model, prevalence variability, Yarvis/Edwards three category, and Slem linear regression. (For additional information, see the review by Ciarlo, Tweed, Shern, Kirkpatrick, & Sachs-Ericsson, 1992.) Yet another technique, spatial smoothing, applied in the study of environmental health–related issues, combines a direct survey and spatial analysis, using information from neighboring areas (Jia, Muennig, & Borawski, 2004). Time series models also can achieve indirect estimates using previously obtained direct survey data (Pfeffermann, 2002).

DATA SOURCES

Each of the analytic methods described in this chapter, of course, relies on the availability of data. Data sources can be classified into three types: nationally representative data sets, selective samples (such as that collected in a randomized trial of a particular intervention), and administrative data (such as Medicare claims or health insurance files). While first providing a brief description of studies using selective samples and administrative data, given the vast number of such studies, this section focuses primarily on nationally representative data sets.

When using any data, it is important to understand where they came from, their original purpose, and whether the proposed use is appropriate. For example, nationally representative data sets may not always provide sufficient detail about population subgroups; in contrast, selective samples or administrative data may not yield estimates that can be generalized to the populations of interest. (See Imai, King, and Stuart [2008] for more discussion of some of these trade-offs.)

Many studies ask and answer research questions by collecting data from a selective sample. Examples include intervention studies such as the Johns Hopkins Center for Prevention and Early Intervention school-based trials (Ialongo et al., 1999) and the Advanced Cognitive Training for Independent and Vital Elderly trial to investigate the effects of cognitive training in older adults (Jobe et al., 2001). Others intensively follow a particular cohort of participants over time, such as the Cache County Study of Memory in Aging (Breitner et al., 1999) and the Great Smoky Mountains Study of mental health service use among children and adolescents in Appalachia (Costello et al., 1996).

Administrative data sources used in public mental health research in the United States include health insurance and Medicare/Medicaid claims files that can provide information on inpatient visits, outpatient visits, and prescriptions filled for individuals in those plans. These data sets often have the benefit of very large sample sizes. Using this type of data, dosReis and colleagues (2008) were able to examine the relationship between continuous antipsychotic treatment and hospitalizations for individuals with schizophrenia. Extensive national mental health registries that link together the administrative sources of data on births, deaths, hospital stays, and crime are available for virtually all individuals in Scandinavian countries, including Denmark and Sweden, and are another important resource. These registries were used in studies by Eaton and colleagues (2004) and Wilcox and colleagues (2010).

Many large surveys have been conducted that provide broad, nationally representative data sets on the prevalence of mental disorders and other public mental health issues (see table 5-3). Most of these surveys are available for use by researchers, sometimes after appropriate clearances or negotiations with the agency or group responsible for initial data collection. Table 5-3 focuses on surveys in the United States, but similar extensive data sources exist in Canada (Gravel & Béland, 2005), the United Kingdom (Jenkins et al., 1997), Australia (Henderson et al., 1993; Jorm, Anstey, Christensen, & Rodgers, 2004), and elsewhere. In fact, the recent World Mental Health 2000 surveys include 28 countries (Demyttenaere et al., 2004).

With a goal of investigating a range of mental disorders across broad populations, many of these data sets are quite diverse in their scope and size. Other data sets, such as the NSDUH (Substance Abuse and Mental Health Services Administration, 2009), focus on particular disorders or behaviors, such as drug abuse and dependence. Still others, such as the Methods for the Epidemiology of Child and Adolescent Mental Disorders (MECA) study (Lahey et al., 1996), focus on the epidemiology of mental disorders in specific populations.

Many of the studies in table 5-3 are representative of the US population or a subset thereof, based on a sampling design that gives each individual in the country some chance of being selected as a subject. A few of the surveys, such as the ECA study (Eaton & Kessler, 1985) and the MECA survey (Lahey et al., 1996), sample from a few geographic areas that are intended to be representative of the United States.

Some of the studies listed, such as the NSDUH, while repeated annually, are technically cross-sectional, since they collect data on different individuals each year. Others, such as the National Longitudinal Surveys conducted by the US Department of Labor (http://www.bls.gov/nls/home.htm), are longitudinal cohort studies, following the same individuals over time. Such longitudinal studies enable researchers to examine more fully both

Table 5-3. US National Data Sets Commonly Used in Public Mental Health

SURVEY	OBJECTIVE	SURVEY PERIOD	TARGET POPULATION
Epidemiologic Catchment Area (ECA) Study[a]	Prevalence of mental disorders and rates of MH service use	1980–1985	US population
National Comorbidity Study (NCS)[a]	Prevalence of mental disorders and rates of MH service use	1990–1992	US household population
National Comorbidity Study—Replication (NCS-R)[a,k]	Prevalence of mental disorders and rates of MH service use	2001–2003	US household population
National Epidemiologic Survey on Alcohol and Related Conditions (NESARC)[b]	Epidemiology of alcohol use disorders and associated health disparities	2001–2005	US household population
National Survey on Drug Use and Health (NSDUH)[c]	Epidemiology of drug use	Annual, 1971–	US household population
National Latino and Asian American Study (NLAAS)[a,c,k]	Mental disorders and MH service use among Latinos and Asian Americans	2002–2003	Latinos and Asian Americans in the US
National Survey of American Life (NSAL)[a,k]	Mental disorders and MH service use among African Americans and Afro-Caribbeans	2001–2003	African American and Afro-Caribbeans in the US
Methods for the Epidemiology of Child and Adolescent Mental Disorders (MECA)[a]	Mental disorders and MH service use among children and adolescents	1991–1992	Children and adolescents in the US
National Ambulatory Medical Care Survey (NAMCS)[d]	Ambulatory medical care use and treatment	Annual, 1973–	Medical care
Midlife Development in the US Survey (MIDUS)[e,f]	Behavioral and psychological factors in physical and mental health	1994–1995	US household population
Youth Risk Behavior Surveillance System (YRBSS)[g]	Health risk behaviors among youth	Biennial, 1991–	High school students
Monitoring the Future (MTF)[h]	Behaviors and attitudes among US youth	Annual, 1975–	8th-, 10th-, and 12th-grade students
National Longitudinal Survey of Youth (NLSY)[i]	Labor force behavior in US	1979–present	US population
Health and Retirement Survey (HRS)[e]	Health behaviors and transitions during and after retirement	Biennial, 1992–	US population

(continued)

Table 5-3. (Continued)

SURVEY	SAMPLE CHARACTERISTICS	SAMPLE SIZE	AGE RANGE (YEARS)	INTERVIEW TOOL	FOLLOW-UP
ECA	Clustered sample of adults living near five university-based sites	20,291	≥18	DIS/DSM-III	Two waves of data collection 12 months apart[j]
NCS	Nationally representative multistage sample	8,098	15–54	UM-CIDI/DSM-III-R	Cross-sectional
NCS-R	Nationally representative multistage sample	9,090	≥18	UM-CIDI/DSM-IV	Cross-sectional
NESARC	Nationally representative sample	43,093	≥18	AUDADIS-IV/DSM-IV	Two waves of data collection (2001–2002, 2004–2005)
NSDUH	Random household sample of nonactive military US civilians	~ 50,000/year	≥12	K6 screen	Cross-sectional, yearly
NLAAS	Nationally representative sample of Latinos and Asian Americans	2,554 Latino; 2,095 Asian American	≥18	WHO-CIDI/DSM-IV	Cross-sectional
NSAL	Nationally representative sample of African American, Afro-Caribbean, and non-Hispanic white individuals	3,570 African American; 1,623 Afro-Caribbean; 1,006 non-Hispanic white	≥18	WHO-CIDI/DSM-IV	Cross-sectional
MECA	Random samples of children at four sites in the US	1,285	9–17	DISC/DSM-III-R	Cross-sectional
NAMCS	Nationally representative sample of patient visits to physician's offices	~ 25,000 visits/year	All ages	Clinical diagnosis	Cross-sectional, yearly

Survey	Sample	N	Age	Instrument	Data collection
MIDUS	Nationally representative random-digit-dial sample of noninstitutionalized household adults	5,900	25–74	Interviewer- and self-administered cognitive and psychological instruments	Two waves of data collection (1994–1995, 2004–2006)
YRBSS	Nationally representative multistage sample of students in private and public schools	~14,000/year	9th- through 12th-grade students	Standardized self-administered school-based survey	Cross-sectional in each year
MTF	Nationally representative stratified multistage clustered area probability sample	~50,000/year	8th-, 10th-, and 12th-grade students	Standardized self-administered school-based survey	Cross-sectional in each year
NLSY	Nationally representative multistage sample	12,686	14–22	Surveys standardized in each year	Annually from 1979 to 1994; biennially since 1994
HRS	Nationally representative stratified multistage clustered area probability sample of retirees	31,022	≥50	Standardized interviewer- and telephone-administered forms	Longitudinal follow-up of existing participants and open recruitment for new participants

For further information about these studies, please refer to http://www.icpsr.umich.edu/. MH = mental health; DIS = Diagnostic Interview Schedule (Anthony et al., 1985); DSM-III = *Diagnostic and Statistical Manual of Mental Disorders*, third edition (APA, 1980); UM-CIDI = University of Michigan Version of the Composite International Diagnostic Interview (Kessler et al., 1994, 1998); DSM-III-R = DSM-III, revised (APA, 1987); DSM-IV = DSM, fourth edition (APA, 1994); AUDADIS-IV = Alcohol Use Disorders and Associated Disabilities Interview Schedule-IV (Grant et al., 2003); K6 screen = 6-item version of a screening instrument for serious mental disorders (SMI; Kessler, 2002, 2003); WHO-CIDI = World Health Organization's Composite International Diagnostic Interview (Robins et al., 1988); DISC = Diagnostic Interview Schedule for Children (Shaffer et al., 2000).

Funded by [a]National Institute of Mental Health, [b]National Institute on Alcohol Abuse and Alcoholism, [c]Substance Abuse and Mental Health Services Administration, [d]National Center for Health Statistics, [e]National Institute on Aging, [f]MacArthur Midlife Research Network, [g]Centers for Disease Control, [h]National Institute on Drug Abuse, [i]US Department of Labor. The Baltimore ECA site was followed up in 1993–1996 and 2004–2005. Participant rosters from all sites were checked against the National Death Index (National Center for Health Statistics, 1997) as recently as 2009 to gather information about mortality. [k]Together, the NCS-R, NLAAS, and NSAL are sometimes referred to as the Collaborative Psychiatric Epidemiology Surveys.

individual change over time and predictors of behaviors and outcomes. For example, such studies can examine the natural history of individuals with bipolar disorder to determine its syndromal stability or the relative amount of time during which an individual experiences depressed, hypomanic, or no symptoms (Judd et al., 2002). Cross-sectional surveys are less expensive and easier to conduct, since they do not follow the same individuals over time. However, they only permit investigation of differences within the groups sampled. Moreover, because they provide no data bearing on how a single individual may change over time, cross-sectional studies provide no insight into the stability of the course of a mental disorder. Nonetheless, cross-sectional studies that employ the same methodology each year, such as the NSDUH, can help describe ecological trends in behaviors and disorders over time.

CONCLUSIONS

This chapter has explored a number of epidemiologic and statistical challenges and solutions associated with asking and answering questions in public mental health. New challenges and opportunities to resolve them will continue to emerge as the field advances.

The dearth of standardized measures for most mental disorders remains an important ongoing challenge to the conduct of public mental health research. As amply demonstrated in this chapter, different studies have employed different measures to collect data, thereby limiting direct comparison of results across surveys and samples (Regier et al., 1998). Greater consistency of measures, achieved, perhaps, through the establishment of a core set of measures, would be an important advance, as would an increased number of statistical methods to combine measures across surveys.

Other challenges that need to be addressed are more central and specific to particular questions within public mental health inquiry. For example, in studying late-life mental health, it becomes more difficult to detect effects of earlier interventions, since individuals have had a vast array of exposures over their lifetimes. Yet another challenge when studying older adults is the issue of competing risks. For example, many individuals do not develop dementia simply because they die of other causes before dementia can become manifest. Genetic analyses, too, pose particular challenges not addressed in detail in this chapter. For example, genetic association studies are particularly affected by the issue of multiple comparisons, and methods have been developed for the situation of testing thousands of genes within one study (Storey & Tibshirani, 2003). (See chapter 8 for more discussion of quantitative methods for genetic analyses in mental health.)

The field of public mental health has contributed to many major advances in statistical methods as researchers have worked to devise solutions to some of its particular challenges. With many challenges remaining in the development of statistical methods for epidemiologic study, it is likely that important statistical advances will continue to be made by ongoing public mental health inquiry.

REFERENCES

Altman, D. G., Schulz, K. F., Moher, D., Egger, M., Davidoff, F., Elbourne, D., & Lang, T. (2001). The revised CONSORT statement for reporting randomized trials: Explanation and elaboration. *Annals of Internal Medicine, 134*(8), 663–694.

American Psychiatric Association. (1980). *Diagnostic and statistical manual of mental disorders* (3rd ed.). Washington, DC: Author.

American Psychiatric Association. (1987). *Diagnostic and statistical manual of mental disorders* (3rd ed., rev.). Washington, DC: Author.

American Psychiatric Association. (1994). *Diagnostic and statistical manual of mental disorders* (4th ed.). Washington, DC: Author.

Angrist, J., Imbens, G., & Rubin, D. (1996). Identification of causal effects using instrumental variables. *Journal of the American Statistical Association, 91,* 444–445.

Anthony, J. C., Folstein, M., Romanoski, A. J., Von Korff, M. R., Newstadt, G. R., Chahal, R., ...Gruenberg, E.M. (1985). Comparison of the lay Diagnostic Interview Schedule and a standardized psychiatric diagnosis. *Archives of General Psychiatry, 42,* 66–675.

Bandeen-Roche, K., Miglioretti, D. L., Zeger, S. L., & Rathouz, P. (1997). Latent variable regression for multiple discrete outcomes. *Journal of the American Statistical Association, 92,* 1375–1386.

Bartholomew, D. J., & Knott, M. (1999). *Latent variable models and factor analysis.* London, UK: Hodder Arnold Publications.

Battese, G. E., Harter, R. M., & Fuller, W. A. (1988). An error-components model for prediction of county crop areas using survey and satellite data. *Journal of the American Statistical Association, 83,* 28–36.

Beck, A. T., Steer, R. A., & Brown, G. K. (1996). *Manual for Beck Depression Inventory-II.* San Antonio, TX: Psychological Corporation.

Benjamini, Y., & Hochberg, Y. (1995). Controlling the false discovery rate: A practical and powerful approach to multiple testing. *Journal of the Royal Statistical Society, 57,* 289–300.

Berkson, J. (1946). Limitations of the application of fourfold table analysis to hospital data. *Biometrics Bulletin, 2*(3), 47–53.

Bickman, L., Guthrie, P. R., Foster, E. M., Lambert, E. W., Summerfelt, W., Breda, C., & Heflinger, C. A. (1995). *Managed care in mental health: The Fort Bragg experiment.* New York, NY: Plenum.

Biglan, A., Ary, D. V., & Wagenaar, A. C. (2000). The value of interrupted time-series experiments for community intervention research. *Prevention Science, 1,* 31–49.

Bock, R. D. (1997). A brief history of item response theory. *Educational Measurement: Issues and Practice, 16,* 21–33.

Bollen, K. A. (2002). Latent variables in psychology and the social sciences. *Annual Review of Psychology, 53,* 605–634.

Boult, C., Reider, L., Frey, K., Leff, B., Boyd, C. M., Wolff, J. L., & Scharfstein, D. (2008). Early effects of "Guided Care" on the quality of health care for multimorbid older persons: A cluster-randomized controlled trial. *Journals of Gerontology, Series A: Biological Sciences and Medical Sciences, 63*(3), 321–327.

Bradshaw, C. P., Koth, C. W., Thornton, L. A., & Leaf, P. J. (2009). Altering school climate through school-wide positive behavioral interventions and supports: Findings from a group-randomized effectiveness trial. *Prevention Science, 10*(2), 100–115.

Breitner, J. C. S., Wyse, B. W., Anthony, J. C., Welsh-Bohmer, K. A., Steffens, D. C., Norton, M., & Khachaturian, A. (1999). APOE-epsilon 4 count predicts age when prevalence of Alzheimer's disease increases—then declines: The Cache County Study. *Neurology, 52*(2), 321–331.

Callahan, C. M., Boustani, M. A., Unverzagt, F. W., Austrom, M. G., Damush, T. M., Perkins, A. J., &

Hendrie, H. C. (2006). Effectiveness of collaborative care for older adults with Alzheimer disease in primary care: A randomized controlled trial. *Journal of the American Medical Association, 295*(18), 2148–2157.

Cannon, M., Huttunen, M., & Murray, R. (2002). The developmental epidemiology of psychiatric disorders. In T. Tsuang and M. Tohen (Eds.), *Textbook in psychiatric epidemiology* (2nd ed., pp. 239–255). New York, NY: John Wiley & Sons.

Ciarlo, J. A., Tweed, D. L., Shern, D. L., Kirkpatrick, L. A., & Sachs-Ericsson, N. (1992). I. Validation of indirect methods to estimate need for mental health services: Concepts, strategy, and general conclusions. *Evaluation and Program Planning, 15,* 115–131.

Collins, L. M., & Wugalter, S. E. (1992). Latent class models for stage-sequential dynamic latent variables. *Multivariate Behavioral Research, 27,* 131–157.

Cook, T. D. (2008). Waiting for life to arrive: A history of the regression-discontinuity design in psychology, statistics and economics. *Journal of Econometrics, 142,* 636–654.

Corballis, M. C., & Traub, R. E. (1970). Longitudinal factor analysis. *Psychometrika, 35,* 79–98.

Costello, E. J., Angold, A., Burns, B. J., Stangl, D. K., Tweed, D. L., Erkanli, A., & Worthman, C. M. (1996). The Great Smoky Mountains study of youth: Goals, design, methods, and the prevalence of DSM-III-R disorders. *Archives of General Psychiatry, 53*(12), 1129–1136.

Curran, P. J., & Hussong, A. M. (2003). The use of latent trajectory models in psychopathology research. *Journal of Abnormal Psychology, 112*(4), 526–544.

Demirtas, H. (2005). Multiple imputation under Bayesianly smoothed pattern-mixture models for nonignorable drop-out. *Statistics in Medicine, 24*(15), 2345–2363.

Demyttenaere, K., Bruffaerts, R., Posada-Villa, J., Gasquet, I., Kovess, V., Lepine, J. P.,...Wang, P. S. (2004). Prevalence, severity, and unmet need for treatment of mental disorders in the World Health Organization World Mental Health Surveys. *Journal of the American Medical Association, 291*(21), 2581–2590.

Diez-Roux, A. (1998). Bringing context back into epidemiology: Variables and fallacies in multilevel analysis. *American Journal of Public Health, 88*(2), 216–222.

Dolan, L. J., Kellam, S. G., Brown, C. H., Werthamer-Larsson, L., Rebok, G. W., Mayer, L. S., ...Wheeler, L. (1993). The short-term impact of two classroom-based preventive interventions on aggressive and shy behaviors and poor achievement. *Journal of Applied Developmental Psychology, 14,* 317–345.

Donner, A., & Klar, N. (2000). *Design and analysis of cluster randomised trials in health research.* London, UK: Arnold.

dosReis, S., Johnson, E., Steinwachs, D., Rohde, C., Skinner, E. A., Fahey, M., & Lehman, A. F. (2008). Antipsychotic treatment patterns and hospitalizations among adults with schizophrenia. *Schizophrenia Research, 101*(1–3), 304–311.

Dunson, D. B. (2003). Dynamic latent trait models for multidimensional longitudinal data. *Journal of the American Statistical Association, 98,* 555–563.

Eaton, W. (1985). The epidemiology of schizophrenia. *Epidemiologic Reviews, 7,* 105–126.

Eaton, W. (1991). Update on the epidemiology of schizophrenia. *Epidemiologic Reviews, 13,* 320–328.

Eaton, W. W., Anthony, J. C., Tepper, S., & Dryman, A. (1992). Psychopathology and attrition in the Epidemiologic Catchment Area surveys. *American Journal of Epidemiology, 135*(9), 1051–1059.

Eaton, W. W., Dryman, A., Sorenson, A., & McCutcheon, A. (1989). DSM-III major depressive disorder in the community: A latent class analysis of data from the NIMH Epidemiologic Catchment Area programme. *British Journal of Psychiatry, 155,* 48–54.

Eaton, W. W., & Kessler, L. G. (1985). *Epidemiologic field methods in psychiatry: The NIMH Epidemiologic Catchment Area program.* New York, NY: Academic Press.

Eaton, W. W., Mortensen, P. B., Agerbo, E., Byrne, M., Mors, O., & Ewald, H. (2004). Coeliac disease and schizophrenia: Population based case control study with linkage of Danish national registers. *British Medical Journal, 328*(7437), 438–439.

Eaton, W. W., Regier, D. A., Locke, B. Z., & Taube, C. A. (1981). The Epidemiologic Catchment Area program of the NIMH. *Public Health Reports, 96*(4), 319–325.

Eldridge, S. M., Ashby, D., & Kerry, S. (2006). Sample size for cluster randomized trials: Effect of coefficient of variation of cluster size and analysis method. *International Journal of Epidemiology, 35,* 1292–1300.

Ensminger, M. E., Anthony, J. C., & McCord, J. (1997). The inner city and drug use: Initial findings from an epidemiological study. *Drug and Alcohol Dependence, 48*(3), 175–184.

Eysenck, H. J. (1992). Four ways five factors are not basic. *Personality and Individual Differences, 13,* 667–673.

Fay, R. E., & Herriot, R. A. (1979). Estimates of income for small places: An application of James-Stein procedures to census data. *Journal of the American Statistical Association, 74,* 269–277.

Flay, B. R. (1986). Efficacy and effectiveness trials (and other phases of research) in the development of health promotion programs. *Preventive Medicine, 15*(5), 451–474.

Flay, B. R., Biglan, A., Boruch, R. F., Gonzalez Castro, F., Gottfredson, D., Kellam, S., ...Ji, P. (2005). Standards of evidence: Criteria for efficacy, effectiveness and dissemination. *Prevention Science, 6*(3), 151–175.

Fleming, J. A., & Hsieh, C.-C. (2002). Introduction to epidemiologic research methods. In M. T. Tsuang & M. Tohen (Eds.), *Textbook in psychiatric epidemiology* (2nd ed., pp. 3–33). New York, NY: John Wiley & Sons.

Folsom, R. E., Shah, B., & Vaish, A. (1999). Substance abuse in states: A methodological report on model based estimates from the 1994–1996 National Household Surveys on Drug Abuse. In *Proceedings of the 1999 Joint Statistical Meetings, American Statistical Association, Survey Research Methods Section* (pp. 371–375). Alexandria, VA: American Statistical Association.

Foster, E. M. (2000). Is more better than less? An analysis of children's mental health services. *Health Services Research, 35*(5, Pt. 2), 1135–1158.

Frangakis, C. E., & Rubin, D. B. (2002). Principal stratification in causal inference. *Biometrics, 58*(1), 21–29.

Furr-Holden, C. D. M., Smart, M. J., Pokorni, J. P., Ialongo, N. S., Holder, H., & Anthony, J. C. (2008). The NIfETy method for environmental assessment of neighborhood-level indicators of alcohol and other drug exposure. *Prevention Science, 9*(4), 245–255.

Gallo, J. J., Anthony, J. C., & Muthén, B. O. (1994). Age differences in the symptoms of depression: A latent trait analysis. *Journal of Gerontology, 49*(6), 251–264.

Ghosh, M., & Rao, J. N. K. (1994). Small area estimation: An appraisal. *Statistical Science, 9,* 55–76.

Gibbons, R. D., Brown, C. H., Hur, K., Marcus, S. M., Bhaumik, D. K., Erkens, J. A., ...Mann, J. J. (2007). Early evidence on the effects of regulators' suicidality warnings on SSRI prescriptions and suicide in children and adolescents. *American Journal of Psychiatry, 164*(9), 1356–1363.

Goldsmith, H. F., Lin, E., Jackson, D. J., Manderscheid, R. W., & Bell, R. A. (1988). The future of mental health needs assessment. In H. F. Goldsmith, E. Lin, R. A. Bell, & D. J. Jackson (Eds.), *Needs assessment: Its future* (pp. 79–93). Washington, DC: US Government Printing Office.

Goldstein, H. (1995). *Multilevel statistical models* (2nd ed.). London, UK: Arnold.

Gonzales, J. F., Placek, P. J., & Scott, C. (1996). Synthetic estimation in followback surveys at the National Center for Health Statistics. In W. L. Schaible (Ed.), *Indirect estimators in U.S. federal programs* (pp. 16–27). New York, NY: Springer.

Graham, J. W. (2009). Missing data analysis: Making it work in the real world. *Annual Review of Psychology, 60*, 549–576.

Grant, B. F., Dawson, D. A., Stinson, F. S., Chou, P. S., Kay, W., & Pickering, R. (2003). The Alcohol Use Disorder and Associated Disabilities Interview Schedule-IV (AUDADIS-IV): reliability of alcohol consumption, tobacco use, family history of depression and psychiatric diagnostic modules in a general population sample. *Drug and Alcohol Dependence, 71*, 7–16.

Gravel, R., & Béland, Y. (2005). The Canadian Community Health Survey: Mental health and well-being. *Canadian Journal of Psychiatry, 50*(10), 573–579.

Grodstein, F., Clarkson, T. B., & Manson, J. E. (2003). Understanding the divergent data on postmenopausal hormone therapy. *New England Journal of Medicine, 348*(7), 645–650.

Gross, A. L., Gallo, J. J., & Eaton, W. W. (2010). Depression and subsequent cancer risk: 24 years of follow-up of the Baltimore Epidemiologic Catchment Area sample. *Cancer Causes and Control, 21*(2), 191–199.

Groves, R. M., Fowler, F. J., Jr., Couper, M. P., Lepkowski, J. M., Singer, E., & Tourangeau, R. (2009). *Survey methodology* (2nd ed.). Hoboken, NJ: John Wiley & Sons.

Harder, V. S., Stuart, E. A., & Anthony, J. C. (2008). Adolescent cannabis problems and young adult depression: Male–female stratified propensity score analyses. *American Journal of Epidemiology, 168*(6), 592–601.

Haviland, A., Nagin, D. S., & Rosenbaum, P. R. (2007). Combining propensity score matching and group-based trajectory analysis in an observational study. *Psychological Methods, 12*(3), 247–267.

Hayden, K. M., Zandi, P. P., Khachaturian, A. S., Szekely, C. A., Fotuhi M., Norton, M. C., ... Welsh-Bohmer, K. A. (2007). Does NSAID use modify cognitive trajectories in the elderly? The Cache County Study. *Neurology, 69*(3), 275–282.

Henderson, A. S., Jorm, A. F., Mackinnon, A. J., Christensen, H., Scott, L. R., Korten, A. E., & Doyle, C. (1993). The prevalence of depressive disorders and the distribution of depressive symptoms in later life: A survey using draft ICD-10 and DSM-III-R. *Psychological Medicine, 23*(3), 719–729.

Henry, K. L., & Huizinga, K. L. (2007). Truancy's effect on the onset of drug use among urban adolescents placed at risk. *Journal of Adolescent Health, 40*(4), e9–e17.

Holzer, C. E., Jackson, D. J., & Tweed, D. (1981). Horizontal synthetic estimation: A strategy for estimating small area health-related characteristics. *Evaluation and Program Planning, 4*, 29–34.

Horvitz, D. G., & Thompson, D. J. (1952). A generalization of sampling without replacement from a finite universe. *Journal of the American Statistical Association, 47*, 663–685.

Ialongo, N., Poduska, J., Werthamer, L., & Kellam, S. (2001). The distal impact of two first grade preventive interventions on conduct problems and disorder in early adolescence. *Journal of Emotional and Behavioral Disorders, 9*, 146–160.

Ialongo, N. S., Werthamer, L., Kellam, S. G., Brown, C. H., Wang, S., & Lin, Y. (1999). Proximal impact of two first-grade preventive interventions on the early risk behaviors for later substance abuse, depression, and antisocial behavior. *American Journal of Community Psychiatry, 27*(5), 599–641.

Imai, K., King, G., & Stuart, E. A. (2008). Misunderstandings among experimentalists and observationalists about causal inference. *Journal of the Royal Statistical Society, Series A, 171*, 481–502.

Insel, T. R. (2006). Beyond efficacy: The STAR*D trial. *American Journal of Psychiatry, 163*(1), 5–7.

Jenkins, R., Bebbington, P., Brugha, T., Farrell, M., Gill, B., Lewis, G., ... Petticrew, M. (1997). The National Psychiatric Morbidity surveys of Great Britain: Strategy and methods. *Psychological Medicine, 27*(4), 765–774.

Jia, H., Muennig, P., & Borawski, E. (2004). Comparison of small-area analysis techniques for estimating county-level outcomes. *American Journal of Preventive Medicine, 26*(5), 453–460.

Jo, B. (2008). Causal inference in randomized trials with mediational processes. *Psychological Methods, 13*(4), 314–336.

Jo, B., Asparouhov, T., Muthén, B. O., Ialongo, N. S., & Brown, C. H. (2008). Cluster randomized trials with treatment noncompliance. *Psychological Methods, 13*(1), 1–18.

Jobe, J. B., Smith, D. M., Ball, K., Tennstedt, S. L., Marsiske, M., Willis, S. L., & Kleinman, K. (2001). ACTIVE: A cognitive intervention trial to promote independence in older adults. *Controlled Clinical Trials, 22*(4), 453–479.

Jorm, A. F., Anstey, K. J., Christensen, H., & Rodgers, B. (2004). Gender differences in cognitive abilities: The mediating role of health state and health habits. *Intelligence, 32*, 7–23.

Judd, L. L., Akiskal, H. S., Schettler, P. J., Endicott, J., Maser, J., Solomon, D. A.,…Keller, M. B. (2002). The long-term natural history of the weekly symptomatic status of bipolar I disorder. *Archives of General Psychiatry, 59*(6), 530–537.

Kellam, S. G., & Anthony, J. C. (1998). Targeting early antecedents to prevent tobacco smoking: Findings from an epidemiologically-based randomized field trial. *American Journal of Public Health, 88*(10), 1490–1495.

Kellam, S. G., Brown, C. H., Poduska, J. M., Ialongo, N. S., Wang, W., Toyinbo, P., & Wilcox, H. C. (2008). Effects of a universal classroom behavior management program in first and second grades on young adult behavioral, psychiatric, and social outcomes. *Drug and Alcohol Dependence, 95*(Suppl. 1), S5–S28.

Kessler, R. C., Andrews, G., Colpe, L. J., Hiripi, E., Mroczek, D. K., Normand S. L.,…Zaslavsky, A. M. (2002). Short screening scales to monitor population prevalences and trends in nonspecific psychological distress. *Psychological Medicine, 32*, 959–976.

Kessler, R., Andrews, G., Mroczek, D., Ustun, B., & Wittchen, H.-U. (1998). The World Health Organization Composite International Diagnostic Interview Short-Form (CIDI-SF). *International Journal of Methods in Psychiatric Research, 7*, 171–185.

Kessler, R. C., Barker, P. R., Colpe, L. J., Epstein, J. F., Gfroerer, J. C., Hiripi, E.,…Zaslavsky, A. M. (2003). Screening for serious mental illness in the general population. *Archives of General Psychiatry, 60*, 184–189.

Kessler, R. C., Berglund, P. A., Walters, E. E., Leaf, P. J., Kouzis, A. C., Bruce, M. L., & Schneier, M. A. (1998). A methodology for estimating the 12-month prevalence of serious mental illness. In R. W. Manderscheid & M. J. Henderson (Eds.), *Mental health, United States, 1998* (pp. 99–109). Rockville, MD: Substance Abuse and Mental Health Services Administration, US Department of Health and Human Services.

Kessler, R. C., Demler, O., Frank, R. G., Olfson, M., Pincus, H. A., Walters, E. E., & Zaslavsky, A. M. (2005). Prevalence and treatment of mental disorders, 1990–2003. *New England Journal of Medicine, 352*(24), 2515–2523.

Kessler, R. C., McGonagle, K. A., Zhao, S., Nelson, C. B., Hughes, M., Eshleman, S.,…Kendler, K. S. (1994). Lifetime and 12-month prevalence of DSM-III-R psychiatric disorders in the United States: Results from the National Comorbidity Survey. *Archives of General Psychiatry, 51*, 8–19.

Kessler, R. C., & Walters, E. E. (2002). The National Comorbidity Survey. In M. T. Tsuang & M. Tohen (Eds.), *Textbook in psychiatric epidemiology* (2nd ed., pp. 343–362). New York, NY: John Wiley & Sons.

Kessler, R. C., Zhao, S., Katz, S. J., Kouzis, A. C., Frank, R. G., Edlund, M., & Leaf, P. J. (1999). Past-year use of outpatient services for psychiatric problems in the National Comorbidity Survey. *American Journal of Psychiatry, 156*(1), 115–123.

Kim, J. O., & Mueller, C. W. (1978). *Factor analysis: Statistical methods and practical issues*. Thousand Oaks, CA: Sage.

Kish, L. (1965). *Survey sampling*. New York, NY: John Wiley & Sons.

Knutson, K., Zhang, W., & Tabnak, F. (2008). Applying the small-area estimation method to estimate a population eligible for breast cancer–detection services. *Preventing Chronic Disease, 5*(1), A10.

Kraemer, H. C., Stice, E., Kazdin, A., Offord, D., & Kupfer, D. (2001). How do risk factors work together? Mediators, moderators, and independent, overlapping and proxy risk factors. *American Journal of Psychiatry, 158*(6), 848–856.

Kuh, D., & Ben-Shlomo, Y. (1997). *A life course approach to chronic disease epidemiology*. New York, NY: Oxford University Press.

Lahey, B. B., Flagg, E. W., Bird, H. R., Schwab-Stone, M. E., Canino, G., Dulcan, M. K.,…Regier, D. A. (1996). The NIMH Methods for the Epidemiology of Child and Adolescent Mental Disorders (MECA) study: Background and methodology. *Journal of the American Academy of Child and Adolescent Psychiatry, 35*(7), 855–864.

Landa, R., & Garrett-Mayer, E. (2006). Development in infants with autism spectrum disorders: A prospective study. *Journal of Child Psychology and Psychiatry, 47*(6), 629–638.

Larson, M. D. (2003). Estimation of small-area proportions using covariates and survey data. *Journal of Statistical Planning and Inference, 112*, 89–98.

Leaf, P. J., German, P. S., Spitznagel, E. L., George, L. K., Landsverk, J., & Windle, C. D. (1985). Sampling: The institutional survey. In W. W. Eaton & L. G. Kessler (Eds.), *Epidemiologic field methods in psychiatry: The NIMH Epidemiologic Catchment Area program* (pp. 49–66). Orlando, FL: Academic Press.

Leoutsakos, J.-M. S., Bandeen-Roche, K., Garrett-Mayer, E., & Zandi, P. P. (2011). Incorporating scientific knowledge into phenotype development: Penalized latent class regression. *Statistics in Medicine, 30*(7), 784–798.

Liang, K. Y., & Zeger, S. L. (1986). Longitudinal data analysis using generalized linear models. *Biometrika, 73,* 13–22.

Lilienfeld, D. E., & Stolley, P. D. (1994). *Foundations of epidemiology.* New York, NY: Oxford University Press.

Lohr, S. L. (2009). *Sampling: Design and analysis* (2nd ed.). Pacific Grove, CA: Duxbury.

Longford, N. T. (2005). *Missing data and small-area estimation.* New York, NY: Springer.

Ludwig, J., & Miller, D. L. (2007). Does Head Start improve children's life chances? Evidence from a regression discontinuity design. *Quarterly Journal of Economics, 122,* 159–208.

MacKinnon, D. P. (2008). *Introduction to statistical mediation analysis.* London, UK: CRC Press.

Malec, D., Sedransk, J., Moriarity, C., & LeClere, F. (1997). Small area inference for binary variables in the National Health Survey. *Journal of the American Statistical Association, 92,* 815–826.

Manton, K. G., Holzer, C. E., III, MacKenzie, E., Spitznagel, E., Forsythe, A., & Jackson, D. (1985). Statistical methods for estimating and extrapolating disease prevalence and incidence rates from multisite study. In W. W. Eaton & R. L. Kessler (Eds.), *Epidemiologic field methods in psychiatry: The NIMH Epidemiologic Catchment Area program* (pp. 351–373). Orlando, FL: Academic Press.

March, J. S., Silva, S. G., Compton, S., Shapiro, M., Califf, R., & Krishnan, R. (2005). The case for practical clinical trials in psychiatry. *American Journal of Psychiatry, 162*(5), 836–846.

Mausner, J. S., & Kramer, S. (1985). *Mausner & Bahn epidemiology: An introductory text* (2nd ed.) Philadelphia, PA: W. B. Saunders.

Maxwell, J. C. (2000). Methods for estimating the number of "hardcore" drug users. *Substance Use and Misuse, 35*(3), 399–420.

McArdle, J. J. (2009). Latent variable modeling of differences and changes with longitudinal data. *Annual Review of Psychology, 60,* 577–605.

McConnell, S., Stuart, E. A., & Devaney, B. (2008). The truncation-by-death problem: What to do in an experimental evaluation when the outcome is not always defined. *Evaluation Research, 32*(2), 157–186.

McCrae, R. R. (1991). The five-factor model and its assessment in clinical settings. *Journal of Personality Assessment, 57*(3), 399–414.

McCrae, R. R., & Costa, P. T. (1992). Four ways five factors are basic. *Personality and Individual Differences, 13,* 653–665.

Menard, C. B., Bandeen-Roche, K. J., & Chilcoat, H. D. (2004). Epidemiology of multiple childhood traumatic events: Child abuse, parental psychopathology and other family-level stressors. *Social Psychiatry and Psychiatric Epidemiology, 39*(11), 857–865.

Messer, S. C., Liu, X., Hoge, C. W., Cowan, D. N., & Engel, C. C. (2004). Projecting mental disorder prevalence from national surveys to populations-of-interest. *Social Psychiatry and Psychiatric Epidemiology, 39*(6), 419–426.

Miranda, J., Chung, J. Y., Green, B. L., Krupnick, J., Siddique, J., Revicki, D. A., & Belin, T. (2003). Treating depression in predominantly low-income young minority women. *Journal of the American Medical Association, 290*(1), 57–65.

Mojtabai, R. (2009). Unmet need for treatment of major depression in the United States. *Psychiatric Services, 60*(3), 297–305.

Murray, D. M. (1998). *Design and analysis of group-randomized trials.* New York, NY: Oxford University Press.

Muthén, B. (2001). Latent variable mixture modeling. In G. A. Marcoulides & R. E. Schumacher (Eds.), *New developments and techniques in structural equation modeling* (pp. 1–24). Philadelphia, PA: Lawrence Erlbaum.

Muthén, B. (2008). Latent variable hybrids: Overview of old and new models. In G. R. Hancock & K. M. Samuelsen (Eds.), *Advances in latent variable mixture models* (pp. 1–24). Charlotte, NC: Information Age Publishing.

Muthén, B., Brown, C. H., Masyn, K., Jo, B., Khoo, S. T., Yang, C. C., . . . Liao, J. (2002). General growth mixture modeling for randomized preventive interventions. *Biostatistics, 3*(4), 459–475.

Muthén, B., & Muthén, L. K. (2000). Integrating person-centered and variable-centered analyses: Growth mixture modeling with latent trajectory classes. *Alcoholism: Clinical and Experimental Research, 24*(6), 882–891.

Muthén, L. K., & Muthén, B. O. (2002). How to use a Monte Carlo study to decide on sample size and determine power. *Structural Equation Modeling, 4,* 599–620.

National Center for Health Statistics. (1997). *National Death Index User's Manual.* Washington, DC: Author.

Netemeyer, R., Bentler, P., Bagozzi, R., Cudeck, R., Cote, J., Lehmann, D.,...Ambler, T. (2001). Structural equations modeling. *Journal of Consumer Psychology, 10*(1–2), 83–100.

Olds, D. L., Kitzman, H., Hanks, C., Cole, R., Anson, E., Sidora-Arcoleo, K.,...Bondy, J. (2007). Effects of nurse home visiting on maternal and child functioning: Age-9 follow-up of a randomized trial. *Pediatrics, 120*(4), e832–e845.

Pasamanick, B., Scarpitti, F. R., & Dinitz, S. (1967). *Schizophrenics in the community: An experimental study in the prevention of hospitalization.* New York, NY: Appleton-Century-Crofts.

Pfeffermann, D. (2002). Small area estimation: New developments and directions. *International Statistical Review, 70*(1), 125–143.

Rao, J. N. K. (2003a). *Small area estimation.* New York, NY: John Wiley & Sons.

Rao, J. N. K. (2003b). Some new developments in small area estimation. *Journal of the Iranian Statistical Society, 2,* 145–169.

Raudenbush, S. W., & Bryk, A. S. (2002). *Hierarchical linear models: Applications and data analysis methods* (2nd ed.). London, UK: Sage.

Regier, D. A., Kaelber, C. T., Rae, D. S., Farmer, M. E., Knauper, B., Kessler, R. C., & Norquist, G. S. (1998). Limitations of diagnostic criteria and assessment instruments for mental disorders: Implications for research and policy. *Archives of General Psychiatry, 55*(2), 109–115.

Regier, D. A., Narrow, W. E., Rae, D. S., Manderscheid, R. W., Locke, B. Z., & Goodwin, F. K. (1993). The de facto U.S. mental and addictive disorders service system: Epidemiologic Catchment Area prospective 1-year prevalence rates of disorders and services. *Archives of General Psychiatry, 50*(2), 85–94.

Robins, J., & Greenland, S. (1986). The role of model selection in causal inference from nonexperimental data. *American Journal of Epidemiology, 123*(3), 392–402.

Robins, L. N., Heizer, J. E., Weissman, M., Orvaschel, H., Gruenberg, E., Berk, J .D., & Regier, D. A. (1984). Lifetime prevalence of specific psychiatric disorders in three sites. *Archives of General Psychiatry, 41*(10), 949–958.

Robins, L. N., Wing, J., Wittchen, H. U., Helzer, J. E., Babor, T. F., Burke, J.,...Towle, L. H. (1988). The composite international diagnostic interview. *Archives of General Psychiatry, 45,* 1069–1077.

Rosenbaum, P. R., & Rubin, D. B. (1983). The central role of the propensity score in observational studies for causal effects. *Biometrika, 70,* 41–55.

Rosner, B. (2006). *Fundamentals of biostatistics.* Belmont, CA: Duxbury Press.

Rost, J., & Langeheine, R. (1997). A guide through latent structure models for categorical data. In J. Rost & R. Langeheine (Eds.), *Applications of latent trait and latent class models in the social sciences* (pp. 13–37). Munster, Germany: Waxmann-Verlag.

Rothwell, P. M. (2005). Clinical trials are too often founded on poor quality pre-clinical research. *Journal of Neurology, 252*(9), 1115.

Rubin, D. B. (1973). Matching to remove bias in observational studies. *Biometrics, 29,* 159–184.

Rubin, D. B. (1976). Inference and missing data. *Biometrika, 63,* 581–592.

Rush, A. J., Fava, M., Wisniewski, S. R., Lavori, P. W., Trivedi, M. H., Sackeim, H. A.,...Niederehe, G. (2004). Sequenced Treatment Alternatives to Relieve Depression (STAR*D): Rationale and design. *Controlled Clinical Trials, 25*(1), 119–142.

Samuels, J., Bienvenu, O. J., Cullen, B., Costa, P. T., Jr., Eaton, W. W., & Nestadt, G. (2004). Personality dimensions and criminal arrest. *Comprehensive Psychiatry, 45*(4), 275–280.

Schafer, J. L., & Graham, J. W. (2002). Missing data: Our view of the state of the art. *Psychological Methods, 7*(2), 147–177.

Schaible, W. L. (Ed.) (1996). *Indirect estimators in U.S. federal programs.* New York, NY: Springer.

Shadish, W. R., Cook, T. D., & Campbell, D. T. (2002). *Experimental and quasi-experimental designs for generalized causal inference.* Boston, MA: Houghton-Mifflin.

Shapiro, S., Skinner, E. A., Kessler, L. G., Von Korff, M., German, P. S., Tischler, G. L.,...Regier, D. A. (1984). Utilization of health and mental health services: Three Epidemiologic Catchment Area sites. *Archives of General Psychiatry, 41*(10), 971–978.

Shaffer, D., Fisher, P., Lucas, C. P., Dulcan, M. K., & Schwab-Stone, M. E. (2000). NIMH Diagnostic Interview Schedule for Children Version IV (NIMH DISC-IV): Description, differences from previous versions, and reliability of some common diagnoses. *Journal of the American Academy of Child Adolescent Psychiatry, 39,* 28–38.

Siddique, J., & Belin, T. R. (2008). Using an approximate Bayesian bootstrap to multiply impute nonignorable missing data. *Computational Statistics and Data Analysis, 53,* 405–415.

Singer, J. D., & Willett, J. B. (2003). *Applied longitudinal data analysis.* New York, NY: Oxford University Press.

Singh, A. C., Stukel, D. M., & Pfeffermann, D. (1998). Bayesian versus frequentist measures of error in small area estimation. *Journal of the Royal Statistical Society: Series B (Statistical Methodology)*, 60, 377.

Stein, L. I., & Test, M. A. (1980). Alternative to mental hospital treatment. I. Conceptual model, treatment program, and clinical evaluation. *Archives of General Psychiatry*, 37(4), 392–397.

Storey, J. D., & Tibshirani, R. (2003) Statistical significance for genome-wide studies. *Proceedings of the National Academy of Sciences of the United States of America*, 100(16), 9440–9445.

Stroup, T. S., McEvoy, J. P., Swartz, M. S., Byerly, M. J., Glick, I. D., Canive, J. M., . . . Lieberman, J. A. (2003). The National Institute of Mental Health Clinical Antipsychotic Trials of Intervention Effectiveness (CATIE) project: Schizophrenia trial design and protocol development. *Schizophrenia Bulletin*, 29(1), 15–31.

Stuart, E. A. (2010). Matching methods for causal inference: A review and a look forward. *Statistical Science*, 25(1), 1–21.

Stuart, E. A., & Green, K. M. (2008). Using full matching to estimate causal effects in nonexperimental studies: Examining the relationship between adolescent marijuana use and adult outcomes. *Developmental Psychology*, 44(2), 395–406.

Stuart, E. A., & Ialongo, N. S. (2010). Matching methods for selection of subjects for follow-up. *Multivariate Behavioral Research*, 45(4), 746–765.

Substance Abuse and Mental Health Services Administration. (2009). *National Survey on Drug Use and Health, 2008* [Computer file]. ICPSR26701-v2. Ann Arbor, MI: Inter-university Consortium for Political and Social Research.

Sudman, S. (1976). *Applied sampling*. New York, NY: Academic Press.

Sugai, G., Horner, R., & Gresham, F. (2001). Behaviorally effective school environments. In M. Shinn, G. Stoner, & H. Walker (Eds.), *Interventions for academic and behavior problems: Preventive and remedial approaches* (pp. 315–350). Silver Spring, MD: National Association of School Psychiatrists.

Tomarken, A. J., & Waller, N. G. (2005). Structural equation modeling: Strengths, limitations, and misconceptions. *Annual Review of Clinical Psychology*, 1, 31–65.

Tunis, S. R., Stryer, D. B., & Clancy, C. M. (2003). Practical clinical trials: Increasing the value of clinical research for decision making in clinical and health policy. *Journal of the American Medical Association*, 290(12), 1624–1632.

Tsuang, M. T., & Tohen, M. (Eds.). (2002). *Textbook in psychiatric epidemiology* (2nd ed.). New York, NY: John Wiley & Sons.

Twigg, L., & Moon, G. (2002). Predicting small area health-related behaviour: A comparison of multilevel synthetic estimation and local survey data. *Social Science and Medicine*, 54(6), 931–937.

Twigg, L., Moon, G., & Jones, K. (2000). Predicting small-area health-related behaviour: A comparison of smoking and drinking indicators. *Social Science and Medicine*, 50(7–8), 1109–1120.

US General Accounting Office. (1994). *Breast conservation versus mastectomy: Patient survival in day-to-day medical practice and in randomized studies* (GAO/PEMD-95-9). Report to the Chairman, Subcommittee on Human Resources and Intergovernmental Relations, Committee on Government Operations, House of Representatives. Washington, DC: Author.

van Belle, G., Fisher, L. D., Heagerty, P. J., & Lumley, T. S. (2004). *Biostatistics: A methodology for the health sciences* (2nd ed.). Hoboken, NJ: John Wiley & Sons.

van der Linden, W. J., & Glas, C. A. W. (Eds.). (2000). *Computerized adaptive testing: Theory and practice*. Dordrecht, Netherlands: Kluwer Academic.

Varnell, S. P., Murray, D. M., Janega, J. B., & Blitstein, J. L. (2004). Design and analysis of group-randomized trials: A review of recent practices. *American Journal of Public Health*, 94(3), 393–399.

Wang, P. S., Lane, M., Olfson, M., Pincus, H. A., Wells, K. B., & Kessler, R. C. (2005). Twelve-month use of mental health services in the United States: Results from the National Comorbidity Survey replication. *Archives of General Psychiatry*, 62(6), 590–592.

Watt, N. F., & Saiz, C. (1991). Longitudinal studies of premorbid development of adult schizophrenia. In E. F. Walker (Ed.), *Schizophrenia: A lifecourse developmental perspective* (pp. 157–192). New York, NY: Academic Press.

West, S. G., Duan, N., Pequegnat, W., Gaist, P., Des Jarlais, D. C., Holtgrave, D., . . . Mullen, P. D. (2008). Alternatives to the randomized controlled trial. *American Journal of Public Health*, 98(8), 1359–1366.

Wilcox, H., Kuramoto, S., Lichtenstein, P., Långström, N., Brent, D., & Runeson, B. (2010). Psychiatric morbidity, violent crime and suicide among children exposed to early parental death: Long-term longitudinal population study in Sweden. *Archives of General Psychiatry*, 49(5), 514–523.

Wright, D., Sathe, N., & Spagnola, K. (2007). *State estimates of substance use from the 2004–2005 National Surveys on Drug Use and Health*.

Rockville, MD: Substance Abuse and Mental Health Services Administration, US Department of Health and Human Services. Available at http://oas.samhsa.gov/states.cfm

You, Y., & Rao, J. N. K. (2003). Pseudo-hierarchical Bayes small area estimation combining unit level models and survey weights. *Journal of Statistical Planning and Inference, 111,* 197–208.

Yu, H., Meng, Y., Mendez-Luck, C., Jhawar, M., & Wallace, S. P. (2007). Small-area estimation of health insurance coverage for California legislative districts. *American Journal of Public Health, 97*(4), 731–737.

Zimmerman, S., Sloane, P. D., Eckert, J. K., Gruber-Baldini, A. L., Morgan, L. A., Hebel, J. R., & Chen, C. K. (2005). How good is assisted living? Findings and implications from an outcomes study. *Journals of Gerontology Series B: Psychological Sciences and Social Sciences, 60*(4), 195–204.

SECTION III

DESCRIPTIVE EPIDEMIOLOGY

6

The Population Dynamics
of Mental Disorders

WILLIAM W. EATON

PIERRE ALEXANDRE

RONALD C. KESSLER

SILVIA S. MARTINS

PREBEN BO MORTENSEN

GEORGE W. REBOK

CARLA L. STORR

KIMBERLY ROTH

Key Points

- Population dynamics of mental disorders is the quantitative description of the natural history of psychopathology

- Natural history includes the precursor and prodromal periods, the incidence, remission, course, and consequences

- The combination of prospective data from the Baltimore Epidemiologic Catchment Area follow-up and the National Comorbidity Survey follow-up allows unparalleled insight into natural history of mental disorders

- Incidence data show that most mental disorders have onsets well before middle age

- About 10–20% of mental disorders endure for decades

- There is extensive comorbidity of mental disorders

- Some mental disorders are associated with raised risk for a variety of later-occurring physical conditions, such as diabetes, heart disease, and stroke

• 125

INTRODUCTION

Population dynamics is the study of changes in the size of populations. When applied to mental disorders, it is a population-level description of the natural history of psychopathology. The three key aspects of the natural history of psychopathology are onset, course, and outcome (Eaton, 2011). The ebb and flow of psychopathology sometimes occur rapidly, as in the brief, acute crescendo of fear involved in a panic attack. More often, however, a mental disorder's course is languid, unfolding over days, weeks, months, years, and even decades. Because a large proportion of individuals with mental disorders do not seek treatment, and those who do may well represent the most severe cases, the natural history of psychopathology is best studied with population-based samples in which individuals are selected from the entire general population, without regard to whether they have received treatment or not. This avoids the well-known treatment-seeking bias (Berkson, 1946) as well as prevalence bias (Cohen & Cohen, 1984). The combination of population-based samples and languid evolution of psychopathology favors the approach of life course epidemiology (Kuh & Ben-Shlomo, 1997).

The following section briefly describes data sources and details the methods used in creating population estimates of mental disorders. The focus then turns to a discussion of the onsets, courses, and outcomes of mental illnesses, based on data from the Baltimore Epidemiologic Catchment Area (ECA) follow-up study (Eaton et al., 1997) and the National Comorbidity Survey (NCS) studies (Kessler, 1994; Kessler et al., 1997).

METHODS AND DATA SOURCES

Data pertinent to the population dynamics of specific mental disorders are expensive to gather. Because a minority of individuals, not necessarily representative of those with a particular disorder, get treatment, a field survey is required to obtain representative data for all but the most severe disorders. Moreover, since some significant mental disorders are relatively rare, to estimate population parameters related to onset, course, and outcome, field surveys must evaluate large numbers of individuals, many of whom may not have a specific sign, symptom, syndrome, or disorder at two or more distinct points in time.

Surveys that establish population estimates for severe mental disorders, such as schizophrenia, bipolar disorder, and dementia, are not useful for a number of reasons. Individuals with these disorders frequently lack insight about and the ability to discuss their health status; typical survey interviewers may lack the clinical skills to work with such individuals. Thus population estimates for these disorders often rely on organizations of health care facilities that coordinate their records, often referred to as surveillance systems or, in the mental health field, as psychiatric case registers. As many as two dozen such psychiatric case registers have existed at one time or another (Baldwin & Evans, 1971; Cleverly & Douglas, 1991; de Salvia, Barbato, Salvo, & Zadro, 1993; Dupont, 1979; Goodman, Rahav, Popper, Ginath, & Pearl, 1984; Hall, Robertson, Dorricott, Olley, & Millar, 1973; Herrman, Baldwin, & Christie, 1983; Kieseppa, Partonen, Kaprio, & Lonnqvist, 2000; Kristjansson, Allebeck, & Wistedt, 1987; Krupinski, 1977; Liptzin & Babigian, 1972; Munk-Jorgensen, Kastrup, & Mortensen, 1993; O'Hare, 1987; Selten & Sijben, 1994; ten Horn, Giel, Gulbinat, & Henderson, 1986; Wing, 1989).

The number of prospective field surveys conducted with sufficiently large samples to estimate incidence rates for mental disorders is small. If a sample with 5,000 person-years of observations is set as a minimum requirement, only a handful of field surveys exist that span a variety of disorders, among them the Stirling County study in Canada (Murphy, Monson, Laird, Sobol, & Leighton, 1998), the Traunstein study in Germany (Fichter, 1990), the Swedish Lundby study (Hagnell, Essen-Moller, Lanke, Ojesjo, & Rorsman, 1990), and the NEMESIS study in the Netherlands (Bijl, van Zessen, Ravelli, de Rijk, & Langendoen, 1998). In the United States, relevant studies include the Baltimore ECA follow-up (Eaton et al., 1997), the follow-up to the NCS (NCS-2) (Kessler,

1995), and the National Epidemiologic Study of Alcohol and Related Conditions (NESARC) (Grant, Moore, Shepard, & Kaplan, 2003).

For the common mental disorders, this chapter presents US data from the Baltimore ECA and both the NCS and NCS-2, which have similar lengths of follow-up. In contrast, as described below, published data from surveillance systems rather than from surveys are presented for particularly severe mental disorders (e.g., schizophrenia, bipolar disorder, and dementia).

• *Baltimore ECA*. In 1981, a probability sample of the 175,211 household residents of eastern Baltimore, ages 18 years and older, was selected for participation in the Baltimore site of the ECA program (Eaton & Kessler, 1985). Persons over age 65 were oversampled purposely by designating all members of a household in that age group for interview, in addition to whoever else in the household was designated in the random selection. In all, of the 4,238 persons who composed the sample, 3,481 completed the interview, an 82% completion rate. As noted in chapter 4, the interview was built around the Diagnostic Interview Schedule (DIS) (Robins, Helzer, Croughan, & Ratcliff, 1981). (Version III of the DIS was used in 1981; version III-R (Robins et al, 1989) was used in both 1993 and 2004.) Over a decade later, primarily in 1993, 1,920 of the 2,633 survivors of those interviewed in 1981 were reinterviewed, with a completion rate of 73%. In 2004 and the first half of 2005, 1,071 (74% of survivors) of those interviewed in 1993 were interviewed yet again. Study attrition was cumulative; thus, for example, the 2004 target sample included only those successfully interviewed in 1993 (Eaton, Kalaydjian, Scharfstein, Mezuk, & Ding, 2007).

• *National Comorbidity Survey*. In 1990–1992, a probability sample of 8,098 individuals in the United States, ages 15–54, was identified to participate in a study designed to estimate the prevalence and the impact of mental and behavioral disturbances (Kessler, 1995). The interview, with a completion rate of 82%, was built around the Composite

International Diagnostic Interview (CIDI: Robins et al., 1988)). (See chapter 4 for a detailed discussion.) The NCS divided the interview into two parts: (1) core diagnostic information elicited from each respondent, and (2) diagnostic assessments and information on risk factors administered to a probability subsample of 5,877 respondents, including all persons found to have any disorder in the first part of the interview, all those ages 15–24, and a random sample of others. In 2001–2003, the NCS-2 successfully reinterviewed 5,001 of the 5,877 original respondents in part 2 (87% of survivors) (Swendsen et al., 2009).

The Baltimore ECA and the NCS complement each other in a number of ways. The Baltimore ECA sample is drawn from a single city; in contrast, the NCS is a national probability sample that allows generalization to the US population as a whole. While lacking respondents under age 18, the Baltimore ECA sample extends further along the life span into old age; the NCS sample includes respondents as young as 15 years, but the oldest respondent at the baseline was 54. The ECA includes obsessive–compulsive disorder, an important disorder not included in the NCS. Despite these differences, the populations studied, assessment instruments used, and diagnostic conventions employed are close enough to permit comparison. In addition, both data sets have sufficiently long follow-ups to generate stable incidence rates by age and sex and to avoid what Murphy and colleagues (2000) describe as the incidence interval effect. Both data sets also contain baseline assessments that allow the samples to be stratified into individuals at risk for onset (i.e., who have never met criteria for diagnosis in their lifetime at the baseline assessment), and those not at risk (who have met criteria for diagnosis sometime at or prior to the baseline).

ONSET

Signs and symptoms potentially related to mental disorders are widespread in the population. Because these symptoms do not always reflect the presence of a mental disorder, the evolution of a normal deviation to a pathologic process is difficult to define and to discern. The absence of firm data on both the concepts themselves and their diagnostic boundaries in the classification system mandates that great care be taken in defining disease onset from an operational perspective. From both clinical and population perspectives, the choice of a particular threshold at which a disorder becomes manifest has significant implications. Clinically, subtle differences in one's approach to treatment may give rise to varied thresholds among clinicians. From the epidemiologic standpoint, such subtle threshold differences may produce widely disparate estimates of a disorder's prevalence and incidence.

With those cautions in mind, one may posit that onset occurs when an individual first enters treatment. A related pair of definitions suggest onset occurs either when a symptom is first noticeable by a clinician or when it is first noticed by the affected individual. Under the operational criteria of the fourth edition of the *Diagnostic and Statistical Manual of Mental Disorders* (DSM-IV) (American Psychiatric Association [APA], 1994), it is possible to conceive of onset as the time at which full criteria are met for the first time in the life of the affected individual. This last definition has been used in a host of population-based studies of the incidence of mental disorders (Eaton, Kramer, Anthony, Chee, & Shapiro, 1989).

The time between occurrence of the earliest causal factor and diagnosis of the disorder is sometimes called the etiologically relevant period (Rothman, 1981), which is often longer for mental disorders than for many physical illnesses. During this period, likely aspects of the etiopathic process—such as risk factors and precursor symptoms—become apparent, sometimes long before a disorder or disease becomes irreversibly pathologic. Precise determination of the time of onset is made easier when onset is linked explicitly to clearly defined pathology. In medicine, pathology generally is conceptualized as abnormal functioning of bodily systems and tissue damage. The 19th-century scientist Virchow defined pathology more broadly as a biological process occurring at the wrong place or wrong time in a manner that contributes to the death of the organism (Leighton & Murphy, 1997). For mental disorders, it is useful to expand that definition to specify that pathology includes not only biological but also psychological and social processes and to include among the ultimate results a decline in both individual and social functioning as well as death (Leighton & Murphy, 1997). Thus one may define pathology as arising when the sociobiological dynamics have become abnormal, signifying a change in the relationship among social and environmental variables as well as in the individual's mental and behavioral processes—a sociobiological metabolism that did not exist prior to onset.

The point at which a disease process becomes irreversible is difficult to observe at the individual level. Examining population-based indicators of the force of morbidity, however, leads to the conceptualization of a continuous course of development toward the manifestation of disease, with an as yet unknown point of irreversibility. At present, even the use of the words *symptom* and *sign* is problematic in the strict medical sense, because one can only hypothesize when a disease begins and it is not possible to ascribe the complaint or behavior to the disease with perfect accuracy. In the end, as suggested elsewhere in this volume, studying the natural history of psychopathology may lead to the conclusion that the concepts of disease and pathology of the infectious disease model are either inappropriate or not useful when one is speaking of mental disorders, suggesting the need for a more explicitly developmental framework (Baltes, Reese, & Lipsitt, 1980; McHugh & Slavney, 1998). The emphasis in the developmental framework is on normally distributed characteristics and continuities in development rather than on the rare examples exhibiting the dichotomies and discontinuities that are found in the disease model.

The prodrome is the period during which some signs or symptoms are present but before diagnostic criteria for a disorder are fully met. It begins at the point of irreversibility, that is, when ultimate diagnosis with the disease is inevitable. Because the prodrome exists only among those eventually diagnosed with the disorder, it can be observed with complete certainty only in a retrospective manner. The presence of subclinical signs or symptoms may help identify individuals at increased risk for developing the disorder. However, given the widespread prevalence of individual signs and symptoms of mental disorders in the general population, many individuals with these early signs and symptoms of disorder likely will not develop the full-blown disorder.

Signs and symptoms from a diagnostic cluster that precede disorder but do not predict the onset of disorder with certainty are referred to here as precursor signs and symptoms. Given current understanding of the onset of mental disorders, few if any signs and symptoms predict onset with certainty; future research may improve the ability to identify and intervene with groups at highest risk for onset based on precursor signs and symptoms. Should such precursors be found, the population-attributable risk (PAR) due to these precursors could be calculated to describe the proportion of new cases that might be prevented with effective screening and early intervention among those with such signs and symptoms. Table 6-1 shows ECA data on the one-year prevalence of the precursor signs and symptoms for major depression and on their relative risk in predicting the onset of depressive disorder during the ECA's first year of follow-up (Eaton, Badawi, & Melton, 1995).

Population-attributable risk (PAR) was estimated based on the prevalence (P) of the precursor and the relative risk (RR) for the disorder, comparing individuals with and without the precursor, using the formula PAR = P(RR − 1)/(P(RR − 1) + 1) (Kleinbaum, Kupper, & Morgenstern, 1982). The term *attributable risk* in this context is slightly different conceptually from other uses because of the limited duration of the follow-up. Therefore the duration of the follow-up is used to condition or qualify the phrasing of the attributable risk (e.g., "sleep problems have a 10-year PAR for depressive disorder"). Sleep problems have the highest relative risk (RR = 7.6) and high prevalence (13.6%). In fact, if a single etiologic pathway existed that connects sleep problems to depressive disorder, its elimination would reduce the subsequent occurrence of depressive disorder by 47%. Depression syndrome (sad mood or anhedonia, plus two or more other symptoms) also has a high relative risk (RR = 5.7). However, because its prevalence is so low (0.5%), its elimination would reduce the subsequent occurrence of depressive disorder by only 2%. The prevention potential inherent in precursor signs and symptoms, as discussed above, has been applied to depression (Dryman & Eaton, 1991; Horwath, Johnson, Klerman, & Weissman, 1992) and is applicable to most disorders.

Table 6-1. One-Year Prevalence of Precursor, Relative Risk, and One-Year Precursor-Attributable Risk for Symptoms of Depressive Disorder

SYMPTOM GROUP	PREVALENCE (%)	RELATIVE RISK	PRECURSOR-ATTRIBUTABLE RISK (%)
Sadness	6.6	7.0	28
Loss of interest	2.2	3.5	5
Weight or appetite	10.4	3.0	17
Sleep problems	13.6	7.6	47
Fatigue	7.9	4.0	19
Psychomotor problems	4.4	5.3	16
Concentration	5.5	6.1	22
Guilt	3.2	10.4	23
Suicidal ideation	12.1	6.8	41
Depression syndrome	0.5	5.7	2

Based on data from four sites of the NIMH Epidemiologic Catchment Area Program.
Source: Eaton et al., 1995.

Comorbidity among mental disorders complicates the study of onset but provides possibilities for prevention. In comorbid cases, it is typical for one disorder to begin earlier than another, yielding the distinction between temporally primary and secondary disorders. Prevention or treatment of early-occurring primary disorders may prevent secondary disorders (Kessler & Price, 1993). Table 6-2 displays how this might happen, using the stem items in the CIDI as potential screens for prevention purposes in the NCS panel.

Positive responses to the stem questions—which, in this interpretation, ask about the presence of precursors—are both prevalent in the population and associated with non-trivial relative risks for the primary disorders 10 years later (see the left side of table 6-2). For example, if persons who responded positively to the stem question for panic disorder ("feeling frightened, anxious or very uneasy in situations in which most people would not be afraid") but who nonetheless did not meet full criteria for a diagnosis of panic disorder in the baseline NCS could have been located and treated with 100% success, and if the relative risk of this predictor was due to the causal effects of the precursor, then 31% of the subsequent onset of panic disorder would have been prevented. Using the same logic, a 100% successful screening and prevention program for major depressive disorder, based on screening for precursors, might prevent as much as 41% of the subsequent onsets.

The right side of table 6-2 shows a similar positive impact of stem items on the full range of secondary disorders considered in the NCS. The row showing 10-year population-attributable risks due to precursors associated with the stem items for major depressive disorder is particularly impressive. By interrupting the etiologic chain from first symptom onset to diagnosable disorder, 44% of panic disorder, 45% of posttraumatic stress disorder, and 37% of drug abuse or dependence might be prevented.

Incidence, the rate at which new cases of a disease occur, is the population equivalent of the crescendo in the process of onset in the individual and expresses the force of morbidity in a population. It is estimated using a numerator of new cases and a denominator of persons at risk for becoming new cases during an articulated period (Lilienfeld & Stolley, 1994). In psychiatric epidemiology, persons at risk are usually defined as those individuals with no history of the disorder over their lifetime up to and including the present. Thus incidence may be termed with greater precision *first lifetime incidence*. Use of the word *rate* demands a specification of a particular time orientation. For example, an annual rate of incidence might be specified as 3 cases per 1,000 persons exposed for 1 year.

Connecting the force of morbidity to individual and environmental characteristics is more likely to identify powerful clues to etiology than are studies of prevalence, in which risk factors can influence the chronicity of pathology as well as its genesis—hence the interest in avoiding so-called prevalence bias (Cohen & Cohen, 1984). Thus this chapter explores the force of morbidity over the life course, with age as the predominant risk factor for disease. Showing how this force changes over the life span may demonstrate the ebb and flow of the risk structure and may help identify etiologic subtypes associated with both environmental and developmentally timed influences. As a result of these findings, primary prevention may be targeted toward peak periods of the force of morbidity and risk.

Estimation of incidence presents certain unusual problems in multiwave field surveys. Once it has been determined that sometime during the lifetime, the full diagnostic criteria were met, the analyst must decide whether to define onset as the first time the criteria were met, the time at which the initial syndromal spell occurred, the time of the first sign or symptom, or the time at which some other criterion occurred. In what follows, consistent with earlier work (Eaton et al., 1997, 2007; Eaton, Kramer, Anthony, Chee, & Shapiro, 1989; Eaton, Kramer, Anthony, Dryman, et al., 1989), onset is defined as the first occurrence of a syndromal spell (the first time symptoms clustered together) in persons who, sometime later, reached full diagnostic criteria. Age of onset is then obtained by asking a question related to a symptom cluster. For example, in the case of depressive disorder, the question

Table 6-2. Prevalence of Precursor, Relative Risk, And Precursor-Attributable Risk for Common Primary and Secondary Mental Disorders

	PREDICTING PRIMARY DISORDER			POPULATION-ATTRIBUTABLE RISK PREDICTING SECONDARY DISORDER					
	LIFETIME PREVALENCE	RELATIVE RISK	PAR	PANIC	ANY PHOBIA	PTSD	MAJOR DEPRESSION	ALCOHOL ABUSE/ DEPENDENCE	DRUG ABUSE/ DEPENDENCE
Panic stem (felt frightened, anxious, or very uneasy)[a]	0.24	2.9	0.31	0.31	0.16	0.22	0.09	0.05	0.16
Any social phobia stem (speaking in public, etc.)[b]	0.29	1.2	0.05	0.15	0.08	0.05	*	0.08	0.10
Any specific phobia stem (heights, flying, etc.)[c]	0.46	2.9	0.47	0.24	0.29	0.22	0.12	0.04	0.08
Any PTSD stem (remembering event, dreams, etc.)[d]	0.33	3.0	0.40	0.21	0.14	0.40	0.12	0.03	0.21
Any MDD stem (sad for two weeks, etc.)[e]	0.49	2.4	0.41	0.44	0.31	0.45	0.41	0.20	0.37
Alcohol stem (started drinking early)[f]	0.13	1.4	0.05	0.00	0.00	0.03	*	0.05	0.24
Any drug stem (sedatives, inhalants, etc.)[g]	0.44	2.9	0.46	0.24	0.08	0.12	0.15	0.26	0.46
Total number of new cases	—	—	—	236	712	215	527	518	191

Based on National Comorbidity Survey (1990–1992) and National Comorbidity Survey Follow-up (2001–2003) (N = 5,001). PAR = population-attributable risk; PTSD = posttraumatic stress disorder; MDD = major depressive disorder.

Disorders recognized based on the following stem items from the Composite International Diagnostic Interview: [a]V301; [b]V402–V406; [c]V501–V510; [d]V6217–V6220; V308–V310; [e]V1817, V1825, V1833, V1841, V1901, V1907, V1913, V1919, V1925); [f]V1801 ≤ 13; [g]V1801 ≤ 13.

*Population-attributable risk not estimable because relative risk was less than 1.0.

might be "When was the first time you felt sad [or respondent's equivalent phrase] for 2 weeks or more and had some of these other problems like [interviewer lists problems mentioned earlier as occurring over the life span, such as lost appetite, sleeplessness, and loss of concentration]?"

Inevitable discrepancies in the timing of syndrome onset across study waves can also complicate the operational definition of onset in multiwave surveys of psychopathology. Respondents' recollections of first onset can vary across waves; a person might first claim no symptoms before baseline and in a later wave recall a prestudy episode. Such conflicting recollections could be due to a slow course of onset or to a heightened awareness of past symptoms following full onset. In such a case, the contradiction is resolved by accepting as correct both the baseline response that no episode had occurred and the follow-up response that an episode did occur, without accepting the cited date of onset. The logic underlying this resolution is that reports closer in time to the event at issue are more likely to be accurate than reports requiring long-term recollection. However, this solution yields a conundrum about dating the onset of an episode that is reported in the follow-up wave to pre-date the baseline. The resolution is to specify such onsets as occurring in the median year between baseline and the later report of onset (usually the age of the respondent at around halfway through the follow-up period). No adjustment is made for the discrepancy in the recalled date of onset.

Since at-risk and not-at-risk groups are defined at the baseline assessment and new cases are defined at follow-up, the analyses presented here might be thought of as grounded in prospective design. At the same time, however, the analyses might be considered retrospective, since respondents are asked to recall the year of the onset during the previous 10 (NCS) or 12 (ECA) years. Thus the analysis, as with many other studies labeled as prospective, might best be described as quasiprospective. This mixed design has a distinct advantage over cross-sectional studies in which age of onset is estimated retrospectively for the entire lifetime of the individual.

In cross-sectional studies, older respondents are more likely to have forgotten episodes from decades earlier in their lives. Further, since individuals with the most severe early episodes are more likely to recall them, the ensuing study bias may estimate fewer episodes and earlier onset than actually occurs. On the other hand, older people, particularly those with cognitive decline, may forget all but the most recent episodes, creating a bias in the opposite direction. Currently, no agreed-upon procedure exists either for estimating or for understanding these biases in cross-sectional studies, supporting the decision to use a quasiprospective approach. It is helpful that the two data sets considered here have roughly similar periods of recall.

At first glance, it may seem problematic to establish a date of onset prior to the youngest age of participants at baseline (15 years in the NCS, 18 in the ECA). However, it can be assumed that no onsets of mental disorders occur before an arbitrarily chosen age—say, 5 years. In this situation, it is an advantage that the youngest age of respondents in the NCS is 15 years. The choice of these ages establishes an equal respondent recall period across all ages, including the youngest. For respondents age 15, it is assumed that onset before the age of 5 is impossible—in effect, age 5 substitutes for the baseline, defining the entire population of 5-year-olds as at risk. For 15-year-old subjects who meet diagnostic criteria, the recalled age of syndromal onset (somewhere between ages 5 and 14) is used to add the case to the numerator at the appropriate age. Similarly, for subjects age 16 years who meet diagnostic criteria at baseline, the recalled age of onset during the prior 10 years (that is, ages 6–15) is used to establish the numerator; for those 17 years old at baseline, the recalled age of onset in the prior 10 years (ages 7–16) is added to the numerator; and so on.

The same procedure is followed for the presentation of ECA data, using 10 years of recall instead of 12 for subjects with diagnosis at baseline. As just noted, this method both establishes an equivalent recall time period for subjects in both studies and reduces the potential recall bias inherent in the better memory of younger respondents. In effect, recall from periods longer than 10 years is not included. This facilitates the ability to estimate the year of age of onset of disorder across the range of ages from 5 through 64 (the oldest follow-up age in the NCS-2 and the entire lifetime in the ECA).

Incidence rate numerators are estimated separately for males and females for each year of life, as described above. The denominators are the total numbers of respondents passing through that same year of life at some point in the follow-up period. Thus, for example, each at-risk respondent with no onset contributes 10 years to the denominators in the NCS. In contrast, each respondent who has experienced onset contributes only the number of years prior to onset, after which their contributions are excluded. Plotted data curves are smoothed with a statistical technique called a kernel (Hastie & Tibshirani, 1990), using 5 years as the window, except for the curves for Alzheimer's dementia, described below.

Neither NCS nor NCS-2 data include all of the mental disorders considered in this chapter, nor do they include respondents age 65 and older. We bridge these gaps using data from the Baltimore ECA follow-up study. Since it is important to know whether the levels of incidence rise or fall in later life, Baltimore ECA data are included with the NCS/NCS-2 data, as seen in figures 6-1 to 6-4. Further, because the NCS did not include the diagnosis of obsessive–compulsive disorder, Baltimore ECA follow-up data are used. The danger inherent in using different data sets is that there are inevitably differences in the assessments, which often include different thresholds for the presence of the disorder, leading to differences in both prevalence and incidence. Because the primary purpose of this chapter is to understand the shape of the force of morbidity over the course of life, we can tolerate overall differences in level.

The curves shown in figures 6-1 through 6-4 visually display the life structure of the force

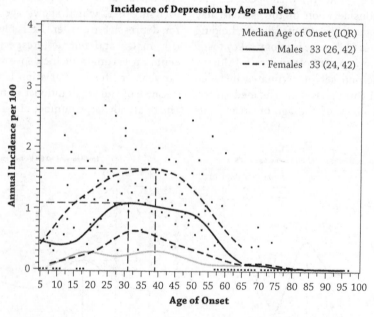

Figure 6-1 Life Course Structure of Depressive Disorder. Each dot represents an estimate of incidence for a particular year of life. Curves up to age 65 are based on smoothing National Comorbidity Survey data over 5-year periods (see text for description). Curves based on Epidemiologic Catchment Area data are shown in gray up to age 65, after which they change to black. Dashed vertical and horizontal lines indicate ages of maximum incidence. IQR = interquartile range.

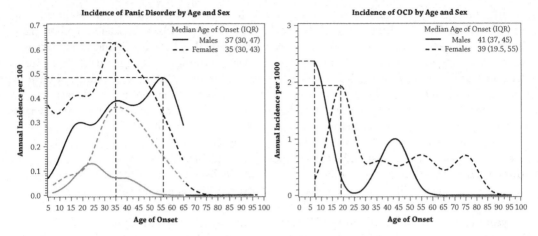

Figure 6-2 Life Course Structure of Panic Disorder and Obsessive–Compulsive Disorder. See figure 6-1 caption for explanation.

of morbidity and include two quantitative estimates from the data. One estimate is the peak incidence of a particular disorder—called the peak force of morbidity. A horizontal line to the ordinate facilitates comparison with other disorders. A vertical line to the abscissa, marking the precise age at which the peak occurs, encourages consideration of forces that may peak at the same stage of a life history, helping to provide clues to disease etiology, a key focus of the field of epidemiology itself (Morris, 1975). The second set of estimates included on figures 6-1 through 6-4 are the median and interquartile range of the age of onset. This

information may help in planning appropriate timing for primary intervention during the life course, the potential of which can be evaluated in part by the proportion of the onsets that take place following the intervention.

The reduction in variation produced by the kernel smoothing procedure is displayed in figure 6-1, which shows age of incidence for depressive disorder. Each blue or red dot (for males and females, respectively) represents an estimate of incidence for a particular year of life. The variation is considerable, because of the small number of new cases and the relatively large number of years of life. The

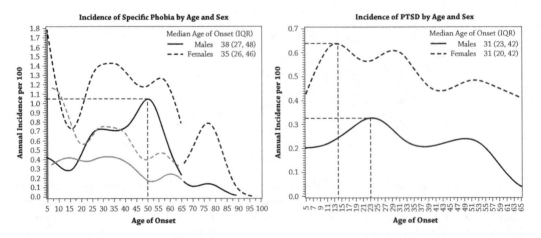

Figure 6-3 Life Course Structure of Specific Phobia and Posttraumatic Stress Disorder. See figure 6-1 caption for explanation.

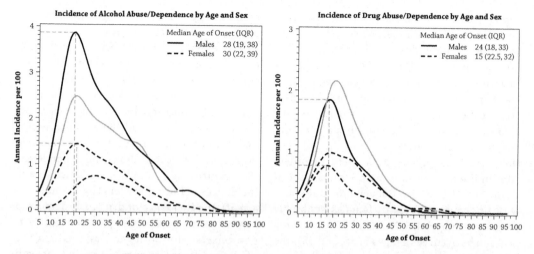

Figure 6-4   Life Course Structure of Substance Disorders. See figure 6-1 caption for explanation.

smoothing procedure estimates an average incidence from a 5-year period, with a point for the midpoint of the 5-year interval. The same process is applied to the average over the 5-year period for the next year of life, with a 5-year average for each subsequent year until the entire life course is completed. While 95% confidence intervals can be estimated for these curves, their breadth makes them of little utility: The lower curve is near the abscissa, and the upper part of the curve is so high that it is off the chart altogether.

Because the data represent the best available estimate, figure 6-1 displays the NCS curves for males and females from ages 5 through 64 in black. The ECA study's onset curves are displayed in gray up to age 65, after which they change to black, representing that the data reflect best estimates for that age range. This same practice of combining the two data sources is applied to other figures where the two sources of data are available (panic disorder in figure 6-2, phobic disorder in figure 6-3, and drug and alcohol disorders in figure 6-4.)

Figure 6-1 elucidates that depression is a disorder of early to middle adulthood. Onset accelerates rapidly after puberty until the dashed vertical and horizontal lines meet at the age of maximum incidence (for males at age 31 and at a rate of incidence of slightly more than 1% per year; for females at age 39 years

and about 1.6% per year). Half of all males and females experience onset before age 33, three-quarters before age 42. The incidence rate then declines sharply until age 65, where it hovers at about 1 or 2 per 1,000 per year until age 75, at which point the Baltimore ECA follow-up found only a handful of new cases.

This decline in the incidence of depressive disorders has confounded some gerontologists, who report many cases of depression in their practices. It could be that the cases seen in clinical practice are recurrences of depression rather than first lifetime episodes. Alternatively, perhaps depression among older adults takes a symptomatic form not delineated in the DSM-IV or captured in the DIS (Gallo, Anthony, & Muthen, 1994). Both the medians and the interquartile ranges found for depression in these quasiprospective analyses are generally consistent with other, fully retrospective analyses of the NCS (Kessler et al., 2005) and the World Mental Health Survey initiative (Kessler et al., 2007) but are about a decade later than the estimated ages of onset in the earliest analyses of depressive disorder as diagnosed according the third edition of the DSM (DSM-III) (APA, 1980) in the ECA program (Christie et al., 1988).

While the anxiety disorders also arise most often in the years between ages 35 and 50 (see figures 6-2 and 6-3), their incidences over the life course are more varied than is the case for depressive disorder. These disorders also have peaks in early childhood. When asked about age of onset, individuals with these disorders often respond that they have had symptoms "my whole life" or "ever since I can remember." The magnitude of this type of response generates substantial peaks very early in life in both NCS and ECA data, suggesting an enduring disposition towards anxiety: a trait. In contrast, the sizable incidences of anxiety disorders later in life may be associated with the social environment of a given developmental stage, with life course curves in females strikingly congruent in both the NCS and ECA (showing peaks in both curves at ages 5, 35, and 55). The ECA also shows a fourth anxiety disorder peak in women, for specific phobias, at about age 75. It may be speculated that the environment becomes more challenging as physical functioning declines, producing new onsets during the later years. For obsessive–compulsive disorder, new occurrences may be the result of cognitive decline, especially a decrease in short-term memory, which stimulates need for checking. These disorders contrast with panic disorder, which loses its force in old age.

Posttraumatic stress disorder is not captured in the ECA program data but has a sizable incidence beginning in adolescence and continuing through middle age in the NCS. The lack of apparent attenuation at age 65 among females suggests the unchanging nature of the environment's potential for trauma.

The substance use disorders—both those linked to alcohol and those for other substances—peak markedly in late adolescence, with a one-year difference between males and females for each disorder (at ages 17 and 18 for drug abuse and dependence among males and females, respectively, and at ages 20 and 21 for alcohol abuse and dependence). (See figure 6-4.) Males have much higher incidences of both disorders than females. By age 50, the incidence of drug disorders drops below one per 1,000 per year—virtually no new onsets—for both genders; the incidence of alcohol disorders does not reach that nadir until about age 75. These results are similar to earlier findings from retrospective explorations of both ECA and NCS data (Christie et al., 1988; Kessler et al., 2005) and to estimates from the World Mental Health Survey initiative (Kessler et al., 2007).

For schizophrenia, bipolar disorder, and dementia, in which lack of insight is common, a diagnosis in a field survey is not as credible as it is for disorders in which lack of insight is rare. For schizophrenia, data from the Danish Psychiatric Case Register are used (Munk-Jorgensen et al., 1993; Pedersen-Carsten, Gotzsche, Moller, & Mortensen, 2006). The curves for schizophrenia in figure 6-5 are

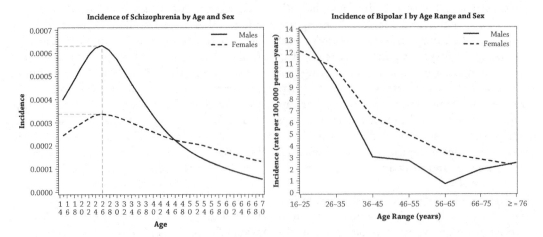

Figure 6-5   Life Course Structure of Schizophrenia and Bipolar Disorder, 1965–1999. Curves for schizophrenia are smoothed based on data from the Danish Psychiatric Case Register. Curves for bipolar disorder are based on data from the Camberwell, England, register and are not smoothed.

kernel-smoothed from point estimates in two year age groups included in a paper by Thorup, Waltoft, Pedersen, Mortensen, and Nordentoft (2007). While the peak age of onset for both males and females is age 26, incidence among males at that age is roughly double that of females (more than 0.60 cases per 1,000 persons per year compared with 0.33 per 1,000 per year, respectively). The gender-based curves cross at age 47 (at about 0.25 cases per 1,000 persons per year); at age 70, the rate for females is more than double that for males of the same age.

For bipolar disorder, also shown in figure 6-5, the Camberwell, England, register is used. Because data from the Camberwell register (Kennedy et al., 2005) are not available as single-year entries, they are not smoothed. The age of onset of bipolar disorder peaks during the early teen years and declines thereafter.

For dementia, figure 6-6 presents an unusual data set that is derived from a systematic review and integration of 18 studies of the incidence of dementia from around the world (Brookmeyer, Johnson, Ziegler-Graham, & Arrighi, 2007; Ziegler-Graham, Brookmeyer, Johnson, & Arrighi, 2008). Data from these

studies were each fitted to linear regressions with the logarithm of incidence as the dependent variable and age as the predictor. The curves shown were drawn using the average of the regression parameters for each sex separately. Virtually no incidence is found before age 65. Thereafter incidence remains below 1% per year for both males and females until about age 80. Beginning in the 80s, the incidence increases at different rates in men and women. The increase is much steeper for females, reaching nearly 20% per year at age 100; rates for males by age 100 are slightly less than half that figure.

COURSE

The symptomatic course of a mental disorder—its natural history—is of considerable interest because it has such a strong effect on prevalence. The preferred analytic framework to explore the natural history of mental disorders is through long-term follow-up of a population-based sample of individuals with known first onsets of illness. Unfortunately, this design is more the exception than the rule. Thus the current discussion takes a practical

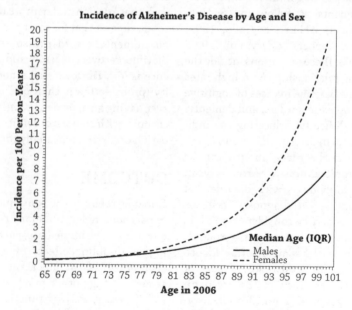

Figure 6-6   **Life Course Structure of Alzheimer's Type Dementia. Curves are based on data derived from 18 studies from around the world (see text for further details). IQR = interquartile range.**

orientation by focusing on the element of chronicity—disease persistence—in prevalent cases.

Table 6-3 shows estimates of the percentages of persons with specific mental disorders at or within one year prior to baseline who, at follow-up, meet the same criteria for the identical disorder. (Because prevalent cases at baseline are more likely to be chronic than a sample of incident cases, the analysis suffers from prevalence bias..) The follow-up periods shown are those found in the ECA and the NCS: 1 year, 10 years, 12 years, and 23 years. The table shows both the baseline prevalence and the number of individuals who represent the numerator of the baseline prevalence. The percentages in the columns on right side of the table are based on the total number of individuals from the baseline prevalence numerator who also participated in the follow-up survey. The table's findings may be compromised, since the success in contacting and interviewing respondents may differ between individuals with a mental disorder at baseline and those who did not meet criteria for disorder at baseline. With few exceptions, studies have found either a small association or no association between the presence of mental disorders at baseline and success in contacting and interviewing respondents at follow-up (Badawi, Eaton, Myllyluoma, Weimer, & Gallo, 1999; Eaton, Anthony, Tepper, & Dryman, 1992; Eaton et al., 2007). Those exceptions include the finding of strong relationships with high rates of death after the baseline in cases of cognitive impairment, drug use disorders, and dementia and with more difficulty in locating the individual at follow-up in drug use disorders.

Should mental disorders, in general, be considered chronic illnesses? After 1 year, about 80% of individuals with disorders at baseline no longer met diagnostic criteria. Those individuals may be considered cured, in remission, or recovered. Among the roughly 20% who still have the same disorder identified at baseline, the persistence of specific disorders ranges from a low of 13% for panic disorder to a high of 49% for alcohol disorder, but most disorders have persistence over this period of 10 (NCS) or 12 (ECA) years of about 15–20%, dropping off slightly after 23

years in the longer ECA follow-up However, obsessive–compulsive disorder appears to be more episodic or short-lived in that persistence drops markedly between year 1 and year 10.

These findings regarding the persistence of specific mental disorders are subject to a variety of interpretations, since they are based on population estimates, not individual medical trajectories. For example, it is possible that a small minority of individuals with a particular disorder at baseline experience a chronic course of illness that emerges annually, including in those years at which follow-up occurs. Alternatively, perhaps at each follow-up point, a totally different 20% sample of baseline cases is experiencing a recurrence. Equally possible, the finding may result from a combination of these natural histories. Unfortunately, available data on prevalent cases and persistence do not permit distinguishing among these possibilities.

The design would benefit from study of cases whose age of onset is taken from the first onset of the given disorder to occur over their lifetime ("first lifetime-incidence") rather than prevalent cases, an analysis that has been conducted only for depressive disorder (Eaton, Shao, et al., 2008), with results not too different from those displayed in table 6-3. Yet even with these design and data weaknesses, analyses do suggest that for most people with a diagnosed mental disorder at some point in their lifetime, recovery is likely and overall persistence is low. However, for a nontrivial minority (probably fewer than one in five of those ever having an episode), the mental disorder is chronic, with courses of remission and exacerbation occurring repeatedly for decades.

OUTCOME

Outcome refers to the consequences or results of psychopathology. In many cases, the consequences can be immediate, such as the impairing or disabling effects of a disorder. This chapter focuses on important, pernicious consequences (e.g., other psychopathology, physical illnesses, loss of functioning, and even death) that arise later in the course of the disorder and are not part of the disorder's defining signs and symptoms.

Table 6-3. Persistence of Selected Common Mental Disorders over Two Decades

| DISORDER | BASELINE PREVALENCE (%) | | PERCENTAGE OF INDIVIDUALS WHO MET CRITERIA IN YEAR PRIOR TO INTERVIEW | | | | |
	ECA	NCS	AFTER 1 YEAR (ECA)	AFTER 10 YEARS (NCS)	AFTER 12 YEARS (ECA)	AFTER 23 YEARS (ECA)
Panic disorder	1.1 (35)	2.1 (144)	13	12	17	8
Social phobia		8.3 (551)		26		NA
Simple phobia	1.0 (34)	8.8 (581)	24	34	28	19
Major depressive disorder	2.9 (96)	8.5 (576)	17	12	13	7
Obsessive–compulsive disorder	2.4 (78)	NA	27	NA	3	24
Drug abuse/dependence	2.5 (83)	3.5 (238)	21	16	18	24
Alcohol abuse/dependence	5.7 (188)	9.6 (694)	49	17	28	15
Personality disorder[a]	8.8 (37)	NA	NA	NA	11	NA
Total	100 (3,481)	100 (5,877)[b]	80 (2,768)	85 (5,001)	55 (1,920)	31 (1,071)

Numbers in parentheses are respondents meeting criteria at baseline; or who were interviewed in follow-up waves. ECA = Baltimore Epidemiologic Catchment Area study and its follow-up; NCS = National Comorbidity Survey and its follow-up; NA = Not available.

[a]Disorder identified in structured psychiatric examination–clinical reappraisal, weighted by inverse of probability of selection, among 294 individuals with data available at both waves.

[b]Number of respondents in part II of NCS baseline survey.

Comorbidity is the occurrence of two or more disorders in a single individual (Feinstein, 1967). Increased interest in narrowly defined mental disorders that has taken place since the introduction of the DSM-III (APA, 1980) has led to a concomitant increased interest in psychiatric comorbidity. Multiple mental disorders may occur simultaneously in the same individual or may arise at different times, giving name to the concept of lifetime comorbidity. Presumably, lifetime comorbidity expresses a genetic diathesis, an early, enduring risk factor, or a long-standing environmental cause. Ultimately, observed patterns of differential comorbidity will contribute to improved nosology. Cross-sectional study of concurrent or lifetime comorbidity focuses on the increase in prevalence for one disorder given the presence of another (Merikangas et al., 1996; Merikangas & Gelernter, 1990; Merikangas et al., 1998). Studies of the natural history of comorbid conditions focus on the issue of risk,

either by exploring respondents' retrospective recall of the relative onset of the disorders or by undertaking a wholly prospective study.

Sizable lifetime comorbidity exists among the mental disorders, as shown in the cross-sectional data from the NESARC baseline survey (Grant et al., 2003). (See table 6-4.) In fact, lifetime comorbidity is more common than the occurrence of a single disorder alone. Notably, all NESARC respondents with bipolar I disorder also reported another lifetime psychiatric comorbidity. Similarly, with the exception of simple phobia and alcohol disorder, past-year comorbidity (not shown) also is more common than the occurrence of any one disorder alone. Because many potentially comorbid mental disorders are not measured in the NESARC, the results displayed in table 6-4 underestimate lifetime psychiatric comorbidity. As the number of disorders in the DSM continues to increase (as discussed in chapter 2), rates of comorbidity also are

Table 6-4. Lifetime Comorbidity of Common Mental Disorders

| | PERCENT WITH | | | | TOTAL NO. OF RESPONDENTS |
	NO OTHER DISORDER	ONE OTHER DISORDER[a]	TWO OTHER DISORDERS[a]	THREE OR MORE OTHER DISORDERS[a]	
Conduct disorder	28.5	32.3	20.0	19.2	415
Major depressive disorder	25.0	29.8	20.9	24.3	6,410
Panic disorder	15.0	19.3	18.4	47.3	2,116
Social phobia	11.7	19.1	19.8	49.4	1,983
Simple phobia	23.4	25.7	17.9	33.0	4,030
Bipolar I disorder	0	5.4	16.9	77.7	935
Alcohol abuse/ dependence	47.7	25.2	12.7	14.4	11,843
Drug abuse/ dependence	5.9	30.1	24.6	39.4	2,063
Personality disorder	19.5	28.7	19.9	31.9	6,295

Based on National Epidemiologic Study of Alcohol and Related Conditions, Wave 1.

[a] Other psychiatric disorders include lifetime major depressive disorder, dysthymia, bipolar I disorder, panic disorder, social phobia, simple phobia, generalized anxiety disorder, alcohol abuse/dependence, drug abuse/dependence, conduct disorder, and personality disorder.

certain to rise. As discussed above, comorbidity among mental disorders frequently is present in their natural histories; some disorders have been found to be common precursors of other mental disorders. With the availability of longitudinal data, these comorbidities may be the subject of etiologic inquiries. For example, Breslau and colleagues (1995) have shown that by accounting for the presence of preexisting, early-life anxiety disorders, the higher prevalence rate of depressive disorder in adult females compared with males is eliminated altogether.

Adolescence and young adulthood mark the peak period of onset for many mental disorders, among them depressive disorder, panic disorder, alcohol disorder, drug use disorder, and schizophrenia. In contrast, many significant, chronic, physical conditions (e.g., heart diseases, cancers, type-2 diabetes and stroke) have peak onsets in midlife or later. Thus physical illness represents another type of comorbidity as well as a possible outcome of psychopathology (Von Korff, Scott, & Gureje, 2009).

Table 6-5 shows the range of later-occurring physical conditions and symptoms that have been linked to antecedent depressive illness, selected for presentation here by virtue of their high prevalence and disabling or fatal consequences. Each relative risk in the table

Table 6-5. Risk of Chronic Medical Conditions Associated with Depression over the Life Course

CONDITION	SOURCE	RELATIVE RISK[a]	CONFIRMING STUDY
Type 2 diabetes	Eaton, Armenian, Gallo, Pratt, & Ford, 1996	2.2	Mezuk, Eaton, Albrecht, & Golden, 2008
Hypertension	Meyer, Armenian, Eaton, & Ford, 2004	2.2	Patten et al., 2009
Heart attack	Pratt et al., 1996	**4.5**	Rugulies, 2002
Stroke	Larson, Owens, Ford, & Eaton, 2001	**2.7**	Ramasubbu & Patten, 2003
Any cancer	Gross, Gallo, & Eaton, 2010	1.0	Oerlemans, van den Akker, Schuurman, Kellen, & Buntinx, 2007
Lung cancer	Gross et al., 2010	0.8	Oerlemans et al., 2007
Breast cancer	Gross et al., 2010	**3.4**	Oerlemans et al., 2007[b]
Colon cancer	Gross et al., 2010	4.3	Oerlemans et al., 2007
Prostate cancer	Gross et al., 2010	1.1	Oerlemans et al., 2007
Arthritis	Eaton, Fogel, & Armenian, 2006	1.3	Not applicable
Osteopenia	Mezuk, Eaton, Golden, Wand, & Lee, 2008	**4.1**[c]	Cizza, Primma, Coyle, Gourgiotis, & Csako, 2010

Based on Baltimore Epidemiologic Catchment Area (ECA) study follow-up, 1981–1996.

[a]Relative risks in boldface are statistically significant at the 0.05 level.

[b]Relative risk for breast cancer in the meta-analysis was 2.5 and significant only for studies with more than 10 years of follow-up (as with the ECA).

[c]Age-adjusted OR estimated from ECA data by Mezuk and colleagues for risk of osteopenia, defined as one or more standard deviations lower in bone mass density than the general population.

was developed through a separate analysis, comparing depressive disorder with other forms of psychopathology and adjusting for other known risk factors for the physical condition. For many conditions, depressive disorder was the only nontrivial predictor of the physical disorder across the range of psychopathology. The relative risks are large enough to place depressive disorder on a par with other known risk factors for major physical problems, such as high cholesterol, family history, hypertension, and obesity as respective risk factors for heart attack, breast cancer, stroke, and type 2 diabetes. Consistent with the developmental approach taken throughout this chapter, subclinical psychopathology (i.e., below a diagnostic threshold) also was found to have a link to the onset of some subsequent physical conditions (not shown). As table 6-5 shows, ECA findings are consistent with those of systematic or meta-analytic literature reviews as well as recent, methodologically credible studies, with the exception that the findings on breast cancer are not entirely consistent with the literature.

Since depressive disorder generally is not treated, despite the availability of effective treatments, and since screening for the disorder is relatively unusual, these data have implications for preventive medicine in the primary care setting. These results show that depression is part of the risk structure for important chronic medical conditions. Varying explanations are possible. One explanation is that depressive disorder raises risk through associated behavioral changes such as weight gain, loss of sleep, and failure to pay attention to regimens that protect from the medical conditions. Another possibility is that the physiological changes that arise with depression, such as alterations in blood platelet reactivity (Musselman et al., 1996) and high levels of cortisol (Rubin, Poland, Leser, Winston, & Blodgett, 1987), may be associated with the increased risk for physical illnesses.

Chronic medical conditions also appear to be strongly associated with schizophrenia, though no single study clearly demonstrates the results. Because the literature is not as well structured, with fewer longitudinal studies, the data presented in table 6-6 are based on cross-sectional associations. Studies selected for inclusion in the table are from well-developed registration systems where

Table 6-6. Chronic Medical Conditions Associated with Schizophrenia

CONDITION	SOURCE	RELATIVE ODDS[a]
Type 2 diabetes	Bresee, Majumdar, Patten, & Johnson, 2010	**1.9**
Hypertension	Bresee et al., 2010	**1.1**
Heart attack	Curkendall, Mo, Glasser, Rose, & Jones, 2004	1.3
Stroke	Lin, Hsiao, Pfeiffer, Hwang, & Lee, 2008	**2.0**[b]
Any cancer	Goldacre, Kurina, Wotton, Yeates, & Seagroat, 2005	1.0
Lung cancer	Goldacre et al., 2005	1.2
Breast cancer	Goldacre et al., 2005	1.0
Colon cancer	Goldacre et al., 2005	0.7
Prostate cancer	Goldacre et al., 2005	0.8
Rheumatoid arthritis	Oken & Schulzer, 1999	**0.3**
Osteopenia	Renn et al., 2009	**1.5**[c]

[a]Relative odds in boldface are statistically significant at the 0.05 level.
[b]Hazard ratio from table 4 of Lin et al., 2008.
[c]Relative odds computed by the authors from data in Renn et al., 2009, tables 1 and 4, for those under 50 years of age with bone mass density more than one standard deviation lower than that of the community; significance based on linear regression model

available and otherwise from studies chosen for their methodological rigor. Those methodologically acceptable studies tend to originate in areas around the world where health care is provided free of charge to the general population, suggesting that the estimates in table 6-6 are likely lower than would be found by similarly methodologically robust studies conducted in the United States.

Nonetheless, schizophrenia appears to pose a similar raised risk for the same chronic physical conditions as with depression. Potential explanations are considerably different, however. The symptoms of schizophrenia often dominate all other health problems and as such are central to treatment by psychiatrists and other mental health professionals. As a result, many of the important physical conditions noted in table 6-6 either may not be prevented or may not be treated early. Even when physical disorders are identified, adherence to treatment and preventive regimens may be more difficult for persons with schizophrenia.

Like depression, schizophrenia appears to be a risk factor for diabetes; however, unlike depression, the mediators for schizophrenia include antipsychotic medications with known side effects of weight gain and diabetes onset. The comorbidity of hypertension, heart attack, and stroke with schizophrenia is lower than

Table 6-7. All-Cause Mortality Associated with Mental Disorders Compared with General Population Sample Without the Disorder

	MEDIAN RELATIVE RISK	INTER-QUARTILE RANGE	NUMBER OF STUDIES FOUND	NUMBER OF STUDIES INCLUDED
Panic disorder	1.9	0.8–3.2	77	4
Social phobia	NA	NA	28	0
Simple phobia	NA	NA	28	0
Major depressive disorder	1.7	1.3–2.2	282	14
Obsessive–compulsive disorder	1.1	1.1–1.7	26	2
Drug abuse/dependence	2.0	1.6–2.1	610	2
Alcohol abuse/dependence	1.8	1.5–2.0	913	7
Personality disorders	4.0	2.8–5.2	111	2
Schizophrenia	2.6	1.9–3.6	832	38
Bipolar disorder	2.6	1.9–9.8	320	3
Dementia (age 60 or over)	2.7	2.0–3.0	2,333	20

NA = Not applicable.

Sources:

Panic disorder: Bruce, Leaf, Rozal, Florio, & Hoff, 1994; Eaton et al., 2007; Grasbeck, Rorsman, Hagnell, & Isberg, 1996; Kouzis, Eaton, & Leaf, 1995.

Major depressive disorder: Bruce et al., 1994; Davidson, Dewey, & Copeland, 1988; Eaton et al., 2007; Gallo et al., 2005; Henderson et al., 1997; Joukamaa et al., 2001; Kouzis et al., 1995; Kua, 1992; Mogga et al., 2006; Murphy et al., 2008; Penninx et al., 1998; Pulska, Pahkala, Laippala, & Kivela, 1997, 1998; Saz et al., 1999.

Obsessive–compulsive disorder: Bruce et al., 1994; Eaton et al., 2007.

Drug abuse/dependence: Eaton et al., 2007; Kouzis et al., 1995.

Alcohol abuse/dependence: Bourgkard et al., 2008; Bruce et al., 1994; Dawson, 2000; Eaton et al., 2007; Kouzis et al., 1995; Rossow & Amundsen, 1997; Vaillant, 1996.

Personality disorders: de Graaf, Bijl, Smit, Ravelli, & Vollebergh, 2000; Meller, Fichter, & Schroppel, 1999.

Schizophrenia: McGrath, Saha, Chant, & Welham, 2008.

Bipolar disorder: Dutta et al., 2007; Laursen, Munk-Olsen, Nordentoft, & Mortensen, 2007; Osby, Brandt, Correia, Ekbom, & Sparen, 2001.

Dementia: Aguero-Torres, Fratiglioni, Guo, Viitanen, & Winblad, 1999; Appelros & Viitanen, 2005; Aronson et al., 1991; Baldereschi et al., 1999; Bonaiuto, Mele, Galluzzo, & Giannandrea, 1995; Engedal, 1996; Guhne, Matschinger, Angermeyer, & Riedel-Heller, 2006; Heeren, van Hemert, & Rooymans, 1992; Hendrie et al., 1995; Johansson & Zarit, 1995; Jorm, Henderson, Kay, & Jacomb, 1991; Juva et al., 1994; Katzman et al., 1994; Liu et al., 1998; Lobo et al., 2000; Skoog, Nilsson, Palmertz, Andreasson, & Svanborg, 1993; Snowdon & Lane, 1995; Tsuji et al., 1995.

for depression. Further, the relative odds are about 1.0—no association—between schizophrenia and either any cancer or specific cancers. Curiously, and for unknown reasons, the relative risk for rheumatoid arthritis actually is smaller among those with schizophrenia than among the general population. The comorbidity of schizophrenia with osteopenia is strong, as is also the case for depression. However, table 6-6 does not include persons over the age of 50, a period during which the odds of osteopenia rise in the general population but, curiously, are level for persons with schizophrenia (Renn et al., 2009).

With these levels of comorbidity, it is not surprising that mental disorders are associated with mortality (death). (See table 6-7.) A systematic review of the literature (Eaton, Martins, et al., 2008) found numerous studies that link mental disorders to mortality. That review revealed strong, replicable associations for only three disorders: major depressive disorder (14 studies), schizophrenia (38 studies), and dementia (20 studies). Reviews of comorbid major depressive disorder and schizophrenia with physical conditions did not include studies addressing the enhanced risk of suicide for persons with these disorders, a contributing factor in their association with mortality. While only a handful of studies exist for other mental disorders, interquartile ranges presented in table 6-7 are narrow enough to suggest heightened risks for mortality among those other disorders as well.

CONCLUSIONS

Perhaps more than in other areas of epidemiologic inquiry, the range of unique issues related to the etiology of mental disorders will benefit from more thorough examination of the illnesses' population dynamics. These disorders have relatively early onsets, opening the potential for courses of disorder that extend across a lifetime. Onset is languid for many disorders, generating particular interest in the precursors and the prodrome and in avenues for screening and early intervention. The mental disorders are highly comorbid with one another, reinforcing the interest in screening for and primary prevention of secondary disorders. The courses

of these disorders are highly varied, with some immediate and permanent recovery and some descent into permanent suffering and disability. A range of outcomes are possible, including the development of chronic physical medical conditions. The etiologically relevant period for these conditions is extended, again offering the possibility of reward for the investigator willing to consider decades of causal action, instead of days, weeks, or months as is the case for many infectious diseases. For these reasons, the epidemiologic study of mental disorders should not be confined to any simple or single parameter, whether prevalence (as in many current cross-sectional studies, as discussed above) or incidence (as in other areas of epidemiology, such as cancer). Rather, the entire range of parameters related to the onset, course, and outcome of mental disorders should be addressed.

ACKNOWLEDGMENTS

Special thanks to Nancy Sampson for help in making estimates from the NCS data for figures 6-1, 6-2, 6-3, and 6-4; to Elizabeth Johnson for make the sex-specific curves in Figure 6-6; and to Jack Samuels for making estimates of persistence of personality disorder in table 6-3.

REFERENCES

Aguero-Torres, H., Fratiglioni, L., Guo, Z., Viitanen, M., & Winblad, B. (1999). Mortality from dementia in advanced age: A 5-year follow-up study of incident dementia cases. *Journal of Clinical Epidemiology, 52*(8), 737–743.

American Psychiatric Association. (1980). *Diagnostic and statistical manual of mental disorders* (3rd ed.). Washington, DC: Author.

American Psychiatric Association. (1994). *Diagnostic and statistical manual of mental disorders* (4th ed.). Washington, DC: Author.

Appelros, P., & Viitanen, M. (2005). What causes increased stroke mortality in patients with pre-stroke dementia? *Cerebrovascular Diseases, 19*(5), 323–327.

Aronson, M. K., Ooi, W. L., Geva, D. L., Masur, D., Blau, A., & Frishman, W. (1991). Dementia: Age-dependent incidence, prevalence, and mortality in the old old. *Archives of Internal Medicine, 151*(5), 989–992.

Badawi, M. A., Eaton, W. W., Myllyluoma, J., Weimer, L. G., & Gallo, J. (1999). Psychopathology and attrition in the Baltimore ECA 15-year follow-up 1981–1996. *Social Psychiatry and Psychiatric Epidemiology, 34*(2), 91–98.

Baldereschi, M., Di, C. A., Maggi, S., Grigoletto, F., Scarlato, G., Amaducci, L., & Inzitari, D. (1999). Dementia is a major predictor of death among the Italian elderly. ILSA Working Group. Italian Longitudinal Study on Aging. *Neurology, 52*(4), 709–713.

Baldwin, J., & Evans, J. H. (1971). The psychiatric case register. *International Psychiatry Clinics, 8*(3), 17–38.

Baltes, P. B., Reese, H. W., & Lipsitt, L. P. (1980). Life-span developmental psychology. *Annual Review of Psychology, 31*, 65–110.

Berkson, J. (1946). Limitations of the application of fourfold table analysis to hospital data. *Biometrics, 2*(3), 47–53.

Bijl, R. V., van Zessen, G., Ravelli, A., de Rijk, C., & Langendoen, Y. (1998). The Netherlands Mental Health Survey and Incidence Study (NEMESIS): Objectives and design. *Social Psychiatry and Psychiatric Epidemiology, 33*(12), 581–586.

Bonaiuto, S., Mele, M., Galluzzo, L., & Giannandrea, E. (1995). Survival and dementia: A 7-year follow-up of an Italian elderly population. *Archives of Gerontology and Geriatrics, 20*(1), 105–113.

Bourgkard, E., Wild, P., Massin, N., Meyer, J. P., Otero, S. C., Fontana, J. M., … Chau, N. (2008). Association of physical job demands, smoking and alcohol abuse with subsequent premature mortality: A 9-year follow-up population-based study. *Journal of Occupational Health, 50*(1), 31–40.

Bresee, L. C., Majumdar, S. R., Patten, S. B., & Johnson, J. A. (2010). Prevalence of cardiovascular risk factors and disease in people with schizophrenia: A population-based study. *Schizophrenia Research, 117*(1), 75–82.

Breslau, N. Schultz, L., & Peterson, E. (1995) Sex differences in depression: a role for preexisting anxiety, *Psychiatry Research, 58*, 1–12.

Brookmeyer, R., Johnson, E., Ziegler-Graham, K., & Arrighi, H. M. (2007). Forecasting the global burden of Alzheimer's disease. *Alzheimer's and Dementia, 3*(3), 186–191.

Bruce, M. L., Leaf, P. J., Rozal, G. P., Florio, L., & Hoff, R. A. (1994). Psychiatric status and 9-year mortality data in the New Haven Epidemiologic Catchment Area Study. *American Journal of Psychiatry, 151*(5), 716–721.

Christie, K. A., Burke, J. D., Regier, D. A., Rae, D. S., Boyd, J. H., & Locke, B. Z. (1988). Epidemiologic evidence for early onset of mental disorders and higher risk of drug abuse in young adults. *American Journal of Psychiatry, 145*(8), 971–975.

Cizza, G., Primma, S., Coyle, M., Gourgiotis, L., & Csako, G. (2010). Depression and osteoporosis: A research synthesis with meta-analysis. *Hormone and Metabolic Research, 42*(7), 467–482.

Cleverly, M., & Douglas, M. (1991). *The Salford mental health register.* Salford, UK: Health Information Unit, Salford Health Authority.

Cohen, P., & Cohen, J. (1984). The clinician's illusion. *Archives of General Psychiatry, 41*(12), 1178–1182.

Curkendall, S. M., Mo, J., Glasser, D. B., Rose, S. M., & Jones, J. K. (2004). Cardiovascular disease in patients with schizophrenia in Saskatchewan, Canada. *Journal of Clinical Psychiatry, 65*(5), 715–720.

Davidson, I. A., Dewey, M. E., & Copeland, J. R. M. (1988). The relationship between mortality and mental disorder: Evidence from the Liverpool longitudinal study. *International Journal of Geriatric Psychiatry, 3*(2), 95–98.

Dawson, D. A. (2000). Alcohol consumption, alcohol dependence, and all-cause mortality 4. *Alcoholism: Clinical and Experimental Research, 24*(1), 72–81.

de Graaf, R., Bijl, R. V., Smit, F., Ravelli, A., & Vollebergh, W. A. M. (2000). Psychiatric and sociodemographic predictors of attrition in a longitudinal study: The Netherlands Mental Health Survey and Incidence Study (NEMESIS). *American Journal of Epidemiology, 152*(11), 1039–1047.

de Salvia, D., Barbato, A., Salvo, P., & Zadro, F. (1993). Prevalence and incidence of schizophrenic disorders in Portogruaro: An Italian case register study. *Journal of Nervous and Mental Disease, 181*(5), 275–282.

Dryman, A., & Eaton, W. W. (1991). Affective symptoms associated with the onset of major depression in the community: Findings from the U.S. NIMH Epidemiologic Catchment Area program. *Acta Psychiatrica Scandinavica, 84*(1), 1–5.

Dupont, A. (1979). Psychiatric case registers as a basis for estimation and monitoring of needs. In H. Hafner (Ed.), *Estimating needs for mental health care: A contribution of epidemiology* (pp. 43–51). New York, NY: Springer-Verlag.

Dutta, R., Boydell, J., Kennedy, N., van Os, J., Fearon, P., & Murray, R. M. (2007). Suicide and other causes of mortality in bipolar disorder: A longitudinal study. *Psychological Medicine, 37*(6), 839–847.

Eaton, W. W. (2011). Studying the natural history of psychopathology, in M. T. Tsuang, M. Tohen, &

P. B. Jones, P. B. (Eds.), *Textbook in psychiatric epidemiology* (pp. 183–220). New York: Wiley-Blackwell.

Eaton, W. W., Anthony, J. C., Gallo, J., Cai, G., Tien, A., Romanoski, A.,…Chen, L. (1997). Natural history of Diagnostic Interview Schedule/DSM major depression: The Baltimore Epidemiologic Catchment Area follow-up. *Archives of General Psychiatry, 54*(11), 993–999.

Eaton, W. W., Anthony, J. C., Tepper, S., & Dryman, A. (1992). Psychopathology and attrition in the Epidemiologic Catchment Area surveys. *American Journal of Epidemiology, 135*(9), 1051–1059.

Eaton, W. W., Armenian, H. K., Gallo, J. J., Pratt, L., & Ford, D. (1996). Depression and risk for onset of type II diabetes: A prospective, population-based study. *Diabetes Care, 19*(10), 1097–1102.

Eaton, W. W., Badawi, M., & Melton, B. (1995). Prodromes and precursors: Epidemiologic data for primary prevention of disorders with slow onset. *American Journal of Psychiatry, 152*(7), 967–972.

Eaton, W., Fogel, J., & Armenian, H. (2006). The consequences of psychopathology in the Baltimore Epidemiologic Catchment Area. In W. Eaton (Ed.), *Medical and psychiatric comorbidity over the course of life* (pp. 21–36). Washington, DC: American Psychiatric Press.

Eaton, W. W., Kalaydjian, A., Scharfstein, D. O., Mezuk, B., & Ding, Y. (2007). Prevalence and incidence of depressive disorder: The Baltimore ECA follow-up, 1981–2004. *Acta Psychiatrica Scandinavica, 116*(3), 182–188.

Eaton, W. W., & Kessler, L. G. (1985). *Epidemiologic field methods in psychiatry: The NIMH Epidemiologic Catchment Area program.* Orlando, FL: Academic Press.

Eaton, W. W., Kramer, M., Anthony, J. C., Chee, E. M. L., & Shapiro, S. (1989). Conceptual and methodological problems in estimation of the incidence of mental disorders from field survey data. In B. Cooper & T. Helgason (Eds.), *Epidemiology and the prevention of mental disorders* (pp. 108–127). London, UK: Routledge.

Eaton, W. W., Kramer, M., Anthony, J. C., Dryman, A., Shapiro, S., & Locke, B. Z. (1989). The incidence of specific DIS/DSM-III mental disorders: Data from the NIMH Epidemiologic Catchment Area program. *Acta Psychiatrica Scandinavica, 79*(2), 163–178.

Eaton, W. W., Martins, S. S., Nestadt, G., Bienvenu, O. J., Clarke, D., & Alexandre, P. (2008). The burden of mental disorders. *Epidemiologic Reviews, 30*, 1–14.

Eaton, W. W., Shao, H., Nestadt, G., Lee, H. B., Bienvenu, O. J., & Zandi, P. (2008). Population-based study of first onset and chronicity in major depressive disorder. *Archives of General Psychiatry, 65*(5), 513–520.

Engedal, K. (1996). Mortality in the elderly: A 3-year follow-up of an elderly community sample. *International Journal of Geriatric Psychiatry, 11*, 467–471.

Feinstein, A. (1967). *Clinical judgement.* Baltimore, MD: Williams & Wilkins.

Fichter, M. M. (1990). *Verlauf psychischer Erkrankungen in der Bevolkerung.* Berlin, Germany: Springer-Verlag.

Gallo, J. J., Anthony, J. C., & Muthen, B. O. (1994). Age differences in the symptoms of depression: A latent trait analysis. *Journal of Gerontology: Psychological Sciences, 49*(6), 251–264.

Gallo, J. J., Bogner, H. R., Morales, K. H., Post, E. P., Ten, H. T., & Bruce, M. L. (2005). Depression, cardiovascular disease, diabetes, and two-year mortality among older, primary-care patients. *American Journal of Geriatric Psychiatry, 13*(9), 748–755.

Goldacre, M. J., Kurina, L. M., Wotton, C. J., Yeates, D., & Seagroat, V. (2005). Schizophrenia and cancer: An epidemiological study. *British Journal of Psychiatry, 187*, 334–338.

Goodman, A. B., Rahav, M., Popper, M., Ginath, Y., & Pearl, E. (1984). The reliability of psychiatric diagnosis in Israel's Psychiatric Case Register. *Acta Psychiatrica Scandinavica, 69*(5), 391–397.

Grant, B. F., Moore, T. C., Shepard, J., & Kaplan, K. (2003). *Source and accuracy statement: Wave 1 National Epidemiologic Survey on Alcohol and Related Conditions.* Bethesda, MD: National Institute on Alcohol Abuse and Alcoholism.

Grasbeck, A., Rorsman, B., Hagnell, O., & Isberg, P. E. (1996). Mortality of anxiety syndromes in a normal population: The Lundby study. *Neuropsychobiology, 33*(3), 118–126.

Gross, A. L., Gallo, J. J., & Eaton, W. W. (2010). Depression and cancer risk: 24 years of follow-up of the Baltimore Epidemiologic Catchment Area sample. *Cancer Causes & Control, 21*(2), 191–199.

Guhne, U., Matschinger, H., Angermeyer, M. C., & Riedel-Heller, S. G. (2006). Incident dementia cases and mortality: Results of the Leipzig Longitudinal Study of the Aged (LEILA75+). *Dementia and Geriatric Cognitive Disorders, 22*(3), 185–193.

Hagnell, O., Essen-Moller, E., Lanke, J., Ojesjo, L., & Rorsman, B. (1990). *The incidence of mental illness over a quarter of a century.* Stockholm, Sweden: Almqvist & Wiksell.

Hall, D., Robertson, N. C., Dorricott, N., Olley, P. C., & Millar, W. M. (1973). The North-East Scottish Psychiatric Case Register—the second phase. *Journal of Chronic Diseases, 26*(6), 375–382.

Hastie, T., & Tibshirani, R. (1990). *Generalized additive models.* New York, NY: Chapman and Hall.

Heeren, T. J., van Hemert, A. M., & Rooymans, H. G. (1992). A community-based study of survival in dementia. *Acta Psychiatrica Scandinavica, 85*(6), 415–418.

Henderson, A. S., Korten, A. E., Jacomb, P. A., Mackinnon, A. J., Jorm, A. F., Christensen, H., & Rodgers, B. (1997). The course of depression in the elderly: A longitudinal community-based study in Australia. *Psychological Medicine, 27*(1), 119–129.

Hendrie, H. C., Osuntokun, B. O., Hall, K. S., Ogunniyi, A. O., Hui, S. L., Unverzagt, F. W., ... Musick, B. (1995). Prevalence of Alzheimer's disease and dementia in two communities: Nigerian Africans and African Americans. *American Journal of Psychiatry, 152*(10), 1485–1492.

Herrman, H., Baldwin, J. A., & Christie, D. (1983). A record-linkage study of mortality and general hospital discharge in patients diagnosed as schizophrenic. *Psychological Medicine, 13*(3), 581–593.

Horwath, E., Johnson, J., Klerman, G., & Weissman, M. (1992). Depressive symptoms as relative and attributable risk factors for first-onset major depression. *Archives of General Psychiatry, 49*(10), 817–823.

Johansson, B., & Zarit, S. H. (1995). Prevalence and incidence of dementia in the oldest old: A longitudinal study of a population-based sample of 84–90-year-olds in Sweden. *International Journal of Geriatric Psychiatry, 10,* 359–366.

Jorm, A. F., Henderson, A. S., Kay, D. W. K., & Jacomb, P. A. (1991). Mortality in relation to dementia, depression and social integration in an elderly community sample. *International Journal of Geriatric Psychiatry, 6,* 5–11.

Joukamaa, M., Heliovaara, M., Knekt, P., Aromaa, A., Raitasalo, R., & Lehtinen, V. (2001). Mental disorders and cause-specific mortality. *British Journal of Psychiatry, 179,* 498–502.

Juva, K., Sulkava, R., Erkinjuntti, T., Makela, M., Valvanne, J., & Tilvis, R. (1994). The prognosis of demented patients: One-year follow-up study of a population sample. *International Journal of Geriatric Psychiatry, 9,* 537–541.

Katzman, R., Hill, L. R., Yu, E. S., Wang, Z. Y., Booth, A., Salmon, D. P., ... Zhang, M. (1994). The malignancy of dementia: Predictors of mortality in clinically diagnosed dementia in a population survey of Shanghai, China. *Archives of Neurology, 51*(12), 1220–1225.

Kennedy, N., Boydell, J., Kalidindi, S., Fearon, P., Jones, P. B., van Os, J., Murray, R. M. (2005). Gender differences in incidence and age at onset of mania and bipolar disorder over a 35-year period in Camberwell, England. *American Journal of Psychiatry, 162*(2), 257–262.

Kessler, R. (1994). The National Comorbidity Survey of the United States. *International Review of Psychiatry, 6,* 365–376.

Kessler, R. C. (1995). The National Comorbidity Survey: Preliminary results and future directions. *International Journal of Methods in Psychiatric Research, 5,* 140–151.

Kessler, R. C., Angermeyer, M., Anthony, J. C., de Graaf, R., Demyttenaere, K., Gasquet, I., ... Ustun, T. B. (2007). Lifetime prevalence and age-of-onset distributions of mental disorders in the World Health Organization's World Mental Health Survey initiative. *World Psychiatry, 6*(3), 168–176.

Kessler, R. C., Anthony, J. C., Blazer, D. G., Bromet, E., Eaton, W. W., Kendler, K., ... Zhao, S. (1997). The U.S. National Comorbidity Survey: Overview and future directions. *Epidemiologia e Psichiatria Sociale, 6*(1), 4–16.

Kessler, R. C., Berglund, P., Demler, O., Jin, R., Merikangas, K. R., & Walters, E. E. (2005). Lifetime prevalence and age-of-onset distributions of DSM-IV disorders in the National Comorbidity Survey Replication. *Archives of General Psychiatry, 62*(6), 593–602.

Kessler, R. C., & Price, R. H. (1993). Primary prevention of secondary disorders: A proposal and agenda. *American Journal of Community Psychology, 21*(5), 607–633.

Kieseppa, T., Partonen, T., Kaprio, J., & Lonnqvist, J. (2000). Accuracy of register- and record-based bipolar I disorder diagnoses in Finland: A study of twins. *Acta Neuropsychiatrica, 12,* 3–106.

Kleinbaum, D. G., Kupper, L. L., & Morgenstern, H. (1982). *Epidemiologic research: Principles and quantitative methods.* Belmont, CA: Lifetime Learning.

Kouzis, A., Eaton, W. W., & Leaf, P. J. (1995). Psychopathology and mortality in the general population. *Social Psychiatry and Psychiatric Epidemiology, 30*(4), 165–170.

Kristjansson, E., Allebeck, P., & Wistedt, B. (1987). Validity of the diagnosis schizophrenia in a psychiatric inpatient register. *Nordic Journal of Psychiatry, 43,* 229–234.

Krupinski, J. (1977). The use of computerized patients' registers in psychiatric epidemiology.

In Shires-Wolf (Ed.), *MEDINFO* (pp. 609–613). North-Holland: IFIP.

Kua, E. H. (1992). A community study of mental disorders in elderly Singaporean Chinese using the GMS-AGECAT package. *Australian and New Zealand Journal of Psychiatry, 26*(3), 502–506.

Kuh, D., & Ben-Shlomo, Y. (1997). *A life-course approach to chronic disease epidemiology.* Oxford, UK: Oxford University Press.

Larson, S., Owens, P., Ford, D., & Eaton, W. (2001). Depressive disorders, dysthymia and risk of stroke: A thirteen year follow-up from the Baltimore ECA. *Stroke, 32*(9), 1979–1983.

Laursen, T. M., Munk-Olsen, T., Nordentoft, M., & Mortensen, P. B. (2007). Increased mortality among patients admitted with major psychiatric disorders: A register-based study comparing mortality in unipolar depressive disorder, bipolar affective disorder, schizoaffective disorder, and schizophrenia. *Journal of Clinical Psychiatry, 68*(6), 899–907.

Leighton, A. H., & Murphy, J. M. (1997). Nature of pathology: The character of danger implicit in functional impairment. *Canadian Journal of Psychiatry, 42*(7), 714–721.

Lilienfeld, D. E., & Stolley, P. D. (1994). *Foundations of epidemiology.* New York, NY: Oxford University Press.

Lin, H. C., Hsiao, F. H., Pfeiffer, S., Hwang, Y. T., & Lee, H. C. (2008). An increased risk of stroke among young schizophrenia patients. *Schizophrenia Research, 101*(1–3), 234–241.

Liptzin, B., & Babigian, H. M. (1972). Ten years experience with a cumulative psychiatric patient register. *Methods of Information in Medicine, 11*(4), 238.

Liu, C. K., Lai, C. L., Tai, C. T., Lin, R. T., Yen, Y. Y., & Howng, S. L. (1998). Incidence and subtypes of dementia in southern Taiwan: Impact of socio-demographic factors. *Neurology, 50*(6), 1572–1579.

Lobo, A., Launer, L. J., Fratiglioni, L., Andersen, K., Di, C. A., Breteler, M. M.,...Hofman, A. (2000). Prevalence of dementia and major subtypes in Europe: A collaborative study of population-based cohorts. Neurologic Diseases in the Elderly Research Group. *Neurology, 54*(11), S4–S9.

McGrath, J., Saha, S., Chant, D., & Welham, J. (2008). Schizophrenia: A concise overview of incidence, prevalence, and mortality. *Epidemiologic Reviews, 30*, 67–76.

McHugh, P. R., & Slavney, P. R. (1998). *The perspectives of psychiatry* (2nd ed.). Baltimore, MD: Johns Hopkins University Press.

Meller, I., Fichter, M. M., & Schroppel, H. (1999). Mortality risk in the octo- and nonagenerians: Longitudinal results of an epidemiological follow-up community study. *European Archives of Psychiatry and Clinical Neurosciences, 249*(4), 180–189.

Merikangas, K. R., Angst, J., Eaton, W., Canino, G., Rubio-Stipec, M., Wacker, H.,...Kupfer, D. (1996). Comorbidity and boundaries of affective disorders with anxiety disorders and substance misuse: Results of an international task force. *British Journal of Psychiatry, 30*(Suppl.), 58–67.

Merikangas, K., & Gelernter, C. S. (1990). Comorbidity for alcoholism and depression. *Psychiatric Clinics of North America, 13*(4), 613–632.

Merikangas, K. R., Mehta, R., Molnar, B. E., Walters, E. E., Swendsen, J. D., Aguilar-Gaziola, S.,...Kessler, R. (1998). Comorbidity of substance use disorders with mood and anxiety disorders: Results of the International Consortium in Psychiatric Epidemiology. *Addictive Behaviors, 23*(6), 893–907.

Meyer, C. M., Armenian, H. K., Eaton, W. W., & Ford, D. E. (2004). Incident hypertension associated with depression in the Baltimore Epidemiologic Catchment area follow-up study. *Journal of Affective Disorders, 83*(2–3), 127–133.

Mezuk, B., Eaton, W. W., Albrecht, S., & Golden, S. (2008). Depression and type 2 diabetes over the lifespan: A meta-analysis. *Diabetes Care, 31*(12), 2383–2390.

Mezuk, B., Eaton, W. W., Golden, S. H., Wand, G., & Lee, B. H. (2008). Depression, antidepressants and bone mineral density in a population-based cohort. *Journal of Gerontology, Biological Sciences, 63*(12), 1410–1415.

Mogga, S., Prince, M., Alem, A., Kebede, D., Stewart, R., Glozier, N., & Hotopf, M. (2006). Outcome of major depression in Ethiopia: Population-based study-1. *British Journal of Psychiatry, 189*, 241–246.

Morris, J. N. (1975). *Uses of epidemiology* (3rd ed.). Edinburgh, UK: Churchill Livingstone.

Munk-Jorgensen, P., Kastrup, M., & Mortensen, P. B. (1993). The Danish psychiatric register as a tool in epidemiology. *Acta Psychiatrica Scandinavica, 370*(Suppl.), 27–32.

Murphy, J. M., Burke, J. D., Jr., Monson, R. R., Horton, N. J., Laird, N. M., Lesage, A.,...Leighton, A. (2008). Mortality associated with depression: A 40-year perspective from the Stirling County study. *Social Psychiatry and Psychiatric Epidemiology, 43*(8), 594–601.

Murphy, J. M., Monson, R., Laird, N., Sobol, A., & Leighton, A. (1998). Identifying depression and anxiety in a 40-year epidemiological investigation: The Stirling County study. *International Journal of Methods in Psychiatric Research, 7*(2), 89–109.

Murphy, J., Monson, R., Laird, N., Sobol, A., & Leighton, A. (2000). Studying the incidence of depression: an 'interval' effect. *International Journal of Methods in Psychiatric Research, 9,* 184–193.

Musselman, D. L., Tomer, A., Manatunga, A. K., Knight, B. T., Poerter, M. R., Kasey, S., … Nemeroff, C. V. (1996). Exaggerated platelet reactivity in major depression. *American Journal of Psychiatry, 153*(10), 1313–1317.

Oerlemans, M. E. J., van den Akker, M., Schuurman, A. G., Kellen, E., & Buntinx, F. (2007). A meta-analysis on depression and subsequent cancer risk. *Clinical Practice and Epidemiology in Mental Health, 3,* 29.

O'Hare, A. (1987). *Three county and St. Loman's psychiatric case registers.* Dublin, Ireland: Cahill Printers.

Oken, R., & Schulzer, M. (1999). At issue: Schizophrenia and rheumatoid arthritis, the negative association revisited. *Schizophrenia Bulletin, 25*(4), 625–638.

Osby, U., Brandt, L., Correia, N., Ekbom, A., & Sparen, P. (2001). Excess mortality in bipolar and unipolar disorder in Sweden. *Archives of General Psychiatry, 58*(9), 844–850.

Patten, S. B., Williams, J. V., Lavorato, D. H., Campbell, N. R., Eliasziw, M., & Campbell, T. S. (2009). Major depression as a risk factor for high blood pressure: Epidemiologic evidence from a national longitudinal study. *Psychosomatic Medicine, 71*(3), 273–279.

Pedersen-Carsten, B., Gotzsche, H., Moller, J. O., & Mortensen, P. B. (2006). The Danish Civil Registration System: A cohort of eight million persons. *Danish Medical Bulletin, 53*(4), 441–449.

Penninx, B., Guralnik, J., Ferrucci, L., Simonsick, E., Deeg, D., & Wallace, R. (1998). Depressive symptoms and physical decline in community-dwelling older persons. *Journal of the American Medical Association, 279*(21), 1720–1726.

Pratt, L. A., Ford, D. E., Crum, R. M., Armenian, H. K., Gallo, J. J., & Eaton, W. W. (1996). Depression, psychotropic medication and risk of heart attack: Prospective data from the Baltimore ECA follow-up. *Circulation, 94*(12), 3123–3129.

Pulska, T., Pahkala, K., Laippala, P., & Kivela, S. L. (1997). Six-year survival of depressed elderly Finns: A community study. *International Journal of Geriatric Psychiatry, 12*(9), 942–950.

Pulska, T., Pahkala, K., Laippala, P., & Kivela, S.L. (1998). Major depression as a predictor of premature deaths in elderly people in Finland: A community study. *Acta Psychiatrica Scandinavica, 97*(6), 408–411.

Ramasubbu, R., & Patten, S. B. (2003). Effect of depression on stroke morbidity and mortality. *Canadian Journal of Psychiatry, 48*(4), 250–257.

Renn, J. H., Yang, N. P., Chueh, C. M., Lin, C. Y., Lan, T. H., & Chou, P. (2009). Bone mass in schizophrenia and normal populations across different decades of life. *BMC Musculoskeletal Disorders, 10,* 1.

Robins, L. N., Helzer, J. E., Croughan, J., & Ratcliff, K. S. (1981). National Institute of Mental Health Diagnostic Interview Schedule: Its history, characteristics, and validity. *Archives of General Psychiatry, 38*(4), 381–389.

Robins, L., Helzer, J., Cottler, L., & Goldring, E. (1989). *NIMH Diagnostic Interview Schedule Version III Revised, Department of Psychiatry,* Washington University-St. Louis.

Robins, L., Wing, J. K., Wittchen, H. U., Helzer, J. E., Babor, T. F., Burke, J., … Towle, L. H. (1988). The Composite International Diagnostic Interview: An epidemiologic instrument suitable for use in conjunction with different diagnostic systems and in different cultures. *Archives of General Psychiatry, 45*(12), 1069–1077.

Rossow, I., & Amundsen, A. (1997). Alcohol abuse and mortality: A 40-year prospective study of Norwegian conscripts. *Social Science and Medicine, 44*(2), 261–267.

Rothman, K. J. (1981). Induction and latent periods. *American Journal of Epidemiology, 114*(2), 253–259.

Rubin, R., Poland, R., Leser, I., Winston, R., & Blodgett, N. (1987). Neuroendocrine aspects of primary endogenous depression, I: Cortisol secretory dynamics in patients and matched controls. *Archives of General Psychiatry, 44*(4), 328–336.

Rugulies, R. (2002). Depression as a predictor for coronary heart disease: A review and meta-analysis. *American Journal of Preventive Medicine, 23*(1), 51–61.

Saz, P., Launer, L. J., Dia, J. L., De-La-Camara, C., Marcos, G., & Lobo, A. (1999). Mortality and mental disorders in a Spanish elderly population. *International Journal of Geriatric Psychiatry, 14*(12), 1031–1038.

Selten, J. P., & Sijben, N. (1994). First admission rates for schizophrenia in immigrants to the Netherlands. The Dutch National Register. *Social Psychiatry and Psychiatric Epidemiology, 29*(2), 71–77.

Skoog, I., Nilsson, L., Palmertz, B., Andreasson, L. A., & Svanborg, A. (1993). A population-based study of dementia in 85-year-olds. *New England Journal of Medicine, 328*(3), 153–158.

Snowdon, J., & Lane, F. (1995). The Botany survey: A longitudinal study of depression and cognitive impairment in an elderly population. *International Journal of Geriatric Psychiatry, 10,* 349–358.

Swendsen, J., Conway, K. P., Degenhardt, L., Dierker, L., Glantz, M., Jin, R.,…Kessler, R. C. (2009). Socio-demographic risk factors for alcohol and drug dependence: The 10-year follow-up of the National Comorbidity Survey. *Addiction, 104*(8), 1346–1355.

ten Horn, C. H., Giel, R., Gulbinat, W. H., & Henderson, J. H. (1986). *Psychiatric case registers in public health—A worldwide inventory 1960–1985.* Amsterdam, Netherlands: Elsevier.

Thorup, A., Waltoft, B. L., Pedersen, C. B., Mortensen, P. B., & Nordentoft, M. (2007). Young males have a higher risk of developing schizophrenia: A Danish register study. *Psychological Medicine, 37*(4), 479–484.

Tsuji, I., Minami, Y., Li, J. H., Fukao, A., Hisamichi, S., Asano, H.,…Shinoda, K. (1995). Dementia and physical disability as competing risks for mortality in a community-based sample of the elderly Japanese. *Tohoku Journal of Experimental Medicine, 176*(2), 99–107.

Vaillant, G. E. (1996). A long-term follow-up of male alcohol abuse. *Archives of General Psychiatry, 53*(3), 243–249.

Von Korff, M. R., Scott, K. M., & Gureje, O. (2009). *Global perspectives on mental–physical comorbidity in the WHO World Mental Health Surveys.* New York, NY: Cambridge University Press.

Wing, J. K. (1989). *Health services planning and research: Contributions from psychiatric case registers.* London, UK: Gaskell.

Ziegler-Graham, K., Brookmeyer, R., Johnson, E., & Arrighi, H. M. (2008). Worldwide variation in the doubling time of Alzheimer's disease incidence rates. *Alzheimer's and Dementia, 4*(5), 316–323.

7

The Relationship of Adult Mental Disorders to Socioeconomic Status, Race/Ethnicity, Marital Status, and Urbanicity of Residence

SILVIA S. MARTINS

JEAN KO

SACHIKO KUWABARA

DIANA CLARKE

PIERRE ALEXANDRE

PETER ZANDI

TAMAR MENDELSON

PREBEN BO MORTENSEN

WILLIAM W. EATON

Key Points

- A comprehensive review of the literature suggests the central importance for adult mental disorders of the variables of socioeconomic status, race/ethnicity, marital status, and urbanicity of residence

- Results are presented from the two best data sets for analyses of important social variables and common adult mental disorders: the Collaborative Psychiatric Epidemiology Surveys and the National Epidemiologic Study of Alcohol and Related Conditions

- For the analysis of schizophrenia, data from the Danish Psychiatric Register are presented

- Low socioeconomic status is associated with schizophrenia, major depressive disorder, anxiety disorders, and substance use disorders

- Blacks and Hispanics have equal or even lower risk for major depressive disorder than Whites, but these groups are at higher risk for chronic or persistent depression than Whites

- Ethnic minorities experience greater alcohol-related problems than Whites

- Being unmarried is associated with a higher prevalence of anxiety disorders, major depressive disorder, bipolar disorder, and schizophrenia

- Schizophrenia is associated with birth or residence in urban areas, but the relationship of urbanicity to other adult mental disorders is unclear

INTRODUCTION

This chapter presents an overview of recent literature and new data on differences in the prevalence of mental disorders across four key social variables: socioeconomic status (SES), race/ethnicity, marital status, and urbanicity. The first variable, SES, refers to the position of individuals, families, or households on one or more dimensions of stratification such as education, income, and wealth (Bollen, Glanville, & Stecklov, 2001). Education and income were chosen as SES indicators in the conduct of this chapter's literature review; education was used as a proxy SES measure for the chapter's data analysis section. While definitions of race/ethnicity vary widely and are the subject of some controversy, from an epidemiologic perspective, the concept generally is defined as a combination of constructs reflecting an individual's physical (phenotypic) and cultural (self-reported race) dimensions as well as one's social identity (ethnicity) (Whaley, 2003). When referring to US studies, this chapter has adopted five broad, commonly used racial/ethnic group descriptors: Whites, Blacks, Hispanics, Native Americans, and Asians (Office of Management and Budget, 1997). Marital status functions as a proxy measure for social cohesion, since research has found marriage to reduce risky, unhealthy behavior and to increase material well-being (Waite, 1996). Urbanicity is a proxy measure for the geographical location and physical environment of a population and is included as a variable because where a person resides can have a direct impact on that individual's health outcomes.

As in other areas of health, population disparities exist in the prevalence, diagnosis, and treatment of mental disorders. Differences in the prevalence of mental disorders can alert public health practitioners to populations at high risk for the disorders and can alert researchers to variables that may confound relationships in observational and clinical studies. Prevalence differences also reflect potential disparities in access to and provision of care, both across and within populations. Not surprisingly, the recently established, US Federal Collaborative for Health Disparities Research identified the reduction of grave disparities across populations in mental health—along with obesity, comorbidities, and the built environment—as a leading health issue that demands immediate policy and program attention (Safran et al., 2009). This chapter focuses on differences in the prevalence of mental disorders in important subgroups of the population as a key element in public mental health efforts to reduce the excess disability and other sequelae associated with mental disorders in the US and around the world.

Data Review Methods

To assess population differences in mental disorders, this review included only general population studies. It did not include studies on disparities in access to mental health care, the focus of chapter 15. Based on a search of the PubMed, PsycINFO, and Scopus databases, a review was conducted of all general population studies published in the past 15 years that included specific, selected matching terms related to specific mental disorders and the four key variables. For instance, of an initial 1,238 studies related to anxiety disorders that met search criteria, 1,088 found not to meet inclusion criteria were dropped. Of the remaining 148 studies retrieved for more detailed exploration, some were dropped either because they were duplicate studies or were not general population studies. Of the initial total, ultimately 75 studies met the search criteria. More details regarding the literature search across major mental disorders are found in table 7-1.

In addition to the literature search, an analysis of population differences among US adults was conducted using data from two nationwide data sets: the Collaborative Psychiatric Epidemiology Surveys (CPES) (Heeringa et al., 2004; Pennell et al., 2004) and the National Epidemiologic Study of Alcohol and Related Conditions (NESARC) (Grant, Moore, Shepard, & Kaplan, 2003; Grant et al., 2004). Both data sets are based on large, nationally representative surveys that measured major mental disorders using diagnostic criteria from the fourth edition of the *Diagnostic and* *Statistical Manual of Mental Disorders* (DSM-IV) (American Psychiatric Association [APA], 1994). Most of the disorder-specific population disparities were analyzed using both the CPES and the NESARC data sets for the purpose of comparison. One caveat is necessary. Because schizophrenia is relatively rare, no field survey data were available for analysis. In their place, data from the population-based register in Denmark were analyzed, since the vast majority of individuals with schizophrenia are in treatment and therefore captured by such a register (Eaton, 1985, 1991). Results of the data analysis are presented following the literature review findings for each major mental disorder.

Most of the disease-specific analyses of CPES and NESARC data focused on 1-year prevalence, in which a disorder was reported as present at the time of the interview or in the immediately prior 12 months. Lifetime prevalence estimates of mental disorders are often less accurate, because they are vulnerable to incomplete recall (Eaton et al., 1997; Parker, 1987; Patten, 2003; Regier et al., 1998; Simon & VonKorff, 1995). In general, recall of more recent events, such as those within the past 12 months, is likely to be less vulnerable

Table 7-1. Population Disparities for Major Mental Disorders: Review of the Literature on General Population Studies

MENTAL DISORDER	NO. OF RETRIEVED ARTICLES MATCHING SEARCH TERMS[a]	FINAL NO. OF ARTICLES SELECTED[b]
Anxiety disorders	1,493	110
Major depressive disorder	5,172	73
Bipolar disorder	131	50
Schizophrenia	2,687	66
Alcohol abuse/dependence	857	64
Drug abuse/dependence	1,048	73

[a]Restricted to articles in English published from January 1993 to October 2008 that were not experimental or on treatments, clinical trials, or interventions. To locate articles, searches were structured as follows.
  Population Disparities: disparities OR differences OR inequalities OR disproportionate OR disadvantage
  AND
  1. Socioeconomic position: socioeconomic OR income OR education OR occupation OR social OR employment status OR type of work OR wealth
  2. Racial/ethnic group: Ethnic OR ethnicity OR racial OR race OR minority
  3. Marital status: Marital status OR marriage OR married
  4. Urbanicity: Urban OR rural OR geographic OR location
[b]After initial review several articles were excluded because studies were duplicated, focused on "at risk" or otherwise specific groups, or were not general population studies.

to such bias (Patten, 2003), although accuracy may vary with age. The 1-year prevalence rates represent a hybrid of both point and period prevalence. Compared with 1-year period prevalence, the hybrid rates suffer from mortality bias—that is, the prevalence numerator does not include persons who enter the study period with the disorder but who die before interview. However, since mental disorders are more chronic than acute and the likelihood of disease-related mortality is not great within a 1-year period, the risk for mortality bias is quite small, further validating the study's use of a 1-year prevalence estimate.

Data Sources

COLLABORATIVE PSYCHIATRIC EPIDEMIOLOGY SURVEYS

The CPES combines data from the National Comorbidity Survey Replication (NCS-R), the National Survey of American Life (NSAL), and the National Latino and Asian American Study (NLAAS) (Heeringa et al., 2004; Pennell et al., 2004), each of which was designed to collect information to estimate the prevalence of mental disorders and mental health service use in a nationally representative sample of the specified population using a complex, stratified sampling design. Using a representative sample of the US population, the NCS-R (data collected between February 2001 and April 2003) sought to estimate the prevalence of mental disorders and mental health service use in the United States (Kessler et al., 2004). The NSAL (data collected between February 2001 and March 2003) was designed to estimate racial/ethnic differences in mental disorders and service use among African Americans, Afro-Caribbean individuals, and White respondents living in the same US communities (Jackson et al., 2004). Similarly, the NLAAS (data collected between May 2002 and November 2003) was designed to estimate the prevalence of mental disorders and service use by Hispanic Americans and Asian Americans living in the United States (Alegria et al., 2007). Response rates were 70.9% for NCS-R, 71.5% for NSAL, and 75.7% for NLAAS. The CPES initiative was possible only because all three studies used the same modified version of the

Composite International Diagnostic Interview to assess mental disorders (Alegria et al., 2007; Heeringa et al., 2004; Jackson et al., 2004; Kessler et al., 2004; Pennell et al., 2004).

The CPES examined a number of sociodemographic variables—age, sex, level of education, racial/ethnic status, and marital status—as factors associated with disparities in past-year prevalence rates of specific adult mental disorders, among them major depressive disorder, bipolar I disorder, panic disorder, social phobia, simple phobia (also called specific phobia), and alcohol or drug abuse or dependence. Diagnoses of the disorders in the CPES surveys were based on the DSM-IV criteria (APA, 1994).

2001–2002 NATIONAL EPIDEMIOLOGIC SURVEY ON ALCOHOL AND RELATED CONDITIONS

The NESARC is a nationally representative survey of noninstitutionalized US civilian individuals, age 18 and older, based on a cross-sectional design and in-person interviews conducted by the US Bureau of the Census under the sponsorship and supervision of the National Institute of Alcohol Abuse and Alcoholism. Details of the sampling frame, interviewing, training, and quality control are described elsewhere (Grant et al., 2003, 2004). The study oversampled young adults, Hispanics, and African Americans. Prevalences were weighted to the 2000 decennial census for age, race, sex, and ethnicity and were further weighted to adjust for sampling probabilities. Study participants were interviewed using the Alcohol Use Disorder and Associated Disabilities Interview Schedule (AUDADIS-IV) (Grant, Dawson, & Hasin, 2001), a structured diagnostic interview designed for use by lay interviewers. Diagnostic methods used in the AUDADIS-IV are described in detail elsewhere (Grant et al., 2004, 2005; Hasin, Goodwin, Stinson, & Grant, 2005). The study achieved an 81% overall response rate.

The sociodemographic variables of interest included age, sex, level of education, racial/ethnic status, marital status, and, unlike in the CPES, urbanicity. The variables were used to examine disparities in the 12-month prevalence of various mental disorders, among them major depressive disorder, bipolar I disorder, panic disorder, social phobia, simple phobia, alcohol abuse or dependence, and drug abuse or dependence. The diagnoses were made consistent with DSM-IV criteria (APA, 1994).

DANISH PSYCHIATRIC REGISTER

The Danish Psychiatric Register (Munk-Jorgensen, Kastrup, & Mortensen, 1993) was used to obtain information on schizophrenia. The register contains data on all admissions to Danish psychiatric inpatient facilities and on outpatient visits to psychiatric departments. Diagnoses in the register are made by physicians using criteria in the 10th revision of the International Classification of Diseases (ICD-10) (World Health Organization, 1992). For schizophrenia, the DSM-IV–comparable F20 ICD code was employed. For analytic purposes, the numerator includes all calendar year 2006 admissions listed on the register with the diagnosis of schizophrenia; the denominator is a random one-in-four sample of residents of Denmark in the same year. Prevalence estimates then weight the denominator to equal the whole population. Danish ethnic differences are limited compared with populations in the United States, so race/ethnic differences are not presented here; further, definitions of some variables in the Danish register differ somewhat from those in the CPES and NESARC.

Data Analysis

To account for the complex sampling schemes of the CPES and NESARC, weighted analyses were conducted using the Sudaan 9.01 and Stata SE 10.0 software packages. Descriptive analyses, including frequency distribution and chi-square, were undertaken to estimate both the overall prevalence of the various disorders and the prevalence by gender, race/ethnicity, marital status, and educational attainment. Logistic regression analyses were conducted to obtain age-adjusted prevalence estimates for the mental disorders of interest.

Data on disparities in the prevalence of mental disorders by education, race/ethnicity,

marital status, and urbanicity are shown in tables 7-2 through 7-5, respectively. The findings are discussed by mental disorder following the literature review for each disorder. Note, however, that because schizophrenia is relatively rare, prevalence rates for this disorder in tables 7-4, 7-11, and 7-15 are presented per 1,000 population instead of per 100 population.[1]

DISORDERS AND THEIR PREVALENCE

This section provides an overview of the major mental disorders and the observed differences in their overall prevalence. The discussion begins with separate explorations of the anxiety disorders, major depressive disorder, bipolar disorder, schizophrenia, alcohol abuse and dependence, and drug abuse and dependence. The sections that follow explore the findings from both the literature review and examination of the NESARC and CPES data sets regarding potential associations between major mental disorders and the four key variables of, educational attainment, race/ethnicity, marital status, and urbanicity.

Anxiety Disorders

With an estimated 1-year prevalence of 18.1% and a lifetime prevalence of 28.8%, anxiety disorders (e.g., panic disorder, social phobia, simple phobia, and obsessive-compulsive disorder) are considered the most common class of mental disorders in the United States (Kessler, Berglund, et al., 2005; Kessler, Chiu, Demler, & Walters, 2005). On a more global level, a World Health Organization (2004) study found that among the 14 countries surveyed, anxiety disorders were the most common disorders in all but one (Ukraine), demonstrating the ubiquitous nature of anxiety disorders around the world. The DSM-IV (APA, 1994) identifies

---

1 In 2006, 2,086 admissions were made to outpatient psychiatric clinics in Denmark, and 4,572,984 residents formed the denominator, yielding a 1-year prevalence of 0.46 per 1,000. This rate is considerably lower than the prevalence of 5 per 1,000 cited in chapter 1, which is based on the findings of McGrath, Saha, Chant, and Welham (2008) and presumably included individuals with schizophrenia who were not in treatment in the given year.

anxiety disorders as encompassing a number of different conditions, each with its own constellation of diagnostic criteria: panic disorder (with and without agoraphobia), agoraphobia without history of panic disorder, specific phobia, social phobia, obsessive–compulsive disorder, posttraumatic stress disorder, acute stress disorder, generalized anxiety disorder, anxiety disorder due to a general medical condition, substance-induced anxiety disorder, and anxiety disorder not otherwise specified. Among these disorders, specific phobia has the greatest lifetime prevalence, with estimates in the range of 6–12%. In contrast, obsessive–compulsive disorder has the lowest lifetime prevalence among the anxiety disorders; estimates consistently are lower than 3% (Kessler, Ruscio, Shear, & Wittchen, 2008).

Mood Disorders

DEPRESSIVE DISORDER

Major depressive disorder is characterized by the cardinal symptoms of sadness or loss of pleasure and interest along with specific somatic symptoms, among them problems with weight, fatigue, sleep, and concentration. To reach diagnostic significance, unremitting symptoms must endure for at least 2 weeks (APA, 1994). As reported in chapter 1, worldwide the 1-year prevalence of major depressive disorder varies from 0.64% to 15.4%, with a median of 5.3% and an interquartile range of 3.6–6.5%.

BIPOLAR DISORDER

Bipolar disorder is defined by the presence of one or more episodes of abnormally elevated energy levels, cognition, and mood (mania) that generally last at least a week, often followed or preceded by one or more episodes of major depression (APA, 1994). Because manic episodes represent such a gross deviation from normal behavior, they generate immediate problems for the affected individual and frequently also for others in the individual's social environment. The median past-year prevalence of bipolar disorder, as noted in chapter 1, is 0.6%, with a relatively small interquartile range of 0.3–1.1%. The symptoms and

characteristics of bipolar disorder I in DSM-IV (APA, 1994) are consistent with the general characterization of what was called manic–depressive illness during the majority of the 20th century. Bipolar disorder II represents a syndrome with considerably less severe levels of mania.

Schizophrenia

Schizophrenia, originally called adolescent dementia by Kraepelin (1893), is characterized by the striking symptoms of visual or auditory hallucinations or delusions, frequently accompanied by chaotic speech or behavior, all of which can be distressing, even frightening, to others. The 1-year median prevalence of the disorder, as reported in chapter 1, is 0.5%, with an interquartile range of 0.3–0.6%.

Alcohol and Drug Use Disorders

ALCOHOL USE DISORDERS

Together, alcohol abuse and dependence are the third leading cause of death in the United States (McGinnis & Foege, 1993) and the fourth leading cause of excess disability worldwide (Murray & Lopez, 1996). These disorders can result in both short- and long-term adverse health consequences. The DSM-IV–related diagnostic criteria for alcohol abuse and dependence (APA, 1994) include the presence of symptoms such as withdrawal and tolerance, alcohol use in dangerous or inappropriate situations, trouble with the law, and a past-year history of alcohol's interfering with obligations at work, school, or home. In 2009, 18.7 million persons in the United States, 7.4% of the population age 12 and older, were found to abuse or be dependent on alcohol (Substance Abuse and Mental Health Services Administration [SAMHSA], 2010). Using data from the NESARC, Cohen, Fein, Arias and Kranzler (2007) found that only 14.6% of individuals with lifetime DSM-IV alcohol abuse or dependence had received treatment.

DRUG USE DISORDERS

The term drug use disorder encompasses both drug abuse and dependence. Drug abuse involves a pattern of use of illegal drugs or misuse of legal drugs that is impairing or disabling. Use of these drugs may lead to criminal penalty in addition to possible physical, social, or psychological harm. Because use of an illegal substance can lead to criminal arrest, use in and of itself is sufficient for the diagnosis of drug abuse. In contrast to drug abuse, drug dependence involves a physiological craving that demands a continuously escalating quantity of the drug to achieve the same desired psychoactive effect, or "high." Moreover, the search for and use of the psychoactive agent comes to dominate the life of the drug-dependent individual.

This chapter does not discuss disparities in drug initiation and drug use per se; rather, it focuses on individuals who have already transitioned from use to abuse or dependence. Thus this review relies on the diagnostic criteria for both drug abuse and dependence found in DSM-IV and ICD-10 and considers both classifications when assessing the prevalence of drug use disorders. One-year prevalence rates for these disorders range from 0.4% in Mexico to 3.6% in the United States, with a median prevalence of 1.8%. According to the 2009 National Survey of Drug Use and Health (SAMHSA, 2010), an estimated 22.5 million persons age 12 or older in the United States were classified with substance dependence or abuse in the year prior to the interview(8.9% of the population age 12 and older). Of these, 3.2 million were classified with dependence on or abuse of both alcohol and illegal drugs, 3.9 million were dependent on or abused illegal drugs but not alcohol, and 15.4 million were dependent on or abused alcohol but not illegal drugs.

Marijuana was the illegal drug with the highest prevalence of past-year dependence or abuse in 2009, followed by nonmedical use of prescription opioids and then by cocaine. Of the 7.1 million persons age 12 or older classified with dependence on or abuse of illegal drugs in 2009, 4.3 million were dependent on or abused marijuana or hashish (1.7% of the total population age 12 or older, and 60.5% of all those classified with illegal drug dependence or abuse), 1.9 million persons were classified with dependence on or abuse of prescription opioids

(0.8% of the total population), and 1.1 million persons were classified with dependence on or abuse of cocaine (0.4% of the total population) (SAMHSA, 2010).

EFFECTS OF SOCIOECONOMIC STATUS ON DISORDER PREVALENCE

Intuitively, one might posit that lower economic status—poverty, lower educational attainment, and lower level of employment—would be associated with a greater risk for major mental disorders, much like trends found for other frequently disabling chronic and acute illnesses. Independent of the specific variables or concepts used to define low SES, several studies have shown that it is associated with schizophrenia, depression, and substance use disorders (Dohrenwend, 2000; Dohrenwend & Dohrenwend, 1969; Dohrenwend et al., 1992). In addition, several authors have sought to examine whether the inverse relationship between mental disorders and SES is due to social selection (downward mobility of the genetically predisposed) or social causation (adversity and stress). Their findings have indicated that social selection is more important in some disorders, such as schizophrenia, while social causation is more important in other disorders, notably depression (Costello, Compton, Keeler & Angold, 2003; Dohrenwend, 2000; Dohrenwend et al., 1992). This section explores just the conjecture of the inverse relationship between SES and psychiatric disorders, based on the literature search described earlier and an assessment of CPES and NESARC data.

Anxiety Disorders

Studies consistently have demonstrated an inverse relationship between anxiety disorder and at least one marker of social or economic disadvantage (Fryers, Melzer, & Jenkins, 2003). The Epidemiologic Catchment Area study (ECA), National Comorbidity Study (NCS), British Psychiatric Morbidity survey, and the Netherlands Mental Health Survey and Incidence Study all showed a significant association between anxiety disorders and most socioeconomic indicators, even after adjustment for age and sex (Bijl, Ravelli, & van Zessen, 1998; Lewis et al., 1998; Muntaner, Eaton, Diala, Kessler, & Sorlie, 1998). Prevalence of anxiety disorders has been found to be higher in groups with less education, greater unemployment, and lower income or material assets.

The ECA data showed groups with lower SES to have a higher prevalence of panic disorder, phobias, and generalized anxiety disorder (Muntaner, Eaton, Miech, & O'Campo, 2004). The ECA data also disclosed a higher prevalence of social phobia, agoraphobia, and obsessive–compulsive disorder among individuals with less education and those of lower socioeconomic class (Eaton & Keyl, 1990; Nestadt, Beinvenu, Cai, Samuels, & Eaton, 1998; Wells, Tien, Garrison, & Eaton, 1994). In prospective analyses low occupational prestige was found to be a risk factor for both panic attacks and panic disorder (Keyl & Eaton, 1990). These general findings about the relationship between SES and anxiety disorder were confirmed in the NCS specifically for generalized anxiety disorder, panic disorder, agoraphobia, simple phobia, and social phobia (Eaton, Kessler, Wittchen, & Magee, 1994; Magee, Eaton, Wittchen, McGonagle, & Kessler, 1996; Wittchen, Zhao, Kessler, & Eaton, 1994). NCS data showed that an anxiety disorder was 2.8 times more common in individuals who had not completed high school than in those with at least a college education, and 2.1 times more common in those with a yearly income under $20,000 than in individuals with a yearly income over $70,000 (Kessler et al., 1994). In particular, social phobia was most prevalent among those of lower education and income as well as among individuals living with their parents. The risk for agoraphobia was more common among homemakers than those working outside the home; it also was inversely related to both income and education (Kessler et al., 1994; Magee et al., 1996).

The estimated prevalence and odds ratios for panic disorder between education levels were consistent across the CPES and NESARC data sets, with CPES data yielding slightly higher prevalence estimates and the NESARC yielding higher odds ratios. (See table 7-2 for findings on anxiety disorders.) According to both data sets, lower levels of education were more strongly associated with panic disorder than were higher levels. The estimated prevalence of social phobia was consistently higher in the CPES across categories of education. Lower levels of education signaled increased risk for social phobia, according to both data sets. As with social phobia, the estimated prevalence of simple phobia was higher in the CPES data than in the NESARC across all levels of education. In both data sets, lower education was strongly associated with simple phobia.

Mood Disorders

Large-scale US surveys generally have found an inverse association between SES and the prevalence of major depressive disorder in adults. The NCS, for example, found education to be inversely associated with prevalence of current major depression (Blazer, Kessler, McGonagle, & Swartz, 1994); education, annual household income, and wealth were inversely associated with prevalence of mood disorders over the previous year (Muntaner et al., 1998). According to the NCS-R, prevalence of past-year depression was associated with poverty and less than a high school education; low income was associated with more severe depression for individuals who experienced past-year major depression (Kessler et al., 2003). ECA follow-up data (Muntaner et al., 1998), as well as data from the Alameda County study (Lynch, Kaplan, & Sema, 1997) and the Healthcare for Communities survey (Gresenz, Sturm, & Tang, 2001) showed a similar inverse association between household income and depressive disorders. Some studies also have found childhood SES to be associated with lifetime risk for depression, independent of later SES and other sociodemographic and psychiatric factors (Gilman, Kawachi, Fitzmaurice, & Buka, 2002, 2003). However, not all US studies have found the prevalence of depression to vary as a function of economic status. (See, for example, Weissman, Bruce, Leaf, Florio, & Holzer, 1991.)

Numerous international studies have reported on the association between economic status and depression (Araya et al., 2001;

Table 7-2. Disparities in Mood and Anxiety Disorders by Socioeconomic Status (as Measured by Education)

	CPES				NESARC			
	LESS THAN HIGH SCHOOL	HIGH SCHOOL	SOME COLLEGE	COLLEGE OR MORE	LESS THAN HIGH SCHOOL	HIGH SCHOOL	SOME COLLEGE	COLLEGE OR MORE
Major depressive disorder (N)	(3,931)	(5,745)	(5,188)	(4,672)	(7,849)	(12,547)	(12,663)	(10,034)
Prevalence (N)[a]	7.64 (282)	6.12 (356)	7.16 (350)	6.16 (276)	7.23 (538)	6.37 (828)	6.91 (903)	5.84 (618)
Odds ratio [CI][b]	1.33 [1.09, 1.62]	0.98 [0.78, 1.24]	1.09 [0.86, 1.38]	1.00	1.33 [1.13, 1.56]	1.09 [0.95, 1.24]	1.12 [0.99, 1.27]	1.00
Panic disorder (N)	(3,931)	(5,745)	(5,185)	(4,671)	(7,849)	(12,547)	(12,663)	(10,034)
Prevalence (N)[a]	3.02 (133)	2.16 (129)	3.05 (139)	1.99 (85)	2.50 (181)	2.09 (266)	2.58 (315)	1.55 (173)
Odds ratio [CI][b]	1.60 [1.15, 2.22]	1.08 [0.84, 1.39]	1.46 [1.06, 2.02]	1.00	1.73 [1.32, 2.25]	1.34 [1.05, 1.70]	1.57 [1.26, 1.95]	1.00
Social phobia (N)	(3,931)	(5,745)	(5,186)	(4,671)	(7,849)	(12,547)	(12,663)	(10,034)
Prevalence (N)[a]	7.04 (257)	6.27 (331)	6.35 (316)	5.34 (217)	3.06 (220)	3.03 (359)	3.01 (362)	1.91 (199)
Odds ratio [CI][b]	1.41 [1.09, 1.84]	1.18 [0.90, 1.54]	1.12 [0.81, 1.54]	1.00	1.71 [1.31, 2.23]	1.60 [1.26, 2.03]	1.52 [1.21, 1.90]	1.00
Simple phobia[c] (N)	(1,292)	(2,687)	(2,666)	(2,353)	(7,849)	(12,547)	(12,663)	(10,034)
Prevalence (N)[a]	11.43 (164)	8.64 (240)	8.31 (224)	16.94 (173)	7.26 (552)	7.07 (880)	7.92 (999)	6.16 (642)
Odds ratio [CI][b]	1.73 [1.26, 2.37]	1.27 [1.04, 1.54]	1.22 [1.01, 1.47]	1.00	1.24 [1.05, 1.46]	1.14 [1.01, 1.29]	1.23 [1.09, 1.40]	1.00

CI = 95% confidence interval.
[a]Row percentage weighted. [b]Adjusted for age and sex. [c]Only available in the NCS-R data, not available in the NLAAS or NSAL.

Stansfeld, Clark, Rodgers, Caldwell, & Power, 2008; Turner & Lloyd, 1999). Lorant and colleagues' (2007) meta-analysis of 51 prevalence studies, 5 incidence studies, and 5 persistence studies not limited to the United States found the association of SES and depression to be characterized by a dose–response relation across the SES spectrum in which income showed stronger associations than education. Low SES is associated with only a slight risk for a new episode of depression (odds ratio = 1.24, $p = 0.004$) and a moderate risk for episode persistence (odds ratio = 2.06, $p < 0.001$) (Lorant et al., 2007). Consistent with those findings, cross-national comparative data on mental disorders collected through the World Health Organization International Consortium in Psychiatric Epidemiology (2000) indicated that SES measures including income, education, and employment were inversely correlated with mood disorders. A more recent, prospective cohort study in Belgium found declines in SES were predictive of increases in depression (Lorant et al., 2007).

Analysis of NESARC and CPES data revealed the estimated prevalences and odds ratios for major depressive disorder to be consistent across the two data sets for education level (see table 7-2). In both data sets, individuals with less than a high school education were more likely than college graduates to have a past-year major depressive disorder.

When it comes to bipolar disorders, a number of clinical studies have found a relationship with higher SES (e.g., Weissman & Myers, 1978; Woodruff, Guze, & Clayton, 1971). In a review of these studies in a seminal textbook on bipolar disorder, Goodwin and Jamison (1990) concluded that "it appears the majority of studies report an association between manic–depressive illness and one or more measures reflecting upper social class." However, later population-based samples revealed a different picture, suggesting that individuals with bipolar disorder in fact were more likely than healthy individuals to have lower levels of education (Canino et al., 1987; Grant et al., 2005; Kessler, Rubinow, Holmes, Abelson, & Zhao, 1997; Merikangas et al., 2007; Weissman et al., 1991), higher levels of unemployment (Merikangas et al., 2007),

or lower incomes (Grant et al., 2005; Jonas, Brody, Roper, & Narrow, 2003; Kessler et al., 1997; Schaffer, Cairney, Cheung, Veldhuizen, & Levitt, 2006). An interesting study conducted using Danish population-based registries provides clues to help reconcile these conflicting findings (Tsuchiya, Agerbo, Byrne, & Mortensen, 2004). It found that parents of cases with bipolar disorder tended to be more highly educated and have greater wealth than the parents of controls. At the same time, however, individuals who were receiving social assistance, pensions, or sickness payments or who were unemployed, had shorter educational histories, or had lower income were at greater risk for bipolar disorder than were controls. Thus bipolar disorder appeared to be associated with a downward drift in SES. The finding is not entirely surprising. Symptoms of bipolar disorder often first arise during adolescence and early adulthood, potentially disrupting educational opportunity and, consequently, the ability to obtain and maintain gainful employment (Dean, Gerner, & Gerner, 2004).

Analyses of CPES and NESARC data found that the estimated prevalence of bipolar I disorder was consistently higher in the NESARC data across levels of education (see table 7-3). In both data sets the odds of bipolar I were higher for those with lower levels of education.

Schizophrenia

The literature exploring the relationship between low SES and higher risk for schizophrenia has a long and extensive history (Dohrenwend & Dohrenwend, 1969; Dohrenwend et al., 1992; Eaton, 1974; Eaton & Harrison, 2001; Jarvis, 1855/1971; Mishler & Scotch, 1963; Goldberg and Morrison, 1963, Turner & Wagenfeld, 1967). Longitudinal studies suggest that the association is due to the effects of disease onset on the ability to compete in the job market. Agerbo, Byrne, Eaton, and Mortensen (2004) found that individuals with schizophrenia were more likely than others to be unemployed, not only at diagnosis but also many years earlier and many years thereafter. Recent Scandinavian studies suggest that if anything, the parents of individuals

Table 7-3. Disparities in Prevalence of Bipolar Disorder by Socioeconomic Status (as Measured by Education)

	CPES				NESARC			
	LESS THAN HIGH SCHOOL	HIGH SCHOOL	SOME COLLEGE	COLLEGE OR MORE	LESS THAN HIGH SCHOOL	HIGH SCHOOL	SOME COLLEGE	COLLEGE OR MORE
Bipolar I disorder (N)	(2,621)	(4,740)	(4,092)	(3,434)	(7,849)	(12,547)	(12,663)	(10,034)
Prevalence (N)[a]	0.69 (24)	0.65 (34)	0.84 (34)	0.19 (8)	1.19 (84)	0.95 (116)	1.05 (142)	0.35 (37)
Odds ratio [CI][b]	3.89 [1.01, 14.9]	3.30 [1.05, 10.3]	3.81 [1.17, 12.4]	1.00	4.06 [2.43, 6.78]	2.80 [1.77, 2.43]	2.71 [1.73, 4.24]	1.00

CI = 95% confidence interval.
[a] Column percentage weighted. [b] Adjusted for age and sex.

with diagnosed schizophrenia are likely to be of higher, not lower, social position (Byrne, Agerbo, Eaton, & Mortensen, 2004). Thus low socioeconomic position is not likely a causal factor for schizophrenia and, while strongly associated with the disorder's prevalence, is not now viewed as a risk factor.

Analyses of Danish register data show that, consistent with the literature, a higher prevalence of schizophrenia is associated with lower levels of educational attainment (see table 7-4). Persons with a high school education or less have about four times the prevalence of schizophrenia as those of higher educational attainment.

Alcohol and Drug Use Disorders

Data from the National Survey of Drug Use and Health (NSDUH) indicate that past-year alcohol abuse and dependence were more prevalent in respondents with family incomes of less than 125% of the federal poverty threshold (9.4%) than among those above that level (7.5%) (SAMHSA, 2005). While individuals of lower SES generally are at greater risk for alcohol dependence, evidence suggests that members of some disadvantaged groups actually are at lower lifetime risk (Anthony, Warner, & Kessler, 1994; Grant et al., 2001). Similarly, while some studies have reported alcohol-related problems to be common among the economically disadvantaged, others have found these problems common among the affluent (Knupfer, 1989). Longitudinal studies have found childhood economic disadvantage to be correlated with adult substance use disorders (Brunswick, Messeri, & Titus, 1992, Poulton et al., 2002). Fothergill and Ensminger (2006) showed low family economic status to be associated with alcohol problems in adulthood. Other studies have found alcohol-related disorders to be more prevalent among adults who experienced socioeconomic disadvantage as children in Europe (Claussen, Davey Smith, & Thelle, 2003; Melchior, Berkman, Niedhammer, Zins, & Goldberg, 2007; Osler, Nordentoft, & Andersen, 2006; Poulton et al., 2002). Melchior and colleagues (2007) found that children in New Zealand who experienced socioeconomic disadvantage were at higher risk of suffering from later alcohol dependence.

Analysis of data from the NCS and the National Longitudinal Alcohol Epidemiologic Study (NLAES) found that respondents with fewer than 12 years of education were 1.5 times more likely to have alcohol dependence than respondents with 16 years or more of education (Grant, 1997). Further, the ECA reports higher levels of education to be associated with lower rates of lifetime prevalence of alcohol abuse and dependence (Helzer, Burnam, & McEvoy, 1991). Using NCS data, Diala, Muntaner, and Walrath (2004) found that although household income was protective against alcohol use and dependence, high

Table 7-4. Disparities in Prevalence of Schizophrenia by Socioeconomic Status (as Measured by Education)

	DANISH PSYCHIATRIC REGISTER				
	LESS THAN HIGH SCHOOL	HIGH SCHOOL	VOCATIONAL	POST HIGH SCHOOL AND BA	POST COLLEGE
Schizophrenia					
Prevalence per 1,000 (N)[a]	0.82 (1,210)	0.79 (252)	0.28 (385)	0.20 (143)	0.22 (48)
Odds ratio [CI][b]	1.00	0.97 [0.85, 1.11]	0.34 [0.31, 0.39]	0.24 [0.20, 0.29]	0.27 [0.20, 0.35]

CI = 95% confidence interval.

[a]Numerator is from all hospital and specialty clinic admissions in Denmark in 2006; denominator from 25% sample of population of Denmark in 2006 (weighted to 100%).

[b]Adjusted for age and sex; 48 cases with missing data excluded.

occupation strata were positively associated with alcohol disorders. While some studies have found a relationship between education level and the onset of alcohol abuse and dependence, the relationship may be explained by a failure to achieve a desired level of education. Thus persons who fail to achieve a sought-for diploma consistently have been found to be at increased risk for alcohol abuse or dependence in adulthood (Crum, Bucholz, Helzer, & Anthony, 1992; Crum, Helzer, & Anthony, 1993).

In Dharan, Nepal, alcohol dependence was found to be more common among individuals with lower levels of education than among more learned individuals (Jhingan, Shyangwa, Sharma, Prasad, & Khandelwal, 2003). However, among women in Sweden, Thundal and Allebeck (1998) found that dissatisfaction with one's level of education, rather than the level of education itself, was associated with an increased prevalence of alcohol abuse and dependence. Divergent results on the impact of SES on the prevalence of alcohol abuse and dependence have been found in a number of Brazilian studies (Almeida Filho et al., 2004; Barros, Botega, Dalgalarrondo, Marín-León, & de Oliveira, 2007; Mendoza-Sassi & Beria, 2003). A study in Puerto Rico found alcohol use disorders to be associated with higher family income and with being employed (Colón, Robles, Canino, & Sahai, 2001).

Studies also have found the prevalence of DSM-IV–diagnosed alcohol dependence to be higher among lower economic groups (Grant, 1997; Hasin, Stinson, Ogburn, & Grant, 2007; Van Oers, Bongers, van de Goor, & Garretsen, 1999). At the same time, evidence suggests that DSM-IV–diagnosed alcohol abuse is positively associated with higher income in adults and educational achievement among college-age youth (Grant, 1997; Hasin et al., 2007; Keyes & Hasin, 2008). A plausible explanation for the findings posits that a diagnosis of current alcohol abuse may not capture the full range of alcohol abusers across all socioeconomic groups (Keyes & Hasin, 2008).

Analysis of CPES data yielded no difference in education level among individuals with past-year alcohol use disorder. In contrast, the NESARC data revealed that those with high school and some college education were more likely to have a past-year alcohol use disorder than were those who were college educated. (See table 7-5.)

In most prevalence studies examined, lifetime and past-year drug use disorders were associated with lower educational attainment (Anthony et al., 1994; Bergen, Gardner, Aggen, & Kendler, 2008; Brugal et al., 1999; Compton, Thomas, Stinson, & Grant, 2007; Grant, 1996; O'Brien & Anthony, 2005; Roberts & Lee, 1993; SAMHSA, 2007; L. A. Warner, Kessler, Hughes, Anthony, & Nelson, 1995). The sole exception, a study reporting data from the 1997 National Survey of Mental Health and Well-Being, found no such association (Hall, Teesson, Lynskey, & Degenhardt, 1999). Indeed, several studies have shown that low educational attainment can be either the cause (Annis & Watson, 1975; Henry & Huizinga, 2007) or the result (Bray, Zarkin, Ringwalt, & Qi, 2000; Ellickson, Bui, Bell, & McGuigan, 1998) of a drug use disorder.

A few studies suggest that individuals of lower educational attainment are at high risk of becoming drug dependent (Grant, 1996; O'Brien & Anthony, 2005) and of experiencing persistent dependence (Grant, 1996) compared with those with higher educational attainment. For instance, O'Brien and Anthony's (2005) analysis of 2001–2002 NSDUH data found that while approximately 5% of recent-onset cocaine users become dependent within 24 months of first use, risk for cocaine dependence was greater among respondents aged 18 years and older who had not graduated from high school than among college graduates. In his analysis of data from the 1991–1992 NLAES, Grant (1996) reported that while individuals with 12 or fewer years of education were less likely to have used drugs compared with the most educated, the former were twice as likely than the latter to become dependent and to persist in their dependence.

When considering income itself, most studies have found lower income levels to be associated with drug use disorders (Compton et al., 2007; Grant, 1996; L. A. Warner et al., 1995). For example, in the 1991–1992 NLAES, respondents in the three lower income groups were more likely to become drug dependent

Table 7-5. Disparities in Prevalence of Alcohol and Drug Disorders by Socioeconomic Status (as Measured by Education)

	CPES				NESARC			
	LESS THAN HIGH SCHOOL	HIGH SCHOOL	SOME COLLEGE	COLLEGE OR MORE	LESS THAN HIGH SCHOOL	HIGH SCHOOL	SOME COLLEGE	COLLEGE OR MORE
Alcohol abuse/ dependence (N)	(3,286)	(4,408)	(3,984)	(3,485)	(7,849)	(12,547)	(12,663)	(10,034)
Prevalence (N)[a]	1.25 (44)	1.55 (55)	1.23 (47)	0.86 (26)	7.04 (461)	8.25 (967)	10.42 (1,180)	7.21 (719)
Odds ratio [CI][b]	1.38 [0.70, 2.70]	1.64 [0.96, 2.78]	1.23 [0.68, 2.25]	1.00	1.19 [0.99, 1.42]	1.27 [1.11, 1.45]	1.44 [1.27, 1.62]	1.00
Drug abuse/ dependence (N)	(3,286)	(4,408)	(3,983)	(3,485)	(7,849)	(12,547)	(12,663)	(10,034)
Prevalence (N)[a]	1.74 (57)	1.78 (69)	1.02 (41)	0.56 (25)	2.34 (150)	2.42 (266)	2.26 (259)	0.98 (102)
Odds ratio [CI][b]	2.41 [1.32, 4.38]	2.38 [1.35, 4.20]	1.26 [0.75, 2.14]	1.00	3.16 [2.23, 4.49]	2.77 [2.05, 3.76]	2.12 [1.59, 2.82]	1.00

CI = 95% confidence interval.
[a]Row percentage weighted. [b]Adjusted for age and sex.

than those in the highest income group (Grant, 1996). Similarly, in the 2001–2002 first wave of the NESARC, lower income level was found to be significantly associated with drug use disorders (Compton et al., 2007). Only a single general population study, in Japan, found that substance use disorders (including alcohol use disorders) were associated with higher income rather than lower-than-average income (Kawakami et al., 2005).

Analyses of both the CPES and NESARC data sets found that lower education levels were significantly associated with past-year drug use disorders (see table 7-5).

EFFECTS OF RACE AND ETHNICITY ON THE PREVALENCE OF DISORDERS

Anxiety Disorders

No consistent association between anxiety disorders and race or ethnicity has been reported in the literature. Some studies have suggested that Black adults may be more likely to experience certain anxiety disorders than other groups (Heurtin-Roberts, Snowden, & Miller, 1997; Neal & Turner, 1991). Thus, Black adults have been found to experience greater rates of agoraphobia than Whites (Brown & Eaton, 1986; Eaton, Dryman, & Weissman, 1991; Neal & Turner, 1991) and specific phobia at three times the rate of Whites (Last & Perrin, 1993; Neal & Turner, 1991). However, other studies posit that at least some of the associations may be attributable to sociodemographic variables that covary with race and ethnicity, such as age, marital status, income, education, and environmental factors (Kessler et al., 1994; Kurz, Malcom, & Cournoyer, 2005; Regier et al., 1993).

Community-based epidemiologic studies in the United States, such as the ECA, the NCS, and the NCS-R, have yielded inconsistent results regarding race- or ethnicity-related differences in the prevalence of anxiety disorder. ECA data, for example, indicated that the prevalence of specific anxiety disorders varies by race and ethnicity (Brown & Eaton, 1986; Eaton et al., 1991; Horwath, Johnson,

& Hornig, 1993; Karno et al., 1989; Robins et al., 1984). In contrast, the NCS found that 12-month prevalence for any anxiety disorder did not differ across racial or ethnic groups (Kessler et al., 1994); and NCS-R data indicated that non-Hispanic Blacks and Hispanics have a significantly lower risk for anxiety disorders than Whites (Kessler, Berglund, et al., 2005). Although analysis of NCS-R data did not find members of disadvantaged ethnic groups to be at increased risk for an anxiety disorder, they were found to experience more persistent disorders when disorders arose (Breslau, Kendler, Su, Aguilar-Gaxiola, & Kessler, 2005).

With regard to specific anxiety disorders, ECA data showed that lifetime prevalence of simple phobia was significantly higher among Blacks than any other racial or ethnic group. Blacks also had a higher lifetime prevalence of social phobia than Whites (Brown & Eaton, 1986; Eaton et al., 1991). These data showed Blacks to be 1.5 times more likely than Whites to report recent phobia (including past-month agoraphobia, social, and simple phobia), even after adjustment for demographic, socioeconomic, and sociocultural factors (Brown, Eaton, & Sussman, 1990). In contrast, Regier et al. (1993) found no significant differences in 1-month prevalence of any anxiety disorder across racial or ethnic groups in the ECA when confounding variables of age, sex, marital status, and SES status were controlled. Data from the ECA's Los Angeles site revealed significant ethnic differences among native Mexican Americans, immigrant Mexican Americans, and Whites in lifetime prevalence for three of six specific anxiety disorders: simple phobia, agoraphobia, and generalized anxiety disorder (Karno et al., 1989). The prevalence of simple phobias was higher among native Mexican Americans than among native Whites or immigrant Mexican Americans, differences that persisted even when controlling for gender, age, and socioeconomic, marital, and employment status. Agoraphobia also was more prevalent among native Mexican Americans than among immigrants, even when controlling for SES. In contrast, Whites recorded high lifetime prevalence of generalized anxiety disorder compared with both native and immigrant Mexican Americans (Karno et al., 1989).

The ECA study yielded no racial differences in the prevalence of panic disorder (Eaton et al., 1991; Horwath et al., 1993; Karno et al., 1989). Findings for other anxiety disorders were less consistent across race and ethnicity.

While the NCS failed to find prevalence differences in panic disorder, simple phobia, and agoraphobia between Black and White adult populations (Kessler et al., 1994), results from the NCS-R indicated that non-Hispanic Blacks and Hispanics have a significantly lower risk for anxiety disorders than Whites (Kessler, Berglund, et al., 2005). These data revealed lower lifetime prevalence for generalized anxiety disorder and social phobia among Hispanics than among Whites and indicated that Blacks have lower lifetime prevalence than Whites for all anxiety disorders (Breslau et al., 2006). In addition, based on survival models that account for differences in age distribution across racial/ethnic groups, an even stronger pattern of lowered risk for anxiety disorders was found among minorities than had been indicated by lifetime prevalence comparisons alone. These survival model–based data showed that non-Hispanic Blacks and Hispanics have significantly lower lifetime risks than Whites for generalized anxiety disorder and social phobia; non-Hispanic blacks have lower lifetime risk for panic disorder than Whites. Further analysis found the lower lifetime risk for anxiety disorders among Hispanics to be attributable entirely to the younger cohort; no significant differences in risk for anxiety were found among the older Hispanics in the study. In contrast, no age differences were found in risk for anxiety disorders among non-Hispanic Blacks (Breslau et al., 2006).

Similarly, a recent analysis of NESARC data found 12-month prevalence of DSM-IV anxiety disorders to be significantly higher among Whites than Blacks (Huang et al., 2006). The prevalence of anxiety among Native Americans was highest, at 15.3%; the 12-month prevalence among Asians was lowest, at 6.9%. Among Hispanics, the prevalence of anxiety disorders was significantly lower (8.8%) than the prevalence among Whites (11.7%) but significantly greater than that of Asians (Huang et al., 2006).

As the foregoing discussion suggests, tremendous variation has been reported across studies, making it difficult to assess the significance of race and ethnicity with respect to anxiety disorders. Reliance on broad racial and ethnic categorizations in both epidemiologic and clinical inquiry into the prevalence of mental disorders may contribute to the literature's often inconsistent findings. Further, some researchers have suggested that race and ethnicity may act as proxies for indicators of socioeconomic disadvantage immigrant status, acculturation, or language proficiency.

Analyses of the CPES and NESARC data showed that with regards to race, estimated odds ratios for panic disorder are slightly higher in the CPES than in the NESARC (see table 7-6). However, with the exception of the association between Asian ethnicity and panic disorder, odds ratios for panic disorder based on the CPES data were not statistically significant at the 5% level; however, they were found to be significant when based on the NESARC data. While prevalences or odds ratios were not estimated for anxiety disorders among Native Americans using CPES data, NESARC estimates for race/ethnicity found that Native Americans were more likely than Whites to have current diagnoses of panic disorder. The estimated prevalences of social phobia from the CPES also were higher for all racial categories than was found in analysis of the NESARC data. Estimated odds ratios were fairly consistent across data sets for social phobia, with the exception of the odds ratio for Asians, which was higher in the NESARC data than the CPES: Although Asians had decreased odds of social phobia compared with Whites in both data sets, the CPES yielded a 61% decreased odds rate (an odds ratio of approximately 0.39) for Asians, whereas NESARC data yielded odds for Asians only 35% lower than the odds for Whites. Consistent with the results for panic disorder and social phobia, the estimated prevalence of simple phobia was also higher in the CPES data than in the NESARC. The CPES also yielded higher odds ratios than the NESARC data for simple phobia, with the exception again of the estimated odds ratio for Asians, which was roughly 0.5 in both the CPES and

Table 7-6. Disparities in Prevalence of Mood and Anxiety Disorders by Race and Ethnicity

	CPES				NESARC				
	WHITE	BLACK	HISPANIC	ASIAN	WHITE	BLACK	NATIVE AMERICAN	HISPANIC	ASIAN
Major depressive disorder (N)	(7,567)	(6,070)	(3,615)	(2,284)	(24,507)	(8,245)	(701)	(8,308)	(1,332)
Prevalence (N)[a]	6.97 (548)	5.42 (327)	6.93 (287)	4.33 (102)	6.88 (1,764)	5.48 (462)	10.50 (77)	5.48 (521)	4.58 (63)
Odds ratio [CI][b]	1.00	0.69 [0.6, 0.8]	0.88 [0.7, 1.04]	0.55 [0.4, 0.76]	1.00	0.71 [0.60, 0.80]	1.56 [1.20, 2.09]	0.71 [0.60, 0.87]	0.6 [0.40, 0.87]
Panic disorder (N)	(7,565)	(6,068)	(3,615)	(2,284)	(24,507)	(8,245)	(701)	(8,308)	(1,332)
Prevalence (N)[a]	2.60 (203)	2.35 (151)	2.59 (104)	1.19 (28)	2.34 (594)	1.58 (140)	4.64 (32)	1.66 (147)	0.89 (12)
Odds ratio [CI][b]	1.00	0.83 [0.6, 1.07]	0.93 [0.7, 1.22]	0.42 [0.25, 0.7]	1.00	0.61 [0.48, 0.80]	1.98 [1.30, 2.98]	0.63 [0.50, 0.81]	0.34 [0.16, 0.80]
Social phobia (N)	(7,566)	(6,068)	(3,615)	(2,284)	(24,507)	(8,245)	(701)	(8,308)	(1,332)
Prevalence (N)[a]	6.74 (533)	5.08 (303)	5.17 (214)	3.0 (71)	3.01 (745)	2.00 (165)	3.56 (30)	1.98 (173)	2.13 (27)
Odds Ratio [CI][b]	1.00	0.68 [0.56, 0.8]	0.65 [0.51, 0.8]	0.39 [0.29, 0.5]	1.00	0.61 [0.48, 0.80]	1.16 [0.70, 1.93]	0.59 [0.47, 0.70]	0.65 [0.40, 0.96]
Simple phobia[c] (N)	(6,696)	(1,230)	(883)	(189)	(24,507)	(8,245)	(701)	(8,308)	(1,332)
Prevalence (N)[a]	8.27 (572)	9.88 (129)	10.02 (91)	4.72 (9)	2.51 (1,841)	7.23 (610)	8.18 (59)	5.65 (502)	4.13 (61)
Odds ratio [CI][b]	1.00	1.11 [0.8, 1.49]	1.14 [0.87, 1.5]	0.50 [0.3, 0.98]	1.00	0.96 [0.80, 1.09]	1.10 [0.80, 1.48]	0.74 [0.60, 0.90]	0.53 [0.40, 0.70]

CI = 95% confidence interval.

[a] Row percentage weighted. [b] Adjusted for age and sex. [c] Only available in the NCS-R data, not available in the NLAAS or NSAL.

NESARC data and was statistically significant in both at the 5% level.

Mood Disorders

Although the disadvantaged status of many racial and ethnic minorities in the United States likely exposes them to more chronic, severe stress than Whites, most studies have found Blacks and Hispanics to be at comparable or even lower risk for major depressive disorder than Whites (Blazer et al., 1994; Breslau et al., 2006; Kessler et al., 2003; Riolo, Nguyen, Greden, & King, 2005; Williams et al., 2007). For instance, disorder-specific analyses of NCS-R data found lifetime prevalence of major depression to be significantly lower among Blacks (10.8%) and Hispanics (13.5%) than among Whites (17.9%) (Breslau et al., 2006). A review of studies comparing lifetime prevalence of major depression among Hispanics and Whites in the United States (Mendelson, Rehkopf, & Kubzansky, 2008) found that of the eight studies meeting inclusion criteria, three reported lower prevalence among Hispanics than Whites and four found no racial/ethnic group differences; one reported higher prevalence among Hispanics in a sample of older adults. Together, these findings suggest that cultural and social factors inherent to some racial and ethnic groups may protect against depression, a finding that warrants further exploration (Breslau et al., 2006; Mendelson et al., 2008).

While most US population-based studies have found a comparable or lower prevalence of depression among racial and ethnic minorities compared with Whites, Blacks and Hispanics both appear to be at higher risk for chronic or persistent depression than Whites(Breslau et al., 2005; Riolo et al., 2005; Williams et al., 2007). In findings from the NCS, Hispanics also were significantly more likely than Whites to experience depression as a comorbidity with one or more other psychiatric disorders (odds ratio = 2.31, 95% confidence interval = [1.29, 4.15]); Blacks showed a trend in the same direction (odds ratio = 1.22, 95% confidence interval = [0.56, 2.65]) (Blazer et al., 1994). Williams and colleagues (2007) most recently reported that despite generally lower prevalence rates, African Americans with depression experienced higher levels of both clinical severity and functional impairment than Whites. Other studies similarly have found more severe symptomatology among Blacks and Hispanics than among Whites (Mendelson et al., 2008; Plant & Sachs-Ericsson, 2004), suggesting the presence of heightened psychological distress that may not be captured fully by the diagnostic nosology.

The considerable heterogeneity within as well as across racial and ethnic categories merits additional attention. Both gender and age often give rise to differences in disease prevalence within a racial or ethnic group. For example, despite the NCS finding of an overall lower prevalence of lifetime major depression among Blacks, the highest lifetime prevalence of depression across all racial and ethnic groups was found among Black females ages 35–44 (Blazer et al., 1994). Hispanics in the NCS-R had lower prevalence than Whites only among those age 43 or younger (Breslau et al., 2006). Use of broad ethnic categories such as "Hispanic" also may obscure within-group variability, since issues such as country of origin, length of US residency, and nativity status all may play a role (Mendelson et al., 2008). For example, data from the National Latino and Asian American study found Puerto Rican Americans to be more likely to experience lifetime depressive disorders than Mexican Americans (Alegria et al., 2007). Finally, a lack of sufficient comparative data reduces the ability to assess the prevalence of depression among a number of underrepresented racial and ethnic minorities in the US population, such as Native Americans and Asian American subgroups.

Analysis of CPES and NESARC data yielded a slightly higher prevalence of major depressive disorder among the CPES Hispanic population than the Hispanic population in the NESARC data (see table 7-6). CPES data also yielded a higher odds ratio for Hispanics than that estimated from the NESARC data; however, the estimated odds ratio associated with being Hispanic in the NESARC data was statistically significant at the 5% level, while the CPES odds ratio was not. No prevalences or odds ratios for any disorders were estimated for Native Americans using the CPES data. However, the NESARC estimates for race found Native Americans to be more likely than Whites to have had a major depressive disorder in the previous year.

Data on the distribution of bipolar disorder across racial and ethnic groups, like those for major depressive disorder, are conflicting. One of the more recent studies (Lloyd et al., 2005) examined the incidence of bipolar disorder in three catchment areas in the United Kingdom and found significantly higher prevalences of bipolar disorder in African-Caribbean, Black African, and mixed-ethnic groups compared with Whites. The NESARC (Grant et al., 2005) also found prevalence differences in racial/ethnic groups compared with Whites: Rates were higher among Native Americans and lower among Asian/Pacific Islanders and Hispanics. Interestingly, no differences were discerned between Whites and Blacks. While the initial NCS study reported small trends toward increased rates of bipolar disorder among non-Whites (Kessler et al., 1997), the finding subsequently was nullified by results of the NCS-R (Merikangas et al., 2007). Several other studies also found no differences in the prevalence of bipolar disorder across racial groups (Jonas et al., 2003; Schaffer et al., 2006). Given the dearth of robust data on the prevalence of bipolar disorder in minority populations, definitive conclusions about differences across these populations are difficult to make.

When CPES and NESARC data were analyzed, the estimated prevalence of bipolar I disorder was consistently higher across racial groups in the NESARC than in the CPES, with the exception that the prevalence estimate for Hispanics was higher in the CPES (see table 7-7). No significant differences in bipolar I disorder were found across racial/ethnic groups in the CPES, while in the NESARC, Hispanics were found to be less likely than Whites to have past-year bipolar I disorder.

Schizophrenia

Ethnic status, often a relatively easy-to-identify characteristic of an individual, indicates a shared history with others. Markers of ethnic status include race, country of origin, and religion. Country of origin has proven to be a consistent risk factor for schizophrenia in the United Kingdom. In the United Kingdom, immigrants from Africa and the Caribbean, as well as their second-generation offspring, have prevalence rates of schizophrenia up to 10 times higher than that found in the general population; the estimated migrant/native-born prevalence ratio for the illness falls between 4 and 5 (McGrath et al., 2004). Results from the Aetiology of and Ethnicity in Schizophrenia and Other Psychoses study confirm that in comparison with White British population, minority status consistently is associated with a higher incidence of schizophrenia, particularly among African-Caribbeans (Incidence Rate Ratio = 9.1) and Black Africans (IRR = 5.8). Most important, the higher prevalence rates in these populations remain significant when controlling for SES (Coid et al., 2008; Kirkbride et al., 2008; Morgan et al., 2006), especially for individuals not born in the United Kingdom.

Because only Black immigrant groups and their second-generation offspring experience a higher prevalence of schizophrenia, this finding likely is not attributable solely to the stresses of immigration. Moreover, since prevalence rates in the countries of origin are not elevated, genetic differences are not likely factors. Suggested causes include the psychological conditions associated with being Black in the United Kingdom or being an émigré from Suriname. Such factors could be associated with discrimination or difficulty planning one's life given the uncertain future often faced by groups at the structural bottom of society (Eaton & Harrison, 2001). One explanation for the second-generation effects relates to the higher prevalence of birth complications often seen in second-generation births, because the better nutrition in the receiving country is transmitted to the fetus, which may be too large for the mother who received weaker nutrition prior to immigration (R. Warner, 1995). Yet another hypothesis is that decreased sunlight in northern climates like those of the Netherlands and the United Kingdom leads to decreased production of vitamin D and thereby puts darker-skinned people

Table 7-7. Disparities in Prevalence of Bipolar Disorder by Race and Ethnicity

	CPES				NESARC				
	WHITE	BLACK	HISPANIC	ASIAN	WHITE	BLACK	NATIVE AMERICAN	ASIAN	HISPANIC
Bipolar I disorder (N)	(7,567)	(6,070)	(1,061)	(189)	(24,507)	(8,245)	(701)	(8,308)	(1,332)
Prevalence (N)[a]	0.57 (44)	0.75 (49)	0.61 (7)	0.00 (0)	0.90 (230)	0.97 (63)	1.72 (16)	0.46 (6)	0.50 (64)
Odds ratio [CI][b]	1.00	1.15 [0.70, 1.95]	0.82 [0.28, 2.40]	NA	1.00	0.90 [0.64, 1.26]	1.83 [0.98, 3.44]	0.43 [0.16, 1.11]	0.47 [0.33, 0.68]

CI = 95% confidence interval. NA = data not available in the data set.
[a]Row percentage weighted. [b]Adjusted for age and sex.

at higher risk for schizophrenia (Kinney et al., 2009; McGrath, 1999).

Alcohol and Drug Use Disorders

Data from the NSDUH (SAMHSA, 2010) indicate that the prevalence of past-year alcohol abuse and dependence was 13.3% among American Indians and Alaska Natives, 8.6% among Hispanics, 7.5% among Whites, 7.0% among Blacks, and 2.6% among Asians, suggesting that disadvantaged ethnic minorities often experience greater alcohol-related problems than Whites (Caetano & Clark, 1998). But looking across the wide array of studies in this area, prevalence findings are not altogether consistent with regard to alcohol abuse and dependence among racial and ethnic groups. Some data analyses have found that Blacks have a significantly higher number of alcohol-related consequences and alcohol dependence symptoms than Whites (Grant, 1997); other studies have found no significant differences between the two groups (Kandel et al., 1997). Early reports from the 1980s found a higher prevalence of alcoholism among Blacks than among Whites (Baskin, Bluestone, & Nelson, 1981; Jones & Gray, 1986), but in later findings from the NCS, Kessler and colleagues (1994) reported that Blacks have a significantly lower prevalence of alcohol use disorders than Whites. The Kessler finding is consistent with the ECA finding that the prevalence of alcohol abuse and dependence among young Whites (ages 18 to 29) was higher than that of young Blacks (Regier et al., 1993).

Considerable heterogeneity has been observed in the prevalence of alcohol abuse and dependence among Hispanic subpopulations. Mexican Americans and Puerto Ricans exhibited higher prevalence rates of alcohol abuse and dependence than Cuban Americans and Hispanics who immigrated from South and Central America(Caetano, Ramisetty-Mikler, & Rodriguez, 2008). NESARC data indicated that the prevalence of alcohol dependence among all Hispanic men was 5.9%, compared with 5.4% for all men; the prevalence among Mexican American men was 9.8% (Grant et al., 2004). These prevalence rates are lower than those found among Hispanics living on

the Mexico–United States border in Texas, for whom the prevalences of alcohol abuse and dependence reach 7% and 14.5%, respectively (Caetano et al., 2008). Reports on ECA data have found Mexican Americans to have a higher (13%) past-year prevalence of alcohol abuse or dependence than Whites (8%) (Burnam et al., 1987). Higher prevalence of lifetime alcohol abuse or dependence also was found among Mexican Americans living in Los Angeles (24%) and Puerto Ricans living in Puerto Rico (12.2%). Among Hispanics in Florida, the prevalence of alcohol abuse and dependence was lower among immigrants than US-born Hispanic Americans (Turner & Gil, 2002). It is important to note that the NCS data yielded no difference in risk for alcohol dependence between Hispanics and Whites (Anthony et al., 1994).

A few studies have found the risk for alcohol dependence to be extremely high in some Native American communities (O'Connell, Novins, Beals, & Spicer, 2005). The NCS, in particular, found alcohol dependence to be significantly higher among Native Americans than Whites (Gilman et al., 2008).

Analyses of CPES and NESARC data show that in the CPES, Asians had lower odds of past-year alcohol use and dependence than Whites (see table 7-8). According to the NESARC, Blacks, Asians, and Hispanics had lower odds of past-year alcohol use and dependence than Whites, while Native Americans were more likely to have past-year alcohol use and dependence than Whites.

While explorations of the prevalence of drug use disorders by race and ethnicity have been undertaken in many countries, the majority of general population survey data in this area come from US studies (Anthony et al., 1994; Beals et al., 1997; Breslau et al., 2006; Colon, Robles, Canino & Sahai, 2001; Chen & Kandel, 2002; Chilcoat & Anthony, 2004; Compton et al., 2007; Costello, Farmer, Angold, Burns, & Erkanli, 1997; Grant, 1996; Kessler et al., 1994; Mitchell, Beals, Novins, & Spicer, 2003; Roberts, Roberts, & Xing, 2006; Smith et al., 2006; Stone, O'Brien, De La Torre, & Anthony, 2007; Swendsen et al., 2008; L. A. Warner et al., 1995). Data from the 2009 NSDUH show that Blacks, Asians, and individuals

Table 7-8. Disparities in Prevalence of Alcohol and Drug Disorders by Race and Ethnicity

	CPES				NESARC				
	WHITE	BLACK	HISPANIC	ASIAN	WHITE	BLACK	NATIVE AMERICAN	HISPANIC	ASIAN
Alcohol abuse/ dependence (N)	(4,180)	(5,546)	(3,259)	(2,178)	(24,507)	(8,245)	(701)	(8,308)	(1,332)
Prevalence (N)[a]	1.30 (73)	1.19 (54)	1.38 (40)	0.17 (5)	8.93 (2,105)	6.86 (481)	12.09 (79)	7.92 (596)	4.54 (66)
Odds ratio [CI][b]	1.00	0.80 [0.49, 1.3]	0.76 [0.4, 1.35]	0.11 [0.04, 0.3]	1.00	0.64 [0.56, 0.70]	1.39 [1.01, 1.90]	0.60 [0.50, 0.72]	0.37 [0.28, 0.50]
Drug abuse/ dependence (N)	(4,180)	(5,545)	(3,259)	(2,178)	(24,507)	(8,245)	(701)	(8,308)	(1,332)
Prevalence (N)[a]	1.34 (74)	1.36 (68)	1.09 (36)	0.76 (14)	1.93 (455)	2.39 (146)	4.92 (33)	1.74 (127)	1.39 (16)
Odds ratio [CI][b]	1.00	0.84 [0.5, 1.28]	0.50 [0.3, 0.82]	0.45 [0.2, 0.94]	1.00	1.03 [0.82, 1.30]	2.66 [1.68, 4.20]	0.58 [0.45, 0.70]	0.54 [0.30, 1.05]

CI = 95% confidence interval. [a]Row percentage weighted. [b]Adjusted for age and sex.

of multiple races or ethnicities in the United States were more likely than Whites to meet criteria for any past-year drug use disorder, even though Blacks were as likely as Whites and Asians were less likely than Whites to be past-year users of any illegal drug. Hispanics, Native Americans, Alaska Natives, and Pacific Islanders had prevalence rates similar to those for Whites (SAMHSA, 2010).

Some studies show that Whites have a higher prevalence of lifetime illegal drug use and dependence than racial/ethnic populations; however, prevalence data on past-year dependence yield a different pattern. Using NCS data and criteria from the revised third edition of the DSM (DSM-III-R) (APA, 1987), Anthony and colleagues (1994) found that compared with Whites, Blacks are less likely to have a history of illegal drug dependence. Yet based on the same data, L. A. Warner and colleagues (1995) reported that among respondents with a lifetime history of dependence, Blacks were significantly more likely than Whites to hmeet criteria for drug dependence with the 12 months prior to the interview; Asians were less likely than Whites to have drug dependence in the prior year. According to NLAES findings, while Whites were more likely to be lifetime drug users, Blacks and Hispanics were respectively 2 and 3.5 times more likely than Whites to have 12-month dependence given dependence in the past (Grant, 1996). Two studies, both using wave 1 NESARC data, found that lifetime and past-year drug use or dependence generally were greater among Native Americans than Whites (Compton et al., 2007; Smith et al., 2006). The same two studies found that lifetime drug use or dependence was lower among Hispanics, African Americans, and Asians than Whites; past-year drug use or dependence was lower among Hispanics than Whites. Similarly, working with NCS-R data, Swendsen and colleagues (2008) found that while individuals classified as "Other" were less likely than Whites to have the opportunity to use drugs, they were more likely to transition to drug abuse once they used drugs.

According to most major epidemiologic prevalence studies of drug use and dependence, Hispanics, the fastest growing population in the United States, currently rank between Blacks and Whites. However, as with other racial and ethnic populations, drug involvement among Hispanics varies by sex, country of origin, nativity, level of acculturation, and other factors (Amaro, Whitaker, Coffman, & Heeren, 1990; Burnam et el., 1987; De la Rosa, Khalsa, & Rouse, 1990; De la Rosa, Vega, & Radisch, 2000; Epstein, Botvin, & Diaz, 2001; Gfroerer & De la Rosa, 1993; Keyes et al., in press; Orozco & Lukas, 2000; Vega et al., 2002; Vega, Alderete, Kolody, & Aguilar-Gaxiola, 1998; Vega, Sribney, Aguilar-Gaxiola, & Kolody, 2004; Vega, Zimmerman, Gil, Warheit, & Apospori, 1993; Wagner-Echeagaray, Schutz, Chilcoat, & Anthony, 1994).

With historical patterns showing Native Americans to have the highest prevalence of drug use and dependence across racial and ethnic groups in the United States, the population warrants particular attention. A comparison of data from the American Indian Service Utilization, Psychiatric Epidemiology, Risk and Protective Factors Project with NCS data found that the prevalence of lifetime, DSM-III-R–diagnosed substance disorder (including both alcohol and drugs of abuse) was comparable between American Indian groups and the general US population (Mitchell et al., 2003). The Substance Abuse and Mental Health Services Administration (2007) reported that in 2002–2005, American Indians and Alaska Natives ages 12 or older were more likely than members of other racial or ethnic groups to have used an illegal drug at least once in the prior year (18.4% vs. 14.6%) and to have a past-year drug use or dependence disorder (5.0% vs. 2.9%); these patterns were consistent within both gender and age groups. While the prevalences of past-year inhalant, pain reliever, tranquilizer, stimulant, and sedative use disorders among American Indians and Alaska Natives were similar to those among members of other racial groups, prevalences were higher among American Indians and Alaska Natives for marijuana, cocaine, and hallucinogen use disorders. Past-year heroin use disorders were more common among members of other racial groups than among American Indians and Alaska Natives (SAMHSA, 2007).

When examining use of and dependence on specific illegal drugs, several studies have found that while Blacks generally have a lower prevalence of drug use and dependence than Whites, they have higher rates of past-year cocaine abuse and dependence (Anthony et al., 1994; Chen & Kandel, 2002; Chilcoat & Anthony, 2004; Grant, 1996). Based on data on 2,349 past-year cocaine users ages 12 and up collected across the 1991–1993 installments of the annual National Household Survey on Drug Abuse (now the NSDUH), Chen and Kandel (2002) found that Black users had a higher prevalence of DSM-IV cocaine dependence compared with Whites (25.5% vs. 11.4%). Moreover, Blacks used cocaine more frequently and by more addictive routes (smoking or injection) than did Whites. Prevalence among Hispanics was intermediate between the two, at 16.7%. Findings from NCS data were similar. Anthony and colleagues (1994) determined that despite similar lifetime and past-year prevalence of cocaine use among Whites and Blacks, the prevalence of cocaine dependence among past-year users was twice as high among Blacks than among Whites or Hispanics. Following the same line of research, Chilcoat and Anthony (2004), analyzing past-year illegal drug dependence data from SAMHSA's annual NSDUH, reported that while Blacks were less likely to use any illegal drug than Whites, Blacks ages 35 or older were more likely to qualify for a diagnosis of drug dependence than Whites (1.3% vs. 0.5%); no differences were found between Hispanics and Whites. These racial and ethnic differences among adults were due primarily to cocaine dependence, for which prevalence among Blacks was several times higher than among non-Hispanic Whites and Hispanics (0.8% vs. 0.1% and 0%, respectively). In fact, cocaine dependence among Blacks exceeded that of any other racial or ethnic population without regard to age (Chilcoat & Anthony, 2004).

Marijuana was the most prevalent drug used by individuals ages 12 and older in the United States in 2009 (SAMHSA, 2010). Based on data from the NLAES and the NESARC, Compton, Grant, Colliver, Glantz, and Stinson (2004) observed that during a 10-year period (1991–1992 through 2001–2002), the prevalence of marijuana use in the United States had remained stable at around 4%. In contrast, the prevalence of marijuana use disorders consistent with DSM-IV diagnostic criteria increased significantly over the same period (from 1.2% to 1.5%). The greatest increases were observed among young adult Hispanic men (from 0.9% to 2.0%) and among Black young adults of both sexes, ages 18–29 (from 1.3% to 2.6% among men and from 0.4% to 1.2% among women). Further, these trends considered together suggest the possibility that the concomitant increase in the potency of delta-9-tetrahydrocannabinol in marijuana during the same time period contributed to the growing prevalence of related disorders (Compton et al., 2004).

Age appears to play a role in the prevalence of marijuana use. Reardon and Buka (2002) found that between the ages of 15 and 17, the incidence of marijuana use disorder is higher among Whites than Blacks or Hispanics. By ages 18–20, however, prevalence rates shift sharply: Onset in Blacks is twice that for Whites and four times that for Hispanics. These findings suggest the transition to adulthood is a time of particularly high risk for Blacks.

Nonmedical use of prescription opioids was the second most prevalent form of drug abuse among current (past month) illegal drug users ages 12 years and older in the United States in 2009, exceeded only by marijuana (SAMHSA, 2010). Only a few studies have examined racial and ethnic differences in the abuse of and dependence on nonmedical prescription drugs (Blanco et al., 2007; Martins, Storr, Zhu, & Chilcoat, 2009; McCabe, Cranford, & West, 2008). Based on an examination of data from both the NLAES and the NESARC, Blanco and colleagues (2007) found that compared with Blacks, Whites were more likely to have a prescription drug use disorder; however, over the 10-year period they studied the protective effect for Blacks decreased. Exploring the same data, McCabe and colleagues (2008) examined trends in both prescription drug abuse disorder and in its co-occurrence with other drug use and dependence. They found that Native Americans experienced a high point prevalence of co-occurring prescription drug use and other substance use disorders. Among Blacks, the prevalence of co-occurrence increased significantly over the decade. In addition, Martins and colleagues (2009) found that among individuals with prescription opioid use disorders, Oxycontin users were more likely to be White or Hispanic than to be Black.

While drug use and dependence generally present differently in adolescents than in adults, only a small number of studies have assessed racial and ethnic differences in these disorders among adolescents. Two reported higher prevalence of drug use and dependence among American Indian youth compared with White youth (Beals et al., 1997; Costello et al., 1997). Kilpatrick and colleagues (2000) found that White youth were three to nine times more likely than Blacks to meet diagnostic criteria for drug use or dependence, but that Hispanics and Native Americans did not differ from Whites in their risk. In a study of 4,175 youth in Houston, Texas, Roberts and colleagues (2006) found that Black youth had a lower risk for any substance use disorder (including both drug and alcohol disorders) than Mexican American or European American youth. No differences were found between European American and Mexican American youth. L. A. Warner, Canino, and Colon (2001) found that lifetime prevalence of drug use or dependence was slightly higher among US adolescents than Puerto Rican adolescents (6.2% vs. 4.1%); however, among lifetime and past-year drug users, the prevalence of drug use and dependence was higher for Puerto Rican youth (lifetime: 49.7% vs. 45.5%; past-year: 55.3% vs. 39.3%).

Analyses of the CPES and NESARC data revealed that in the CPES, Hispanics and Asians had half the odds of non-Hispanic Whites for past-year drug use or dependence. NESARC data showed Native Americans to be almost three times more likely to have past-year drug use or dependence than Whites. (See table 7-8.)

EFFECTS OF MARITAL STATUS ON THE PREVALENCE OF DISORDERS

Anxiety Disorders

Being unmarried, divorced, or separated has been associated with a higher prevalence of anxiety disorders. Several studies have described markedly higher prevalence rates of anxiety disorders among separated or divorced individuals than among individuals in other marital status categories (Davidson, Hughes, George, & Blazer, 1993; Kessler, Berglund, et al., 2005; Magee et al., 1996; Regier et al., 1993; Schneier, Johnson, Hornig, Liebowitz, & Weissman, 1992). The ECA found marital status to be one of the most powerful correlates of anxiety disorder and of overall risk for mental disorder: Separated or divorced people were twice as likely as married people to have anxiety disorders after controlling for age, gender, race/ethnicity, and SES (Regier et al., 1993). General population surveys in Australia, the Netherlands, Germany, and the United States have found that unmarried persons have odds ratios for anxiety disorders of 0.9–5.1 compared with married persons (Baumeister & Harter, 2007). The NCS-R also found marital disruption to be associated with anxiety disorders (Kessler, Berglund, et al., 2005).

Analyses of CPES and NESARC data found that the estimated prevalence of panic disorder among individuals who either had never married or no longer were married was higher in the CPES data than the NESARC (see table 7-9). Similarly, for panic disorder, the estimated odds ratios associated with being no longer married were higher in the CPES than in the NESARC data. Data from the CPES and the NESARC yielded the finding that panic disorder is significantly associated with being formerly married. The estimated prevalence of social phobia was consistently higher in the CPES than the NESARC, without regard to marital status. The estimated odds ratio of social phobia among individuals who were no longer married compared with the odds for the married group was 1.81 in the CPES data, statistically significant at the 5% level. In contrast, the estimated odds ratio of social phobia among those no longer married was only 1.15 in the NESARC data, only marginally different from the married group and not statistically significant. Odds ratios for social phobia among the never married group were not statistically significant in either data set. As with social phobia, the estimated prevalence of simple phobia was consistently higher in the CPES

Table 7-9. Disparities in Prevalence of Mood and Anxiety Disorders by Marital Status

	CPES			NESARC		
	MARRIED/ COHABITATING	SEPARATED/ DIVORCED/ WIDOWED	NEVER MARRIED	MARRIED/ COHABITATING	SEPARATED/ DIVORCED/ WIDOWED	NEVER MARRIED
Major depressive disorder (N)	(10,520)	(4,363)	(4,353)	(22,081)	(11,117)	(9,895)
Prevalence (N)[a]	5.05 (510)	9.10 (365)	8.70 (389)	5.20 (1,112)	9.78 (966)	7.78 (809)
Odds ratio [CI][b]	1.00	2.12 [1.73, 2.60]	1.26 [1.02, 1.55]	1.00	2.15 [1.90, 2.43]	1.21 [1.08, 1.36]
Panic disorder (N)	(10,519)	(4,361)	(4,652)	(22,081)	(11,117)	(9,895)
Prevalence (N)[a]	1.94 (198)	3.98 (147)	2.67 (141)	1.97 (421)	2.88 (299)	2.16 (215)
Odds ratio [CI][b]	1.00	2.25 [1.60, 3.15]	1.02 [0.71, 1.47]	1.00	1.61 [1.34, 1.94]	0.83 [0.65, 1.06]
Social phobia (N)	(10,520)	(4,361)	(4,652)	(22,081)	(11,117)	(9,895)
Prevalence (N)[a]	5.03 (488)	7.56 (286)	8.00 (347)	2.57 (531)	2.83 (293)	3.20 (316)
Odds ratio [CI][b]	1.00	1.81 [1.48, 2.22]	1.14 [0.94, 1.38]	1.00	1.15 [0.99, 1.37]	1.05 [0.86, 1.29]
Simple phobia[c] (N)	(5,167)	(1,934)	(1,897)	(22,081)	(11,117)	(9,895)
Prevalence (N)[a]	7.99 (429)	10.18 (201)	8.62 (171)	7.04 (1,525)	7.68 (819)	6.92 (729)
Odds ratio [CI][b]	1.00	1.36 [1.13, 1.63]	0.82 [0.62, 1.07]	1.00	1.10 [0.99, 1.22]	0.98 [0.88, 1.10]

CI = 95% confidence interval.

[a]Column percentage weighted. [b]Adjusted for age and sex. [c]Only available in the NCS-R data, not available in the NLAAS or NSAL.

data than in the NESARC for all categories of marital status. In the CPES the association of simple phobia with being formerly married was stronger than in the NESARC.

Mood Disorders

Research by Gove, Hughes, and Style Briggs (1983) on the relation between marital status and mental health improved on earlier correlational studies that had failed to control for possible confounders. Their analysis of data from a national probability sample in the United States found that without regard to living arrangement, married individuals enjoy better mental health than unmarried individuals (Hughes & Gove, 1981). While there is a common belief that men may derive more mental health benefits from marriage than women, Gove and colleagues (1983) found the strength of the marriage–mental health relation to be comparable across the sexes. Individuals who had never married reported better mental health and lower distress than those who had been divorced or widowed (Gove et al., 1983). A later population-based study found that consistent with the earlier research, divorced individuals experience significantly higher levels of distress than married individuals or those who have never married (Hope, Rodgers, & Power, 1999). The quality of marriage also has been found to exert an influence: Higher marital adjustment and satisfaction are predictive of lower levels of depression (Holt-Lunstad, Birmingham, & Jones, 2008).

Recent population-based studies examining the relationship between marital status and depressive disorders among parents have reported similar findings (DeKlyen, Brooks-Gunn, McLanahan, & Knab, 2006). The incidence of major depressive episodes for both mothers and fathers was lower among married parents than among unmarried parents. Parents who were neither romantically involved nor cohabiting—generally either divorced or separated—were found to experience the highest incidence of depression and were significantly more depressed than cohabiting parents and noncohabiting, romantically involved parents. The association between marital status and depression for mothers was somewhat attenuated but still persisted when controlling for sociodemographic factors such as age, race, and SES. In contrast, the relationship became stronger for fathers in adjusted models (DeKlyen, Brooks-Gunn, McLanahan, & Knab, 2006). Analysis of the NCS found that separated or divorced mothers were at greater risk for major depression and dysthymia than married and never-married mothers (Afifi, Cox, & Enns, 2006). The Health and Retirement study found that among individuals ages 51–61, married couples, with or without children, had the fewest depressive symptoms; single women living with children had the greatest number of depressive symptoms (Hughes & Waite, 2002).

Beyond the United States, research data also indicate an association between marital status and depression. Analysis of nationally representative data from Canada suggests that single mothers are almost twice as likely to have experienced a depressive episode as their married peers (15.4% vs. 6.8%) (Cairney, Thorpe, Rietschlin, & Avison, 1999). Single mothers were twice as likely to have had a depressive episode as women without dependent children according to the 2000 National Psychiatric Morbidity Study in the United Kingdom (Cooper et al., 2008). However, the study also found no significant differences in risk for depression among single mothers, partnered mothers, and other women when sociodemographic factors were controlled.

The estimated prevalences and odds ratios for major depressive disorder were consistent across the CPES and NESARC data sets for marital status (see table 7-9). In both data sets, individuals who never married or were no longer married were more likely to have past-year major depressive disorder than married individuals.

Epidemiologic studies almost uniformly show individuals with bipolar disorder to be more likely either never to have been married or to have been married previously (Grant et al., 2005; Kessler et al., 1997; Merikangas et al., 2007; Weissman et al., 1991). While marriage may be protective against bipolar disorder, it is more likely that the disorder disrupts the ability to form stable relationships, resulting in an unmarried status among many individuals with bipolar disorder.

Analyses of the CPES and NESARC data sets by marital status found the estimated prevalence of bipolar I disorder to be consistently higher in the NESARC data (see table 7-10). In the CPES, unmarried respondents (no longer married or never married) were more likely than married respondents to have past-year bipolar I disorder; this was true only for those no longer married in the NESARC.

Schizophrenia

Unmarried status is a well-established risk factor for schizophrenia (Eaton, 1975). Agerbo and colleagues (2004) found that compared with the general population, individuals with schizophrenia are more likely to be single as many as 20 years prior to diagnosis, with relative odds of about 4. The relative odds of being single with schizophrenia, compared to being married, are more than 15 at the time of first admission to treatment and remain high for decades thereafter. The effect is greater for males, perhaps because disease onset for males most often occurs during the years of marriage planning. Similar to SES, marital status plays a small role, if any, in the etiologic chain of causes leading to schizophrenia; however, it is predicted to be associated with the prevalence of schizophrenia (Agerbo et al., 2004).

Analysis of Danish register data shows a strong relationship between marital status and schizophrenia (see table 7-11). Individuals who have never married have 15 times the prevalence rate and divorced individuals 10 times the prevalence rate of those who are married. Individuals who are widowed have only a minimally increased prevalence of schizophrenia.

Alcohol and Drug Use Disorders

The Substance Abuse and Mental Health Services Administration (2005) has found that among the US adult population, 16.0% of individuals who never married met the criteria for alcohol abuse or dependence in the prior year, compared with 10.0% of those who were divorced or separated, 4.6% of those who were married, and 1.3% of those who were widowed. Other research has similarly disclosed that marital status and living arrangement have an effect on alcohol-related problems; for example, alcohol abuse and dependence were found to be most common among unmarried persons (Alonso et al., 2004; Klose & Jacobi, 2004).

Examining ECA data, Crum and colleagues (1993) found that never having been married, becoming separated or divorced, and being widowed were associated with increased risk of alcohol abuse and dependence. Later, using follow-up ECA data, Crum, Chan, Chen, Storr, and Anthony (2005) found single status to be a strong predictor of alcohol dependence. A study based on data from the New Haven ECA site found marital dissatisfaction at baseline to be associated significantly with a diagnosis of alcohol use disorder at follow-up; dissatisfied spouses were 3.7 times more likely than satisfied spouses to have a later diagnosis of

Table 7-10. Disparities in Prevalence of Bipolar Disorder by Marital Status

	CPES			NESARC		
	MARRIED/ COHABITATING	SEPARATED/ DIVORCED/ WIDOWED	NEVER MARRIED	MARRIED/ COHABITATING	SEPARATED/ DIVORCED/ WIDOWED	NEVER MARRIED
Bipolar I disorder (N)	(7,451)	(3,702)	(3,734)	(22,081)	(11,117)	(9,895)
Prevalence (N)[a]	0.38 (38)	0.78 (27)	0.97 (35)	0.67 (146)	1.09 (118)	1.28 (115)
Odds ratio [CI][b]	1.00	2.81 [1.37, 5.75]	1.24 [0.58, 2.67]	1.00	2.27 [1.61, 3.20]	1.09 [0.74, 1.40]

CI = 95% confidence interval.
[a]Column percentage weighted. [b]Adjusted for age and sex.

Table 7-11. Disparities in Prevalence of Schizophrenia by Marital Status at Admission

	DANISH PSYCHIATRIC CASE REGISTER				
	MARRIED AND LIVING WITH SPOUSE	COHABITATING	UNMARRIED LIVING ALONE	DIVORCED LIVING ALONE	WIDOWED LIVING ALONE
Schizophrenia					
Prevalence per 1000 (N)[a]	0.09 (197)	0.20 (115)	1.37 (1,502)	1.00 (310)	0.14 (38)
Odds ratio [CI][b]	1.00	2.16 [1.72, 2.72]	14.98 [12.92, 17.38]	10.48 [9.07, 12.96]	1.49 [1.05, 2.10]

CI = 95% confidence interval.

[a]Numerator is from all hospital and specialty clinic admissions in Denmark in 2006; denominator from 25% sample of population of Denmark in 2006 (weighted to 100%).

[b]Adjusted for age and sex.

alcohol use disorder (Whisman, Uebelacker, & Bruce, 2006).

In Sweden, alcohol abuse and dependence were found to be associated with either poor communication with one's spouse or having never been married (Thundal & Allebeck, 1998). A history of multiple divorces also significantly increased the risk of alcohol abuse and dependence (Thundal & Allebeck, 1998). In a nationally representative Finnish survey, Joutsenniemi and colleagues (2007) found that respondents living alone or cohabiting were more likely to have alcohol abuse or dependence than married respondents. An Iceland-based study found high prevalence rates of alcohol dependence among widowed, separated, or divorced individuals ages 55–57 (Stefansson, Lindal, Björnsson, & Guomundsdottir, 1994); alcohol dependence was most common among widowers and divorcés in a Nepal township (Jhingan et al., 2003). Results from other countries also confirm that single parents, persons living alone, and persons living with someone other than a partner have high prevalences of alcohol abuse and dependence (Bijl et al., 1998; Colon et al., 2001; Klose & Jacobi, 2004; Sundquist & Frank, 2004; Wang & El-Guebaly, 2004).

A number of longitudinal studies have found that acquiring both a spousal and a parental role appears to have beneficial effects on the risk for alcohol abuse and dependence (Chilcoat & Breslau, 1996; Prescott & Kendler,

2000). Also, alcohol abuse has been associated with lower odds of marriage and higher odds of divorce (Cheung, 1998; Chilcoat & Breslau, 1996), though not all studies support these findings (Power, Rodgers, & Hope, 1999).

Analyses of CPES and NESARC data found that the prevalence of past-year alcohol use and dependence was higher in both data sets among individuals no longer married (i.e., separated, divorced, or widowed) than among married persons, and higher still among those who had never married (see table 7-12).

Findings regarding marital status and alcohol disorders are mirrored in the relationship of marital status to drug use and dependence. In general, individuals who have never married or who are no longer married (divorced, separated, or widowed) are more likely to be dependent on illegal drugs (Compton et al., 2007; Grant, 1996; McCabe et al., 2008). In the NLAES data (Grant, 1996) the lifetime and 12-month prevalences of DSM-IV–diagnosed drug dependence were 2.9% and 0.8%, respectively; but persistence of dependence was three times more likely among individuals who never married than among married respondents. Those previously but no longer married also were at increased risk of dependence. More recently, Compton and colleagues (2007) found that those who no longer were married or who had never married were more likely to have lifetime drug use or dependence than married respondents. Analyses of the CPES

Table 7-12. Disparities in Prevalence of Alcohol and Drug Disorders by Marital Status

	CPES			NESARC		
	MARRIED/ COHABITATING	SEPARATED/ DIVORCED/ WIDOWED	NEVER MARRIED	MARRIED/ COHABITATING	SEPARATED/ DIVORCED/ WIDOWED	NEVER MARRIED
Alcohol abuse/ dependence (N)	(8,075)	(3,322)	(3,766)	(22,081)	(11,117)	(9,895)
Prevalence (N)[a]	0.73 (62)	1.16 (36)	2.71 (74)	6.05 (1,237)	8.09 (740)	15.86 (1350)
Odds ratio [CI][b]	1.00	2.42 [1.32, 4.46]	2.01 [1.33, 3.03]	1.00	2.35 [2.06, 2.67]	1.41 [1.27, 1.56]
Drug abuse/ dependence (N)	(8,075)	(3,322)	(3,765)	(22,081)	(11,117)	(9,895)
Prevalence (N)[a]	0.59 (62)	0.82 (31)	3.58 (99)	1.02 (201)	1.70 (142)	45.15 (434)
Odds ratio [CI][b]	1.00	2.73 [1.56, 4.77]	1.94 [1.25, 3.01]	1.00	3.06 [2.35, 3.98]	1.96 [1.59, 2.42]

CI = 95% confidence interval.
[a]Column percentage weighted. [b]Adjusted for age and sex.

and NESARC data show that in both surveys, the prevalence of past-year drug use disorder was higher among individuals no longer married than among married respondents, and even higher among those who had never married (see table 7-12).

EFFECTS OF URBANICITY ON THE PREVALENCE OF DISORDERS

Anxiety Disorders

Urban–rural differences in the prevalence of common mental illnesses such as the anxiety disorders have been reported in the literature. However, while a number of studies have investigated the prevalence of psychiatric disorders in rural compared with urban communities, few have used reliable diagnostic procedures to define specific disorders. Moreover, urban–rural comparisons most often have been made across rather than within studies (Judd et al., 2002). Judd and colleagues (2002) identified three studies that used reliable diagnostic processes and made urban–rural comparisons. Of them, only one, conducted in Korea, found differences between urban and rural settings, specifically that agoraphobia and panic disorder were more common in rural than urban residences (Lee et al., 1990a). On the whole, however, a strong association does not appear to exist between location of residence and anxiety disorder.

In the United States, data from the ECA and the NCS yielded only small differences in the prevalence of mental disorders between rural and urban settings, but only two of the five ECA sites (Durham and St. Louis) had sufficient populations to allow examination of such differences. The results of the ECA comparisons were not consistent across diagnostic categories. While increased 1-year and lifetime prevalences of generalized anxiety disorder were observed in urban areas, the finding was not statistically significant (Blazer et al., 1985; Blazer, Hughes, George, Swartz, & Boyer, 1991).

Data from the NCS were examined at the county level, distinguishing among major metropolitan counties (major metropolitan areas), urbanized counties not in the major metropolitan areas (other urban areas), and rural counties. The effects of urbanicity at the county level generally were not statistically significant. However, major metropolitan residents were more likely than rural residents to show comorbidity with other psychiatric disorders in the 12 months prior to the interview (Kessler et al., 1994).

In a household survey in the United Kingdom, a higher prevalence of psychiatric morbidity was found in urban areas than in rural areas; however, when social differences were considered, the higher prevalence among urban residents remained significant only for neurotic disorder (Paykel, Abbot, Jenkins, Brugha, & Meltzer, 2000). The Australian National Survey of Mental Health and Well-being found no differences in the prevalence of anxiety disorders based on urbanicity (Andrews, Henderson, & Hall, 2001).

Analyses of NESARC data showed no difference in urbanicity for panic disorder (see table 7-13). However, respondents with social phobia and simple phobia appeared more likely to live in rural than urban areas.

Mood Disorders

Urban living has long been hypothesized to carry a greater risk for major depressive disorder than living in rural areas (Dohrenwend & Dohrenwend, 1974), perhaps due to greater social isolation, physical danger, and other psychosocial stressors found in urban settings. Nonetheless, a review of urban–rural differences in the prevalence of mental disorders concluded that no such distinction is apparent in most studies; urbanicity is a much poorer predictor of depression prevalence than sociodemographic factors (Judd et al., 2002). Such findings must be approached with caution, however, since methodological shortcomings and inconsistencies in the categorization of urban and rural regions are a significant limitation in this area of research (Judd et al., 2002; Kovess-Masféty, Alonso, de Graaf, & Demyttenaere, 2005).

In the United States, analysis of data from the North Carolina subset of the ECA suggested that the prevalence of major

Table 7-13. Disparities in Prevalence of Mood and Anxiety Disorders by Urbanicity

	NESARC		
	URBAN	SUBURBAN	RURAL
Major depressive disorder (N)	(1,5002)	(20,295)	(7,796)
Prevalence (N)[a]	7.13 (113)	5.95 (1,236)	7.16 (538)
Odds ratio [CI][b]	1.00	0.84 [0.75, 0.95]	1.05 [0.9, 1.23]
Panic disorder (N)	(15,002)	(20,295)	(7,796)
Prevalence (N)[a]	2.36 (350)	2.11 (420)	2.03 (165)
Odds ratio [CI][b]	1.00	0.92 [0.77, 1.09]	0.91 [0.72, 1.14]
Social phobia (N)	(15,002)	(20,295)	(7,796)
Prevalence (N)[a]	2.58 (377)	2.53 (497)	3.57 (266)
Odds ratio [CI][b]	1.00	1.01 [0.83, 1.22]	1.46 [1.15, 1.86]
Simple Phobia (N)	(15,002)	(20,295)	(7,796)
Prevalence (N)[a]	6.80 (1,044)	6.93 (1,392)	8.14 (637)
Odds ratio [CI][b]	1.00	1.02 [0.87, 1.19]	1.21 [1.00, 1.47]

CI = 95% confidence interval.
[a]Column percentage weighted. [b]Adjusted for age and sex.

depression was two to three times higher in urban areas than in rural areas, even after controlling for sociodemographic factors (Blazer et al., 1985; Cromwell, George, Blazer, & Landerman, 1986). In contrast, neither the NCS (Blazer et al., 1994; Kessler et al., 1994) nor the NCS-R (Kessler et al., 2003) found that urbanicity and region of the United States were significantly associated with either current or lifetime prevalence of major depressive disorder. Analysis of nationally representative data from the 1999 National Health Interview Survey found the unadjusted prevalence of depression to be slightly but significantly higher in rural areas (6.1%) than in urban settings (5.2%) (Probst et al., 2006). The authors interpreted those regional differences in the prevalence of depressive illness as reflecting poor health status, chronic disease, and poverty, which are more common in rural areas. Few studies appear to have undertaken an explicit examination of geographic differences in prevalence rates of depression among youth, though Costello, Keeler, and Angold (2001) did report that the prevalence of depressive disorders among their rural

sample was comparable to that reported in surveys of youth in urban areas over the prior two decades.

While findings beyond the United States have been mixed, the majority of studies have reported no rural–urban differences in depression, including studies conducted in Canada (Parikh, Wasylenki, Goering, & Wong, 1996), Korea (Lee et al., 1990b), New Zealand (Romans-Clarkson, Walton, Herbison, & Mullen, 1990), and France (Kovess-Masféty, Lecoutour, & Delavelle, 2005). Analysis of data from the 1998–1999 Canadian National Population Health Survey yielded a higher prevalence of major depression in urban areas than in rural communities after controlling for sociodemographic factors (Wang, 2004). However, the opposite was true among White and nonimmigrant individuals, highlighting the complexity of urban–rural distinctions. Urban–rural differences in the prevalence of depression were found in two of six countries assessed in the European Study of the Epidemiology of Mental Disorders. Controlling for sociodemographic factors, rural areas in France were characterized by a higher prevalence of depressive disorder than urban areas;

the opposite pattern was found in Belgium; and no rural–urban differences were found in Germany, Italy, Spain, and the Netherlands (Kovess-Masféty, Alonso, et al., 2005).

Analyses of the NESARC data showed no differences in urbanicity for major depressive disorder (see table 7-13).

Differences across sociodemographic groups in the prevalence of bipolar disorder do not appear to be as stark as they are for schizophrenia, as discussed below. Thus while the two major epidemiologic studies of psychiatric disorders in the United States (the ECA and the NCS) found trends toward elevated prevalence of bipolar disorder in urban areas compared with rural areas, the trends were not statistically significant (Kessler et al., 1997; Robins et al., 1984). Similarly, a Danish study using population-based registries to establish a cohort of over two million individuals found an increased prevalence of bipolar disorder in one of three provincial Danish cities with more than 100,000 inhabitants (Mortensen, Pedersen, Melbye, Mors, & Ewald, 2003). However, as in the ECA and NCS findings, little evidence was found for an urbanicity-related risk for bipolar disorder, again in stark contrast to findings regarding schizophrenia (Pedersen & Mortensen, 2001). Other epidemiologic studies in the United States (Grant et al., 2005) Canada (Parikh et al., 1996) and Puerto Rico (Canino et al., 1987) found no difference in the prevalence of bipolar disorder across geographic density–related settings.

Analyses of NESARC data showed that individuals with past-year bipolar I disorder were more likely to be living in rural than in urban areas (see table 7-14).

Schizophrenia

In the 1930s, Faris and Dunham (1939) showed that while the homes of individuals first admitted for the treatment of manic–depressive illness (roughly equivalent to our diagnosis of bipolar disorder) were distributed more or less randomly throughout Chicago, admissions for the treatment of schizophrenia tended to reside more in the center of the city, with decreasing prevalence as one moved outward into more affluent zones. This and similar findings (Eaton, 1974) were interpreted to result from the choice of city living by individuals who later would develop schizophrenia. Subsequent European prospective studies conducted well prior to onset in late adolescence (Lewis, David, & Andreasson, 1992), or even at birth (Marcelis, Navarro-Mateu, Murray, Selten, & Van Os, 1998), found the relative risk for schizophrenia to be about two to four times higher among those born in urban areas than among those born elsewhere. The underlying biological processes associated with urban residence remain unclear. Increased relative risk does not appear to be the result of differences in obstetric complications between urban and rural areas (Eaton, Mortensen, & Frydenberg, 2000), though it might be connected to differences during infancy in factors such as breastfeeding (McCreadie, 1997). The increased relative risk might also be related to differences in the physical environment, such as a higher concentration of lead in the soil and air in cities; differences in the cultural environment, for example, in expectations to leave the family of origin and define a new life plan (Eaton & Harrison, 2001); crowding, which might give rise to the spread of infections (Torrey &

Table 7-14. Disparities in Prevalence of Bipolar Disorder by Urbanicity

	NESARC		
	URBAN	SUBURBAN	RURAL
Bipolar I disorder (*N*)	(15,002)	(20,295)	(7,796)
Prevalence (*N*)[a]	0.88 (138)	0.78 (154)	1.09 (87)
Odds ratio [CI][b]	1.00	0.96 [0.70, 1.29]	1.39 [1.02, 1.91]

CI = 95% confidence interval.
[a]Column percentage weighted. [b]Adjusted for age and sex.

Table 7-15. Disparities in Prevalence of vwSchizophrenia by Urbanicity at Birth

	DANISH PSYCHIATRIC REGISTER				
	TOWNS WITH LESS THAN 10,000	CITIES WITH 10,000–100,00	CITIES WITH MORE THAN 100,000	COPENHAGEN SUBURB	COPENHAGEN
Schizophrenia					
Prevalence per 1000 (N)[a]	0.28 (416)	0.45 (557)	0.60 (319)	0.44 (266)	1.08 (604)
Risk ratio [CI][b]	1.00	1.64 [1.45, 1.87]	2.16 [1.86, 2.49]	1.59 [1.36, 1.86]	3.92 [3.42, 4.44]

CI = 95% confidence interval.
[a]Numerator is from all hospital and specialty clinic admissions in Denmark in 2006; denominator is from 25% sample of population of Denmark in 2006 (weighted to 100%).
[b]Adjusted for age and sex.

Yolken, 1995, 1998); or a host of other factors, including possible interaction of urbanicity with genetic risk and cognitive social capital (Van Os, Pedersen, & Mortensen, 2004).

Analysis of Danish register data shows that urbanicity at birth is strongly associated with schizophrenia (see table 7-15). Persons born in the large capital city of Copenhagen were found to have about four times the prevalence of schizophrenia as those born in small towns.

Alcohol and Drug Use Disorders

Findings on rural–urban differences in the prevalence of alcohol abuse and dependence are not conclusive. In an ECA-related study in the Piedmont of North Carolina, alcohol abuse and dependence were found to be more common in rural areas (Blazer et al., 1985). However,

no significant differences in the prevalence of alcohol abuse and dependence were found between subjects in the rural Michigan Upper Peninsula and more urban Lower Michigan (Steele, Sesney, & Kreher, 1999).

In a study in the United Kingdom, urban subjects were found to have a higher prevalence of alcohol dependence than rural subjects, with semirural (suburban) subjects between the two. These urban–rural differences in alcohol dependence lost their statistical significance after adjustments were made for living circumstances and life stress (Paykel et al., 2000). Individuals in Denmark had a higher prevalence of alcohol abuse than those living in Greenland, but no differences were detected between those living in large and small cities in Greenland (Madsen, Gronbaek, Bjerregaard, & Becker, 2005). Living in an urban area in Finland was found to be associated with a

Table 7-16. Disparities in Prevalence of Alcohol and Drug Disorders by Urbanicity

	NESARC		
	URBAN	SUBURBAN	RURAL
Alcohol abuse/dependence (N)	(15,002)	(20,295)	(7,796)
Prevalence (N)[a]	9.07 (1,237)	7.97 (1,473)	8.81 (617)
Odds ratio [CI][b]	1.00	0.95 [0.83, 1.09]	1.11 [0.94, 1.32]
Drug abuse/dependence (N)	(15,002)	(20,295)	(7,796)
Prevalence (N)[a]	2.26 (301)	1.88 (341)	1.92 (135)
Odds ratio [CI][b]	1.00	0.95 [0.77, 1.16]	1.01 [0.76, 1.33]

CI = 95% confidence interval.
[a]Column percentage weighted. [b]Adjusted for age and sex.

higher excess risk of alcohol dependence than rural living (Joutsenniemi et al., 2007). The prevalence of alcohol dependence in the rural Riverland region in South Australia was higher than in nonrural regions of the area (Clayer et al., 1995). In Nepal, alcohol dependence was found to be more common among individuals in the urban area of the Matwali community (Jhingan et al., 2003) than among those in the countryside.

Analyses of the NESARC data showed no significant differences in alcohol use or dependence related to urbanicity (see table 7-16).

Only a few general population studies have reported on urban–rural differences in drug use and dependence (Anthony et al., 1994; Diala et al., 2004; SAMHSA, 2007; L. A. Warner et al., 1995). One reason is that in an effort to protect respondent confidentiality, most US general population studies do not disclose county-level drug abuse–related data. Studies reporting on this issue generally have found that individuals living in rural areas are less likely to meet diagnostic criteria for a drug use or dependence disorder than those living in urban areas.

Using data from the NCS, Anthony and colleagues (1994) showed that respondents living in metropolitan areas were more likely to have a history of drug dependence than those living in rural areas. Based on the same data, L. A. Warner's group (1995) reported a significant association between urbanicity and lifetime drug use, albeit not with lifetime dependence or the persistence of dependence. Also analyzing NCS data, Diala and colleagues (2004) found that both rural and urban Blacks were less likely to report lifetime drug use disorders than Whites. Rural college graduates were less likely to report drug use disorders than rural residents with fewer years of education. In contrast, metropolitan college graduates were more likely to report drug use disorders than metropolitan residents with less education. Data from Australia's National Survey of Mental Health and Well-Being (Hall et al., 1999) showed Australian-born respondents living in capital cities to be more likely to have an ICD-10–diagnosable drug use or dependence disorder than those living elsewhere in Australia. Analyses of NESARC data did not show any significant differences in drug use or dependence based on urbanicity. (See table 7-16.)

CONCLUSION

This chapter has explored differences in the prevalences of major mental disorders in the general population across four major social variables: SES, race/ethnicity, marital status, and urbanicity. Table 7-17 summarizes the strength of the associations found between these social variables and mental disorders in the CPES and NESARC data.

Associations between mental disorders and these four key social variables vary with the mental disorder under study. Major depressive disorder is associated consistently with lower SES across studies, possibly due to greater persistence among those with lower SES. Bipolar disorder is associated with lower SES, possibly due to a downward drift in SES. Individuals with bipolar disorder are more likely to have never married or to have formerly been married. Alcohol use disorders, too, have been found more commonly among unmarried individuals. Both birth in an urban area and unmarried status have been closely associated with the prevalence of schizophrenia. Most studies show that drug use disorders are associated with lower educational attainment. In some cases, differences in disorders across variables are not as striking, as for anxiety disorders and bipolar I disorder, in which differences in prevalence across racial/ethnic groups are inconsistent. Similarly, alcohol use disorders have been associated with both low and high socioeconomic position. For most mental disorders, associations with urbanicity remain unresolved and in need of further research.

The four social variables examined in this chapter (SES, race/ethnicity, marital status, and urbanicity) can play different roles when associated with mental disorders. In some cases, these social factors can be risk factors for a mental disorder; in others they can be consequences of a mental disorder (e.g., low educational attainment secondary to a childhood disorder). Also, these social variables can interact with one another and act as confounders, mediators, or moderators in the

Table 7-17. Summary of Associations Between Mental Disorders and Population Disparities

DISORDER	EDUCATION			RACE/ETHNICITY		MARITAL STATUS			URBANICITY	
	CPES	NESARC	DENMARK	CPES	NESARC	CPES	NESARC	DENMARK	NESARC	DENMARK
Major depression	+	+	*	+	+	++	++	*	+	*
Panic disorder	++	++	*	+	++	++	++	*	−	*
Social phobia	+	++	*	++	++	++	−	*	+	*
Simple phobia	++	+	*	++	++	+	−	*	−	*
Schizophrenia	*	*	+++	*	*	*	*	+++	*	+++
Bipolar I	+++	+++	*	+	−	+++	++	*	+	*
Alcohol disorder	−	+	*	++	++	++	++	*	−	**
Drug disorder	++	+++	*	+	+++	++	+++	*	−	*

* Data not obtained.
+ Significant weak association (odds ratio < 1.5).
++ Significant moderate association (odds ratio = 1.5–2.5).
+++ Significant strong association (odds ratio > 1.5).
− Nonsignificant.

association of specific mental disorders with specific social factors. Finally, it is important to keep in mind that disparities in the prevalence of mental and behavioral disorders exist and that more studies are needed to better understand and diminish these disparities by lowering prevalence in high risk groups.

REFERENCES

Afifi, T. O., Cox, B. J., & Enns, M. W. (2006). Mental health profiles among married, never-married, and separated/divorced mothers in a nationally representative sample. *Social Psychiatry and Psychiatric Epidemiology, 41*(2), 122–129.

Agerbo, E., Byrne, M., Eaton, W., & Mortensen, P. B. (2004). Marital and labor market status in the long run in schizophrenia. *Archives of General Psychiatry, 61*(1), 28–33.

Alegria, M., Mulvaney-Day, N., Torres, M., Polo, A., Cao, Z., & Canino, G. (2007). Prevalence of psychiatric disorders across Latino subgroups in the United States. *American Journal of Public Health, 97*(1), 68–75.

Almeida Filho, N., Lessa, I., Magalhães, L., Araújo, M. J., Aquino, E., Kawachi, I., & James, S. A. (2004). Alcohol drinking patterns by gender, ethnicity, and social class in Bahia, Brazil. *Revista de Saude Publia, 38*(1), 45–54.

Alonso, J., Angermeyer, M. C., Bernert, S., Bruffaerts, R., Brugha, T. S., Bryson, H., ... Vollebergh, W. A. (2004). Prevalence of mental disorders in Europe: Results from the European Study of the Epidemiology of Mental Disorders (ESEMeD) project. *Acta Psychiatrica Scandinavica, 420*(Suppl.), 21–27.

Amaro, H., Whitaker, R., Coffman, G., & Heeren, T. (1990). Acculturation and marijuana and cocaine use: Findings from HHANES 1982–84. *American Journal of Public Health, 80*(Suppl.), 54–60.

American Psychiatric Association. (1987). *Diagnostic and statistical manual of mental disorders* (3rd ed., rev.). Washington, DC: Author.

American Psychiatric Association. (1994). *Diagnostic and statistical manual of mental disorders* (4th ed.). Washington, DC: Author.

Andrews, G., Henderson, S., & Hall, W. (2001). Prevalence, comorbidity, disability, and service utilization: Overview of the Australian National Mental Health Survey. *British Journal of Psychiatry, 178*, 145–153.

Annis, H., & Watson, C. (1975). Drug use and school dropout: A longitudinal study. *Canadian Counsellor, 9*, 155–161.

Anthony, J. C., Warner, L. A., & Kessler, R. C. (1994). Comparative epidemiology of dependence on tobacco, alcohol, controlled substances, and inhalants: Basic findings from the National Comorbidity Survey. *Experimental and Clinical Psychopharmacology, 2*, 244–268.

Araya, R., Rojas, G., Fritsch, J., Solis, J., Signorelli, A., & Lewis, G. (2001). Common mental disorders in Santiago, Chile: Prevalence and socio-demographic correlates. *British Journal of Psychiatry, 178*, 228–233.

Barros, M. B., Botega, N. J., Dalgalarrondo, P., Marín-León, L., & de Oliveira, H. B. (2007). Prevalence of alcohol abuse and associated factors in a population-based study. *Revista de Saude Publica, 41*(4), 502–509.

Baskin, D., Bluestone, H., & Nelson, M. (1981). Ethnicity and psychiatric diagnosis. *Journal of Clinical Psychology, 37*(3), 529–537.

Baumeister, H., & Harter, M. (2007). Prevalence of mental disorders based on general population surveys. *Social Psychiatry and Psychiatric Epidemiology, 42*(7), 537–546.

Beals, J., Piasecki, J., Nelson, S., Jones, M., Keane, E., Dauphinais, P., ... Manson, S. M. (1997). Psychiatric disorder among American Indian adolescents: Prevalence in Northern Plains youth. *Journal of the American Academy of Child and Adolescent Psychiatry, 36*(9), 1252–1259.

Bergen, S. E., Gardner, C. O., Aggen, S. H., & Kendler, K. S. (2008). Socioeconomic status and social support following illicit drug use: Causal pathways or common liability? *Twin Research and Human Genetics, 11*(3), 266–274.

Bijl, R. V., Ravelli, A., & van Zessen, G. (1998). Prevalence of psychiatric disorder in the general population: Results of the Netherlands Mental Health Survey and Incidence Study (NEMESIS). *Social Psychiatry and Psychiatric Epidemiology, 33*(12), 587–595.

Blanco, C., Alderson, D., Ogburn, E., Grant, B. F., Nunes, E. V., Hatzenbuehler, M. L., & Hasin, D. S. (2007). Changes in the prevalence of non-medical prescription drug use and drug use disorders in the United States: 1991–1992 and 2001–2002. *Drug and Alcohol Dependence, 90*(2–3), 252–260.

Blazer, D., George, L. K., Landerman, R., Pennybacker, M., Melville, M. L., Woodbury, M., ... Locke, B. (1985). Psychiatric disorders: A rural/urban comparison. *Archives of General Psychiatry, 42*(7), 651–656.

Blazer, D., Hughes, D., George, L. K., Swartz, M., & Boyer, R. (1991). Generalized anxiety disorder. In L. N. Robins, & D. A. Regier (Eds.), *Psychiatric* disorders in America (pp. 180–203). New York: Free Press.

Blazer, D., Kessler, R. C., McGonagle, K. A., & Swartz, M. S. (1994). The prevalence and distribution of major depression in a national community sample: The National Comorbidity Survey. *American Journal of Psychiatry, 151*(7), 979–986.

Bollen, K. A., Glanville, J. L., & Stecklov, G. (2001). Socioeconomic status and class in studies of fertility and health in developing countries. *Annual Review of Sociology, 27,* 153–185.

Bray, J. W., Zarkin, G. A., Ringwalt, C., & Qi, J. (2000). The relationship between marijuana initiation and dropping out of high school. *Health Economics, 9*(1), 9–18.

Breslau, J., Aguilar-Gaxiola, S., Kendler, K. S., Su, M., Williams, D., & Kessler, R. C. (2006). Specifying race-ethnic differences in risk for psychiatric disorder in a U.S. national sample. *Psychology and Medicine, 36*(1), 57–68.

Breslau, J., Kendler, K. S., Su, M., Aguilar-Gaxiola, S., & Kessler, R. C. (2005). Lifetime risk and persistence of psychiatric disorders across ethnic groups in the United States. *Psychological Medicine, 35*(3), 317–327.

Brown, D. R., & Eaton, W. W. (1986, September). *Racial differences in risk factors for phobic disorders.* Paper presented at the 114th meeting of the American Public Health Association, Las Vegas, NV.

Brown, D. R., Eaton, W. W., & Sussman, L. (1990). Racial differences in the prevalence of phobic disorders. *Journal of Nervous and Mental Disease, 178*(7), 434–441.

Brugal, M. T., Domingo-Salvany, A., Maguire, A., Cayla, J. A., Villalbi, J. R., & Hartnoll, R. (1999). A small area analysis estimating the prevalence of addiction to opioids in Barcelona, 1993. *Journal of Epidemiology and Community Health, 53*(8), 488–494.

Brunswick, A. F., Messeri, P., & Titus, S. (1992). Predictive factors in adult substance abuse: A prospective study of African-American adolescents. In M. Glantz & R. Pickens (Eds.), *Vulnerability to abuse* (pp. 419–472). Washington, DC: American Psychological Association.

Burnam, M. A., Hough, R. L., Escobar, J. I., Karno, M., Timbers, D. M., Telles, C. A., & Locke, B. Z. (1987). Six-month prevalence of specific psychiatric disorders among Mexican Americans and Whites in Los Angeles. *Archives of General Psychiatry, 44*(8), 687–694.

Byrne, M., Agerbo, E., Eaton, W. W., & Mortensen, P. B. (2004). Parental socio-economic status and risk of first admission with schizophrenia: A Danish national register–based study. *Social Psychiatry and Psychiatric Epidemiology, 39*(2), 87–96.

Caetano, R., & Clark, C. L. (1998). Trends in alcohol-related problems among Whites, Blacks, and Hispanics: 1984–1995. *Alcoholism Clinical and Experimental Research, 22*(2), 534–538.

Caetano, R., Ramisetty-Mikler, S., & Rodriguez, L. A. (2008). The Hispanic Americans Baseline Alcohol Survey (HABLAS): Rates and predictors of alcohol abuse and dependence across Hispanic national groups. *Journal of Studies on Alcohol and Drugs, 69*(3), 441–448.

Cairney, J., Thorpe, C., Rietschlin, J., & Avison, W. R. (1999). 12-month prevalence of depression among single and married mothers in the 1994 National Population Health Survey. *Canadian Journal of Public Health, 90*(5), 320–324.

Canino, G. J., Bird, H. R., Shrout, P. E., Rubio-Stipec, M., Bravo, M., Martinez, R.,...Guevara, L. M. (1987). The prevalence of specific psychiatric disorders in Puerto Rico. *Archives of General Psychiatry, 44*(8), 727–735.

Chen, K., & Kandel, D. (2002). Relationship between extent of cocaine use and dependence among adolescents and adults in the United States. *Drug and Alcohol Dependence, 68*(1), 65–85.

Cheung, Y. B. (1998). Can marital selection explain the differences in health between married and divorced people? From a longitudinal study of a British birth cohort. *Public Health, 112*(2), 113–117.

Chilcoat, H., & Anthony, J. (2004). Drug use and dependence. In I. Livingston (Ed.), *Handbook of Black American health policies and issues behind disparities in health* (2nd ed.). Westport, CT: Greenwood Publishing.

Chilcoat, H. D., & Breslau, N. (1996). Alcohol disorders in young adulthood: Effects of transitions into adult roles. *Journal of Health and Social Behavior, 37*(4), 339–349.

Claussen, B., Davey Smith, G., & Thelle, D. (2003). Impact of childhood and adulthood socioeconomic position on cause specific mortality: The Oslo Mortality Study. *Journal of Epidemiology and Community Health, 57*(1), 40–45.

Clayer, J. R., McFarlane, A. C., Bookless, C. L., Air, T., Wright, G., & Czechowicz, A. S. (1995). Prevalence of psychiatric disorders in rural South Australia. *Medical Journal of Australia, 163*(3), 124–125, 128–129.

Cohen, E., Fein, R., Arias, A., & Kranzler, H. R. (2007). Alcohol treatment utilization: Findings from the National Epidemiologic Survey on Alcohol and Related Conditions. *Drug and Alcohol Dependence, 86*(2–3), 214–221.

Coid, J. W., Kirkbride, J. B., Barker, D., Cowden, F., Stamps, R., Yang, M., & Jones, P. B. (2008). Raised incidence rates of all psychoses among migrant groups: Findings from the East London First Episode of Psychosis study. *Archives of General Psychiatry, 65*(11), 1250–1258.

Colón, H. M., Robles, R. R., Canino, G., & Sahai, H. (2001). Prevalence and correlates of DSM-IV substance use disorders in Puerto Rico. *Boletín de la Asociación Médica de Puerto Rico, 93*(1–12), 12–22.

Compton, W. M., Grant, B. F., Colliver, J. D., Glantz, M. D., & Stinson, F. S. (2004). Prevalence of marijuana use disorders in the United States: 1991–1992 and 2001–2002. *Journal of the American Medical Association, 291*(17), 2114–2121.

Compton, W. M., Thomas, Y. F., Stinson, F. S., & Grant, B. F. (2007). Prevalence, correlates, disability, and comorbidity of DSM-IV drug abuse and dependence in the United States: Results from the National Epidemiologic Survey on Alcohol and Related Conditions. *Archives of General Psychiatry, 64*(5), 566–576.

Cooper, C., Bebbington, P. E., Meltzer, H., Bhugra, D., Brugha, T., Jenkins, R.,…King, M. (2008). Depression and common mental disorders in lone parents: Results of the 2000 National Psychiatric Morbidity Survey. *Psychological Medicine, 38*(3), 335–342.

Costello, E. J., Compton, S. N., Keeler, G., & Angold, A. (2003). Relationship between poverty and psychopathology: A natural experiment. *Journal of the American Medical Association, 290*(15), 2023–2029.

Costello, E. J., Farmer, E. Z. M., Angold, A., Burns, B. J., & Erkanli, A. (1997). Psychiatric disorders among American-Indian and White youth in Appalachia: The Great Smoky Mountains study. *American Journal of Public Health, 87*(5), 827–832.

Costello, E. J., Keeler, G. P., & Angold, A. (2001). Poverty, race/ethnicity, and psychiatric disorder: A study of rural children. *American Journal of Public Health, 91*(9), 1494–1498.

Cromwell, B. A., Jr., George, L. K., Blazer, D., & Landerman, R. (1986). Psychosocial risk factors and urban/rural differences in the prevalence of major depression. *British Journal of Psychiatry, 149*, 307–314.

Crum, R. M., Bucholz, K. K., Helzer, J. E., & Anthony, J. C. (1992). The risk of alcohol abuse and dependence in adulthood: The association with educational level. *American Journal of Epidemiology, 135*(9), 989–999.

Crum, R. M., Chan, Y.-F., Chen, L.-S., Storr, C. L., & Anthony, J. C. (2005). Incidence rates for alcohol dependence among adults: Prospective data from the Baltimore Epidemiologic Catchment Area follow-up survey, 1981–1996. *Journal of Studies on Alcohol, 66*(6), 795–804.

Crum, R. M., Helzer, J. E., & Anthony, J. C. (1993). Level of education and alcohol abuse and dependence in adulthood: A further inquiry. *American Journal of Public Health, 83*(6), 830–837.

Davidson, J. R., Hughes, D. C., George, L. K., & Blazer, D. G. (1993). The epidemiology of social phobia: Findings from the Duke Epidemiological Catchment Area study. *Psychological Medicine, 23*(3), 709–718.

Dean, B. B., Gerner, D., & Gerner, R. H. (2004). A systematic review evaluating health-related quality of life, work impairment, and healthcare costs and utilization in bipolar disorder. *Current Medical Research and Opinion, 20*(2), 139–154.

DeKlyen, M., Brooks-Gunn, J., McLanahan, S., & Knab, J. (2006). The mental health of married, cohabiting, and non-coresident parents with infants. *American Journal of Public Health, 96*(10), 1836–1841.

De La Rosa, M. R., Khalsa, J. H., & Rouse, B. A. (1990). Hispanics and illicit drug use: A review of recent findings. *International Journal of the Addictions, 25*(6), 665–691.

De La Rosa, M., Vega, R., & Radisch, M. A. (2000). The role of acculturation in the substance abuse behavior of African-American and Latino adolescents: Advances, issues, and recommendations. *Journal of Psychoactive Drugs, 32*(1), 33–42.

Diala, C. C., Muntaner, C., & Walrath, C. (2004). Gender, occupational, and socioeconomic correlates of alcohol and drug abuse among U.S. rural, metropolitan, and urban residents. *American Journal of Drug and Alcohol Abuse, 30*(2), 409–428.

Dohrenwend, B. P. (2000). The role of adversity and stress in psychopathology: Some evidence and its implications for theory and research. *Journal of Health and Social Behavior, 41*(1), 1–19.

Dohrenwend, B. P., & Dohrenwend, B. S. (1969). *Social status and psychological disorder: A causal inquiry.* New York, NY: John Wiley & Sons.

Dohrenwend, B. P., & Dohrenwend, B. S. (1974). Psychiatric disorders in urban settings. In G. Caplan & S. Arieti (Eds.), *American handbook of psychiatry. Child and adolescent psychiatry: Sociocultural and community psychiatry* (pp. 424–449). New York, NY: Basic Books.

Dohrenwend, B. P., Levav, I., Shrout, P. E., Schwartz, S., Naveh, G., Link, B. G.,…Stueve, A. (1992). Socioeconomic status and psychiatric disorders: The causation–selection issue. *Science, 255*(5047), 946–952.

Eaton, W. W. (1974). Residence, social class, and schizophrenia. *Journal of Health and Social Behavior, 15*(4), 289–299.

Eaton, W. W. (1975). Marital status and schizophrenia. *Acta Psychiatrica Scandinavica, 52*(5), 320–329.

Eaton, W. (1985). The epidemiology of schizophrenia. *Epidemiologic Reviews, 7,* 105–126.

Eaton, W. (1991). Update on the epidemiology of schizophrenia. *Epidemiologic Reviews, 13,* 320–328.

Eaton, W. W., Anthony, J. C., Gallo, J., Cai, G., Tien, A., Romanoski, A., & Lyketsos, C. (1997). Natural history of Diagnostic Interview Schedule/ DSM-IV major depression. The Baltimore Epidemiological Catchment Area follow-up. *Archives of General Psychiatry, 54*(11), 993–999.

Eaton, W. W., Dryman, A., & Weissman, M. M. (1991). Panic and phobia. In L. N. Robins & D. A. Regier (Eds.), *Psychiatric disorders in America: The Epidemiologic Catchment Area Study* (pp. 155–179). New York, NY: Free Press.

Eaton, W. W., & Harrison, G. (2001). Life chances, life planning, and schizophrenia: A review and interpretation of research on social deprivation. *International Journal of Mental Health, 30,* 58–81.

Eaton, W. W., Kessler, R. C., Wittchen, H. & Magee, W. J. (1994). Panic and panic disorder in the United States. *American Journal of Psychiatry, 151*(3), 413–420.

Eaton, W. W., & Keyl, P. M. (1990). Risk factors for the onset of DIS/DSM-II agoraphobia in a prospective, population-based study. *Archives of General Psychiatry, 47*(9), 819–824.

Eaton, W. W., Mortensen, P. B., & Frydenberg, M. (2000). Obstetric complications, urbanization, and psychosis. *Schizophrenia Research, 43*(2–3), 117–123.

Ellickson, P., Bui, K., Bell, R., & McGuigan, K. (1998). Does early drug use increase the risk of dropping out of high school? *Journal of Drug Issues, 28*(2), 357–381.

Epstein, J. A., Botvin, G. J., & Diaz, T. (2001). Linguistic acculturation associated with higher marijuana and polydrug use among Hispanic adolescents. *Substance Use & Misuse, 36*(4), 477–499.

Faris, R. E., & Dunham, W. (1939). *Mental disorders in urban areas.* Chicago, IL: University of Chicago Press.

Fothergill, K., & Ensminger, M. E. (2006). Childhood and adolescent antecedents of drug and alcohol problems: A longitudinal study. *Drug and Alcohol Dependence, 82*(1), 61–76.

Fryers, T., Melzer, D., & Jenkins, R. (2003). Social inequalities and the common mental disorders. *Social Psychiatry and Psychiatric Epidemiology, 38*(5), 229–237.

Gfroerer, J., & De La Rosa, M. (1993). Protective and risk factors associated with drug use among Hispanic youth. *Journal of Addictive Diseases, 12*(2), 87–107.

Gilman, S. E., Breslau, J., Conron, K. J., Koenen, K. C., Subramanian, S. V., & Zaslavsky, A. M. (2008). Education and race-ethnicity differences in the lifetime risk of alcohol dependence. *Journal of Epidemiology and Community Health, 62*(3), 224–230.

Gilman, S. E., Kawachi, I., Fitzmaurice, G. M., & Buka, S. L. (2002). Socioeconomic status in childhood and the lifetime risk of major depression. *International Journal of Epidemiology, 31*(2), 359–367.

Gilman, S. E., Kawachi, I., Fitzmaurice, G. M., & Buka, S. L. (2003). Family disruption in childhood and risk of adult depression. *American Journal of Psychiatry, 160*(5), 939–946.

Goldberg, E. M., & Morrison, S. L. (1963). Schizophrenia and social class. *British Journal of Psychiatry, 109,* 785–802.

Goodwin, F. K., & Jamison, K. R. (1990). *Manic-depressive illness.* New York, NY: Oxford University Press.

Gove, W. R., Hughes, M., & Style Briggs, C. (1983). Does marriage have positive effects on psychological well-being of the individual? *Journal of Health and Social Behavior, 24*(2), 122–131.

Grant, B. F. (1996). Prevalence and correlates of drug use and DSM-IV drug dependence in the United States: Results of the National Longitudinal Alcohol Epidemiologic Survey. *Journal of Substance Abuse, 8*(2), 195–210.

Grant, B. F. (1997). Prevalence and correlates of alcohol use and DSM-IV alcohol dependence in the United States: Results of the National Longitudinal Alcohol Epidemiologic Survey. *Journal of Studies on Alcohol, 58*(5), 464–473.

Grant, B. F., Dawson, D. A., & Hasin, D. S. (2001). *The Alcohol Use Disorders and Associated Disabilities Interview Schedule—version for DSM-IV (AUDADIS-IV).* Bethesda, MD: National Institute on Alcohol Abuse and Alcoholism.

Grant, B. F., Moore, T. C., Shepard, J., & Kaplan, K. (2003). *Source and accuracy statement for wave 1 of the 2001–2002 National Epidemiologic Survey on Alcohol and Related Conditions.* Bethesda, MD: National Institute on Alcohol Abuse and Alcoholism.

Grant, B. F., Stinson, F. S., Dawson, D. A., Chou, S. P., Dufour, M. C., Compton, W.,...Kaplan, K. (2004). Prevalence and co-occurrence of substance use disorders and independent mood and anxiety disorders: Results from the National Epidemiologic Survey on Alcohol and Related Conditions. *Archives of General Psychiatry, 61*(8), 807–816.

Grant, B. F., Stinson, F. S., Hasin, D. S., Dawson, D. A., Chou, S. P., Ruan, W. J., & Huang, B. (2005). Prevalence, correlates, and comorbidity of bipolar I disorder and Axis I and II disorders: Results from the National Epidemiologic Survey on Alcohol and Related Conditions. *Journal of Clinical Psychiatry, 66*(10), 1205–1215.

Gresenz, C. R., Sturm, R., & Tang, L. (2001). Income and mental health: Unraveling community and individual level relationships. *Journal of Mental Health Policy and Economics, 4*(4), 197–203.

Hall, W., Teesson, M., Lynskey, M., & Degenhardt, L. (1999). The 12-month prevalence of substance use and ICD-10 substance use disorders in Australian adults: Findings from the National Survey of Mental Health and Well-Being. *Addiction, 94*(10), 1541–1550.

Hasin, D. S., Goodwin, R. D., Stinson, F. S., & Grant, B. F. (2005). Epidemiology of major depressive disorder: Results from the National Epidemiologic Survey on Alcoholism and Related Conditions. *Archives of General Psychiatry, 62*(10), 1097–1106.

Hasin, D. S., Stinson, F. S., Ogburn, E., & Grant, B. F. (2007). Prevalence, correlates, disability, and comorbidity of DSM-IV alcohol abuse and dependence in the United States: Results from the National Epidemiologic Survey on Alcohol and Related Conditions. *Archives of General Psychiatry, 64*(7), 830–842.

Heeringa, S. G., Wagner, J., Torres, M., Duan, N., Adams, T., & Berglund, P. (2004). Sample designs and sampling methods for the Collaborative Psychiatric Epidemiology Studies (CPES). *International Journal of Methods in Psychiatric Research, 13*(4), 221–240.

Helzer, J. E., Burnam, A., & McEvoy, L. T. (1991). Alcohol abuse and dependence. In L. N. Robins & D. A. Regier (Eds.), *Psychiatric disorders in America: The Epidemiologic Catchment Area Study* (pp. 81–115). New York, NY: Free Press.

Henry, K. L., & Huizinga, D. H. (2007). Truancy's effect on the onset of drug use among urban adolescents placed at risk. *Journal of Adolescent Health, 40*(4), 358.e9–358.17.

Heurtin-Roberts, S., Snowden, L., & Miller, L. (1997). Expressions of anxiety in African Americans: Ethnography and the Epidemiological Catchment Area studies. *Culture, Medicine and Psychiatry, 21*(3), 337–363.

Holt-Lunstad, J., Birmingham, W., & Jones, B. Q. (2008). Is there something unique about marriage? The relative impact of marital status, relationship quality, and network social support on ambulatory blood pressure and mental health. *Annals of Behavioral Medicine, 35*(2), 239–244.

Hope, S., Rodgers, B., & Power, C. (1999). Marital status transitions and psychological distress: Longitudinal evidence from a national population sample. *Psychological Medicine, 29*(2), 381–389.

Horwath, E., Johnson, J., & Hornig, C. (1993). Epidemiology of panic disorders in African Americans. *American Journal of Psychiatry, 150*(3), 465–469.

Hu, Y. R., & Goldman, N. (1990). Mortality differentials by marital status: An international comparison. *Demography, 27*(2), 233–250.

Huang, B., Grant, B. F., Dawson, D. A., Stinson, F. S., Chou, S. P., Saha, T. D.,...Pickering, R. P. (2006). Race-ethnicity and the prevalence and co-occurrence of *Diagnostic and Statistical Manual of Mental Disorders, IV,* alcohol and drug use disorders and Axis I and II disorders: United States, 2001 to 2002. *Comprehensive Psychiatry, 47*(4), 252–257.

Hughes, M., & Gove, W. (1981). Living alone, social integration, and mental health. *American Journal of Sociology, 87*(1), 48–74.

Hughes, M. E., & Waite, L. J. (2002). Health in household context: Living arrangements and health in late middle age. *Journal of Health and Social Behavior, 43*(1), 1–21.

Jackson, J. S., Torres, M., Caldwell, C. H., Neighbors, H. W., Nesse, R. M., Taylor, R. J.,...Williams, D. R.(2004). The National Survey of American Life: A study of racial, ethnic and cultural influences on mental disorders and mental health. *International Journal of Methods in Psychiatry Research, 13*(4), 196–207.

Jarvis, E. (1971). *Insanity and idiocy in Massachusetts: Report of the Commission on Lunacy, 1855.* Boston, MA: Harvard University Press. (Original work published 1855)

Jhingan, H. P., Shyangwa, P., Sharma, A., Prasad, K. M. R., & Khandelwal, S. K. (2003). Prevalence of alcohol dependence in a town in Nepal as assessed by the CAGE questionnaire. *Addiction, 98*(3), 339–343.

Jonas, B. S., Brody, D., Roper, M., & Narrow, W. E. (2003). Prevalence of mood disorders in a national sample of young American adults. *Social Psychiatry and Psychiatric Epidemiology, 38*(11), 618–624.

Jones, B. E., & Gray, B. A. (1986). Problems in diagnosing schizophrenia and affective disorders among Blacks. *Hospital and Community Psychiatry*, 37(1), 61–65.

Joutsenniemi, K., Martelin, T., Kestilä, L., Martikainen, P., Pirkola, S., & Koskinen, S. (2007). Living arrangements, heavy drinking and alcohol dependence. *Alcohol and Alcoholism*, 42(5), 480–491.

Judd, F. K., Jackson, H. J., Komiti, A., Murray, G., Hodgins, G., & Fraser, C. (2002). High prevalence disorders in urban and rural communities. *Australian and New Zealand Journal of Psychiatry*, 36, 104–113.

Kandel, D. B., Johnson, J. G., Bird, H. R., Canino, G., Goodman, S. H., Lahey, B. B.,…Schwab-Stone, M.(1997). Psychiatric disorders associated with substance abuse among children and adolescents: Findings from the Methods for the Epidemiology of Child and Adolescent Mental Disorders (MECA) study. *Journal of Abnormal Child Psychology*, 25, 121–132.

Karno, M., Golding, J. M, Burnam, M. A., Hough, R. L., Escobar, J. I., Wells, K. M, & Boyer, R. (1989). Anxiety disorders among Mexican Americans and Whites in Los Angeles. *Journal of Nervous and Mental Disease*, 177(4), 202–209.

Kawakami, N., Takeshima, T., Ono, Y., Uda, H., Hata, Y., Nakane, H.,…Kikkawa, T. (2005). Twelve-month prevalence, severity, and treatment of common mental disorders in communities in Japan: Preliminary finding from the World Mental Health Japan survey 2002–2003. *Psychiatry and Clinical Neurosciences*, 59(4), 441–452.

Kessler, R. C., Berglund, P., Chiu, W. T., Demler, O., Heeringa, S., Hiripi, E.,…Zheng, H. (2004). The U.S. National Comorbidity Survey Replication (NCS-R): Design and field procedures. *International Journal of Methods in Psychiatry Research*, 13(2), 69–92.

Kessler, R. C., Berglund, P., Demler, O., Jin, R., Koretz, D., Merikangas, K. R.,…Wang, P. S. (2003). The epidemiology of major depressive disorder: Results from the National Comorbidity Survey Replication (NCS-R). *Journal of the American Medical Association*, 289(23), 3095–3105.

Kessler, R. C., Berglund, P., Demler, O., Jin, R., Merikangas, K. R., & Walters, E. E. (2005). Lifetime prevalence and age-of-onset distributions of DSM-IV disorders in the National Comorbidity Survey Replication. *Archives of General Psychiatry*, 62(6), 593–602.

Kessler, R. C., Chiu, W. T., Demler, O., & Walters, E. E. (2005). Prevalence, severity, and comorbidity of 12-month DSM-IV disorders in the National Comorbidity Survey Replication. *Archives of General Psychiatry*, 62(6), 617–627.

Kessler, R. C., McGonagle, K. A., Zhao, S., Nelson, C. B., Hughes, M., Eshleman, S.,…Kendler, K. S. (1994). Lifetime and 12-month prevalence of DSM-III-R psychiatric disorders in the United States: Results from the National Comorbidity Survey. *Archives of General Psychiatry*, 51(1), 8–19.

Kessler, R. C., Rubinow, D. R., Holmes, C., Abelson, J. M., & Zhao, S. (1997). The epidemiology of DSM-III-R bipolar I disorder in a general population survey. *Psychological Medicine*, 27(5), 1079–1089.

Kessler, R. C., Ruscio, A. M., Shear, K., & Wittchen, H. U. (2008). Epidemiology of anxiety disorders. In M. M. Antony & M. B. Stein (Eds.), *Oxford handbook of anxiety and related disorders* (pp. 19–33). New York, NY: Oxford University Press.

Keyes, K. M., & Hasin, D. S. (2008). Socio-economic status and problem alcohol use: The positive relationship between income and the DSM-IV alcohol abuse diagnosis. *Addiction*, 103(7), 1120–1130.

Keyes, K. M., Martins, S. S., Hatzenbuehler, M. L., Bates, L. M., Blanco, C., & Hasin, D. S. (2012). Mental health service utilization for psychiatric disorders among Latinos living in the United States: The role of ethnic subgroup, ethnicity of social network, perceived discrimination and ethnic identification. *Social Psychiatry and Psychiatric Epidemiology*, 47(3), 383–394.

Keyl, P. M., & Eaton, W. W. (1990). Risk factors for the onset of panic disorder and other panic attacks in a prospective, population-based study. *American Journal of Epidemiology*, 131(2), 301–311.

Kilpatrick, D. G., Acierno, R., Saunders, B., Resnick, H. S., Best, C. L., & Schnurr, P. P. (2000). Risk factors for adolescent substance abuse and dependence: Data from a national sample. *Journal of Consulting and Clinical Psychology*, 68(1), 19–30.

Kinney, D. K., Teixeira, P., Hsu, D., Napoleon, S. C., Crowley, D. J., Miller, A.,…Huang, E. (2009). Relation of schizophrenia prevalence to latitude, climate, fish consumption, infant mortality, and skin color: A role for prenatal vitamin D deficiency and infections? *Schizophrenia Bulletin*, 35(3), 582–595.

Kirkbride, J. B., Barker, D., Cowden, F., Stamps, R., Yang, M., Jones, P. B., & Coid, J. W. (2008). Psychoses, ethnicity and socio-economic status. *British Journal of Psychiatry*, 193, 18–24.

Klose, M., & Jacobi, F. (2004). Can gender differences in the prevalence of mental disorders be explained by sociodemographic factors? *Archives of Women's Mental Health*, 7(2), 133–148.

Knupfer, G. (1989). The prevalence in various social groups of eight different drinking patterns, from abstainers to frequent drunkenness: Analysis of 10 U.S. surveys combined. *British Journal of Addiction*, 84(11), 1305–1318.

Kovess-Masféty, V., Alonso, J., de Graaf, R., & Demyttenaere, K. (2005). A European approach to rural–urban differences in mental health: The ESEMeD 2000 comparative study. *Canadian Journal of Psychiatry*, 50(14), 926–936.

Kovess-Masféty, V., Lecoutour, X., & Delavelle, S. (2005). Mood disorders and urban/rural settings: Comparisons between two French regions. *Social Psychiatry and Psychiatric Epidemiology*, 40(8), 613–618.

Kraepelin, E. (1893). *Psychiatrie: Ein kurzes Lehruch fur Studerende und Aerzte* (4th ed.). Leipzig, Germany: Abel Verlag.

Kurz, B., Malcom, B., & Cournoyer, D. (2005). In the shadow of race: Immigrant status and mental health. *Affilia*, 20(4), 434–447.

Last, C. G., & Perrin, S. (1993). Anxiety disorders in African-American and Caucasian American children. *Journal of Abnormal Child Psychology*, 21(2), 153–164.

Lee, C. K., Kwak, Y. S., Yamamoto, J., Rhee, H., Kim, Y. S., Han, J. H., ... Lee, Y. H. (1990a). Psychiatric epidemiology in Korea, Part I: Gender and age differences in Seoul. *Journal of Nervous and Mental Disease*, 178(4), 242–246.

Lee, C. K., Kwak, Y. S., Yamamoto, J., Rhee, H., Kim, Y. S, Han, J. H., ... Lee, Y. H. (1990b). Psychiatric epidemiology in Korea, Part II: Urban and rural differences. *Journal of Nervous and Mental Disease*, 178(4), 247–252.

Lewis, G., Bebbington, P. E., Brugha, T., Farrell, M., Gill, B., Jenkins, R., & Meltzer, H. (1998). Socioeconomic status, standard of living, and neurotic disorder. *Lancet*, 352(9128), 605–609.

Lewis, G., David, A., & Andreasson, S. A. P. (1992). Schizophrenia and city life. *Lancet*, 340(8812), 137–140.

Lloyd, T., Kennedy, N., Fearon, P., Kirkbride, J., Mallett, R., Leff, J., ... Jones, P. B. (2005). Incidence of bipolar affective disorder in three UK cities: Results from the AESOP study. *British Journal of Psychiatry*, 186, 126–131.

Lorant, V., Croux, C., Welch, S., Deliege, D., Mackenbach, J., & Ansseau, M. (2007). Depression and socio-economic risk factors: Seven-year longitudinal population study. *British Journal of Psychiatry*, 190, 293–298.

Lynch, J. W., Kaplan, G. A., & Shema, S. J. (1997). Cumulative impact of sustained economic hardship on physical, cognitive, psychological, and social functioning. *New England Journal of Medicine*, 337(26), 1889–1895.

Madsen, M. H., Gronbaek, M., Bjerregaard, P., & Becker, U. (2005). Urbanization, migration, and alcohol use in a population of Greenland Inuit. *International Journal of Circumpolar Health*, 64(3), 234–245.

Magee, W. J., Eaton, W. W., Wittchen, H., McGonagle, K. A., & Kessler, R. C. (1996). Agoraphobia, simple phobia, and social phobia in the National Comorbidity Survey. *Archives of General Psychiatry*, 53(2), 159–168.

Marcelis, M., Navarro-Mateu, F., Murray, R., Selten, J.-P., & Van Os, J. (1998). Urbanization and psychosis: A study of 1942–1978 birth cohorts in the Netherlands. *Psychological Medicine*, 28(4), 871–879.

Martins, S. S., Storr, C. L., Zhu, H., & Chilcoat, H. D. (2009). Correlates of extramedical use of OxyContin versus other analgesic opioids among the U.S. general population. *Drug and Alcohol Dependence*, 99(1–3), 58–67.

McCabe, S. E., Cranford, J. A., & West, B. T. (2008). Trends in prescription drug abuse and dependence, co-occurrence with other substance use disorders, and treatment utilization: Results from two national surveys. *Addictive Behaviors*, 33(10), 1297–1305.

McCreadie, R. G. (1997). The Nithsdale Schizophrenia Surveys 16: Breast-feeding and schizophrenia: Preliminary results and hypotheses. *British Journal of Psychiatry*, 170, 334–337.

McGinnis, J. M., & Foege, W. H. (1993). Actual causes of death in the United States. *Journal of the American Medical Association*, 270(18), 2207–2212.

McGrath, J. (1999). Hypothesis: Is low prenatal vitamin D a risk-modifying factor for schizophrenia? *Schizophrenia Research*, 40(3), 173–177.

McGrath, J., Saha, S., Chant, D., & Welham, J. (2008). The epidemiology of schizophrenia: A concise overview of incidence, prevalence and mortality. *Epidemiologic Reviews*, 30, 67–76.

McGrath, J., Saha, S., Welham, J., El, S. O., MacCauley, C., & Chant, D. (2004). A systematic review of the incidence of schizophrenia: The distribution of rates and the influence of sex, urbanicity, migrant status and methodology. *BMC Medicine*, 2, 13.

Melchior, M., Berkman, L. F., Niedhammer, I., Zins, M., & Goldberg, M. (2007). The mental health effects of multiple work and family demands: A prospective study of psychiatric sickness absence in the French GAZEL study. *Social Psychiatry and Psychiatric Epidemiology, 42*(7), 573–582.

Mendelson, T., Rehkopf, D., & Kubzansky, L. D. (2008). Depression among Latinos in the United States: A meta-analytic review. *Journal of Consulting and Clinical Psychology, 76*(3), 355–366.

Mendoza-Sassi, R. A., & Beria, J. U. (2003). Prevalence of alcohol use disorders and associated factors: A population-based study using AUDIT in Southern Brazil. *Addiction, 98*(6), 799–804.

Merikangas, K. R., Akiskal, H. S., Angst, J., Greenberg, P. E., Hirschfeld, R. M., Petukhova, M., & Kessler, R. C. (2007). Lifetime and 12-month prevalence of bipolar spectrum disorder in the National Comorbidity Survey Replication. *Archives of General Psychiatry, 64*(5), 543–552.

Mishler, E. G., & Scotch, N. A. (1963). Sociocultural factors in the epidemiology of schizophrenia. *Psychiatry, 26,* 313–351.

Mitchell, C. M., Beals, J., Novins, D. K., & Spicer, P. (2003). Drug use among two American Indian populations: Prevalence of lifetime use and DSM-IV substance use disorders. *Drug and Alcohol Dependence, 69*(1), 29–41.

Morgan, C., Dazzan, P., Morgan, K., Jones, P., Harrison, G., Leff, J.,...Fearon, P. (2006). First episode psychosis and ethnicity: Initial findings from the AESOP study. *World Psychiatry, 5*(1), 40–46.

Mortensen, P. B., Pedersen, C. B., Melbye, M., Mors, O., & Ewald, H. (2003). Individual and familial risk factors for bipolar affective disorders in Denmark. *Archives of General Psychiatry, 60*(12), 1209–1215.

Munk-Jorgensen, P., Kastrup, M., & Mortensen, P. B. (1993). The Danish psychiatric register as a tool in epidemiology. *Acta Psychiatrica Scandinavica, 370*(Suppl.), 27–32.

Murray, C. J. L., & Lopez, A. D. (1996). *The global burden of disease.* Cambridge, MA: Harvard University Press.

Muntaner, C., Eaton, W. W., Diala, C., Kessler, R. C., & Sorlie, P. D. (1998). Social class, assets, organizational control and the prevalence of common groups of psychiatric disorders. *Social Science and Medicine, 47*(12), 2043–2053.

Muntaner, C., Eaton, W. W., Miech, R., & O'Campo, P. (2004). Socioeconomic position and major mental disorders. *Epidemiologic Reviews, 26,* 53–62.

Neal, A. M., & Turner, S. M. (1991). Anxiety disorders research with African-Americans: Current status. *Psychological Bulletin, 109*(3), 400–410.

Nestadt, G., Bienvenu, O. J., Cai, G., Samuels, J., & Eaton, W. W. (1998). Incidence of obsessive–compulsive disorders in adults. *Journal of Nervous and Mental Disease, 186*(7), 401–406.

O'Brien, M. S., & Anthony, J. C. (2005). Risk of becoming cocaine dependent: Epidemiological estimates for the United States, 2000–2001. *Neuropsychopharmacology, 30*(5), 1006–1018.

O'Connell, J. M., Novins, D. K., Beals, J., & Spicer, P. (2005). Disparities in patterns of alcohol use among reservation-based and geographically dispersed American Indian populations. *Alcoholism, Clinical and Experimental Research, 29*(1), 107–116.

Office of Management and Budget. (1997). *Revisions to the standards for the classification of federal data on race and ethnicity.* Washington, DC: Executive Office of the President. Retrieved from http://whitehouse.gov/omb/fedreg_1997standards

Orozco, S., & Lukas, S. (2000). Gender differences in acculturation and aggression as predictors of drug use in minorities. *Drug and Alcohol Dependence, 59*(2), 165–172.

Osler, M., Nordentoft, M., & Andersen, A. N. (2006). Childhood social environment and risk of drug and alcohol abuse in a cohort of Danish men born in 1953. *American Journal of Epidemiology, 163*(7), 654–661.

Parikh, S. V., Wasylenki, D., Goering, P., & Wong, J. (1996). Mood disorders: Rural/urban differences in prevalence, health care utilization, and disability in Ontario. *Journal of Affective Disorders, 38*(1), 57–65.

Parker, G. (1987). Are the lifetime prevalence estimates in the ECA study accurate? *Psychological Medicine, 17*(2), 275–282.

Patten, S. B. (2003). Recall bias and major depression lifetime prevalence. *Social Psychiatry and Psychiatric Epidemiology, 38*(6), 290–296.

Paykel, E. S., Abbot, R., Jenkins, R., Brugha, T. S., & Meltzer, H. (2000). Urban–rural mental health differences in Great Britain: Findings from the National Morbidity Survey. *Psychological Medicine, 30*(2), 269–280.

Pedersen, C. B., & Mortensen, P. B. (2001). Evidence of a dose–response relationship between urbanicity during upbringing and schizophrenia risk. *Archives of General Psychiatry, 58*(11), 1039–1046.

Pennell, B. E., Bowers, A., Carr, D., Chardoul, S., Cheung, G. Q., Dinkelmann, K.,...Torres, M. (2004).The development and implementation of the National Comorbidity Survey Replication, the National Survey of American Life, and the National Latino and Asian-American Survey. *International Journal of Methods in Psychiatric Research, 13*(4), 241–269.

Plant, E. A., & Sachs-Ericsson, N. (2004). Racial and ethnic differences in depression: The roles of social support and meeting basic needs. *Journal of Consulting and Clinical Psychology, 72*(1), 41–52.

Poulton, R., Caspi, A., Milne, B. J., Thomson, W. M., Taylor, A., Sears, M. R., & Moffitt, T. E. (2002). Association between children's experience of socioeconomic disadvantage and adult health: A life-course study. *Lancet, 360*(9346), 1640–1645.

Power, C., Rodgers, B., & Hope, S. (1999). Heavy alcohol consumption and marital status: Disentangling the relationship in a national study of young adults. *Addiction, 94*(10), 1477–1487.

Prescott, C. A., & Kendler, K. S. (2000). Influence of ascertainment strategy on finding sex differences in genetic estimates from twin studies of alcoholism. *American Journal of Medical Genetics, 96*(6), 754–761.

Probst, J. C., Laditka, S. B., Moore, C. G., Harun, N., Powell, M. P., & Baxley, E. G. (2006). Rural–urban differences in depression prevalence: Implications for family medicine. *Family Medicine, 38*(9), 653–660.

Reardon, S.F., & Buka, S.L. (2002). Differences in onset and persistence of substance abuse and dependence among Whites, Blacks, and Hispanics. *Public Health Reports, 117*(Suppl. 1), s51–s59.

Regier, D. A., Farmer, M. E., Rae, D. S., Myers, J. K., Kramer, M., Robins, L. N.,...Locke, B. Z. (1993). One-month prevalence of mental disorders in the United States and sociodemographic characteristics: The Epidemiologic Catchment Area study. *Acta Psychiatrica Scandinavica, 88*(1), 35–47.

Regier, D. A., Kaelber, C. T., Rae, D. S., Farmer, M. E., Knauper, B., Kessler, R. C., & Norquist, G. S. (1998). Limitations of diagnostic criteria and assessment instruments for mental disorders. *Archives of General Psychiatry, 55*(2), 109–115.

Riolo, S. A., Nguyen, T. A., Greden, J. F., & King, C. A. (2005). Prevalence of depression by race/ethnicity: Findings from the National Health and Nutrition Examination Survey III. *American Journal of Public Health, 95*(6), 998–1000.

Roberts, R. E., & Lee, E. S. (1993). Occupation and the prevalence of major depression, alcohol, and drug abuse in the United States. *Environmental Research, 61*(2), 266–278.

Roberts, R. E., Roberts, C. R., & Xing, Y. (2006). Prevalence of youth-reported DSM-IV psychiatric disorders among African-, European-, and Mexican-American adolescents. *Journal of the American Academy of Child and Adolescent Psychiatry, 45*(11), 1329–1337.

Robins, L. N., Helzer, J. E., Weissman, M. M., Orvaschel, H., Gruenberg, E., Burke, J. D., Jr., & Regier, D. A. (1984). Lifetime prevalence of specific psychiatric disorders in three sites. *Archives of General Psychiatry, 41*(10), 949–958.

Robins, L. N., & Regier, D. A. (Eds.). (1991). *Psychiatric disorders in America.* New York, NY: Free Press.

Romans-Clarkson, S. E., Walton, V. A., Herbison, P., & Mullen, P. E. (1990). Psychiatric morbidity among women in urban and rural New Zealand: Psychosocial correlates. *British Journal of Psychiatry, 156*, 85–91.

Safran, M. A., Mays, R. A., Jr., Huang, L. N., McCuan, R., Pham, P. K., Fisher, S. K.,...Trachtenberg, A. (2009). Mental health disparities. *American Journal of Public Health, 99*(11), 1962–1966.

Schaffer, A., Cairney, J., Cheung, A., Veldhuizen, S., & Levitt, A. (2006). Community survey of bipolar disorder in Canada: Lifetime prevalence and illness characteristics. *Canadian Journal of Psychiatry, 51*(1), 9–16.

Schneier, F. R., Johnson, J., Hornig, C. D., Liebowitz, M. R., & Weissman, M. M. (1992). Social phobia: Comorbidity and morbidity in an epidemiological sample. *Archives of General Psychiatry, 49*(4), 282–288.

Simon, G. E., & VonKorff, M. (1995). Recall of psychiatric history in cross-sectional surveys: Implications for epidemiologic research. *Epidemiologic Reviews, 17*(1), 221–227.

Smith, S. M., Stinson, F. S., Dawson, D. A., Goldstein, R., Huang, B., & Grant, B. F. (2006). Race/ethnic differences in the prevalence and co-occurrence of substance use disorders and independent mood and anxiety disorders: Results from the National Epidemiologic Survey on Alcohol and Related Conditions. *Psychological Medicine, 36*(7), 987–998.

Stansfeld, S. A., Clark, C., Rodgers, B., Caldwell, T., & Power, C. (2008). Childhood and adulthood socio-economic position and midlife depressive and anxiety disorders. *British Journal of Psychiatry, 192*, 152–153.

Steele, R. S., Sesney, J. W., & Kreher, N. E. (1999). The prevalence of alcohol abuse and dependence in two geographically distinct regions in Michigan: An UPRNet study. *Wisconsin Medical Journal, 98*(1), 54–57.

Stefansson, J. G., Lindal, E., Björnsson, J. K., & Guomundsdottir, A. (1994). Period prevalence rates of specific mental disorders in an Icelandic cohort. *Social Psychiatry and Psychiatric Epidemiology, 29*(3), 119–125.

Stone, A. L., O'Brien, M. S., De La Torre, A., & Anthony, J. C. (2007). Who is becoming hallucinogen dependent soon after hallucinogen use starts? *Drug and Alcohol Dependence, 87*(2–3), 153–163.

Substance Abuse and Mental Health Services Administration. (2005). *Results from the 2004 National Survey on Drug Use and Health: National findings.* Rockville, MD: Substance Abuse and Mental Health Services Administration, US Department of Health and Human Services.

Substance Abuse and Mental Health Services Administration. (2007). *Results from the 2006 National Survey on Drug Use and Health: National findings.* Rockville, MD: Substance Abuse and Mental Health Services Administration, US Department of Health and Human Services.

Substance Abuse and Mental Health Services Administration. (2010). *Results from the 2009 National Survey on Drug Use and Health: National findings.* Rockville, MD: Substance Abuse and Mental Health Services Administration, US Department of Health and Human Services.

Sundquist, K., & Frank, G. (2004). Urbanisation and hospital admission rates for alcohol and drug abuse: A follow-up study of 4.5 million women and men in Sweden. *Addiction, 99*(10), 1298–1305.

Swendsen, J., Anthony, J. C., Conway, K. P., Degenhardt, L., Dierker, L., Glantz, M.,…Merinkangas, K. R. (2008). Improving targets for the prevention of drug use disorders: Sociodemographic predictors of transitions across drug use stages in the National Comorbidity Survey Replication. *Preventive Medicine, 47*(6), 629–634.

Thundal, K. L., & Allebeck, P. (1998). Abuse of and dependence on alcohol in Swedish women: Role of education, occupation and family structure. *Social Psychiatry and Psychiatric Epidemiology, 33*(9), 445–450.

Torrey, E., & Yolken, R. (1995). At issue: Could schizophrenia be a viral zoonosis transmitted from house cats? *Schizophrenia Bulletin, 21*(2), 167–171.

Torrey, E. F., & Yolken, R. H. (1998). At issue: Is household crowding a risk factor for schizophrenia? *Schizophrenia Bulletin, 24*(3), 321–324.

Tsuchiya, K. J., Agerbo, E., Byrne, M., & Mortensen, P. B. (2004). Higher socio-economic status of parents may increase risk for bipolar disorder in the offspring. *Psychological Medicine, 34*(5), 787–793.

Turner, R. J., & Gil, A. G. (2002). Psychiatric and substance use disorders in South Florida: Racial/ethnic and gender contrasts in a young adult cohort. *Archives of General Psychiatry, 59*(1), 43–50.

Turner, R. J., & Lloyd, D. A. (1999). The stress process and the social distribution of depression. *Journal of Health and Social Behavior, 40*(4), 374–404.

Turner, R. J., & Wagenfeld, M. O. (1967). Occupational mobility and schizophrenia. *American Sociological Review, 32*(1), 104–113.

Van Oers, J. A., Bongers, I. M., van de Goor, L. A., & Garretsen, H. F. (1999). Alcohol consumption, alcohol-related problems, problem drinking, and socioeconomic status. *Alcohol and Alcoholism, 34*(1), 78–88.

Van Os, J., Pedersen, C. B., & Mortensen, P. B. (2004). Confirmation of synergy between urbanicity and familial liability in the causation of psychosis. *American Journal of Psychiatry, 161*(12), 2312–2314.

Vega, W. A., Aguilar-Gaxiola, S., Andrade, L., Bijl, R., Borges, G., Caraveo-Anduaga, J. J.,…Wittchen, H. U. (2002). Prevalence and age of onset for drug use in seven international sites: Results from the International Consortium of Psychiatric Epidemiology. *Drug and Alcohol Dependence, 68*(3), 285–297.

Vega, W. A., Alderete, E., Kolody, B., & Aguilar-Gaxiola, S. (1998). Illicit drug use among Mexicans and Mexican-Americans in California: The effects of gender and acculturation. *Addiction, 93*(12), 1839–1850.

Vega, W. A., Sribney, W. M., Aguilar-Gaxiola, S., & Kolody, B. (2004). Twelve-month prevalence of DSM-III-R psychiatric disorders among Mexican Americans: Nativity, social assimilation, and age determinants. *Journal of Nervous and Mental Disease, 192*(8), 532–541.

Vega, W. A., Zimmerman, R., Gil, A., Warheit, G. J., & Apospori, E. (1993). Acculturation strain theory: Its application in explaining drug use behavior among Cuban and other Hispanic youth. *NIDA Research Monograph, 130*, 144–166.

Wagner-Echeagaray, F. A., Schutz, C. G., Chilcoat, H. D., & Anthony, J. C. (1994). Degree of acculturation and the risk of crack cocaine smoking among Hispanic Americans. *American Journal of Public Health, 84*(11), 1825–1827.

Waite, L. J. (1996). Social science finds: "Marriage matters." *The Responsive Community, 6*, 26–36.

Wang, J. L. (2004). Rural–urban differences in the prevalence of major depression and associated impairment. *Social Psychiatry and Psychiatric Epidemiology, 39*(1), 19–25.

Wang, J., & El-Guebaly, N. (2004). Sociodemographic factors associated with comorbid major depressive episodes and alcohol dependence in the general population. *Canadian Journal of Psychiatry, 49*(1), 37–44.

Warner, L. A., Canino, G., & Colon, H. M. (2001). Prevalence and correlates of substance use disorders among older adolescents in Puerto Rico and the United States: A cross-cultural comparison. *Drug and Alcohol Dependence, 63*(3), 229–243.

Warner, L. A., Kessler, R. C., Hughes, M., Anthony, J. C., & Nelson, C. B. (1995). Prevalence and correlates of drug use and dependence in the United States: Results from the National Comorbidity Survey. *Archives of General Psychiatry, 52*(3), 219–229.

Warner, R. (1995). Time trends in schizophrenia: Changes in obstetric risk factors with industrialization. *Schizophrenia Bulletin, 21*(3), 483–500.

Weissman, M. M., Bruce, M. L., Leaf, P. J., Florio, L. P., & Holzer, C. E. (1991). Affective disorders. In L. N. Robins & D. A. Regier (Eds.), *Psychiatric disorders in America: The Epidemiologic Catchment Area Study* (pp. 53–80). New York, NY: Free Press.

Weissman, M. M., & Myers, J. K. (1978). Affective disorders in a U.S. urban community: The use of research diagnostic criteria in an epidemiological survey. *Archives of General Psychiatry, 35*(11), 1304–1311.

Wells, J. C., Tien, A. Y., Garrison, R., & Eaton, W. W. (1994). Risk factors for the incidence of social phobia as determined by the Diagnostic Interview Schedule in a population-based study. *Acta Psychiatrica Scandinavica, 90*(2), 84–90.

Whaley, A. L. (2003). Ethnicity/race, ethics and epidemiology. *Journal of the National Medical Association, 95*(8), 743–745.

Whisman, M. A., Uebelacker, L. A., & Bruce, M. L. (2006). Longitudinal association between marital dissatisfaction and alcohol use disorders in a community sample. *Journal of Family Psychology, 20*(1), 164–167.

Williams, D. R., Gonzalez, H. M., Neighbors, H., Nesse, R., Abelson, J. M., Sweetman, J., & Jackson, J. S. (2007). Prevalence and distribution of major depressive disorder in African Americans, Caribbean Blacks, and Whites: Results from the National Survey of American Life. *Archives of General Psychiatry, 64*(3), 305–315.

Wittchen, H., Zhao, S., Kessler, R. C., & Eaton, W. W. (1994). DSM-III-R generalized anxiety disorder in the National Comorbidity Survey. *Archives of General Psychiatry, 51*(5), 355–364.

Woodruff, R. A., Jr., Guze, W. B., & Clayton, P. J. (1971). Unipolar and bipolar primary affective disorder. *British Journal of Psychiatry, 119*(548), 33–38.

World Health Organization. (1992). *International statistical classification of diseases and related health problems* (10th rev.). Geneva, Switzerland: Author.

World Health Organization. (2004). Prevalence, severity, and unmet need for treatment of mental disorders in the World Mental Health Organization World Mental Health Surveys. *Journal of the American Medical Association, 291*(21), 2581–2590.

World Health Organization International Consortium in Psychiatric Epidemiology (ICPE). (2000). Cross-national comparisons of the prevalences and correlates of mental disorders. *Bulletin of the World Health Organization, 78*(4), 413–426.

SECTION IV

Mechanisms of Risk

8

Genes as a Source of Risk for Mental Disorders

PETER P. ZANDI

HOLLY C. WILCOX

LULU DONG

SANDY CHON

BRION MAHER

Key Points

- Family, twin, and adoption studies consistently demonstrate that genetic factors are an important contributor to the etiology of common mental and behavioral disorders

- The risk of disease in first-degree relatives of someone who is affected, compared with the risk in the general population, is called the recurrence risk and it ranges from as low as 4 for Alzheimer's disease up to 150 for autism

- Twin studies have shown that heritability of common mental and behavioral disorders—the proportion of variability in risk of disease due to variation in genetic factors—ranges from a low of 40% for depression up to 90% for autism.

- Genome-wide linkage, association, and expression studies have been widely used, but the genes that contribute to susceptibility for mental and behavioral disorders still are largely unknown

- A major challenge in studying the genetics of mental and behavioral disorders is the difficulty of defining phenotypes according to an accepted "gold standard" measure

- The genetic architecture of mental and behavioral disorders is very complex, with numerous genes contributing to susceptibility independently and interactively with each other and with environmental factors

- Sequencing of the human genome and the ensuing genomics revolution hold great promise for advancing our understanding of the etiology of mental and behavioral disorders

- Sequencing the entire genomes of populations of individuals will be possible soon and will allow important advances in understanding of the genetics of mental and behavioral disorders

INTRODUCTION

Sir Francis Galton, the prolific polymath with a keen interest in human variation, was the first to coin the phrase "nature versus nurture" to describe the long-running, sometimes acrimonious debate about the relative importance of those two influences in determining human behavior. Today, that phrase has been supplanted by "genes versus environment." Most serious scholars interested in studying disturbances of human behavior today no longer debate whether it is genes *or* environment. Instead, they seek to explain how genes *and* environment interact to give rise to such disturbances. While both are vitally important components of a complex etiologic equation, this chapter focuses specifically on the genetic contribution.

The genomics revolution, ushered in by the launch of the Human Genome Project in 1990, has transformed the ability to study the genetic contribution to human behavior. The simple yet monumental goal of the Human Genome Project was to determine the DNA sequence across the entire human genome. The effort required a concerted $300 million effort by an international group including 16 publicly funded sites and one private venture (Marshall, 2000). On June 26, 2000, Francis Collins and Craig Venter, the two scientists who had led competing efforts to complete the job, stood together to announce that a rough draft of the sequence had been completed (International Human Genome Mapping Consortium, 2001; Venter et al., 2001). The achievement, justifiably lauded as a landmark in science, in reality only marked the beginning of the revolution.

The next, perhaps even more daunting steps were to catalogue how the DNA sequence varies from one individual to the next and to describe what the DNA sequence does. Major initiatives spun off from the Human Genome Project have set out to complete these important tasks, among them the HapMap Project (International HapMap Consortium, 2003), which aims to identify and catalogue DNA sequence variation in major populations around the world, and the ENCODE project, which seeks to characterize all functional elements across the DNA sequence (ENCODE Project Consortium, 2007). These efforts have laid the foundation for fulfilling the ultimate goal of the revolution: to explain how variation in the DNA sequence relates to differences in human health, from well-being to pathology.

This chapter explores the current understanding of how genetic factors contribute to human mental health in general, and in particular how they lead to disturbances that can affect public mental health in significant ways. It begins with an explanation of some basic genetic concepts crucial to understanding how genetic factors can influence human mental health. It then describes the leading research paradigm used to investigate the role of genetic factors and highlights a number of discoveries made in implementing this paradigm. The chapter closes with a discussion of the challenges that remain to better understanding how genetic factors contribute to mental health and why ongoing research in this area is crucial.

BASIC GENETIC CONCEPTS

Every cell in the human body has a nucleus that contains genetic material packaged in units called chromosomes (see figure 8-1). Each human cell includes 23 pairs of chromosomes, one set inherited from the mother, the

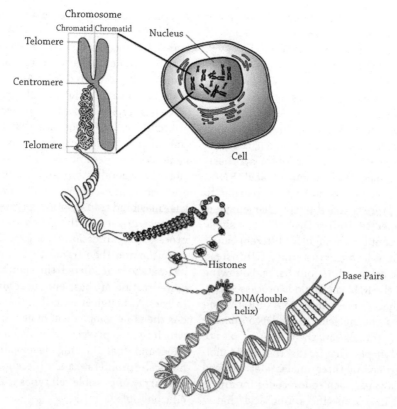

Figure 8-1 **Eukaryotic Cell. Picture shows nucleus containing DNA material packaged into chromosomes.**

From Access Excellence @ the National Health Museum: http://www.accessexcellence.org/RC/VL/GG/chromosome.php. Courtesy: National Human Genome Research Institute.

other from the father. A cell with the full complement of chromosomes is said to be diploid. Twenty-two pairs are referred to as autosomes (non–sex-related chromosomes) and labeled chromosomes 1 through 22. The 23rd pair of chromosomes are the sex chromosomes containing the genetic material that determines the sex of the individual. Two X chromosomes yield a female, while an X and a Y chromosome yield a male. Together, the 23 pairs of chromosomes constitute the human genome.

Each chromosome is composed of a deoxyribonucleic acid (DNA) molecule tightly wound around packing proteins, called histones. The DNA molecule itself has a double helix structure formed by two "backbones," or strands made of alternating sugar and phosphate molecules, that run in opposite directions parallel to each other. Attached to a carbon atom

within each sugar molecule in the backbone is one of four *bases*: adenine (A), thymine (T), cytosine (C), and guanine (G). A single sugar and phosphate molecule together with one of the four bases is known as a *nucleotide*. The two strands are joined together like a zipper due to bonding between the bases of each nucleotide on opposite strands. Due to their physiochemical properties, an A base on one strand always pairs with a T on the other strand and a G always pairs with a C, in a process known as complementary base pairing. The sequence of these paired bases conveys the fundamental information of the genetic code.

The DNA molecule carries out three basic functions that compose what is referred to as the central dogma of biology: replication, transcription, and translation. During *replication*, the DNA molecule duplicates itself, forming two copies with identical nucleotide sequences, achieved by taking advantage of complementary base pairing (noted above). Each backbone, or strand, of the parent DNA molecule acts as template upon which a complementary strand of DNA is synthesized with the aid of enzymes called DNA polymerases, yielding two new, identical, double-stranded DNA molecules. During *transcription*, the DNA molecule serves as a template for the synthesis of a single molecule of ribonucleic acid (RNA), again using complementary base pairing to direct the process, aided by another enzyme, RNA polymerase. Unlike DNA, RNA is single stranded, contains a slightly different sugar molecule, and incorporates uracil (U) instead of thymine as one of its four bases. Following synthesis, the RNA molecule is processed further into mature messenger RNA (mRNA) and then leaves the nucleus to undergo *translation*. During translation, the mRNA couples to a *ribosomal complex* that "reads" the mRNA molecule in groups of three nucleotides (termed *codons*) at a time. Each codon codes for and is translated into a specific amino acid that is bonded with others in a polypeptide chain.

This conversion key from codon to amino acid forms the universal genetic code common to all living organisms. It is the genetic code that dictates how the sequence of DNA nucleotides is first transcribed and then translated into a linear sequence of amino acids to form a polypeptide that will become a protein. The human body contains 20 distinct standard amino acids, each with slightly different physiochemical properties. The linear sequence of these amino acids determines how the polypeptide chain folds in on itself to form a fully realized, three-dimensional structure with specific domains that govern the ultimate functions the nascent protein will carry out in the body.

The functional unit of a DNA molecule is the *gene*. The traditional conception is that one gene codes for one protein. In eukaryotic organisms (animals), such as humans, genes are organized into multiple alternating *exons* and *introns*. While the entire gene is transcribed into an RNA molecule, through posttranscriptional processing, RNA sequences complementary to the introns are spliced out, and those complementary to the exons are stitched together to form a mature mRNA ready to be translated into a polypeptide. Because exons may be stitched together in various combinations, multiple related mRNAs can be generated from a single primary RNA transcript.

Genes typically contain *promoter regions*, stretches of DNA sequence that bind to the "machinery" necessary for transcribing the gene. Within these promoter regions and possibly elsewhere within and around the gene are other, noncoding regulatory sequences that may bind transcription factors that either enhance or repress the gene's transcriptional process. The expression of the gene (i.e., its transcription and then translation into a protein) ultimately is regulated through the complex orchestration of these enhancer and repressor factors. Although every cell in the human body has the same complement of genes, the ways in which their expression is turned on or off over time and space during development control how cells proliferate and differentiate into the vast array of possible cell types with their specific physiologic roles.

The human genome contains anywhere from 20,000 to 25,000 genes (International Human Genome Sequencing Consortium, 2004). However, given possible splice variants, even a relatively limited number of genes can generate a much greater number of proteins, greatly expanding the complexity of the repertoire of functions that can be carried out (Xing & Lee, 2006). Only around 5% of the DNA sequence in the genome is estimated to have a function. Perhaps less than 2% codes for amino acids that are synthesized into proteins (i.e., coding sequences), while the remaining 3% controls the expression of genes or is responsible for other, related functions (i.e., noncoding regulatory sequences). The other 95% of the genome has been referred to as "junk DNA," likely a misnomer since the functional significance of these sequences is still being explored (Pheasant & Mattick, 2007).

The information stored in DNA is passed from one cell to another through the process of *mitosis* and from one organism to the next through *meiosis*. In mitosis, which occurs during an organism's development, the set of chromosomes in the nucleus undergoes a cycle of replication in which an identical copy of the entire set is created. The cell then divides, forming two daughter cells, each containing one of the identical sets of chromosomes. Hence like the parent cell, both daughter cells are diploid. In contrast, meiosis occurs during sexual reproduction. The sex cell undergoes two rounds of division. In the first round, the chromosomes replicate; then homologous chromosomes (the pair from the mother and the pair from the father) line up and exchange genetic material in a process called recombination. This shuffles the genetic material between the maternal and paternal chromosomes. The homologous chromosomes then segregate into separate daughter cells that subsequently undergo a second round of division. This second round gives rise to four cells, referred to as *gametes*, that are haploid (i.e., that have half the full complement of chromosomes). Then, during sexual reproduction, a gamete from the male joins with a gamete from the female, forming a diploid zygote that, through the process of mitosis, will go on to become a developing organism.

In meiosis, the multiple rounds of cell division may give rise to mutation events, introducing errors into the DNA sequence that may be transmitted from parent to offspring. These mutation events may occur at the chromosomal level. For example, nondisjunction events (in which the chromosome pairs do not separate properly) may occur during meiosis, with the result that the offspring inherits an abnormal copy of a chromosome. Because many genes on a chromosome may be affected by such an event, the phenotypic consequences in the offspring often are significant.. A common nondisjunction event is trisomy 21, in which an individual inherits an extra copy of all or part of chromosome 21, resulting in Down syndrome. Other, lesser mutations may occur that affect smaller stretches of chromosomes. These may involve deletions or duplications of chromosomal segments or translocations between segments of different chromosomes. The phenotypic consequences range widely, depending on how many and which specific genes are affected by the event. A body of evidence is amassing that copy number variants like deletions or duplications may play a role

in psychiatric disorders like autism or schizophrenia (Cook & Scherer, 2008).

Mutations also may occur at the DNA sequence level, affecting only one or a few base pairs. Such mutations include microsatellite repeats, in which a small number of base pairs are repeated multiple times along the DNA sequence, and single-nucleotide polymorphisms (SNPs), in which a single base pair is altered. SNPs are the most common variants in the human genome. In fact, over 90% of the genetic variation in the human population can be explained by the estimated 10 million SNPs in the genome (International HapMap Consortium, 2003). While affecting only a single base pair, SNPs can have significant phenotypic consequences, depending on the location of the alteration. If an SNP occurs in a nonfunctional region of the genome, then of course the mutation will have no apparent phenotypic consequence. However, if the mutation occurs within the coding sequence of a gene, altering the encoded amino acid, the functioning of the resulting protein may be disrupted, leading to observable phenotypic consequences. For example, sickle cell anemia, a disease of considerable public health importance, is caused by a single SNP in the hemoglobin gene. The SNP leads the amino acid glutamic acid to be replaced by valine. As a result, hemoglobin aggregates in red blood cells and distorts them into a sickle shape that decreases their elasticity.

The specific variants at a particular sequence site at which a mutation has occurred are referred to as *alleles*. Given that DNA includes two copies of each chromosome, individuals will have a pair of alleles at each site, referred to as a genotype. The pair of alleles may have additive effects on a phenotype, or the effects of one allele may predominate over the other. A dominant allele is one in which only one copy is necessary to produce a particular phenotype; in contrast, a recessive allele requires two copies to produce the phenotype.

If the phenotypic effect of an allele confers some survival advantage to the individual, its frequency in the population will increase. If, on the other hand, the allele lowers reproductive fitness, its frequency will decrease or remain low in the population. A mutation that has introduced an allele that rises to a level in the population greater than 1% is commonly referred to as a *polymorphism*. If an allele is neutral with respect to reproductive fitness and several other assumptions are met, then its frequency in the population will remain constant from one generation to the next. The proportion of homozygotes and heterozygotes at the locus can be estimated by the binomial formula $a^2 + 2ab + b^2$, in which a and b are the frequency of the two alleles. This is known as Hardy-Weinberg equilibrium, one of the most important theorems in population genetics.

THE RESEARCH PARADIGM

The goal of genetic epidemiology is to understand how variation in the human genome is related to susceptibility to disease. It seeks to explain how differences in the genomic sequence from one individual to the next influence who becomes ill and who does not in the population. To achieve this goal, genetic epidemiologists follow the research paradigm shown in figure 8-2.

The paradigm lays out a series of questions to be addressed sequentially, beginning with the basic question "What is the phenotype of interest?" where a phenotype can be any measurable characteristic of the disease. The answer is not as simple as it may appear; without a well-described phenotype that can be measured with reliability and validity, it may be impossible to adequately correlate genotypes with it. The second question asks, "What evidence demonstrates that genetic factors contribute to variability in the phenotype?" To answer this question, genetic epidemiologists have turned to family, twin, and adoption studies. These studies not only provide evidence of the genetic contribution to the phenotype but also can help quantify the magnitude of that contribution. If the evidence suggests that genetic factors contribute only to a small proportion of the variability in the phenotype, the study may proceed no further, saving valuable resources and time. If, however, evidence suggests that genetic factors contribute to a meaningful proportion of the phenotype, it makes sense to move forward to ask, "How is the phenotype transmitted from one generation to the next?" Segregation studies can provide clues about the genetic model underlying the phenotype that in turn can help inform efforts to answer the next question: "What genes are responsible and where are they located in the genome?"

Linkage and association studies are the two main designs used to answer these questions and to map the relevant genes. Once specific genes are identified, one final question must be addressed: "How do these genes interact with environmental factors to determine the expression of the phenotype in the population?" Epidemiologic studies, and in particular prospective cohort studies, are best suited to exploring this final question.

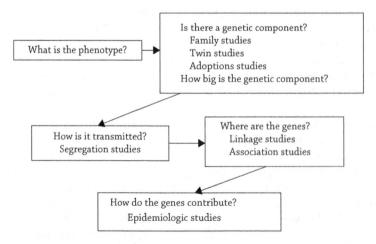

Figure 8-2   **The Genetic Epidemiology Research Paradigm.**

What Is the Phenotype?

Defining the phenotype is particularly challenging for mental disorders, largely because, in contrast to physical disorders, no "gold standard" measures exist. For example, well-validated, biologically grounded measures exist for conditions such as diabetes, heart disease, and cancer. In contrast, in many cases, comparable measures are not yet available for the study of mental disorders. The introduction of modern diagnostic classification systems such as the *Diagnostic and Statistical Manual of Mental Disorders* series (American Psychiatric Association, 1952, 1968, 1980, 1987, 1994) has clearly helped establish more reliable diagnostic procedures that have facilitated research into the named mental disorders. While the validity of these systems remains in question, this chapter nevertheless first focuses on the genetics of disorders as they have been conceptualized by these systems, saving for later discussion of the impact of the widely debated limitations of the nosology on scientific discovery.

Do Genetic Factors Contribute to the Disorder?

FAMILY STUDIES

Family studies can help assess whether and the extent to which genetic factors contribute to a disorder. The logic underlying family studies posits that if a disorder is genetically determined, genetically related individuals in families should have higher concordance for the disorder. On average, first-degree relatives (i.e., parents, siblings or offspring) share 50% of their alleles across the genome, while the percentage of shared alleles is less for more distantly related individuals. The level of allele sharing decreases as one moves out on the family tree until it reaches the same as that among unrelated individuals. As a result, disorders with a genetic component tend to aggregate in families.

A number of approaches can help determine if a particular disorder aggregates in families. Most simply, one might identify individuals with and without the disorder in question (cases and controls, respectively) and ask them

if any of their relatives have the disorder. The presence of a genetic component can be gleaned by comparing rates of the disorder among relatives of cases and controls. However, this approach relies on reports by cases and controls about the experiences of their relatives. Such self-reported information may be unreliable and, worse, biased in ways that skew the observed associations. For example, compared with controls, individuals with the disorder may pay more attention to it, be more motivated to know about its occurrence among relatives, and consequently report it more frequently when it exists.

Direct assessment of the relatives of the ascertained cases of the disorder and controls represents a more rigorous approach, providing a more unbiased estimate of what is called the recurrence risk ratio. A widely used metric in genetic epidemiology, the recurrence risk ratio is the relative risk of disease in relatives of people with the disorder (cases) compared with that in relatives of unaffected controls (or, more generally, in the population). It provides an estimate of the degree to which a disorder aggregates in families and can be related to the effect size of genetic factors on the disorder (Risch, 1990). Appendix Tables 8-1 through 8-12 present summary findings from seminal family studies for the major mental disorders of public health interest.

These findings provide substantial evidence of familial aggregation: Relatives of people with a given disorders are at increased risk for the disorder compared with the relatives of unaffected controls or in the general population. Reasonable estimates of the recurrence risk ratios for these disorders vary, ranging from a two- to fivefold increased risk for Alzheimer's disease (Breitner, Silverman, Mohs, & Davis, 1988; Lautenschlager et al., 1996) to as high as a 30- to 150-fold increased risk for autism (Newschaffer, Fallin, & Lee, 2002). Such estimates are consistent with the notion that genetic factors play an important contributing role in susceptibility to these mental disorders.

TWIN STUDIES

Although evidence from family studies suggests genetic contributions to the major

Table 8-1. Obsessive–Compulsive Disorder: Summary of Findings from Family, Twin, and Adoption Studies

FAMILY STUDIES	FIRST-DEGREE RELATIVES		DIAGNOSTIC CRITERIA	MORBIDITY RISK IN FIRST-DEGREE RELATIVES[a]	
	CASES (N)	CONTROLS (N)		CASES (%)	CONTROLS (%)
Carey & Gottesman (1981)[b]	15	15	DSM-III	87	47
Insel, Hoover, & Murphy (1983)[c]	54	—	FH of treatment	0.0	—
Rasmussen & Tsuang (1986)	88	—	FH	5	—
McKeon & Murray (1987)[d]	149	151	ICD-8, RDC	0.7	0.7
Pitman, Green, Jenike, & Mesulam (1987)	75	86	FH	8.0	1
Bellodi, Sciuto, Diaferia, Ronchi, & Smeraldi (1992)	234	—	DSM-III-R, FH	3.6	—
Black, Noyes, Goldstein, & Blum (1992)	120	129	DSM-III	2.6	2.4
Fyer et al. (1993)	148	—	DSM-III	7.0	—
Nicolini, Weissbecker, Mejía, & Sánchez de Carmona (1993)	268	—	DSM-III-R, FH	4.9	—
Pauls, Alsobrook, Goodman, Rasmussen, & Leckman (1995)	466	113	DSM-III-R, FH	10.3	1.9
Sciuto, Pasquale, & Bellodi (1995)	445	—	DSM-III-R, FH	5.6	—
Nestadt et al. (2000)	326	297	DSM-IV	11.7	2.7
Grados et al. (2001)	323	289	DSM-IV	15.5	5.2
Black, Gaffney, Schlosser, & Gabel (2003)[e]	43	35	DSM-III-R	23.3	2.9

TWIN STUDIES	MZ PAIRS (N)	DZ PAIRS (N)	DIAGNOSTIC CRITERIA	MZ CONCORDANCE[F] (%)	DZ CONCORDANCE[F] (%)
Carey & Gottesman (1981)[b]	15	15	DSM-III	87	47
Torgersen (1983)	3	9	DSM-III	0	0
Andrews, Stewart, Allen, & Henderson (1990)	186	260	DSM-III	0	0
Bolton, Rijsdijk, O'Connor, Perrin, & Eley (2007)	1,599	3,063	DSM-IV	57	22
Adoption Studies					
None					

DSM = Diagnostic and Statistical Manual of Mental Disorders; DSM-III = DSM, 3rd ed. (American Psychiatric Association [APA], 1980); DSM-III-R = DSM-III, revised (APA, 1987); DSM-IV = DSM, 4th ed. (APA, 1994); FH = family history; ICD-8 = International Classification of Diseases, 8th revision (WHO, 1968); RDC = Research Diagnostic Criteria (Spitzer & Robins, 1978); MZ = monozygotic; DZ = dizygotic.

[a]Values are unadjusted in Insel et al. (1983), Rasmussen & Tsuang (1986), McKeon & Murray (1987), Pitman et al. (1987), Fryer et al. (1993), Nicolini et al. (1993), Nestadt et al. (2000), and Grados et al. (2001). Values in remaining studies were age-adjusted by the Stromgren method.

[b]Obsessional symptoms or features. [c]Rate in parents only. [d]Used diagnosis of obsessive–compulsive neurosis. [e]Rate in offspring only. [f]All concordance rates are pairwise calculations.

Table 8-2. Panic Disorder: Summary of Findings from Family, Twin, and Adoption Studies

FAMILY STUDIES	FIRST-DEGREE RELATIVES		DIAGNOSTIC CRITERIA	MORBIDITY RISK IN FIRST-DEGREE RELATIVES[a]	
	CASES (N)	CONTROLS (N)		CASES (%)	CONTROLS (%)
Crowe, Noyes, Pauls, & Slymen (1983)	278	262	DSM-III, FH	17.3	1.8
Noyes et al. (1986)	241	113	DSM-III, FH	17.3	4.2
Hopper, Judd, Derrick, & Burrows (1987)	519	—	FH	11.6	—
Maier, Lichtermann, Minges, Oehrlein, & Franke (1993)	174	309	DSM-III-R	7.9	2.3
Mendlewicz, Papadimitriou, & J., W. (1993)	122	130	RDC	13.2	0.9
Weissman (1993)	141	255	DSM-III, FH	10.6	0.7
Goldstein et al. (1994)	141	225	DSM-III-R	16.4	1.8
Fyer et al. (1996)	236	380	DSM-III-R	10	3

TWIN STUDIES	MZ PAIRS (N)	DZ PAIRS (N)	DIAGNOSTIC CRITERIA	MZ CONCORD-ANCE[b] (%)	DZ CONCORD-ANCE[b] (%)	HERITABILITY (%)
Torgersen (1983)	13	16	DSM-III	31	0	—
Kendler, Neale, Kessler, Heath, & Eaves (1993)	NR	NR	DSM-III-R	24	11	14-19
Skre, Onstad, Torgersen, Lygren, & Kringlen (1993)	12	18	DSM-III-R	42	17	—
Perna, Caldirola, Arancio, & Bellodi (1997)	26	34	DSM-IV	73	0	—
Scherrer et al. (2000)	1,867	1,495	DSM-III-R	39	13–17 (FF), 33–43	
Kendler, Gardner, & Prescott (2001)	1,412	2,380	DSM-III-R	31 (F), 39 (M)	5 (MM), 20 (DZO)	

ADOPTION STUDIES

None

DSM = Diagnostic and Statistical Manual of Mental Disorders; DSM-III = DSM, 3rd ed. (American Psychiatric Association [APA], 1980); DSM-III-R = DSM-III, revised (APA, 1987); DSM-IV = DSM, 4th ed. (APA, 1994); FH = family history; RDC = Research Diagnostic Criteria (Spitzer & Robins, 1978); MZ = monozygotic; DZ = dizygotic; NR = not reported; F = female; M = male; DZO = dizygotic, opposite-sex twins.
[a]Risk is unadjusted in the studies by Noyes et al. (1986), Hopper et al. (1987), and Fyer et al. (1996). Risk was estimated by the Kaplan-Meier method in the Weissman (1993) and Goldstein et al. (1994) studies and was age-adjusted by the Stromgren method in all other studies.
[b]All concordance rates are proband-wise calculations with the exception of those for Perna et al (1997), which are pairwise calculations.

Table 8-3. Major Depression: Summary of Findings from Family Studies

FAMILY STUDIES	FIRST-DEGREE RELATIVES		DIAGNOSTIC CRITERIA	MORBIDITY RISK IN FIRST-DEGREE RELATIVES[a]	
	CASES (N)	CONTROLS (N)		CASES (%)	CONTROLS (%)
Tsuang, Winokur, & Crowe (1980)	340	—	Feighner et al. (1972), FH	12	—
Mendlewicz & Baron (1981)	248	—	Feighner et al. (1972)	21.4	—
Gershon et al. (1982)	133	208	RDC	16.6	5.8
Perris, Perris, Ericsson, & Von Knorring (1982)	88 (P), 148 (S)	—	ICD-9, DSM-III	21.7 (P), 14.8 (S)	—
Weissman, Kidd, & Prusoff (1982)	810	521	RDC, FH	1 (M), 3 (F)	4 (M), 9 (F)
Winokur, Tsuang, & Crowe (1982)	305	344	DSM-II, Feighner et al. (1972)	11.2	7.3
Leckman et al. (1984)[b]	810	521	RDC, DSM-III, FH	14.9	5.6
Weissman et al. (1984)	974	521	RDC, FH	16.8–18.4	5.9
Merikangas, Leckman, Prusoff, Pauls, & Weissman (1985)	639	418	RDC, FH	15	—
Bland, Newman, & Orn (1986)	763	—	Feighner et al. (1972)	8.6	—
Weissman et al. (1986)[a]	1,331 total	—	RDC, FH	14.9	—
McGuffin, Katz, & Bebbington (1987)	315	—	PSE, FH	24.7	—
Price, Kidd, & Weissman (1987)	433	—	RDC, DSM-III	23	—
Stancer, Persad, Wagener, & Jorna (1987)	282	—	Feighner et al. (1972), FH	24.4	—
Kupfer, Frank, Carpenter, & Neiswanger (1989)	726	—	RDC, FH	20.7	—
Maier et al. (1991)	190	139	RDC, FH	17.3	7.9
Heun & Maier (1993)	306	221	RDC, FH	19	7.7
Maier, Lichtermann, Minges, Hallmayer, et al. (1993)	697	—	RDC, FH	21.6	—

FH = family history; RDC = Research Diagnostic Criteria (Spitzer & Robins, 1978); ICD-9 = International Classification of Diseases, 9th revision (WHO, 1979); DSM-III = Diagnostic and Statistical Manual of Mental Disorders, 3rd ed. (American Psychiatric Association, 1980); P = parents, S = siblings; M = males, F = females; PSE = present-state examination.

[a]Values from Mendlewicz & Baron (1981), Gershon et al. (1982), Winokur et al. (1982), Weissman et al. (1984), McGuffin et al. (1987), Stancer et al. (1987), and Kupfer et al. (1989) were age-adjusted using the Stromgren method. Values from Bland et al. (1986) and Maier et al. (1993) were age-adjusted using the Kaplan-Meier method. Values from Tsuang et al. (1980), and Perris et al. (1982) were age-adjusted by the Weinberg method. Values from Maier et al. (1991) were age-adjusted using the Stromgren-Weinberg method. All remaining studies report unadjusted rates.

[b]Rates determined by proportional hazards model, controlling for age, sex, and interview status.

Table 8-4. Major Depression: Summary of Findings from Twin and Adoption Studies

TWIN STUDIES	MZ PAIRS (N)	DZ PAIRS (N)	POPULATION	DIAGNOSTIC CRITERIA	MZ CONCORDANCE[a] (%)	DZ CONCORDANCE[a] (%)	HERITABILITY (%)
Bertelsen, Harvald, & Hauge (1977)	35	17	Population-based and psychiatric registries	Kraepelin	43	18	—
Torgersen (1986)	151 pairs total		Hospital based	DSM-III	27	12	54
Englund & Klein (1990)	7	5	Hospital based	RDC	28.6	0	—
Andrews et al. (1990)	29	53	Population based	DSM-III	12.9	17.2	—
McGuffin, Katz, & Rutherford (1991)	84	130	Hospital based	DSM-III	53	28	43
Kendler, Neale, Kessler, Heath, & Eaves (1992)	1,033 F pairs		Population based	DSM-III, DSM-III-R, RDC	48[b]	42[b]	33–45
Kendler Pedersen, Johnson, Neale, & Mathe (1993)	43	106	Hospital and population based	DSM-III-R	39.1	23.6	—
McGuffin, Katz, Watkins, & Rutherford (1996)	68	109	Hospital based	DSM-III, DSM-III-R, DSM-IV	62[c]	28[c]	48
Lyons et al. (1998)	268	266	Vietnam Era Twin Registry	DSM-III-R	22.5	14	36

Bierut et al. (1999)	1,323	755 same sex, 584 opposite sex	Volunteer based	DSM-IV	38 (F), 20 (M)	23 (MM), 25 (FF), 22 (FM), 36 (MF)	44
Kendler & Prescott (1999)	1,373	997 same sex, 1,415 opposite sex	Population based	DSM-III-R	47.4 (F), 41.4 (M)	34.2 (MM), 42.6 (FF), 34.7 (FM), 45.8 (MF)	34
Kendler, Gatz, Gardner, & Pedersen (2006)	4,091	11,402	Population based	DSM-III-R	44 (F), 31 (M)	16 (FF), 11 (MM), 11 (DZO)	38

ADOPTEES STUDY DESIGN	CASES (N)	CONTROLS (N)	DIAGNOSTIC CRITERIA	RATE IN CASE ADOPTEES (%)	RATE IN CONTROL ADOPTEES (%)
Cadoret (1978)	83	43	Feighner et al. (1972)	67	9
Adoptees Family Design	Biological Relatives (N)	Adoptive Relatives (N)		Rate in Biological Relatives (%)	Rate in Adoptive Relatives (%)
Wender et al. (1986)	387[d]	180[d]	DSM-III, RDC	2.1	0.6

MZ = monozygotic; DZ = dizygotic; DSM = Diagnostic and Statistical Manual of Mental Disorders; DSM-III = DSM, 3rd ed. (American Psychiatric Association [APA], 1980); DSM-III-R = DSM-III, revised (APA, 1987); DSM-IV = DSM, 4th ed. (APA, 1994); RDC = Research Diagnostic Criteria (Spitzer & Robins, 1978); F = female; M = male; FM = opposite-sex twins with female as proband and male as cotwin; MF = opposite-sex twins with male as proband and female as cotwin; DZO = dizygotic, opposite-sex twins. [a]Using DSM-III-R criteria. [b]Ignoring missing cases. [c]Relatives of probands with unipolar disorder, bipolar disorder, neurotic depression, or affect reaction.

[d]All concordance rates are probandwise calculations.

Table 8-5. Bipolar Disorder: Summary of Findings from Family, Twin, and Adoption Studies

FAMILY STUDIES	TYPE	FIRST-DEGREE RELATIVES CASES (N)	CONTROLS (N)	DIAGNOSTIC CRITERIA	MORBIDITY RISK IN FIRST-DEGREE RELATIVES[a] CASES (%)	CONTROLS (%)
Mendlewicz, Linkowski, & Wilmotte (1980)	BP	—	—	Winokur et al. (1969)	18.7	—
Tsuang et al. (1980)	BP	160	—	Feighner et al. (1972), FH for mania	1.9	—
Baron, Gruen, Asnis, & Kane (1982)	BP	135	—	RDC, FH	14.5	—
Gershon et al. (1982)	BP I	441	217	RDC	4.5	0
	BP II	16	208	RDC	4.5	0.5
Winokur et al. (1982)	BP	196	344	DSM-II, Feighner et al. (1972)	1.5	0.3
Coryell, Endicott, Reich, Andreasen, & Keller (1984)	BP I	278	—	RDC	2.9	—
	BP II	111	—	RDC	9.8	—
Fieve, Go, Dunner, & Elston (1984)	BP	1,309	—	RDC	6.6	—
Tsuang, Faraone, & Fleming (1985)	BP	218	517	ICD-9	2.8	0.2
Andreasen et al. (1987)	BP I	569	—	RDC	3.9	—
	BP II	267	—	RDC	8.2	—
Dwyer & DeLong (1987)	BP	71	—	RDC	14.1	—
Rice et al. (1987)	BP	557	—	RDC, FH	5.7	—
Strober et al. (1988)	BP	115	—	RDC	14.8	—
Pauls, Morton, & Egeland (1992)	BP I	408	—	RDC, FH	8.7	—
Heun & Maier (1993)	BP I	166	221	RDC, FH	3.6	0.5
	BP II	115	221	RDC, FH	6.1	0.5
Maier, Lichtermann, Minges, Hallmayer, et al. (1993)	BP	389	419	RDC	7.0	1.8
Sadovnick et al. (1994)	BP I	781	—	DSM-III-R, FH	3.5	—

	TYPE						
Wals et al. (2001)[b]	BP	140	—	DSM-IV	3.0	—	—
Lichtenstein et al. (2009)	BP	40,487 total	—	ICD-8,9,10	6.4 (offspring) 7.9 (sibling)	—	—
Baek et al. (2011)	BP I	237	—	DSM-IV	3.4	—	—
	BP II	137	—	DSM-IV	3.0	—	—

TWIN STUDIES	TYPE	MZ PAIRS (N)	DZ PAIRS (N)	DIAGNOSTIC CRITERIA	MZ CONCORDANCE[c] (%)	DZ CONCORDANCE[c] (%)	HERITABILITY (%)
Allen, Cohen, Pollin, & Greenspan (1974)	BP	15	34	DSM-II	20	0	33
Bertelsen et al. (1977)	BP	34	37	Kraepelin, 1913	62	8	—
Torgersen (1986)	BP	151 total	—	DSM-III	75	0	—
Kendler, Pedersen, et al. (1993)	BP	13	22	DSM-III-R	38.5	4.5	—
Kendler, Pedersen, Neale, & Mathe (1995)	BP	154	326	DSM-III-R	39	5	79
Cardno et al. (1999)	Mania	22	27	RDC	36.4	7.4	84
McGuffin et al. (2003)	BP	30	37	DSM-IV	40	5.4	85
Kieseppa, Partonen, Haukka, Kaprio, & Lönnqvist (2004)	BP I	7	26	DSM-IV	43	6	93
Edvardsen et al. (2008)	BP I	8	13	DSM-III-R	25	0	73
	BP II	13	12	DSM-III-R	23.1	16.7	58

ADOPTEES FAMILY DESIGN	TYPE	BIOLOGICAL RELATIVES (N)	ADOPTIVE RELATIVES (N)	DIAGNOSTIC CRITERIA	RATE IN BIOLOGICAL RELATIVES (%)	RATE IN ADOPTIVE RELATIVES (%)
Mendlewicz & Rainer (1977)	BP	57	57	Feighner et al. (1972)	7.0	1.8
Wender et al. (1986)	BP	387[d]	180[d]	DSM-III, RDC	5.2	2.8

BP = bipolar; FH = family history; RDC = Research Diagnostic Criteria (Spitzer & Robins, 1978); DSM = Diagnostic and Statistical Manual of Mental Disorders; DSM-II = DSM, 2nd ed. (American Psychiatric Association [APA], 1968); DSM-III = DSM, 3rd ed. (APA, 1980); DSM-III-R = DSM-III, revised (APA, 1987); DSM-IV = DSM, 4th ed. (APA, 1994); ICD = International Classification of Diseases; ICD-8 = ICD, 8th revision (WHO, 1968); ICD-9 = ICD, 9th revision (WHO, 1979); ICD-10 = ICD, 10th revision (WHO, 1993); MZ = monozygotic; DZ = dizygotic.

[a] Values are unadjusted in Gershon et al. (1982), Tsuang et al. (1985), Andreasen et al. (1987), Dwyer & DeLong (1987), Strober et al. (1988), Heun & Maier (1993), Wals et al. (2001), Lichtenstein et al. (2009), and Baek et al. (2011). Values in Pauls et al. (1992) were age-adjusted using the Kaplan-Meier method. Values in Mendlewicz et al. (1980) and Tsuang et al. (1980) were age-adjusted with the Weinberg method. Values in Sadovnick et al. (1994) were age-adjusted using maximum likelihood. Values in all other studies were age-adjusted based on the Strömgren method.

[b] Offspring only. [c] All concordance rates are proband-wise calculations except those for Allen et al. (1974) and Cardno et al. (1999), which are pairwise. [d] Relatives of probands with either unipolar disorder, bipolar disorder, neurotic depression, or affect reaction.

Table 8-6. Schizophrenia: Summary of Findings from Family, Twin, and Adoption Studies

FAMILY STUDIES	FIRST-DEGREE RELATIVES		DIAGNOSTIC CRITERIA	MORBIDITY RISK IN RELATIVES[a]	
	CASES (N)	CONTROLS (N)		CASES (%)	CONTROLS (%)
Mendlewicz, Linkowski, & Wilmotte (1980)	—	—	Feighner et al. (1972)	16.9	—
Tsuang et al. (1980)	362	—	Feighner et al. (1972), FH	5.5	—
Abrams & Taylor (1983)	125	—	RDC	1.6	—
Guze, Cloninger, Martin, & Clayton (1983)	111	1,076	Feighner et al. (1972)	3.6	0.6
Baron et al. (1985)	329	337	RDC, DSM-III	5.8	0.6
Frangos, Athanassenas, Tsitourides, Katsanou, & Alexandrakou (1985)	478	536	DSM-III, FH	3.97	0.74
Kendler, Gruenberg, & Tsuang (1985)	703	931	DSM-III	3.7	0.2
Jorgensen et al. (1987)	151	—	DSM-III	9.3	—
Coryell & Zimmerman (1988)	72	160	DSM-III	1.4	0
Gershon et al. (1988)	97	349	RDC	3.1	0.6
Maier, Hallmayer, Minges, & Lichtermann (1990)	463	294	RDC	5	0.3
Maj, Starace, & Pirozzi (1991)	68	43	DSM-III-R, FH	8.8	0
Kendler, McGuire, et al. (1993)	276	428	DSM-III-R	6.5	0.5
Maier, Lichtermann, Minges, Hallmayer, et al. (1993)	589	—	RDC	5.1	—
Parnas et al. (1993)[b]	207	104	DSM-III-R	16.2	1.9

				MZ	DZ	
Varma, Zain, & Singh (1997)	530	—	DSM-III, FH	16.9		—
Asarnow et al. (2001)	102	122	DSM-III-R, FH	2.2		0
Chang et al. (2002)	234	—	DIGS	2.5[c], 3.9[d]		—
Maier et al. (2002)	449	312	DSM-III-R, FH	5		0.8
Somnath, Janardhan Reddy, & Jain (2002)	282	212	DSM-IV	7.8		0.4
Lichtenstein et al. (2009)	40,487 total		ICD-8,9,10	9.9 (offspring), 9.0 (sibling)		—

TWIN STUDIES	MZ PAIRS (N)	DZ PAIRS (N)	DIAGNOSTIC CRITERIA	MZ CONCORD-ANCE[E] (%)	DZ CONCORD-ANCE[E] (%)	HERITABILITY (%)
Feighner et al. (1972)	22	33	RDC	47	11	71
Farmer, McGuffin, & Gottesman (1987)	26	34	DSM-III	48	10	85
Onstad, Skre, Torgersen, & Kringlen (1991)	31	28	DSM-III-R	48	4	—
Tsujita et al. (1992)	18	7	DSM-III-R	50	14	—
Klaning (1996)	13	17	ICD-10	44	11	—
Cannon, Kaprio, Lonnqvist, Huttunen, & Koskenvuo (1998)	67	187	ICD-8, DSM-III-R	46	9	—
Franzek & Beckmann (1998)	22	23	DSM-III-R	79	17	83
Cardno et al. (1999)	40	50	DSM-III-R	43	0	84
	43	50	ICD-10	42	2	83
	42	56	RDC	41	5	82

(continued)

Table 8-6. (Continued)

ADOPTEES STUDY DESIGN	CASES (N)	CONTROLS (N)	DIAGNOSTIC CRITERIA	RATE IN CASE ADOPTEES (%)	RATE IN CONTROL ADOPTEES (%)
Lowing, Mirsky, & Pereira (1983)	39	39	DSM-III	2.6	0
Tienari et al. (2003)	137	192	DSM-III-R	5.1	1.6

ADOPTEES FAMILY DESIGN		BIOLOGICAL RELATIVES (N)	ADOPTIVE RELATIVES (N)	DIAGNOSTIC CRITERIA	RATE IN BIOLOGICAL RELATIVES (%)	RATE IN ADOPTIVE RELATIVES (%)
Kendler Gruenberg, & Kinney (1994)	P Case	178	41	DSM-III	2.3	—
	P Ctrls	162	54	DSM-III	2.3	—
	N Case	209	—	DSM-III	3.3	—
	N Ctrls	299	—	DSM-III	0.3	—
Kety et al. (1994)	P Case	172	42	DSM-II	4.7	0
	P Ctrls	155	51	DSM-II	0	0
	C Case	108	40	DSM-II	5.6	0
	C Ctrls	113	62	DSM-II	9	0
	N Case	279	111	DSM-II	5	0
	N Ctrls	234	117	DSM-II	0.4	0

FH = family history; RDC = Research Diagnostic Criteria (Spitzer & Robins, 1978); DSM = Diagnostic and Statistical Manual of Mental Disorders; DSM-II = DSM, 2nd ed. (American Psychiatric Association [APA], 1968); DSM-III = DSM, 3rd ed. (APA, 1980); DSM-III-R = DSM, 3rd ed., revised (APA, 1987); DSM-IV = DSM, 4th ed. (APA, 1994); DIGS = Diagnostic Interview for Genetic Studies; ICD = International Classification of Diseases; ICD-8 = ICD, 8th revision (WHO, 1968); ICD-9 = ICD, 9th revision (WHO, 1979); ICD-10 = ICD, 10th revision (WHO, 1993); MZ = monozygotic; DZ = dizygotic; P = National sample; N = National sample; C = Copenhagen sample.

[a]Values are unadjusted in Guze et al. (1983), Jorgensen et al. (1987) Parnas et al. (1993), Varma et al. (1997), and Lichtenstein et al. (2009). Values in Kendler, McGuire, et al. (1993) and Asarnow et al. (2001) were age-adjusted by the Kaplan-Meier method. Values in Frangos et al. (1985), Maj et al. (1991), Maier, Lichtermann, Minges, Hallmayer, et al. (1993), Maier et al. (2002), and Somnath et al. (2002) were age-adjusted by the Weinberg method. Values in remaining studies were age-adjusted by the Stromgren method. [b]Kaplan-Meier method estimate. [c]Weinberg method estimate. [d]All concordance rates are proband-wise calculations.

[b]Values are for schizophrenia in the adopted-away offspring of mothers with and without schizophrenia. [c]Values are for schizophrenia in the adopted-away offspring of mothers with and without schizophrenia.

Table 8-7. Alzheimer's Disease: Summary of Findings from Family Studies

FAMILY STUDIES	FIRST-DEGREE RELATIVES		DIAGNOSTIC CRITERIA	AGE-ADJUSTED MORBIDITY RISK IN FIRST-DEGREE RELATIVES	
	CASES (N)	CONTROLS (N)		CASES (%)	CONTROLS (%)
Heston, Mastri, Anderson, & White (1981)	—	—	Autopsy and medical records, family informants	15.1 siblings, 17.7 parents, 7.0 second-degree[a]	5.5[a]
Heyman et al. (1983)	1,278	254	History of cognitive decline before age 75, evidence from medical records	13.9 siblings, 14.4 parents[b]	1 relative with dementia
Breitner & Folstein (1984)	440	253	DSM-III for dementia	55.3 for siblings and children of agraphic AD probands, 57.6 for siblings and children of aphasic/apractic AD probands[c]	12.2[c]
Mohs, Breitner, Silverman, & Davis (1987)	244	211	NINCDS-ADRDA	45.9[d]	12.1[e]
Breitner, Silverman, Mohs, & Davis (1988)	366	100	NINCDS-ADRDA	49.3[f]	9.8[g]
Huff, Auerbach, Chakravarti, & Boller (1988)	250	232	NINCDS-ADRDA	45[h]	11[i]
R. L. Martin, Gerteis, & Gabrielli (1988)	130 first-degree, 239 second-degree	144 first-degree, 289 second-degree	NINCDS-ADRDA, CDR	40.8 first-degree[j], 9.8 second-degree[k]	23.3 first-degree,[j] 17.4 second-degree[c]
Zubenko, Huff, Beyer, Auerbach, & Teply (1988)	211	210	NINCDS-ADRDA	48.9[l]	10.2[l]
Farrer, O'Sullivan, Cupples, Growdon, & Myers (1989)	967	572	NINCDS-ADRDA	39 maximum,[m] 24% weighted[m,n]	29 maximum,[c] 16 weighted[c,n]
Korten et al. (1993)	460	650	NINCDS-ADRDA	32,[o] 81[h]	13[o]
Silverman et al. (1994)	621	640	NINCDS-ADRDA	24.8[d]	10[e]

DSM-III = Diagnostic and Statistical Manual of Mental Disorders, 3rd ed. (American Psychiatric Association, 1980); AD = Alzheimer's disease (Morris, 1993); NINCDS-ADRDA = National Institute of Neurological and Communicative Disorders and Stroke—Alzheimer's Disease and Related Disorders Association; CDR = Clinical Dementia Rating.

[a]By age 84. [b]By age 90. [c]By age 75. [d]By age 86. [e]By age 87. [f]By age 85. [g]By age 99. [h]By age 98. [i]By age 83. [j]By age 82. [k]By age 90–95 interval. [l]By age 93. [m]Estimate obtained by weighting pos-sible AD cases to have 50% risk of actually having AD. [o]By age 88.

Table 8-8. Alzheimer's Disease: Summary of Findings from Twin Studies

TWIN STUDIES	MZ PAIRS (N)	DZ PAIRS (N)	AGE AT ASSESSMENT (YEARS)	POPULATION	AD PREVALENCE (%)	DIAGNOSTIC CRITERIA	MZ CONCORDANCE[a] (%)	DZ CONCORDANCE[a] (%)	HERITABILITY (%)
Nee et al. (1987)	17	5	57–85, 70	Recruited from ADRDA, families of patients, Mothers of Twins Club, and physicians	—	NINCDS-ADRDA	58.3	57.1	—
Breitner et al. (1995)	17	17	62–73	National Academy of Sciences registry of veteran twins	0.42	DSM-III-R, or CERAD and NIA criteria for postmortem diagnosis	21.1	11.1	—
Raiha, Kaprio, Koskenvuo, Rajala, & Sourander (1996)	51	43	—	Finland birth registry linked to discharge diagnosis of dementia	5.3 MZ, 2.3 DZ[b]	NINCDS-ADRDA, DSM-III-R	31.3	9.3	—
Bergem, Engedal, & Kringlen (1997)	12	26	79	Norway birth registry	—	NINCDS-ADRDA, DSM-III-R	83	46	55–61[c]
Gatz et al. (1997)	10	30	77–78	Sweden birth registry	3.3	NINCDS-ADRDA, DSM-III-R	66.7	21.9	74
Gatz et al. (2006)	1083	3,142	75–79	Sweden twin registry	—	NINCDS-ADRDA, DSM-IV	45 (M), 58 (F)	19 (MM), 41 (FF), 21 (DZO)	58–79

AD = Alzheimer's disease; MZ = monozygotic; DZ = dizygotic; ADRDA = Alzheimer's Disease and Related Disorders Association; NINCDS = National Institute of Neurological and Communicative Disorders and Stroke; DSM = Diagnostic and Statistical Manual of Mental Disorders; DSM-III-R = DSM, 3rd ed., revised (American Psychiatric Association [APA], 1987); DSM-IV = DSM, 4th ed. (APA, 1994);CERAD = Consortium to Establish a Registry for Alzheimer's Disease; NIA = National Institute of Aging; M = male; F = female; DZO = dizygotic, opposite-sex twins.
[a]All concordance rates are proband-wise calculations. [b]Age-adjusted cumulative incidence. [c]Depending on the percentage of positive cases included in sample.

Table 8-9. Attention Deficit Hyperactivity Disorder: Summary of Findings from Family Studies

FAMILY STUDIES	FIRST-DEGREE RELATIVES		DIAGNOSTIC CRITERIA	MORBIDITY RISK IN RELATIVES[A]	
	CASES (N)	CONTROLS (N)		CASES (%)	CONTROLS (%)
Cantwell (1972)	50 (F) 50 (M)	50 (F) 50 (M)	HACS	4 (F) 15 (M)	0.0 (F) 2.0 (M)
Welner, Welner, Stewart, Palkes, & Wish (1977)	47 (F) 42 (M)	50 (F) 54 (M)	HACS	9 (F) 26 (M)	6 (F) 9 (M)
Biederman et al. (1986)	75	73	DSM-III	31.5	5.7
Biederman, Faraone, Keenan, Knee, & Tsuang (1990)	264	92	DSM-III	25.1	4.6
Biederman et al. (1992)	454	368	DSM-III-R	16	3
Biederman et al. (1995)	84	—	DSM-III-R	57	—
Samuel et al. (1999)	37	52	DSM-III-R, DSM-IV	12 (DSM-III-R), 16 (DSM-IV)	0 (DSM-III-R), 2 (DSM-IV)
Faraone et al. (2000)	417	369	DSM-III-R, DSM-IV	21	4
Smalley et al. (2000)	256	—	DSM-IV	55	—
Biederman et al. (2008)	743 total	—	DSM-III-R	52	—
Lee et al. (2008)	200	47	DSM-IV	62	2
Monuteaux et al. (2008)	417	—	DSM-III-R	77	—
Biederman et al. (2009)	291	285	DSM-III-R	23	11

F = females; M = males; HACS = hyperactive child syndrome (Stewart, Pitts, Craig, & Dieruf, 1966; Morrison & Stewart, 1973); DSM = Diagnostic and Statistical Manual of Mental Disorders; DSM-III = DSM, 3rd ed. (American Psychiatric Association [APA], 1980); DSM-III-R = DSM-III, revised (APA, 1987); DSM-IV = DSM, 4th ed. (APA, 1994).

[a] Values are unadjusted in Cantwell (1972), Welner et al. (1977), Biederman et al. (1986, 1995), Smalley et al. (2000), and Lee et al. (2008). Values in Biederman et al. (2008, 2009) and Monuteaux et al. (2008) were age-adjusted using Cox models. Values in Biederman et al. (1990, 1992) were age-adjusted using the Kaplan-Meier method. Values in Samuel et al. (1999) and Faraone et al. (2000) were age-adjusted using Huber's formula.

Table 8-10. Attention Deficit Hyperactivity Disorder: Summary of Findings from Twin and Adoption Studies

TWIN STUDIES	MZ PAIRS (N)	DZ PAIRS (N)	DIAGNOSTIC CRITERIA	MZ CONCORDANCE[a] (%)	DZ CONCORDANCE[a] (%)	HERITABILITY (%)
Willerman (1973)	54	39	HARS	92	60	77
R. Goodman & Stevenson (1989)	285 pairs total		Rutter (1967)	51	27 (MM), 30 (FM), 17 (MF), 13 (FF)	64
Gillis, Gilger, Pennington, & DeFries (1992)	84	62	DICA-P	79	32	87–98
Stevenson (1992)	91	105	Rutter (1967)	66	28	76
Edelbrock, Rende, Plomin, & Thompson (1995)	99	82	CBCL-AP	68	29	66
Schmitz, Fulker, & Mrazek (1995)	129	270	CBCL-AP	74	20	65
Thapar, Hervas, & McGuffin (1995)	226	334	Rutter (1967)	71 (M), 58 (F)	22 (MM), 5 (FF), 23 (DZO)	88
Gjone, Stevenson, & Sundet (1996)	526	389	CBCL-AP	77.8 (M), 73.4(F)	44.9 (M), 73.4 (F)	66.3 (M), 75.2 (F)
Silberg et al. (1996)	612	585	DSM-III-R	57.9 (M), 57.0 (F)	0.6 (MM), 21.2 (FF), 10.5 (DZO)	—
Eaves et al. (1997)	588	546	DSM-III-R	62 (M), 52 (F)	25 (MM), 23 (FF), 28 (DZO)	62 (M), 54 (F)
Levy, Hay, McStephen, Wood, & Waldman (1997)	849	1,089	DSM-III-R	82.4	37.9	75–91
Sherman, Iacono, & McGue (1997)	194	94	DSM-III-R	69	42	69

Nadder, Silberg, Eaves, Maes, & Meyer (1998)	377	523	CAPA	44 (M), 31 (F)	5 (M), 11 (F), 8 (DZO)	61
Rhee, Waldman, Hay, & Levy (1999)	1,034	1,009	DSM-III-R	80	31 (MM), 39 (FF), 29 (DZO)	85–90
Coolidge, Thede, & Young (2000)	140	84	DSM-IV	87	18	82
Hudziak, Rudiger, Neale, Heath, & Todd (2000)	220	271	CBCL-AP	69 (M), 66 (F)	26 (MM), 20 (FF)	68 (M), 60 (F)
Thapar, Harrington, Ross, & McGuffin (2000)	731	1,189	DuPaul (1981) ADHD rating scale	52	28	79
Willcutt, Pennington, & DeFries (2000)[b]	215	158	DSM-III	72	46	78
N. Martin, Scourfield, & McGuffin (2002)	278	378	SDQ hyperactivity scale, Conners (1969) scale	55 SDQ, 73 Conners	4 SDQ, 25 Conners	72
Rietveld, Hudziak, Bartels, van Beijsterveldt, & Boomsma (2003)	4,106	6,728	CBCL-AP	70 (M), 70 (F)	20 (MM), 30 (FF), 28 (DZO)	68–76
Kuntsi et al. (2004)	625	491	DSM-IV	64	20	—
Larsson, Larsson, & Lichtenstein (2004)	796	1,259	DSM-III-R	63 (F), 74 (M)	39 (MM), 35 (FF), 26 (MF), 26 (FM)	61 (F), 74 (M)
McLoughlin, Ronald, Kuntsi, Asherson, & Plomin (2007)	2,226	3,996	DSM-IV	88 (M), 88 (F)	50 (MM), 53 (FF), 52 (DZO)	—
Polderman et al. (2007)	224	337	CBCL-AP, SWAN/HI, SWAN/AD	67 (CBCL-AP), 91 (SWAN/HI), 85 (SWAN/AD)	25 (CBCL-AP), 43 (SWAN/HI), 38 (SWAN/AD)	73 (CBCL-AP), 90 (SWAN/HI), 82 (SWAN/AD)

(continued)

Table 8-10. (Continued)

TWIN STUDIES	MZ PAIRS (N)	DZ PAIRS (N)	DIAGNOSTIC CRITERIA	MZ CONCORDANCE[a] (%)	DZ CONCORDANCE[a] (%)	HERITABILITY (%)
Wood, Rijsdijk, Saudino, Asherson, & Kuntsi (2008)	150	224	Conners (1969) scale	78	40	77
Bornovalova, Hicks, Iacono, & McGue (2010)	685	384	DICA-R, DSM-III-R	72	28	73
Greven, Rijsdijk, & Plomin (2011)	2,013	3,568	DSM-IV	89 (M), 88 (F)	46 (MM), 53 (FF), 47 (DZO)	76

ADOPTEES FAMILY DESIGN	BIOLOGICAL RELATIVES (N)	ADOPTIVE RELATIVES (N)	DIAGNOSTIC CRITERIA	RATE IN BIOLOGICAL RELATIVES (%)	RATE IN ADOPTIVE RELATIVES (%)
Morrison & Stewart (1973)	59	35	HACS	7.5	2.1
Cantwell (1975)	109	91	HACS	20.2	3.3
Sprich et al. (2000)	198 P 112 S	50 P 12 S	DSM-III-R DSM-III-R	18 P 31 S	6 P 8 S

MZ = monozygotic; DZ = dizygotic; HARS = Werry-Weiss-Peters Home Activity Rating Scale (Werry, 1968); M = male; F = female; FM = opposite-sex twins with female as proband and male as cotwin; MF = opposite-sex twins with male as proband and female as cotwin; DICA-P = Diagnostic Interview for Children and Adolescents—Parent Interview (Herjanic & Reich, 1982); CBCL-AP = Child Behavior Checklist—Attention Problem scale (Achenbach et al., 1991); DZO = dizygotic, opposite-sex twins; DSM = Diagnostic and Statistical Manual of Mental Disorders; DSM-III = DSM, 3rd ed. (American Psychiatric Association [APA], 1980); DSM-III-R = DSM-III, revised (APA, 1987); DSM-IV = DSM, 4th ed. (APA, 1994); CAPA = Child and Adolescent Psychiatric Assessment (Angold & Costello, 2000); ADHD = attention deficit hyperactivity disorder; SDQ = Strengths and Difficulties Questionnaire (Goodman, 1997); SWAN/HI = Strengths and Weaknesses of ADHD Symptoms and Normal Behavior scale, Hyperactivity/Impulsivity (nine DSM-IV items); SWAN/AD = Strengths and Weaknesses of ADHD Symptoms and Normal Behavior scale, Attention Deficit (nine DSM-IV items); DICA-R = Diagnostic Interview for Children and Adolescents—Revised (Reich, 2000); HACS = hyperactive child syndrome (Morrison & Stewart, 1973; Stewart et al., 1966); P = parents; S = siblings.

[a]All concordance rates are proband-wise calculations. [b]Extreme hyperactivity/impulsivity.

Table 8-11. Conduct Disorder: Summary Findings from Family, Twin, and Adoption Studies

FAMILY STUDIES	CASES (N)	CONTROLS (N)	DIAGNOSTIC CRITERIA	MORBIDITY RISK IN FIRST-DEGREE RELATIVES	
				CASES (%)	CONTROLS (%)
Faraone, Biederman, Keenan, & Tsuang (1991)	24[a]	26	DSM-III	38	5

TWIN STUDIES[b]	MZ PAIRS (N)	DZ PAIRS (N)	DIAGNOSTIC CRITERIA	MZ CORRELATION[c]	DZ CORRELATION[c]	HERITABILITY (%)
Eaves et al. (1997)	300	184	DSM-III	0.66 (M), 0.68 (F)[d]	0.38 (M), 0.37 (F), 0.32 (DZO)[d]	69 (M), 31 (F)[d]
Slutske et al. (1997)	396 (M), 930 (F)	231 (M), 533 (F), 592 (DZO)	DSM-III	0.70 (M), 0.68 (F)	0.37 (M), 0.48 (F), 0.34 (DZO)	65 (M), 43 (F)
Young, Stallings, Corley, Krauter, & Hewitt (2000)	175	162	DSM-IV	0.35	0.17	34
Goldstein, Prescott, & Kendler (2001)	347	211	DSM-IV	0.39[e] 0.41[f]	0.16[e] 0.23[f]	38[e] 36[f]

ADOPTEES STUDIES DESIGN	CASES (N)	CONTROLS (N)	DIAGNOSTIC CRITERIA	RATE IN CASE ADOPTEES (%)	RATE IN CONTROL ADOPTEES (%)
Cadoret, Yates, Troughton, Woodworth, & Stewart (1996)[g]	28	74	DSM-III	75	17

DSM = Diagnostic and Statistical Manual of Mental Disorders; DSM-III = DSM, 3rd ed. (American Psychiatric Association [APA], 1980); DSM-IV = DSM, 4th ed. (APA, 1994); MZ = monozygotic; DZ = dizygotic; M = male; F = female; DZO = dizygotic, opposite-sex twins.

[a] Cases met DSM-III criteria for both attention deficit disorder and conduct disorder.

[b] Twin studies included here are published studies on DSM-III or DSM-IV conduct disorder or conduct disorder symptoms. For the broad phenotype of antisocial behavior/criminality/aggression, see Rhee & Waldman (2002).

[c] Within-pair twin correlations.

[d] Twin correlations and heritability estimate based on mother interview; Eaves et al. (1997) also reported twin correlations and heritability estimates based on father interview, child interview, mother questionnaires, father questionnaires, child questionnaires, and teacher questionnaires.

[e] Conduct disorder symptoms, onset < age 15. [f] Conduct disorder symptoms, onset < age 18. [g] All adoptees were female.

Table 8-12. Autism Spectrum Disorder: Summary Findings from Family, Twin, and Adoption Studies

FAMILY STUDIES	FIRST-DEGREE RELATIVES		DIAGNOSTIC CRITERIA	MORBIDITY RISK IN FIRST-DEGREE RELATIVES	
	CASES (N)	CONTROLS (N)		CASES (%)	CONTROLS (%)
Bolton et al. (1994)	99	36	ICD-10, DSM-III-R, FH	2.9[a]	0
Pickles et al. (1995)	99	36	ICD-10, DSM-III-R, FH	0 for parents; 5 (M), 0 (F) for siblings[b]	0 for parents and siblings[b]

TWIN STUDIES	MZ PAIRS (N)	DZ PAIRS (N)	DIAGNOSTIC CRITERIA	MZ CONCORDANCE[c] (%)	DZ CONCORDANCE[c] (%)	HERITABILITY (%)
Folstein & Rutter (1977)	11	10 DZS	Rutter (1971)	36	0	—
Ritvo, Freeman, Mason-Brothers, Mo, & Ritvo (1985)	23	10 DZS, 7 DZO	RDC, DSM-III	96	24	—
Steffenburg et al. (1989)	11	10 DZS, 1 triplet	DSM-III-R	91	0	—
Bailey et al. (1995)	25	20 DZS, 2 triplet	ICD-10	60	0	—
Le Couteur et al. (1996)	28	20 DZS	DSM-IV, ICD-10	73 (A), 78 (ASD)	0 (A), 10 (ASD)	—
Taniai, Nishiyama, Miyachi, Imaeda, & Sumi (2008)	19	14 DZS, 12 DZO	DSM-IV	93	31	73 (M), 87 (F)
Rosenberg et al. (2009)	67	120 DZS, 90 DZO	DSM-IV	88	31	-
Hallmayer et al. (2011)	40 (M, A)	31 (M, A)	DSM-IV[d]	58	21	37 (A)
	7 (F, A)	10 (F, A)		60	27	
	45 (M, ASD)	45 (M, ASD)		77	31	38 (ASD)
	9 (F, ASD)	13 (F, ASD)		50	36	

Adoption Studies
None

ICD-10 = International Classification of Diseases, 10th revision (WHO, 1993); DSM = Diagnostic and Statistical Manual of Mental Disorders; DSM-III = DSM, 3rd ed. (American Psychiatric Association [APA], 1980); DSM-III-R = DSM-III, revised (APA, 1987); DSM-IV = DSM, 4th ed. (APA, 1994); FH = family history; M = male; F = female; MZ = monozygotic; DZ = dizygotic; DZS = dizygotic, same-sex twins; DZO = dizygotic, opposite-sex twins; RDC = Research Diagnostic Criteria (Spitzer & Robins, 1978); A = strict autism (narrow definition); ASD = autism spectrum disorder (broad definition).
[a] Around 6% showed pervasive developmental disorder (PDD). [b] Rates were for the relatives of the probands having autism or PDD. [c] Concordance rates are pairwise concordance.
[d] Twin pairs were initially identified using records that indicate DSM-IV diagnosis of ASD; the combination of Autism Diagnostic Interview - Revised (Lord et al., 1994) and Autism Diagnostic Observation Schedule (Lord et al., 1989) also generates DSM-IV diagnosis of ASD.

mental disorders, it does not constitute proof, since families share the same environment as well as genes. The familial aggregation typically observed for these disorders actually may be more the product of environmental than of genetic factors. Other study designs must be implemented in efforts to tease apart the relative contribution of these two factors. Twin and adoption studies can be informative in this regard.

The logic underlying twin studies is simple. If genetic factors contribute to a disorder, then monozygotic (identical) twins, who share 100% of their alleles, should be more concordant for the disorder than dizygotic (fraternal) twins who, like other siblings, share only 50% of their alleles. A fundamental assumption of twin studies is that since twins, whether monozygotic or dizygotic, share a common environment, any difference in concordance for a disorder must be the product of differences in shared genetic makeup.

However, these assumptions about twin studies have been questioned. Some researchers posit that monozygotic twins share more of a common environment than dizygotic twins (Richardson & Norgate, 2005). For example, monozygotic twins typically are more physically and temperamentally similar than dizygotic twins and as a result may be treated the same by others. Environmental differences between the two types of twins may emerge even earlier. In the intrauterine environment, monozygotic twins typically share a common chorion (fetal sack) while dizygotic twins are dichorionic. If intrauterine factors play a role in the mental disorder in question, the common intrauterine environment may contribute to an observed excess of concordance for the disorder in monozygotic compared with dizygotic twins.

Even if the equal-environment assumption does not exactly hold, twin studies of major mental disorders have been pursued actively and have proven useful. Given the relative rarity of both twinning and major mental disorders, it is logistically challenging to carry out well-conducted twin studies of mental disorders. Fortunately, a number of Scandinavian countries, such as Sweden and Denmark, include specialized twin registries as part of their national medical registries, enabling them to amass large samples of twins and to follow them over time. Used widely to study mental disorders, these twin registries have yielded rates of concordance for a number of mental disorders in both monozygotic and dizygotic twins, from which estimates of heritability for the disorders have been calculated.

Heritability is another common metric in genetic epidemiology that has been used to measure how much genetic factors may contribute to a disorder. A phenotype's overall variance can be divided into variance related to environmental factors and to genetic factors. In its broadest sense, heritability is the proportion of total variance in a phenotype contributed by genetic factors. Genetic variance itself can be further divided into variance related to additive effects of all alleles on the manifestation of disorder and variance resulting from dominance effects between alleles. In its more narrow sense, heritability is defined as the proportion of a phenotype's total variance due only to the additive genetic effects. Broad-sense heritability can be calculated through studies that compare monozygotic and dizygotic twins, while narrow-sense heritability can be calculated from family studies comparing parents and offspring. While comparable, the two measures provide slightly different pictures of the phenotype's underlying genetic architecture.

Tables 8-1 to 8-12 summarize key findings from a number of twin studies of major mental disorders. These estimates, like those from family studies, suggest that genetic factors play a significant role in susceptibility to the corresponding disorders, with significantly greater concordance rates among monozygotic twins than among dizygotic twins. Based on these twin studies, reasonable estimates of the heritability of these disorders range from as low as 30–40% for depression (Sullivan, Neale, & Kendler, 2000) to as high as 90% for autism (Folstein & Rosen-Sheidley, 2001).

Some caution is necessary with respect to the interpretation of heritability. Because heritability is a population-based concept, estimates of it do not indicate the extent to which a disorder is caused by genes in an individual. For example, the estimate of heritability for schizophrenia of around 80% (Sullivan, Kendler, & Neale, 2003) does not mean that genetics accounts for 80% of an individual's schizophrenia. Moreover, estimates of hereditability can vary across populations in ways that cannot be explained solely by sampling variability. Thus in a highly homogeneous environment, a population's heritability estimates might be very high simply because any variability in the susceptibility to the disorder must be due to genetic factors. Further, hereditability does not account either for inaccuracies in the equal-environment assumption or for gene–environment interactions that might play an important role in mental disorders.

ADOPTION STUDIES

Adoption studies provide another means by which to tease apart the relative contributions of genetic and environmental factors to the manifestation of a mental disorder. Adoptions create situations in which genetically related individuals are raised in different family environments and, at the same time, genetically unrelated individuals are raised in the same family environments. Concordances for disorders among the former provide estimates of the genetic contribution to a disorder, while concordances among the latter provide estimates of the environmental contribution.

Two adoption study designs have been used to examine mental disorders. The first is the *adoptees study* method. In this design, rates of a disorder are compared between the adopted-away children of parents with the disorder and adopted-away children whose parents do not have the disorder. Typically, the adopted-away children of mothers are studied because it is easier to track parental relationships with mothers than with fathers. In the second design, the *adoptees family method*, the rates of disorder in biological and adoptive relatives of adoptees with the disorder are compared with the rates in biological and adoptive relatives of adoptees without the disorder. If rates are greater among the biological relatives of affected adoptees than among the biological relatives of unaffected adoptees, genetic influences are suggested. If, however, the rates are greater among the adoptive relatives of affected adoptees than the adoptive relatives of unaffected adoptees, environmental influences are suggested.

While adoption studies can provide powerful inferences about the relative contribution of genetic factors to a disorder, they also have important limitations. First, selective placement of children into adoptive homes similar to their biological homes (e.g., in socioeconomic status or educational background) may bias potential inferences: Genetic influences on a disorder might exaggerate observed similarities between adoptive relatives; alternatively, environmental influences might exaggerate observed similarities between biological relatives. Second, early-life environmental factors (possibly including the intrauterine environment) may influence the trajectory of a disorder before the child is adopted away. As a result, observed similarities between adopted-away children and their biological parents actually may be due to early-life environmental factors rather than to genetic factors, as one might be led to conclude from the premise of adoption studies. Finally, the genetic and environmental influences observed in adoption may not be generalizable to a broader population.

Despite these limitations, adoption studies have helped advance understanding of the genetics of mental disorders. Tables 8-1 to 8-12 provide a précis of the findings of key adoption studies of major mental disorders of public health interest. As with twin studies, many logistical challenges must be overcome to conduct adoption studies; as a result, few have been conducted. Indeed, of the mental disorders considered here, not one adoption study has been conducted on obsessive–compulsive disorder, panic disorder, Alzheimer's disease, or autism spectrum disorders. Studies reporting on other mental disorders consistently have found higher concordance rates among biological relatives than among adoptive relatives, providing further support for the important role of genetic factors in susceptibility to schizophrenia, bipolar disorder, and major depression.

How is the Disorder Transmitted from One Generation to the Next?

Once evidence shows that genetic factors play an important role in susceptibility to a disorder, the next question is "What is the underlying genetic model that explains how the disorder is transmitted from one generation to the next?" Several competing genetic models of inheritance may be explored. At one end of the spectrum is a Mendelian model, in which the disorder is the product of a single gene transmitted according to the *first law of the segregation of a pair of alleles*, delineated by Gregor Mendel in his seminal experiments with the garden pea plant in the late 1800s. The Mendelian models encompass the autosomal dominant, autosomal recessive, X-linked dominant, and X-linked recessive models, each of which leads to a distinctive familial pattern of transmission. Autosomal dominant disorders, for example, tend to appear in each generation, affecting offspring of an affected parent approximately 50% of the time. These kinds of disorders are not transmitted from unaffected parents. In contrast, autosomal recessive disorders typically are seen in siblings of an affected individual but not in the parents, and the recurrence risk in siblings is approximately 1 in 4. Both autosomal dominant and autosomal recessive disorders affect males and females equally, which helps to distinguish them from the X-linked disorders. At the opposite extreme of the spectrum of Mendelian models is the polygenic model, under which a disorder is caused by numerous genes, each contributing a vanishingly small and equal additive effect.

Segregation studies can help test which genetic model might best explain the inheritance of a disorder. In such a study, family medical histories are collected from individuals with the disorder of interest, and the patterns of transmission of the disorder within the families are noted. The models are then compared to determine which is most consistent with the observed data. Assumptions from each model, translated into mathematical equations, are used to make predictions about familial transmission of the disorder. The most parsimonious model that generates predictions closest to the observed transmission is declared the "winner" and offered as the best explanation for the data.

Segregation studies of psychiatric disorders have met with limited success. The consensus from such studies is that while the inheritance of a psychiatric disorder in a small subset of families may be due to a single Mendelian gene, the overwhelming majority of that particular disorder in a population cannot be explained by simple genetic models. Rather, transmission appears to be considerably more complex and probably is best explained by a multifactorial model in which disease susceptibility is the product of both independent and interaction effects of a number of genes and a host of environmental factors.

Where Are Susceptibility Genes?

With evidence from family, twin, and adoption studies that genetic factors contribute to a disorder as well as clues to the underlying model of inheritance, a sufficient rationale exists to initiate a search for specific susceptibility genes. The goal is to identify the genes in which sequence variation contributes to the risk for developing the disorder in question. Two main study designs are employed: linkage studies and association studies. Both designs use genetic markers, specific locations on the human genome with known allelic variation in the population in question. While any type of sequence variation may act as a genetic marker, markers typically are either microsatellites (regular repeats of nucleotide sequences) or SNPs (single-base-pair variants). These markers can help pinpoint the identities and locations of the sequence variants that are causally related to the disorder of interest.

Linkage studies either take a model-based (parametric) approach or an allele-sharing (nonparametric) approach. In the former, multiple families with significant numbers of affected relatives are identified and genotyped (i.e., have their genotypes determined) at select genetic markers. A test statistic (typically a Log of Odds (LOD) score) is calculated for each marker as a measure of whether the marker's alleles cosegregate with the disorder in each family at a rate greater than would be expected by chance given Mendel's *second law of independent assortment* between two genetic loci. The higher the LOD score, the more likely the marker is linked to and therefore located proximate to the disease-causing gene. This approach is considered model based because calculation of the LOD score statistic relies on the specification of a genetic model.

The allele-sharing approach was developed to overcome challenges inherent in delineating the correct genetic model with which to calculate the linkage statistic for etiologically complex disorders. This approach requires smaller family constellations and uses pairs of affected relatives as the basic unit of analysis. Affected relative pairs are genotyped at specific genetic markers, and then a test statistic (such as the nonparametric linkage score) is calculated. The test statistic assesses whether the markers' alleles are "identical by descent" (i.e., come from the same common ancestor) more often than would be expected by chance given Mendel's first law. The higher the allele-sharing statistic for a given marker, the greater the evidence that the marker is linked to the disease-causing gene. Because this calculation does not require specification of a genetic model, it is referred to as model free.

In contrast to linkage studies, association studies capitalize on linkage disequilibrium to directly test for associations between markers' alleles and disease. Linkage disequilibrium is a concept that not only encompasses linkage between two loci but also indicates that specific alleles of the two loci are both in phase (i.e., on the same chromosomes) and transmitted together from one generation to the next more than would be expected by chance given the frequencies of the two alleles in the population.

Association studies may either be population based or family based. In the former, affected individuals (cases) and individuals without the disorder (controls) are identified. They are then genotyped at specific genetic markers, and a test statistic (e.g., an odds ratio) is calculated to determine if the distribution of alleles of the markers differs significantly between the cases and controls. Such tests of association can be confounded by population stratification, in which the racial/ethnic backgrounds of cases and controls may differ in systematic ways that could result in spurious associations between case status and genetic markers that simply differ across racial/ethnic groups.

To overcome this potential limitation, a family-based alternative study method has been proposed. In this approach, trios of parents and their affected offspring are collected and genotyped at genetic markers of interest. A test statistic (such as the transmission disequilibrium test) is calculated to assess whether the alleles of the marker are transmitted from heterozygous parents to the affected offspring more than expected by chance given Mendel's first law. Since parents and offspring are essentially matched on racial/ethnic background, such tests of association are immune to population stratification confounds. This approach has been extended beyond trios to arbitrary pedigree structures.

Association studies, whether population or family based, typically are more powerful than linkage studies in detecting loci (Risch & Merikangas, 1996) with common risk variants (allele frequencies greater than 5%) and modest effects on disease (relative risks less than 2.0). However, because linkage disequilibrium decays more rapidly than linkage as a function of distance, the genetic markers need to be closer to the disease-related locus for a study to detect an association signal than they do for a study to detect a linkage signal. Thus greater coverage of markers across a region is needed to retain the advantages of association studies over linkage studies. Linkage studies, on the other hand, may be better suited for identifying loci with rare risk variants (allele frequencies less than 1%) that are highly penetrant (relative risk greater than 2.0) or are characterized by extensive allelic heterogeneity with several risk variants across the locus contributing to disease (Clerget-Darpoux & Elston, 2007).

Both linkage and association studies can be used to conduct targeted or genome-wide searches for susceptibility genes. Targeted searches survey for linkage or association across specific regions in the genome or in candidate genes thought to be biologically relevant to the disorder. In contrast, genome-wide searches use positional cloning to scan the entire genome in an atheoretical fashion to pinpoint the location of susceptibility genes. Because a genome-wide search is more exhaustive and not constrained by existing knowledge, it can reveal entirely new etiologic mechanisms underlying a disorder, but often at considerable financial cost.

Genome-wide linkage studies have been used for the past several decades, but with limited success in mapping genes for complex mental disorders. It is not until only very recently that genome-wide association studies (GWASs) have become possible. Completion of the Human Genome Project resulted in the identification of millions of SNPs across the genome that can serve as markers in GWASs. Concurrently, development of high-throughput genotyping technologies has made it possible

to assay these polymorphisms in thousands of samples in a cost-effective manner. The emergence of GWASs has revolutionized the field of human disease genetics as a whole, and now these methods are being applied throughout the study of complex mental disorders. Indeed, an ambitious initiative, referred to as the Psychiatric GWAS Consortium, has been established for five major disorders, and activities of these GWASs have now been underway since its establishment (Cichon et al., 2009). These studies are being applied to search for susceptibility genes in mental disorders where previous efforts largely failed. A new generation of genome-wide association studies and genome-wide linkage studies have been applied to search for susceptibility genes in mental disorders where genes in mental disorders has been limited to specific conditions. Three genes for early-onset dis-

ease are relatively rare and account for less than 1% of the disease in the population (Ertekin-Taner, 2007). The fourth gene is APOE. The risk allele in this gene (referred to as ε4) is relatively common in the population and is known to increase the risk of the more common forms

of the disease in a dose-dependent fashion. Compared with individuals without the high-risk allele, carriers of one ε4 allele have around a three-fold increased risk of Alzheimer's disease and those with two copies have up to a 14-fold increased risk, with effects varying markedly by age and racial/ethnic background (Farrer et al., 1997). The APOE gene has been estimated to account for anywhere from 20% to 70% of Alzheimer's disease in the population (Ertekin-Taner, 2007).

A wide range of other candidate genes have been implicated in the other major mental disorders of public health interest. However, consistent evidence for the role of these genes in disease risk has not been forthcoming, making it impossible to draw a definitive link between gene and mental disorder. New bioinformatics resources have recently been developed to amass published genetic association studies of major mental disorders and support meta-analyses to create an ongoing, systematic review of the genes that may play a role in susceptibility to specific mental disorders. The research community can freely access these resources to keep up to date with the accumulating evidence and monitor progress in the field. Examples include such online sources as AlzGene for Alzheimer's disease (http://www.alzgene.org/), Metamoodics for major depression and bipolar disorder (http://metamood-ics.igm.jhmi.edu/metamoodics/), and SzGene for schizophrenia (http://www.schizophrenia-forum.org/res/sczgene/default.asp).

Although only a few susceptibility genes for mental disorders have been conclusively identified to date, a clearer picture of the genetic architecture underlying these disorders is beginning to emerge from the search for susceptibility genes. Consistent with findings from earlier segregation studies, the picture looks very complex. A recent GWAS of schizophrenia (International Schizophrenia Consortium, 2009) has provided compelling evidence for a considerable polygenic contribution to mental disorders in which risk is due to the composite influence of hundreds or even thousands of common variants with modest effect sizes that individually are difficult to detect. At the same time, several other GWASs of schizophrenia (International Schizophrenia

Consortium, 2008; Stefansson et al., 2008) and autism (Sebat et al., 2007) have recently yielded intriguing evidence that rare structural variations, defined as small genomic duplications or deletions, with large effect sizes may also contribute to the occurrence of those disorders, at least in some pedigrees (McClellan, Susser, & King, 2007). Thus given the totality of evidence, it is likely that the genetic contributions to mental disorders are due to a mix of many common genetic variants with modest effect sizes on risk and rare variants with larger effect sizes and that multiple strategies will be needed to elucidate the multiple genetic pathways to disorder.

How Do the Genes Interact with Other Factors in the Population?

Once susceptibility genes have been identified, the next step is to understand how they interact with other genetic and environmental factors to result in the expression of the disorder across different populations, times, and places. Epidemiologically informed study designs are best suited for this purpose—particularly prospective studies, in which temporal relationships between exposures and outcomes can be readily established.

Perhaps the most widely studied mental illness–related gene–environment interaction is the putative interaction between a promoter polymorphism in 5-HTT (the serotonin transporter gene) and early-life environmental stressors in the pathway to clinically significant depressive illness. The 5-HTT gene encodes an integral membrane protein that transports the neurotransmitter serotonin from synaptic spaces back into presynaptic neurons and is a target of a class of antidepressants, the selective serotonin reuptake inhibitors. The promoter of this gene contains a repeat-length polymorphism with two relatively common alleles (typically designated as *short* and *long*) shown to differentially influence expression of the gene (Lesch et al., 1996).

While a number of studies have investigated the potential association of this polymorphism with depression, the results have been mixed. A now classic prospective study by Caspi and colleagues (2003) further examined this association in a population-based cohort followed from birth through adulthood. The study searched for evidence of an interaction between the 5-HTT gene and early-life stress in the pathway to depression. These researchers found that compared with individuals who were homozygous for the long allele, carriers of the short allele were significantly more vulnerable to depression when exposed to early-life stress, providing a compelling demonstration of a gene–environment interaction that potentially could explain the previous inconsistent findings on the association between 5-HTT and depression.

The study's findings were widely heralded, and numerous subsequent studies sought to replicate the findings and expand the scope to related conditions. However, reporting on a recent systematic meta-analysis of these studies, Risch and colleagues (2009) concluded the evidence failed to support the original study's finding of an interaction between 5-HTT and early-life stress. Subsequently, several investigators (e.g., Caspi et al., 2010) have disputed the meta-analysis's conclusion, arguing that the null finding might be the product of important heterogeneity between studies. They suggested that studies with more objective measures of early-life stress consistently showed a significant interaction, while several larger studies, given heavier weight in the meta-analysis, failed to find any interaction because of the use of less rigorous self-reports of early stress. As a result, the jury is still out on whether the putative interaction between 5-HTT and early-life stress is real, and studies are ongoing to establish its etiologic relevance. The initial report by Caspi and colleagues (2003) continues to motivate the search for other gene–environment interactions in mental disorders and to serve as a useful template for the conduct of future inquiry.

THE CHALLENGES AHEAD

Despite an increasingly powerful set of tools available to the research community as a result of the genomics revolution, the effort to characterize the genetic factors that may play a significant role in major mental disorders has been challenging. There are two main reasons for this difficulty. The first is that the genetic architecture of these disorders is clearly quite complex. While single genes acting in a Mendelian fashion may contribute to a small proportion of mental disorders in the population, the overwhelming majority of risk to these disorders appears to be the product of many genes acting independently (genetic heterogeneity) and interactively (genetic epistasis), in concert with environmental factors. The relevant variants in these genes likely have a wide range of effects on disease, with multiple rarer variants having larger risk effects, but only in certain subsets of the population, and more common variants having exceedingly small marginal effects on risk in the broader population. Such complexity makes it difficult to identify a single specific genetic factor that contributes to the overall architecture of susceptibility.

The second reason that identifying genetic factors associated with mental disorders is difficult is the inherent uncertainty in measuring phenotypes related to mental disorders. As discussed earlier, no gold standard diagnostic measures exist for most mental disorders; thus the validity of existing measures remains unclear. Complicating the picture, many mental disorders span a continuum of severity and are accompanied by a range of related conditions. Autism, for example, presents as a spectrum of phenotypically related conditions ranging from core autism to broader pervasive developmental disorders. Although a familial relationship appears to exist across these conditions (Newschaffer et al., 2002), it remains to be seen whether they are genetically related. Some researchers have even posited that autism is a continuously distributed trait in the population and that its discrete characterization is artificial (Constantino & Todd, 2003).

It also remains unclear whether all of the disorders are distinct or are in some way etiologically related. Often there is significant overlap between disorders that initially were conceptualized as distinct. For example, ever since the work of Emil Kraepelin, bipolar disorder and schizophrenia have been treated as distinct disorders. However, some researchers (e.g., Crow, 1995) have argued that an etiologic overlap exists between these disorders and that treating them as separate is not valid. Finally, while most mental disorders manifest with heterogeneous clinical features and a wide array of comorbidities, the extent to which the diverse presentations reflect different etiologic entities remains unknown. Clearly, the inability to operationalize valid measures has hindered efforts to associate genetic factors with specific phenotypic entities.

New Approaches

Investigators are pursuing new approaches that use the latest technologies to overcome the many challenges in studying the genetics of complex mental disorders. One of the most promising of these is large-scale DNA sequencing using next-generation sequencing technologies. Recent advances in the scale of DNA sequencing are making it feasible to sequence whole *exomes* (the complete exon content of the genome) or entire genomes in relatively large samples. Using these approaches, an investigator can examine case–control frequency differences for moderately rare (frequency of 1–5%) or very rare (frequency less than 1%) variants that are not adequately assessed by traditional GWASs. In addition, large multiplex pedigrees previously collected for linkage analysis may be reexamined via sequencing to search for rare sequence variants shared among affected pedigree members. As the ability to sequence entire genomes for less than $1,000 per subject becomes a reality in the foreseeable future, the application of sequencing approaches to exploring the impact of rare variations on complex human behavior phenotypes will become commonplace.

Another promising approach focuses on the role of epigenetics in disease risk. Epigenetics has been defined as heritable influences, other than the actual sequence bases (A, C, T, and G), that affect gene expression and ultimately disease risk. Although there are several classes of epigenetic changes, the focus here is on DNA methylation. Briefly, DNA methylation refers to the addition of a methyl group to cytosine in areas of the genome that are enriched with C and G nucleotides. While the technical details of methylation are beyond the scope of this chapter, the impact of DNA methylation may be central to understanding how gene expression is regulated. Important regions of many genes are potential targets of methylation, including the promoter region. As discussed earlier, the promoter region contains binding sites that allow the transcriptional machinery of the cell to transcribe a gene to RNA. Thus methylation is a mechanism by which the expression of a gene can be reduced or silenced. Importantly, all of the somatic cells in the body, regardless of the function they perform, contain the same complement of DNA and hence the same genes. Moreover, an individual's cells contain the same complement of DNA before and after the onset of a disease. What regulatory mechanisms of gene expression allow the same DNA to lead to different cell types and also to lead to disease in someone who was previously well is among the most important unanswered questions in biology. For decades, scientists have recognized the impact of methylation during development in imprinting (the selective expression of a gene inherited from one parent versus the other) and in X chromosome inactivation (the silencing of one of the X chromosomes in females).

Recently the importance of methylation on a wider scale has become apparent. New, array-based technologies are making it possible to assess the role of variation in methylation at sites throughout the genome. By using such technologies, investigators will soon be able to answer many pressing questions about methylation: Does methylation, or some other epigenetic phenomenon, explain some of the heritability of human disease that common or rare genetic variation does not? Is methylation a marker for the impact of the environment on specific genes? Is methylation a primary mechanism in the regulation of gene expression? Does methylation present a potential target for a next generation of therapeutic agents in mental disorders?

Rationale For Further Research

Despite the challenges ahead, the motivation remains strong to continue investigating how genetic factors contribute to mental disorders. By identifying genetic factors that contribute to the etiology of a disorder, researchers can open a rare window into the biological pathways that, when disturbed, are responsible for the onset of illness. More rational interventions for both treatment and prevention are possible with a clearer understanding of the relevant molecular pathways. The value of this approach is seen most apparently in Alzheimer's disease. The discovery of the three autosomal dominant genes for this disorder transformed the understanding of the pathogenic mechanisms involved in the disease, sparking efforts to intervene in those mechanisms. Further, by resolving the genetic architecture of different psychiatric disorders, it may be possible to develop a clearer nosology of how those disorders are related to one another. Finally, identification of specific genetic factors contributing to mental disorders may give rise to better means of predicting who is at risk for these disorders, ultimately helping to direct interventions to those individuals who would benefit the most.

REFERENCES

Abrams, R., & Taylor, M. A. (1983). The genetics of schizophrenia: A reassessment using modern criteria. *American Journal of Psychiatry, 140*, 171–175.

Achenbach, T. M., Howell, C. T., Quay, H. C., Conners, C. K. (1991) National survey of problems and competencies among four- to sixteen-year-olds: parents' reports for normative and clinical samples. Monographs of the Society for Research in Child Development.

Allen, M. G., Cohen, S., Pollin, W., & Greenspan, S. I. (1974). Affective illness in veteran twins: A diagnostic review. *American Journal of Psychiatry, 131*, 1234–1239.

American Psychiatric Association. (1952). *Diagnostic and statistical manual of mental disorders.* Washington, DC: Author.

American Psychiatric Association. (1968). *Diagnostic and statistical manual of mental disorders* (2nd ed.). Washington, DC: Author.

American Psychiatric Association. (1980). *Diagnostic and statistical manual of mental disorders* (3rd ed.). Washington, DC: Author.

American Psychiatric Association. (1987). *Diagnostic and statistical manual of mental disorders* (3rd ed., rev.). Washington, DC: Author.

American Psychiatric Association. (1994). *Diagnostic and statistical manual of mental disorders* (4th ed.). Washington, DC: Author.

Andreasen, N. C., Rice, J., Endicott, J., Coryell, W., Grove, W. M., & Reich, T. (1987). Familial rates of affective disorder: A report from the National Institute of Mental Health Collaborative Study. *Archives of General Psychiatry, 44*, 461–469.

Andrews, G., Stewart, G., Allen, R., & Henderson, A. S. (1990). The genetics of six neurotic disorders: A twin study. *Journal of Affective Disorders, 19*, 23–29.

Angold, A. & Costello, E. J. (2000). The child and adolescent psychiatric (CAPA). *Journal of American Academy of Child and Adolescent Psychiatry, 39*, 39–48.

Asarnow, R. F., Nuechterlein, K. H., Fogelson, D., Subotnik, K. L., Payne, D. A., Russell, A.T.,…Kendler, K. S. (2001). Schizophrenia and schizophrenia-spectrum personality disorders in the first-degree relatives of children with schizophrenia: The UCLA family study. *Archives of General Psychiatry, 58*, 581–588.

Baek, J. H., Park, D. Y., Choi, J., Kim, J. S., Choi, J. S., Ha, K.,…Hong, K. S. (2011). Differences between bipolar I and bipolar II disorders in clinical features, comorbidity, and family history. *Journal of Affective Disorders, 131*, 59–67.

Bailey, A., Le Couteur, A., Gottesman, I., Bolton, P., Simonoff, E., Yuzda, E., & Rutter, M. (1995). Autism as a strongly genetic disorder: Evidence from a British twin study. *Psychological Medicine, 25*, 63–77.

Baron, M., Gruen, R., Asnis, L., & Kane, J. (1982). Schizoaffective illness, schizophrenia and affective disorders: Morbidity risk and genetic transmission. *Acta Psychiatrica Scandinavica, 65*, 253–262.

Baron, M., Gruen, R., Rainer, J. D., Kane, J., Asnis, L., & Lord, S. (1985). A family study of schizophrenic and normal control probands: Implications for the spectrum concept of schizophrenia. *American Journal of Psychiatry, 142*, 447–455.

Bellodi, L., Sciuto, G., Diaferia, G., Ronchi, P., & Smeraldi, E. (1992). Psychiatric disorders in the families of patients with obsessive–compulsive disorder. *Psychiatry Research, 42*, 111–120.

Bergem, A. L., Engedal, K., & Kringlen, E. (1997). The role of heredity in late-onset Alzheimer disease and vascular dementia: A twin study. *Archives of General Psychiatry, 54*, 264–270.

Bertelsen, A., Harvald, B., & Hauge, M. (1977). A Danish twin study of manic–depressive disorders. *British Journal of Psychiatry, 130*, 330–351.

Biederman, J., Faraone, S. V., Keenan, K., Benjamin, J., Krifcher, B., Moore, C.,…Tsuang, M. T. (1992). Further evidence for family-genetic risk factors in attention deficit hyperactivity disorder: Patterns of comorbidity in probands and relatives in psychiatrically and pediatrically referred samples. *Archives of General Psychiatry, 49*, 728–738.

Biederman, J., Faraone, S. V., Keenan, K., Knee, D., & Tsuang, M. T. (1990). Family-genetic and psychosocial risk factors in DSM-III attention deficit disorder. *Journal of the American Academy of Child and Adolescent Psychiatry, 29*, 526–533.

Biederman, J., Faraone, S. V., Mick, E., Spencer, T., Wilens, T., Kiely, K.,…Warburton, R. (1995). High risk for attention deficit hyperactivity disorder among children of parents with childhood onset of the disorder: A pilot study. *American Journal of Psychiatry, 152*, 431–435.

Biederman, J., Munir, K., Knee, D., Habelow, W., Armentano, M., Autor, S.,…Waternaux, C. (1986). A family study of patients with attention deficit disorder and normal controls. *Journal of Psychiatric Research, 20*, 263–274.

Biederman, J., Petty, C. R., Monuteaux, M. C., Mick, E., Clarke, A., Ten Haagen, K., & Faraone, S. V. (2009). Familial risk analysis of the association between attention-deficit/hyperactivity disorder and psychoactive substance use disorder in female adolescents: A controlled study. *Journal of Child Psychology and Psychiatry, 50*, 352–358.

Biederman, J., Petty, C. R., Wilens, T. E., Fraire, M. G., Purcell, C. A., Mick, E.,…Faraone, S. V. (2008). Familial risk analyses of attention deficit hyperactivity disorder and substance use disorders. *American Journal of Psychiatry, 165*, 107–115.

Bierut, L. J., Heath, A. C., Bucholz, K. K., Dinwiddie, S. H., Madden, P. A., Statham, D.J.,…Martin, N. G. (1999). Major depressive disorder in a community-based twin sample: Are there different genetic and environmental contributions for men and women? *Archives of General Psychiatry, 56*, 557–563.

Black, D. W., Gaffney, G. R., Schlosser, S. & Gabel, J. (2003). Children of parents with obsessive-compulsive disorder—a 2-year follow-up study. *Acta Psychiatrica Scandinavica, 107*, 305–313.

Black, D. W., Noyes, R., Jr., Goldstein, R. B., & Blum, N. (1992). A family study of obsessive–compulsive disorder. *Archives of General Psychiatry, 49*, 362–368.

Bland, R. C., Newman, S. C., & Orn, H. (1986). Recurrent and non-recurrent depression: A family study. *Archives of General Psychiatry, 43*, 1085–1089.

Bolton, P., Macdonald, H., Pickles, A., Rios, P., Goode, S., Crowson, M.,…Rutter, M. (1994). A case-control family history study of autism. *Journal of Child Psychology and Psychiatry, 35*, 877–900.

Bolton, D., Rijsdijk, F., O'Connor, T. G., Perrin, S., & Eley, T. C. (2007). Obsessive–compulsive disorder, tics and anxiety in 6-year-old twins. *Psychological Medicine, 37,* 39–48.

Bornovalova, M. A., Hicks, B. M., Iacono, W. G., & McGue, M. (2010). Familial transmission and heritability of childhood disruptive disorders. *American Journal of Psychiatry, 167,* 1066–1074.

Breitner, J. C., & Folstein, M. F. (1984). Familial Alzheimer dementia: A prevalent disorder with specific clinical features. *Psychological Medicine, 14,* 63–80.

Breitner, J. C., Silverman, J. M., Mohs, R. C., & Davis, K. L. (1988). Familial aggregation in Alzheimer's disease: Comparison of risk among relatives of early- and late-onset cases, and among male and female relatives in successive generations. *Neurology, 38,* 207–212.

Breitner, J. C., Welsh, K. A., Gau, B. A., McDonald, W. M., Steffens, D. C., Saunders, A. M., . . . Page, W. F. (1995). Alzheimer's disease in the National Academy of Sciences–National Research Council Registry of Aging Twin Veterans. III. Detection of cases, longitudinal results, and observations on twin concordance. *Archives of Neurology, 52,* 763–771.

Cadoret, R. J. (1978). Evidence for genetic inheritance of primary affective disorder in adoptees. *American Journal of Psychiatry, 135,* 463–466.

Cadoret, R. J., Yates, W. R., Troughton, E., Woodworth, G., & Stewart, M. A. (1996). An adoption study of drug abuse/dependency in females. *Comprehensive Psychiatry, 37,* 88–94.

Cannon, T. D., Kaprio, J., Lonnqvist, J., Huttunen, M., & Koskenvuo, M. (1998). The genetic epidemiology of schizophrenia in a Finnish twin cohort: A population based modeling study. *Archives of General Psychiatry, 55,* 67–74.

Cantwell, D. P. (1972). Psychiatric illness in the families of hyperactive children. *Archives of General Psychiatry, 27,* 414–417.

Cantwell, D. P. (1975). Genetics of hyperactivity. *Journal of Child Psychology and Psychiatry, 16,* 261–264.

Cardno, A. G., Marshall, E. J., Coid, B., Macdonald, A. M., Ribchester, T. R., Davies, N. J., . . . Murray, R.M. (1999). Heritability estimates for psychotic disorders: The Maudsley twin psychosis series. *Archives of General Psychiatry, 56,* 162–168.

Carey, G., & Gottesman, I. (1981). *Twin and family studies of anxiety, phobic, and obsessive disorders.* New York: Raven Press.

Caspi, A., Sugden, K., Moffitt, T. E., Taylor, A., Craig, I. W., Harrington, H., . . . Poulton, R. (2003). Influence of life stress on depression: Moderation by a polymorphism in the *5-HTT* gene. *Science, 301,* 386–389.

Caspi, A., Hariri, A.R., Holmes, A., Uher, R., Moffitt, T.E. (2010). Genetic sensitivity to the environment: the case of the serotonin transporter gene and its implications for studying complex disease traits. *American Journal of Psychiatry, 167,* 509–527.

Chang, C. J., Chen, W. J., Liu, S. K., Cheng, J. J., Yang, W. C., Chang, H .J., . . . Hwu, H. G. (2002). Morbidity risk of psychiatric disorders among the first-degree relatives of schizophrenia patients in Taiwan. *Schizophrenia Bulletin, 28,* 379–392.

Cichon, S., Craddock, N., Daly, M., Faraone, S. V., Gejman, P. V., Kelsoe, J., . . . Sullivan, P. F. (2009). Genomewide association studies: History, rationale, and prospects for psychiatric disorders. *American Journal of Psychiatry, 166,* 540–556.

Clerget-Darpoux, F., & Elston, R. C. (2007). Are linkage analysis and the collection of family data dead? Prospects for family studies in the age of genome-wide association. *Human Heredity, 64,* 91–96.

Conners, C. K. (1969). A teacher rating scale for use in drug studies with children. *American Journal of Psychiatry, 126,* 884–888.

Constantino, J. N., & Todd, R. D. (2003). Autistic traits in the general population: A twin study. *Archives of General Psychiatry, 60,* 524–530.

Cook, E. H., Jr ., & Scherer, S. W. (2008). Copy-number variations associated with neuropsychiatric conditions. *Nature, 455,* 919–923.

Coolidge, F. L., Thede, L. L., & Young, S. E. (2000). Heritability and the comorbidity of attention deficit hyperactivity disorder with behavioral disorders and executive function deficits: A preliminary investigation. *Developmental Neuropsychology, 17,* 273–287.

Coryell, W., Endicott, J., Reich, T., Andreasen, N., & Keller, M. (1984). A family study of bipolar II disorder. *British Journal of Psychiatry, 145,* 49–54.

Coryell, W., & Zimmerman, M. (1988). The heritability of schizophrenia and schizoaffective disorder: A family study. *Archives of General Psychiatry, 45,* 323–327.

Crow, T. J. (1995). A continuum of psychosis, one human gene, and not much else—the case for homogeneity. *Schizophrenia Research, 17,* 135–145.

Crowe, R. R., Noyes, R., Pauls, D. L., & Slymen, D. (1983). A family study of panic disorder. *Archives of General Psychiatry, 40,* 1065–1069.

DuPaul, G. J. (1981). Parent and teacher ratings of ADHD symptoms: Psychometric properties in a community-based sample. *Journal of Clinical Child Psychology, 20,* 245–253.

Dwyer, J. T., & Delong, G. R. (1987). A family history study of twenty probands with childhood manic–depressive illness. *Journal of the American Academy of Child and Adolescent Psychiatry, 26,* 176–180.

Eaves, L. J., Silberg, J. L., Meyer, J. M., Maes, H. H., Simonoff, E., Pickles, A.,...Hewitt, J. K. (1997). Genetics and developmental psychopathology: 2. The main effects of genes and environment on behavioral problems in the Virginia Twin Study of adolescent behavioral development. *Journal of Child Psychology and Psychiatry, 38,* 965–980.

Edelbrock, C., Rende, R., Plomin, R., & Thompson, L. A. (1995). A twin study of competence and problem behavior in childhood and early adolescence. *Journal of Child Psychology and Psychiatry, 36,* 775–785.

Edvardsen, J., Torgersen, S., Roysamb, E., Lygren, S., Skre, I., Onstad, S., & Oien, P. A. (2008). Heritability of bipolar spectrum disorders: Unity or heterogeneity? *Journal of Affective Disorders, 106,* 229–240.

ENCODE Project Consortium. (2007). Identification and analysis of functional elements in 1% of the human genome by the ENCODE pilot project. *Nature, 447,* 799–816.

ENCODE Project Consortium. (2007). Identification and analysis of functional elements in 1% of the human genome by the ENCODE pilot project. *Nature, 447,* 799–816.

Englund, S. A., & Klein, D. N. (1990). The genetics of neurotic-reactive depression: A reanalysis of Shapiro's (1970) twin study using diagnostic criteria. *Journal of Affective Disorders, 18,* 247–252.

Ertekin-Taner, N. (2007). Genetics of Alzheimer's disease: A centennial review. *Neurological Clinics, 25,* 611–667.

Faraone, S. V., Biederman, J., Keenan, K., & Tsuang, M. T. (1991). Separation of DSM-III attention deficit disorder and conduct disorder: Evidence from a family-genetic study of American child psychiatric patients. *Psychological Medicine, 21,* 109–121.

Faraone, S. V., Biederman, J., Mick, E., Williamson, S., Wilens, T., Spencer, T.,...Zallen, B. (2000). Family study of girls with attention deficit hyperactivity disorder. *American Journal of Psychiatry, 157,* 1077–1083.

Farmer, A. E., McGuffin, P., & Gottesman, I. I. (1987). Twin concordance for DSM-III schizophrenia: Scrutinizing the validity of the definition. *Archives of General Psychiatry, 44,* 634–641.

Farrer, L. A., Cupples, L. A., Haines, J. L., Hyman, B., Kukull, W. A., Mayeux, R.,...van Duijn, C. M. (1997). Effects of age, sex, and ethnicity on the association between apolipoprotein E genotype and Alzheimer disease. *Journal of the American Medical Association, 278,* 1349–1356.

Farrer, L. A., O'Sullivan, D. M., Cupples, L. A., Growdon, J. H., & Myers, R. H. (1989). Assessment of genetic risk for Alzheimer's disease among first-degree relatives. *Annals of Neurology, 25,* 485–493.

Feighner, J. P., Robins, E., Guze, S. B., Woodrugge R. A., Winokur, G., & Munoz, R. (1972). Diagnostic criteria for use in psychiatric research. *Archives of General Psychiatry, 26,* 57–67.

Fieve, R. R., Go, R., Dunner, D. L., & Elston, R. (1984). Search for biological/genetic markers in a long-term epidemiological and morbid risk study of affective disorders. *Journal of Psychiatric Research, 18,* 425–445.

Folstein, S. E., & Rosen-Sheidley, B. (2001). Genetics of autism: Complex aetiology for a heterogeneous disorder. *National Review of Genetics, 2,* 943–955.

Folstein, S., & Rutter, M. (1977). Infantile autism: A genetic study of 21 twin pairs. *Journal of Child Psychology and Psychiatry, 18,* 297–321.

Frangos, E., Athanassenas, G., Tsitourides, S., Katsanou, N., & Alexandrakou, P. (1985). Prevalence of DSM III schizophrenia among the first-degree relatives of schizophrenic probands. *Acta Psychiatrica Scandinavica, 72,* 382–386.

Franzek, E., & Beckmann, H. (1998). Different genetic background of schizophrenia spectrum psychoses: A twin study. *American Journal of Psychiatry, 155,* 76–83.

Fyer, A., Mannuzza, S., Chapman, T. F., Liebowitz, M. R., Aronowitz, B., & Klein, D. F. (1993, March). Familial transmission of obsessive–compulsive disorder [Abstract]. Paper presented at the 1st International OCD Conference, Capri, Italy.

Fyer, A. J., Mannuzza, S., Chapman, T. F., Lipsitz, J., Martin, L. Y., & Klein, D. F. (1996). Panic disorder and social phobia: Effects of comorbidity on familial transmission. *Anxiety, 2*(4), 173–178.

Gatz, M., Pedersen, N. L., Berg, S., Johansson, B., Johansson, K., Mortimer, J. A.,...Ahlbom, A. (1997). Heritability for Alzheimer's disease: The study of dementia in Swedish twins. *Journals of Gerontology. Series A, Biological Sciences and Medical Sciences, 52,* M117–M125.

Gatz, M., Reynolds, C. A., Fratiglioni, L., Johansson, B., Mortimer, J. A., Berg, S.,...Pedersen, N. L. (2006). Role of genes and environments for explaining Alzheimer disease. *Archives of General Psychiatry, 63,* 168–174.

Gershon, E. S., DeLisi, L. E., Hamovit, J., Nurnberger, J. I., Jr., Maxwell, M. E., Schreiber, J.,...

Guroff, J. J. (1988). A controlled family study of chronic psychoses: Schizophrenia and schizoaffective disorder. *Archives of General Psychiatry, 45,* 328–336.

Gershon, E. S., Hamovit, J., Guroff, J. J., Dibble, E., Leckman, J. F., Sceery, W., ... Bunney, W. E. , Jr. (1982). A family study of schizoaffective, bipolar I, bipolar II, unipolar, and normal control probands. *Archives of General Psychiatry, 39,* 1157–1167.

Gillis, J. J., Gilger, J. W., Pennington, B. F., & DeFries, J. C. (1992). Attention deficit disorder in reading-disabled twins: Evidence for a genetic etiology. *Journal of Abnormal Child Psychology, 20,* 303–315.

Gjone, H., Stevenson, J., & Sundet, J. M. (1996). Genetic influence on parent-reported attention-related problems in a Norwegian general population twin sample. *Journal of the American Academy of Child and Adolescent Psychiatry, 35,* 588–598.

Goldstein, R. B., Prescott, C. A., & Kendler, K. S. (2001). Genetic and environmental factors in conduct problems and adult antisocial behavior among adult female twins. *Journal of Nervous and Mental Disease, 189,* 201–209.

Goldstein, R. B., Weissman, M. M., Adams, P. B., Horwath, E., Lish, J. D., Charney, D., ... Wickramaratne, P. J. (1994). Psychiatric disorders in relatives of probands with panic disorder and/or major depression. *Archives of General Psychiatry, 51,* 383–394.

Goodman, R. (1997). The strengths and difficulties questionnaire: a research note. *Journal of Child Psychology and Psychiatry, 38,* 581–586.

Goodman, R., & Stevenson, J. (1989). A twin study of hyperactivity—II. The aetiological role of genes, family relationships and perinatal adversity. *Journal of Child Psychology and Psychiatry, 30,* 691–709.

Grados, M. A., Riddle, M. A., Samuels, J. F., Liang, K. Y., Hoehn-Saric, R., Bienvenu, O. J., ... Nestadt, G. (2001). The familial phenotype of obsessive-compulsive disorder in relation to tic disorders: The Hopkins OCD family study. *Biological Psychiatry, 50,* 559–565.

Greven, C., Rijsdijk, F. V., & Plomin, R. (2011). A twin study of ADHD symptoms in early adolescence: Hyperactivity–impulsivity and inattentiveness show substantial genetic overlap but also genetic specificity. *Journal of Abnormal Child Psychology, 39,* 265–275.

Guze, S. B., Cloninger, C. R., Martin, R. L., & Clayton, P. J. (1983). A follow-up and family study of schizophrenia. *Archives of General Psychiatry, 40,* 1273–1276.

Hallmayer, J., Cleveland, S., Torres, A., Phillips, J., Cohen, B., Torigoe, T., ... Risch, N. (2011). Genetic heritability and shared environmental factors among twin pairs with autism. *Archives of General Psychiatry, 68*(11), 1095–1102.

Heun, R., & Maier, W. (1993). The distinction of bipolar II disorder from bipolar I and recurrent unipolar depression: Results of a controlled family study. *Acta Psychiatrica Scandinavica, 87,* 279–284.

Herjanic, B., & Reich, W. (1982). Development of a structured psychiatric interview for children: Agreement between child and parent on individual symptoms. *Journal of Abnormal Child Psychology, 10,* 307–324.

Heston, L. L., Mastri, A. R., Anderson, V. E., & White, J. (1981). Dementia of the Alzheimer type: Clinical genetics, natural history, and associated conditions. *Archives of General Psychiatry, 38,* 1085–1090.

Heyman, A., Wilkinson, W. E., Hurwitz, B. J., Schmechel, D., Sigmon, A. H., Weinberg, T., ... Swift, M. (1983). Alzheimer's disease: Genetic aspects and associated clinical disorders. *Annals of Neurology, 14,* 507–515.

Hopper, J. L., Judd, F. K., Derrick, P. L., & Burrows, G. D. (1987). A family study of panic disorder. *Genetic Epidemiology, 4,* 33–41.

Hudziak, J. J., Rudiger, L. P., Neale, M. C., Heath, A. C., & Todd, R. D. (2000). A twin study of inattentive, aggressive, and anxious/depressed behaviors. *Journal of the American Academy of Child and Adolescent Psychiatry, 39,* 469–476.

Huff, F. J., Auerbach, J., Chakravarti, A., & Boller, F. (1988). Risk of dementia in relatives of patients with Alzheimer's disease. *Neurology, 38,* 786–790.

Insel, T. R., Hoover, C., & Murphy, D. L. (1983). Parents of patients with obsessive–compulsive disorder. *Psychological Medicine, 13,* 807–811.

International HapMap Consortium. (2003). The International HapMap Project. *Nature, 426,* 789–796.

International Human Genome Mapping Consortium. (2001). A physical map of the human genome. *Nature, 409,* 934–941.

International Human Genome Sequencing Consortium. (2004). Finishing the euchromatic sequence of the human genome. *Nature, 431,* 931–945.

International Schizophrenia Consortium. (2008). Rare chromosomal deletions and duplications increase risk of schizophrenia. *Nature, 455,* 237–241.

International Schizophrenia Consortium. (2009). Common polygenic variation contributes to risk of schizophrenia and bipolar disorder. *Nature, 460*, 748–752.

Jorgensen, A., Teasdale, T. W., Parnas, J., Schulsinger, F., Schulsinger, H., & Mednick, S. A. (1987). The Copenhagen High-Risk Project: The diagnosis of maternal schizophrenia and its relation to offspring diagnosis. *British Journal of Psychiatry, 151*, 753–757.

Kendler, K. S., Gardner, C. O., & Prescott, C. A. (2001). Panic syndromes in a population-based sample of male and female twins. *Psychological Medicine, 31*, 989–1000.

Kendler, K. S., Gatz, M., Gardner, C. O., & Pedersen, N. L. (2006). A Swedish national twin study of lifetime major depression. *American Journal of Psychiatry, 163*, 109–114.

Kendler, K. S., Gruenberg, A. M., & Kinney, D. K. (1994). Independent diagnoses of adoptees and relatives as defined by DSM-III in the provincial and national samples of the Danish Adoption Study of Schizophrenia. *Archives of General Psychiatry, 51*, 456–468.

Kendler, K. S., Gruenberg, A. M., & Tsuang, M. T. (1985). Psychiatric illness in first-degree relatives of schizophrenic and surgical control patients: A family study using DSM-III criteria. *Archives of General Psychiatry, 42*, 770–779.

Kendler, K. S., McGuire, M., Gruenberg, A. M., O'Hare, A., Spellman, M., & Walsh, D. (1993). The Roscommon Family Study. I. Methods, diagnosis of probands, and risk of schizophrenia in relatives. *Archives of General Psychiatry, 50*, 527–540.

Kendler, K. S., Neale, M. C., Kessler, R. C., Heath, A. C., & Eaves, L. J. (1992). A population-based twin study of major depression in women: The impact of varying definitions of illness. *Archives of General Psychiatry, 49*, 257–266.

Kendler, K. S., Neale, M. C., Kessler, R. C., Heath, A. C., & Eaves, L .J. (1993). Panic disorder in women: A population-based twin study. *Psychological Medicine, 23*, 397–406.

Kendler, K. S., Pedersen, N., Johnson, L., Neale, M. C., & Mathe, A. A. (1993). A pilot Swedish twin study of affective illness, including hospital- and population-ascertained subsamples. *Archives of General Psychiatry, 50*, 699–700.

Kendler, K. S., Pedersen, N. L., Neale, M. C., & Mathe, A. A. (1995). A pilot Swedish twin study of affective illness including hospital- and population-ascertained subsamples: Results of model fitting. *Behavior Genetics, 25*, 217–232.

Kendler, K. S., & Prescott, C. A. (1999). A population based twin study of lifetime major depression in men and women. *Archives of General Psychiatry, 56*, 39–44.

Kety, S. S., Wender, P. H., Jacobsen, B., Ingraham, L. J., Jansson, L., Faber, B., & Kinney, D. K. (1994). Mental illness in the biological and adoptive relatives of schizophrenic adoptees: Replication of the Copenhagen Study in the rest of Denmark. *Archives of General Psychiatry, 51*, 442–455.

Kieseppa, T., Partonen, T., Haukka, J., Kaprio, J., & Lönnqvist, J. (2004). High concordance of bipolar I disorder in a nationwide sample of twins. *American Journal of Psychiatry, 161*, 1814–1821.

Klaning, U. (1996). *Schizophrenia in twins: Incidence and risk factors* (Unpublished doctoral dissertation). University of Aarhus, Denmark.

Korten, A. E., Jorm, A. F., Henderson, A. S., Broe, G. A., Creasey, H., & McCusker, E. (1993). Assessing the risk of Alzheimer's disease in first-degree relatives of Alzheimer's disease cases. *Psychological Medicine, 23*, 915–923.

Kraepelin, E. (1913) Psychiatria, VIII Auflage. Leipzig: Barth.

Kuntsi, J., Eley, T. C., Taylor, A., Hughes, C., Asherson, P., Caspi, A., & Moffitt, T. E. (2004). Co-occurrence of ADHD and low IQ has genetic origins. *American Journal of Medical Genetics, 124B*, 41–47.

Kupfer, D. J., Frank, E., Carpenter, L. L., & Neiswanger, K. (1989). Family history in recurrent depression. *Journal of Affective Disorders, 17*, 113–119.

Larsson, J. O., Larsson, H., & Lichtenstein, P. (2004). Genetic and environmental contributions to stability and change of ADHD symptoms between 8 and 13 years of age: A longitudinal twin study. *Journal of the American Academy of Child and Adolescent Psychiatry, 43*, 1267–1275.

Lautenschlager, N. T., Cupples, L. A., Rao, V. S., Auerbach, S. A., Becker, R., Burke, J.,…Farrer, L.A. (1996). Risk of dementia among relatives of Alzheimer's disease patients in the MIRAGE study: What is in store for the oldest old? *Neurology, 46*, 641–650.

Leckman, J. F., Weissman, M. M., Prusoff, B. A., Caruso, K. A., Merikangas, K. R., Pauls, D. L., & Kidd, K. K. (1984). Subtypes of depression: Family study perspective. *Archives of General Psychiatry, 41*(9), 833–838.

Le Couteur, A., Bailey, A., Goode, S., Pickles, A., Robertson, S., Gottesman, I., & Rutter, M. (1996). A broader phenotype of autism: The clinical spectrum in twins. *Journal of Child Psychology and Psychiatry, 37*, 785–801.

Lee, S. I., Schachar, R. J., Chen, S. X., Ornstein, T. J., Charach, A., Barr, C., & Ickowicz, A. (2008). Predictive validity of DSM-IV and ICD-10 criteria for ADHD and hyperkinetic disorder. *Journal of Child Psychology and Psychiatry, 49*, 70–78.

Lesch, K. P., Bengel, D., Heils, A., Sabol, S. Z., Greenberg, B. D., Petri, S.,...Murphy, D. L. (1996). Association of anxiety-related traits with a polymorphism in the serotonin transporter gene regulatory region. *Science, 274*, 2294–2295.

Levy, F., Hay, D. A., McStephen, M., Wood, C., & Waldman, I. (1997). Attention-deficit hyperactivity disorder: A category or a continuum? Genetic analysis of a large-scale twin study. *Journal of the American Academy of Child and Adolescent Psychiatry, 36*, 737–744.

Lichtenstein, P., Yip, B. H., Björk, C., Pawitan, Y., Cannon, T. D., Sullivan, P. F., & Hultman, C. M. (2009). Common genetic determinants of schizophrenia and bipolar disorder in Swedish families: A population-based study. *Lancet, 373*, 234–239.

Lord, C., Rutter, M., Goode S., Heemsbergen, J., Jordan, H., Mawhood, L., Schopler, E. (1989). Autism diagnostic observation schedule: A standardized observation of communicative and social behavior. *Journal of Autism and Developmental Disorders, 19*, 185–212.

Lord, C., Rutter, M., Le Couteur A. (1994). Autism Diagnostic Interview - Revised: A revised version of a diagnostic interview for caregivers of individuals with possible pervasive developmental disorders. *Journal of Autism and Developmental Disorders, 24*, 659–685.

Lowing, P. A., Mirsky, A. F., & Pereira, R. (1983). The inheritance of schizophrenia spectrum disorders: A reanalysis of the Danish adoptee study data. *American Journal of Psychiatry, 140*, 1167–1171.

Lyons, M. J., Eisen, S. A., Goldberg, J., True, W., Lin, N., Meyer, J.M.,...Tsuang, M. T. (1998). A registry-based twin study of depression in men. *Archives of General Psychiatry, 55*, 468–472.

Maier, W., Hallmayer, J., Minges, J., & Lichtermann, D. (1990). Morbid risks in relatives of affective, schizoaffective, and schizophrenic patients—results of a family study. In A. Marneros & M. T. Tsuang (Eds.), *Affective and schizoaffective disorders: Similarities and differences* (pp. 201–207). New York, NY: Springer-Verlag.

Maier, W., Lichtermann, D., Franke, P., Heun, R., Falkai, P., & Rietschel, M. (2002). The dichotomy of schizophrenia and affective disorders in extended pedigrees. *Schizophrenia Research, 57*, 259–266.

Maier, W., Lichtermann, D., Minges, J., Heun, R., Hallmayer, J., & Klinger, T. (1991). Unipolar depression in the aged: Determinants of familial aggregation. *Journal of Affective Disorders, 23*, 53–61.

Maier, W., Lichtermann, D., Minges, J., Hallmayer, J., Heun, R., Benkert, O., & Levinson, D. F. (1993). Continuity and discontinuity of affective disorders and schizophrenia: Results of a controlled family study. *Archives of General Psychiatry, 50*, 871–883.

Maier, W., Lichtermann, D., Minges, J., Oehrlein, A., & Franke, P. (1993). A controlled family study in panic disorder. *Journal of Psychiatric Research, 27*, 79–87.

Maj, M., Starace, F., & Pirozzi, R. (1991). A family study of DSM-III-R schizoaffective disorder, depressive type, compared with schizophrenia and psychotic and non-psychotic major depression. *American Journal of Psychiatry, 148*, 612–616.

Marshall, E. (2000). Rival genome sequencers celebrate a milestone together. *Science, 288*, 2294–2295.

Martin, N., Scourfield, J., & McGuffin, P. (2002). Observer effects and heritability of childhood attention-deficit hyperactivity disorder symptoms. *British Journal of Psychiatry, 180*, 260–265.

Martin, R. L., Gerteis, G., & Gabrielli, W. F., Jr. (1988). A family-genetic study of dementia of Alzheimer type. *Archives of General Psychiatry, 45*, 894–900.

McClellan, J. M., Susser, E., & King, M. C. (2007). Schizophrenia: A common disease caused by multiple rare alleles. *British Journal of Psychiatry, 190*, 194–199.

McGuffin, P., Katz, R., & Bebbington, P. (1987). Hazard, heredity and depression: A family study. *Journal of Psychiatric Research, 21*, 365–375.

McGuffin, P., Katz, R., & Rutherford, J. (1991). Nature, nurture and depression: A twin study. *Psychological Medicine, 21*, 329–335.

McGuffin, P., Katz, R., Watkins, S., & Rutherford, J. (1996). A hospital-based twin register of the heritability of DSM-IV unipolar depression. *Archives of General Psychiatry, 53*, 129–136.

McGuffin, P., Rijsdijk, F., Andrew, M., Sham, P., Katz, R., & Cardno, A. (2003). The heritability of bipolar affective disorder and the genetic relationship to unipolar depression. *Archives of General Psychiatry, 60*, 497–502.

McKeon, P., & Murray, R. (1987). Familial aspects of obsessive–compulsive neurosis. *British Journal of Psychiatry, 151*, 528–534.

McLoughlin, G., Ronald, A., Kuntsi, J., Asherson, P., & Plomin, R. (2007). Genetic support for the dual nature of attention deficit hyperactivity disorder: Substantial genetic overlap between the inattentive and hyperactive–impulsive components. *Journal of Abnormal Child Psychology, 35*, 999–1008.

Mendlewicz, J., & Baron, M. (1981). Morbidity risks in subtypes of unipolar depressive illness: Differences between early and late onset forms. *British Journal of Psychiatry, 139*, 463–466.

Mendlewicz, J., Linkowski, P., & Wilmotte, J. (1980). Relationship between schizoaffective illness and affective disorders or schizophrenia: Morbidity risk and genetic transmission. *Journal of Affective Disorders, 2*, 289–302.

Mendlewicz, J., Papadimitriou, G., & Wilmotte, J. (1993). Family study of panic disorder: Comparison with generalized anxiety disorder, major depression and normal subjects. *Psychiatric Genetics, 3*, 73–78.

Mendlewicz, J., & Rainer, J. D. (1977). Adoption study supporting genetic transmission in manic–depressive illness. *Nature, 268*, 327–329.

Merikangas, K. R., Leckman, J. F., Prusoff, B. A., Pauls, D. L., & Weissman, M. M. (1985). Familial transmission of depression and alcoholism. *Archives of General Psychiatry, 42*, 367–372.

Mohs, R. C., Breitner, J. C., Silverman, J. M., & Davis, K. L. (1987). Alzheimer's disease: Morbid risk among first-degree relatives approximates 50% by 90 years of age. *Archives of General Psychiatry, 44*, 405–408.

Monuteaux, M. C., Faraone, S. V., Hammerness, P., Wilens, T. E., Fraire, M., & Biederman, J. (2008). The familial association between cigarette smoking and ADHD: A study of clinically referred girls with and without ADHD, and their families. *Nicotine & Tobacco Research, 10*, 1549–1558.

Morris, J.C. (1993). The Clinical Dementia Rating (CDR): current versions and scoring results. *Neurology, 43*, 2412–2414.

Morrison, J. R., & Stewart, M. A. (1973). The psychiatric status of the legal families of adopted hyperactive children. *Archives of General Psychiatry, 28*, 888–891.

Nadder, T. S., Silberg, J. L., Eaves, L. J., Maes, H. H., & Meyer, J. M. (1998). Genetic effects on ADHD symptomatology in 7- to 13-year-old twins: Results from a telephone survey. *Behavior Genetics, 28*, 83–99.

Nee, L. E., Eldridge, R., Sunderland, T., Thomas, C. B., Katz, D., Thompson, K. E.,...Cohen, R. (1987). Dementia of the Alzheimer type: Clinical and family study of 22 twin pairs. *Neurology, 37*, 359–363.

Nestadt, G., Samuels, J., Riddle, M., Bienvenu, O. J., 3rd, Liang, K. Y., LaBuda, M.,...Hoehn-Saric, R. (2000). A family study of obsessive–compulsive disorder. *Archives of General Psychiatry, 57*, 358–363.

Newschaffer, C. J., Fallin, D., & Lee, N. L. (2002). Heritable and nonheritable risk factors for autism spectrum disorders. *Epidemiologic Reviews, 24*, 137–153.

Nicolini, H., Weissbecker, K., Mejía, J. M., & Sánchez de Carmona, M. (1993). Family study of obsessive compulsive disorder in a Mexican population. *Archives of Medical Research, 24*, 193–198.

Noyes, R., Jr., Crowe, R. R., Harris, E. L., Hamra, B. J., McChesney, C. M., & Chaudhry, D. R. (1986). Relationship between panic disorder and agoraphobia: A family study. *Archives of General Psychiatry, 43*, 227–232.

Onstad, S., Skre, I., Torgersen, S., & Kringlen, E. (1991). Twin concordance for DSM-III-R schizophrenia. *Acta Psychiatrica Scandinavica, 83*, 395–401.

Parnas, J., Cannon, T. D., Jacobsen, B., Schulsinger, H., Schulsinger, F., & Mednick, S. A. (1993). Lifetime DSM-III-R diagnostic outcomes in the offspring of schizophrenic mothers: Results from the Copenhagen High-Risk Study. *Archives of General Psychiatry, 50*, 707–714.

Pauls, D. L., Alsobrook, J. P., 2nd, Goodman, W., Rasmussen, S., & Leckman, J. F. (1995). A family study of obsessive–compulsive disorder. *American Journal of Psychiatry, 152*, 76–84.

Pauls, D. L., Morton, L. A., & Egeland, J. A. (1992). Risks of affective illness among first-degree relatives of bipolar I old-order Amish probands. *Archives of General Psychiatry, 49*, 703–708.

Perna, G., Caldirola, D., Arancio, C., & Bellodi, L. (1997). Panic attacks: A twin study. *Psychiatry Research, 66*, 69–71.

Perris, C., Perris, H., Ericsson, U., & Von Knorring, L. (1982). The genetics of depression: A family study of unipolar and neurotic-reactive depressed patients. *Archiv für Psychiatrie und Nervenkrankheiten, 232*, 137–155.

Pheasant, M., & Mattick, J. S. (2007). Raising the estimate of functional human sequences. *Genome Research, 17*, 1245–1253.

Pickles, A., Bolton, P., Macdonald, H., Bailey, A., Le Couteur, A., Sim, C. H., & Rutter, M. (1995). Latent-class analysis of recurrence risk for complex phenotypes with selection and measurement error: A twin and family history study of autism. *American Journal of Human Genetics, 57*, 717–726.

Pitman, R. K., Green, R. C., Jenike, M. A., & Mesulam, M. M. (1987). Clinical comparison of Tourette's disorder and obsessive–compulsive disorder. *American Journal of Psychiatry, 144*, 1166–1171.

Polderman, T. J, Derks, E. M., Hudziak, J. J., Verhulst, F. C., Posthuma, D., & Boomsma, D. I. (2007). Across the continuum of attention skills: A twin study of the SWAN ADHD rating scale. *Journal of Child Psychology and Psychiatry, 48,* 1080–1087.

Price, R. A., Kidd, K. K., & Weissman, M. M. (1987). Early onset (under age 30 years) and panic disorder as markers for etiologic homogeneity in major depression. *Archives of General Psychiatry, 44,* 434–440.

Raiha, I., Kaprio, J., Koskenvuo, M., Rajala, T., & Sourander, L. (1996). Alzheimer's disease in Finnish twins. *Lancet, 347,* 573–578.

Rasmussen, S. A., & Tsuang, M. T. (1986). Clinical characteristics and family history in DSM-III obsessive compulsive disorder. *American Journal of Psychiatry, 143,* 317–322.

Reich, W. (2000) Diagnostic interview for children and adolescents (DICA). *Journal of the American Academy of Child and Adolescent Psychiatry, 39,* 59–66.

Rhee, S. H., & Waldman, I. D. (2002). Genetic and environmental influences on antisocial behavior: A meta-analysis of twin and adoption studies. *Psychological Bulletin, 128,* 490–529.

Rhee, S. H., Waldman, I. D., Hay, D. A., & Levy, F. (1999). Sex differences in genetic and environmental influences on DSM-III-R attention-deficit/hyperactivity disorder. *Journal of Abnormal Psychology, 108,* 24–41.

Rice, J., Reich, T., Andreasen, N. C., Endicott, J., Van Eerdewegh, M., Fishman, R.,...Klerman, G. L. (1987). The familial transmission of bipolar illness. *Archives of General Psychiatry, 44,* 441–447.

Richardson, K., & Norgate, S. (2005). The equal environments assumption of classical twin studies may not hold. *British Journal of Educational Psychology, 75,* 339–350.

Rietveld, M. J., Hudziak, J. J., Bartels, M., van Beijsterveldt, C. E., & Boomsma, D. I. (2003). Heritability of attention problems in children: I. Cross-sectional results from a study of twins, age 3–12 years. *American Journal of Medical Genetics, 117B,* 102–113.

Risch, N. (1990). Linkage strategies for genetically complex traits. II. The power of affected relative pairs. *American Journal of Human Genetics, 46,* 229–241.

Risch, N., Herrell, R., Lehner, T., Liang, K. Y., Eaves, L., Hoh, J.,...Merikangas, K. R. (2009). Interaction between the serotonin transporter gene (*5-HTTLPR*), stressful life events, and risk of depression. *Journal of the American Medical Association, 301,* 2462–2471.

Risch, N., & Merikangas, K. (1996). The future of genetic studies of complex human diseases. *Science, 273,* 1516–1517.

Ritvo, E. R., Freeman, B. J., Mason-Brothers, A., Mo, A., & Ritvo, A. M. (1985). Concordance for the syndrome of autism in 40 pairs of afflicted twins. *American Journal of Psychiatry, 142,* 74–77.

Rosenberg, R. E., Law, J. K., Yenokyan, G., McGready, J., Kaufmann, W. E., & Law, P. A. (2009). Characteristics and concordance of autism spectrum disorders among 277 twin pairs. *Archives of Pediatrics and Adolescent Medicine, 163,* 907–914.

Rutter, M. (1967) A children's behaviour questionnaire for completion by teachers: preliminary findings. *Journal of Child Psychology and Psychiatry, 8,* 1–11.

Rutter, M. (1971). The description and classification of infantile autism. In: D. W. Churchill, G. D. Alpern, M. K. de Meyer, Eds., *Infantile Autism* (pp. 8–28). Springfield, IL: C. C. Thomas.

Sadovnick, A. D., Remick, R. A., Lam, R., Zis, A. P., Yee, I. M., Huggins, M. J., & Baird, P. A. (1994). Mood Disorder Service Genetic Database: Morbidity risks for mood disorders in 3,942 first-degree relatives of 671 index cases with single depression, recurrent depression, bipolar I, or bipolar II. *American Journal of Medical Genetics, 54,* 132–140.

Samuel, V. J., George, P., Thornell, A., Curtis, S., Taylor, A., Brome, D.,...Biederman, J. (1999). A pilot controlled family study of DSM-III-R and DSM-IV ADHD in African-American children. *Journal of the American Academy of Child and Adolescent Psychiatry, 38,* 34–39.

Scherrer, J. F., True, W. R., Xian, H., Lyons, M. J., Eisen, S. A., Goldberg, J.,...Tsuang, M. T. (2000). Evidence for genetic influences common and specific to symptoms of generalized anxiety and panic. *Journal of Affective Disorders, 57,* 25–35.

Schmitz, S., Fulker, D. W., & Mrazek, D. A. (1995). Problem behavior in early and middle childhood: An initial behavior genetic analysis. *Journal of Child Psychology and Psychiatry, 36,* 1443–1458.

Sciuto, G., Pasquale, L., & Bellodi, L. (1995). Obsessive compulsive disorder and mood disorders: A family study. *American Journal of Medical Genetics, 60,* 475–479.

Sebat, J., Lakshmi, B., Malhotra, D., Troge, J., Lese-Martin, C., Walsh, T.,...Wigler, M. (2007). Strong association of de novo copy number mutations with autism. *Science, 316,* 445–449.

Sherman, D. K., Iacono, W. G., & McGue, M. K. (1997). Attention-deficit hyperactivity disorder dimensions: A twin study of inattention and impulsivity–hyperactivity. *Journal of* the American Academy of Child and Adolescent Psychiatry, 36, 745–753.

Silberg, J., Rutter, M., Meyer, J., Maes, H., Hewitt, J., Simonoff, E.,…Eaves, L. (1996). Genetic and environmental influences on the covariation between hyperactivity and conduct disturbance in juvenile twins. Journal of Child Psychology and Psychiatry, 37, 803–816.

Silverman, J. M., Raiford, K., Edland, S., Fillenbaum, G., Morris, J. C., Clark, C. M.,…Heyman, A. (1994). The Consortium to Establish a Registry for Alzheimer's Disease (CERAD). Part VI. Family history assessment: A multicenter study of first-degree relatives of Alzheimer's disease probands and non-demented spouse controls. Neurology, 44, 1253–1259.

Skre, I., Onstad, S., Torgersen, S., Lygren, S., & Kringlen, E. (1993). A twin study of DSM-III-R anxiety disorders. Acta Psychiatrica Scandinavica, 88, 85–92.

Slutske, W. S., Heath, A. C., Dinwiddie, S. H., Madden, P. A., Bucholz, K. K., Dunne, M. P.,…Martin, N. G. (1997). Modeling genetic and environmental influences in the etiology of conduct disorder: A study of 2,682 adult twin pairs. Journal of Abnormal Psychology, 106, 266–279.

Smalley, S. L., McGough, J. J., Del'Homme, M., NewDelman, J., Gordon, E., Kim, T.,…McCracken, J. T. (2000). Familial clustering of symptoms and disruptive behaviors in multiplex families with attention-deficit/hyperactivity disorder. Journal of the American Academy of Child and Adolescent Psychiatry, 39, 1135–1143.

Somnath, C. P., Janardhan Reddy, Y. C., & Jain, S. (2002). Is there a familial overlap between schizophrenia and bipolar disorder? Journal of Affective Disorders, 72, 243–247.

Sprich, S., Biederman, J., Crawford, M. H., Mundy, E., Saraone, S. V. (2000). Adoptive and biological families of children and adolescents with ADHD. Journal of the American Academy of Child and Adolescent Psychiatry, 39, 1432–1437.

Spitzer, R. L. & Robins E. (1978) Research diagnostic criteria: rationale and reliability. Archives of General Psychiatry, 35, 773–782.

Stancer, H. C., Persad, E., Wagener, D. K., & Jorna, T. (1987). Evidence for homogeneity of major depression and bipolar affective disorder. Journal of Psychiatric Research, 21, 37–53.

Stefansson, H., Rujescu, D., Cichon, S., Pietiläinen, O. P., Ingason, A., Steinberg, S.,…Stefansson, K. (2008). Large recurrent microdeletions associated with schizophrenia. Nature, 455, 232–236.

Steffenburg, S., Gilberg, C., Hellgren, L., Andersson, L., Gillberg, I. C., Jakobsson, G., & Bohman, M. (1989). A twin study of autism in Denmark, Finland, Iceland, Norway, and Sweden. Journal of Child Psychology and Psychiatry, 30, 405–416.

Stevenson, J. (1992). Evidence for a genetic etiology in hyperactivity in children. Behavior Genetics, 22, 337–344.

Stewart, M. A., Pitts, F. N., Jr., Craig, A. G., & Dieruf, W. (1966). The hyperactive child syndrome. American Journal of Orthopsychiatry, 36, 861–867.

Strober, M., Morrell, W., Burroughs, J., Lampert, C., Danforth, H., & Freeman, R. (1988). A family study of bipolar I disorder in adolescence: Early onset of symptoms linked to increased familial loading and lithium resistance. Journal of Affective Disorders, 15, 255–268.

Sullivan, P. F., Kendler, K. S., & Neale, M. C. (2003). Schizophrenia as a complex trait: Evidence from a meta-analysis of twin studies. Archives of General Psychiatry, 60, 1187–1192.

Sullivan, P. F., Neale, M. C., & Kendler, K. S. (2000). Genetic epidemiology of major depression: Review and meta-analysis. American Journal of Psychiatry, 157, 1552–1562.

Taniai, H., Nishiyama, T., Miyachi, T., Imaeda, M., & Sumi, S. (2008). Genetic influences on the broad spectrum of autism: Study of proband-ascertained twins. American Journal of Medical Genetics, 147B, 844–849.

Thapar, A., Harrington, R., Ross, K., & McGuffin, P. (2000). Does the definition of ADHD affect heritability? Journal of the American Academy of Child and Adolescent Psychiatry, 39, 1528–1536.

Thapar, A., Hervas, A., & McGuffin, P. (1995). Childhood hyperactivity scores are highly heritable and show sibling competition effects: Twin study evidence. Behavior Genetics, 25, 537–544.

Tienari, P., Wynne, L. C., Laksy, K., Moring, J., Nieminen, P., Sorri, A.,…Wahlberg, K. E. (2003). Genetic boundaries of the schizophrenia spectrum: Evidence from the Finnish adoptive family study of schizophrenia. American Journal of Psychiatry, 160, 1587–1594.

Torgersen, S. (1983). Genetic factors in anxiety disorders. Archives of General Psychiatry, 40, 1085–1089.

Torgersen, S. (1986). Genetic factors in moderately severe and mild affective disorders. Archives of General Psychiatry, 43, 222–226.

Tsuang, M. T., Faraone, S. V., & Fleming, J. A. (1985). Familial transmission of major affective disorders: Is there evidence supporting the distinction between unipolar and bipolar disorders? British Journal of Psychiatry, 146, 268–271.

Tsuang, M. T., Winokur, G., & Crowe, R. R. (1980). Morbidity risks of schizophrenia and affective disorders among first-degree relatives of patients with schizophrenia, mania, depression and surgical conditions. *British Journal of Psychiatry, 137*, 497–504.

Tsujita, T., Okazaki, Y., Fujimaru, K., Minami, Y., Mutoh, Y., Maeda, H.,…Nakane, Y. (1992). *Twin concordance rate of DSM-III-R schizophrenia in a new Japanese sample.* Paper presented at the Seventh International Congress on Twin Studies, Tokyo, Japan.

Varma, S. L., Zain, A. M., & Singh, S. (1997). Psychiatric morbidity in the first-degree relatives of schizophrenic patients. *American Journal of Medical Genetics, 74*, 7–11.

Venter, J. C., Adams, M. D., Myers, E. W., Li, P. W., Mural, R. J., Sutton, G. G.,…Zhu, X. (2001). The sequence of the human genome. *Science, 291*, 1304–1351.

Wals, M., Hillegers, M. H., Reichart, C. G., Ormel, J., Nolen, W. A., & Verhulst, F. C. (2001). Prevalence of psychopathology in children of a bipolar parent. *Journal of the American Academy of Child and Adolescent Psychiatry, 40*, 1094–1102.

Weissman, M. M. (1993). Family genetic studies of panic disorder. *Journal of Psychiatric Research, 27*, 69–78.

Weissman, M. M., Gershon, E. S., Kidd, K. K., Prusoff, B. A., Leckman, J. F., Dibble, E.,… Guroff, J. J. (1984). Psychiatric disorders in the relatives of probands with affective disorders: The Yale University–National Institute of Mental Health Collaborative Study. *Archives of General Psychiatry, 41*, 13–21.

Weissman, M. M., Kidd, K. K., & Prusoff, B. A. (1982). Variability in rates of affective disorders in relatives of depressed and normal probands. *Archives of General Psychiatry, 39*, 1397–1403.

Weissman, M. M., Merikangas, K. R., Wickramaratne, P., Kidd, K. K., Prusoff, B. A., Leckman, J. F., & Pauls, D. L. (1986). Understanding the clinical heterogeneity of major depression using family data. *Archives of General Psychiatry, 43*, 430–434.

Welner, Z., Welner, A., Stewart, M., Palkes, H., & Wish, E. (1977). A controlled study of siblings of hyperactive children. *Journal of Nervous and Mental Disease, 165*, 110–117.

Wender, P., Kety, S. S., Rosenthal, D., Schulsinger, F., Ortmann, J., & Lunde, I. (1986). Psychiatric disorders in the biological and adoptive families of adopted individuals with affective disorders. *Archives of General Psychiatry, 43*, 923–929.

Werry, J.S. (12968) Developmental hyperactivity. *Pediatric Clinics of North America, 15*, 581–599.

Willcutt, E. G., Pennington, B. F., & DeFries, J. C. (2000). Etiology of inattention and hyperactivity/impulsivity in a community sample of twins with learning difficulties. *Journal of Abnormal Child Psychology, 28*, 149–159.

Willerman, L. (1973). Activity level and hyperactivity in twins. *Child Development, 44*, 288–293.

Winokur, G., Clayton, P., Reich, T. (1969) Manic-depressive illness. St. Louis, MO: Mosby.

Winokur, G., Tsuang, M., & Crowe, R. R. (1982). The Iowa 500: Affective disorder in relatives of manic and depressed patients. *American Journal of Psychiatry, 139*, 209–212.

Wood, A., Rijsdijk, F., Saudino, K. J., Asherson, P., & Kuntsi, J. (2008). High heritability for a composite index of children's activity level measures. *Behavior Genetics, 38*, 266–276.

World Health Organization (1968). ICD-8 classification of mental and behavioral disorders - diagnostic criteria for research. World Health Organization.

World Health Organization (1979). ICD-9 classification of mental and behavioral disorders - diagnostic criteria for research. World Health Organization.

World Health Organization (1993). ICD-10 classification of mental and behavioral disorders - diagnostic criteria for research. World Health Organization.

Xing, Y., & Lee, C. (2006). Alternative splicing and RNA selection pressure—evolutionary consequences for eukaryotic genomes. *Nature Reviews Genetics, 7*, 499–509.

Young, S. E., Stallings, M. C., Corley, R. P., Krauter, K. S., & Hewitt, J. K. (2000). Genetic and environmental influences on behavioral disinhibition. *American Journal of Medical Genetics, 96*, 684–695.

Zubenko, G. S., Huff, F. J., Beyer, J., Auerbach, J., & Teply, I. (1988). Familial risk of dementia associated with a biologic subtype of Alzheimer's disease. *Archives of General Psychiatry, 45*, 889–893.

9

Mental Disorders Across the Life Span and the Role of Executive Function Networks

MICHELLE C. CARLSON

DANA ELDRETH

YI-FANG CHUANG

WILLIAM W. EATON

Key Points

- From an evolutionary perspective the prefrontal cortex (PFC) is the newest region of the brain and is responsible for integrating the past and present in anticipation of future rewards and threats

- The PFC is the locus of executive function and the regulation of many prosocial behaviors

- Executive function is a key domain of cognition that is related to vulnerability to mental disorders over the life course

- During developmental windows in both PFC maturation and decline, the brain may be more biologically vulnerable to environmental stressors that act as risk factors for mental illnesses

- Certain mental disorders, such as attention deficit hyperactivity disorder, schizophrenia, and depression, and progressive neurologic disorders such as Huntington's disease and Alzheimer's disease arise during periods tied to the development of executive functions over the life course

- Biomarkers developed from research in neuroimaging, genetics, and neurochemistry improve accuracy of diagnoses, help explain pathogenesis and pathophysiology, and predict prognosis

- Therapies and rehabilitation strategies used to improve planning and problem solving may be helpful in a range of mental and behavioral disorders with deficits in executive function

- Older adults at high risk for executive dysfunction maintain great potential for brain plasticity and cognitive resilience

INTRODUCTION

The brain is the organ from which all behavior emanates, whether functional or dysfunctional. Mental disorders often arise as the result of chronic brain dysfunctions. Understanding the etiologies and common pathways to mental disorders merits a life span examination of development of the prefrontal cortex (PFC), the longest developing and behaviorally most complex region of the brain. From an evolutionary perspective, the PFC is the newest region of the brain and is responsible for integrating the past and present in anticipation of future rewards and threats. It further represents the locus in regulating many prosocial behaviors. The life course perspective offered in this chapter links the development of this crucial regional network and the onset of numerous brain–behavior disorders, from youth through late life, providing a novel framework from which to build an understanding of common pathways through which multiple etiologies affect mental health. Identification of common pathways will offer novel and synergistic perspectives into early detection of those individuals who are most vulnerable to mental disorders and at the same time will guide primary and secondary prevention and treatment interventions targeting components of executive function and dysfunction.

This chapter begins by defining executive functions and their importance to prosocial behavior and independent functioning. It then describes how these functions develop concomitantly with prefrontal brain growth through childhood and adolescence and decline in late life. Next the chapter reviews specific mental disorders that arise during these developmental windows and the executive dysfunctions common to those disorders. The disorders considered, which occur in early, mid-, and later life, include attention deficit hyperactivity disorder, schizophrenia, depression, generalized anxiety disorder, Huntington's disease, Parkinson's disease, and possibly Alzheimer's disease. The chapter concludes by highlighting the importance of imaging and biomarkers, methods that will continue to elucidate brain–behavior relationships and so aid early detection, prognosis, and treatment. Use of these tools may yield insight into whether developmental lags or noxious exposures at various stages of prefrontal maturation lead to pleiotropic phenotypes or disorders. At the fundamental public health level, better understanding the intersection of PFC development and the etiology of mental illness may help inform the design of increasingly effective therapeutic programs that extend beyond the treatment of individual disorders by incorporating a common approach to target executive dysfunctions more broadly. These programs could both enrich and buffer executive function over the life course, particularly in persons with mental disorders, who may be particularly vulnerable to age-related developmental declines in executive function.

DEVELOPMENT AND EXECUTIVE FUNCTION

A general overview of normative brain–behavior development and how declines in executive function late in life mirror patterns of growth during youth provides a foundation on which an understanding of behavioral disorders cross the life course can be built. Executive function, a key domain of cognition, appears particularly vulnerable to mental disorders over the life course. This is likely due in part to the PFC's long developmental window from infancy through emerging adulthood, and optimally requires intact development and integration of complex networks within the PFC. The PFC is a large area that is functionally divided into three regions and parallel circuits: the orbitofrontal cortex (the most ventral part of the PFC), the dorsolateral cortex (DLPFC), and the anterior cingulate cortex (ACC) (Cummings, 1993). The PFC represents a "top down" region that regulates the limbic network, including both the hippocampus and the amygdala, which are respectively responsible for memory and acquisition of emotional memory. Top-down executive regulation of these limbic regions by the PFC involves integration of the past, present, and anticipated future gains in the execution of goal-directed behavior. In day-to-day operational terms, executive processes generally involve the initiation, planning, coordination, and sequencing of actions toward the completion of a goal (Baddeley, Bressi, Della Sala, Logie, & Spinnler, 1991; Baddeley, Logie, Bressi, Della Sala, & Spinnler, 1986; Meyer & Kleras, 1997; Norman & Shallice, 1986; Shallice, 1994; West, 1996). Psychometric tasks have been used to identify and separate complex components of executive function according to:

- task switching and set shifting, as when one flexibly responds to a new work priority or a delay
- inhibition of distracting or irrelevant information in the environment and in memory, as when trying to locate in a crowd your friend in the green sweater
- working memory, in which one manipulates stored information, as when mentally calculating one's portion of a group dinner bill.

These component abilities have been extensively mapped to specific prefrontal structures using lesion studies (e.g., Drewe, 1975) and, more recently, through advanced neuroimaging

techniques (e.g., Bush, Whalen, Shin, & Rauch, 2006; D'Esposito et al., 1995; Smith & Jonides, 1999). As a result, they can provide valuable insight into the pathophysiology of mental disorders.

These executive abilities have been associated in imaging studies primarily with the activation of a number of prefrontal regions, such as the DLPFC and the ACC (Botvinick, Nystrom, Fissell, Carter, & Cohen, 1999; C. S. Carter, Mintun, & Cohen, 1995 Casey, Giedd, & Thomas, 2000; Hazeltine, Bunge, Scanlon, & Gabrieli, 2003; Hazeltine, Poldrack, & Gabrieli, 2000; Pardo, Pardo, Janer, & Raichle, 1990; Rafal et al., 1996). The ontogeny of the PFC lags behind that of the brain's sensory regions. Maturation remains incomplete until one's early 20s (Gogtay et al., 2004), presumably because the development of the complex integrative functions supported by the PFC follows maturation of simpler and sensory-specific networks (Garon, Bryson, & Smith, 2008). Total gray matter volume increases through childhood and decreases (or is "pruned") after puberty (Giedd et al., 1999; Sowell, Thompson, Tessner & Toga, 2001). In comparison, white matter tissue, which provides connections across gray matter regions, grows progressively from posterior to anterior regions into adulthood (Giedd et al., 1999; Jernigan et al., 1991; Paus et al., 1999). During the PFC's more protracted developmental period, both frontal-striatal-thalamic and frontal–cerebellar networks that mediate inhibitory control of attention mature steadily from childhood to adulthood (Casey, Getz, & Galvan, 2008; Rubia, Smith, Taylor, & Brammer, 2007), concomitantly with age-associated increases in prefrontal activity (Bunge, Dudukovic, Thomason, Vaidya, & Gabrieli, 2002; Durston and Casey, 2006; Rubia et al., 2000; Tamm, Menon, & Reiss, 2002). Motor-based inhibitory abilities mediated by the more rapidly maturing parietal cortex develop by adolescence; more complex, executive inhibitory abilities mediated by the prefrontal lobes continue to develop into adulthood (Adleman et al., 2002; Casey, Thomas, Davidson, Kunz, & Franzen, 2002). Maturation of executive inhibitory control in adulthood may account for the partial resolution of behavioral impulsivity and hyperactivity symptoms common to disorders such as attention deficit hyperactivity disorder (ADHD), the first disorder that will be reviewed in this chapter.

DEVELOPMENTAL DECLINES IN EXECUTIVE FUNCTION

The late-developing PFC is more vulnerable than other brain regions to the effects of aging, a finding that led Fuster (1989) to coin the phrase "last in, first out." Substantial age-related deficits have been observed in each of the executive control abilities mentioned above. For example, with increasing age, older adults show, difficulties in tasks requiring the inhibition of prepotent, or well-practiced, responses, such as the Stroop task, during which one must inhibit a rapidly available response, reading the name of a color, in favor of naming the conflicting color of the ink the word is printed in (Kramer & Atchley, 2000; Nieuwenhuis, Ridderinkhof, de Jong, Kok, & van der Molen, 2000; Olincy, Ross, Young, & Freedman, 1997). Similarly, age-related reductions in activity of the DLPFC have been associated with poorer response inhibition (Milham et al., 2002). Age-related decreases in DLPFC activation, and corresponding increases in ACC activation, have been interpreted as representing a decrease in the DLPFC's ability to exert control over the capacity to maintain attention, making older adults more susceptible to environmental distraction (Banich et al., 2000, 2001; MacDonald, Cohen, Stenger, & Carter, 2000; Milham et al., 2002).

In longitudinal observations of older, community-dwelling adults, the task-switching component of prefrontally mediated executive function has been shown to decline earlier than verbal memory (Carlson, Xue, Zhou, & Fried, 2009), suggesting that interventions targeting executive function could delay and thereby mitigate memory declines that may lead to dementia. Consistent with this finding that executive declines precede declines in memory, in vivo studies of the aging human brain reliably demonstrate disproportionately greater loss of cortical volume in the frontal and prefrontal regions than in the parietal and temporal areas

responsible for memory formation and language (Buckner, 2004; Madden, 2000; Raz, 2000; Resnick, Pham, Kraut, Zonderman, & Davatzikos, 2003). Further, connecting white matter also undergoes substantial decay in the later stages of the life course, with the largest deterioration occurring in prefrontal regions and in tracts leading to and from the anterior brain regions (K. M. Kennedy et al., 2009). One study linked such reductions in the integrity of connective white matter tissue, with slower performance on visual target detection tasks in older individuals (Madden et al., 2004).

The functional consequences of decreased executive control over distraction appear to include decreased capacity to perform instrumental activities of daily living among aging adults and individuals with progressive mental disorders as well as among those with vascular dementia and Parkinson's disease (Boyle et al., 2003; Cahn et al., 1998; Cahn-Weiner, Boyle, & Malloy, 2002; Cahn-Weiner, Ready, & Malloy, 2003; Cahn-Weiner et al., 2007; Royall, Palmer, Chiodo, & Polk, 2004, 2005). Thus executive functions are an important potential target for community and clinical intervention.

BIOLOGICAL WINDOWS OF VULNERABILITY TO MENTAL DISORDERS

The brain may be particularly vulnerable to the onset of mental disorders at particular stages of PFC development and decline across the life span. During such developmental windows in both PFC maturation and decline, the brain may be more biologically vulnerable to environmental stressors that act as risk factors for mental illnesses. This interaction between biological vulnerability, or diathesis, and environmental stressors is summarized as the diathesis–stress model, described in detail in chapter 10 and most commonly applied to the onset of schizophrenia (Bleuler, 1963; Rosenthal, 1963). Many mental disorders, including ADHD, schizophrenia, depression, and generalized anxiety disorder, and neurodegenerative dementias such as Huntington's disease, Parkinson's disease, and Alzheimer's disease are associated with deficits in inhibitory control and with dysfunction of supporting frontostriatal (Huntington's and Parkinson's disease) and mesolimbic (Alzheimer's disease) pathways. We now turn to a review of each of these disorders in the context of their relationship to brain developmental milestones.

Attention Deficit Hyperactivity Disorder

Attention deficit hyperactivity disorder is a heterogeneous developmental disorder with clinical features that include inattention, difficulty completing tasks, impulsivity, and hyperactivity, all of which interfere with performance at school or work (American Psychiatric Association [APA], 2000). The prevalence rate for ADHD is estimated to be 5.3% worldwide (Polanczyk, deLima, Horta, Biederman, & Rohde, 2007). As cited in chapter 1, a median 1-year prevalence rate of 2.60% was reported in 21 studies of ADHD. Estimates in school-age children in the United States range from 3% to 7% (APA, 2000). Of the associated symptoms, impulsivity and hyperactivity sharply decline with age from childhood through adolescence into early adulthood (Biederman, Mick, & Farone, 2000), coinciding with the maturation of the PFC (Diamond, 2002). Given increased independence in adolescence, young people with ADHD appear more likely to engage in risky behaviors such as smoking (Lambert & Hartsough, 1998), unprotected sex (Barkley, 1998), alcohol and drug use (Barkley, 1998), and criminal behavior (Satterfield & Schell, 1997). Onset and remission of selected ADHD symptoms during frontal lobe development highlight the brain's vulnerability and plasticity during these critical windows (Barkley, 1997).

The frontostriatal circuits are key targets of ADHD investigation. This network encompasses the PFC, the ACC, and the subcortical striatum (caudate and putamen). ADHD is associated with deficits in inhibitory control, an executive function largely orchestrated by the ACC (Bush, Luu, & Posner, 2000) and the DLPFC (Garavan, Ross, & Stein, 1999; Rubia, Smith, Brammer, & Taylor, 2003). Some researchers postulate that ADHD is associated with a maturational delay of approximately three years (Shaw et al., 2007) in prefrontal regions that regulate inhibitory control, attention, and perception of time (Castellanos et al., 2002; Rubia et al., 2007). Coinciding with this lag are inefficient recruitment of prefrontal areas within the frontostriatal circuit and cerebellum in both boys (Castellanos et al., 1996) and girls (Castellanos et al., 2001), as well as striatal brain volume reductions, primarily in boys (A. Qiu et al., 2009). Reduced prefrontal volume also has been observed in children with ADHD (Castellanos et al., 1996). During cognitive tasks involving response inhibition, adolescents with ADHD have been found to experience diminished recruitment of the frontostriatal network (Bush, Valera, & Seidman, 2005; Casey et al., 1997; Durston, 2003). Other studies of inhibitory control in ADHD have found prefrontal hyperactivity (Schulz et al., 2005) along with striatal hypoactivity (Vaidya et al., 1998), which may reflect either inefficient compensatory mechanisms or dysregulated neural networks (Gatzke-Kopp & Beauchaine, 2007).

In addition to the frontostriatal network, altered mesolimbic–cortical dopamine circuitry may contribute to cognitive symptoms of ADHD such as inattentiveness, impulsivity, hyperactivity, and executive dysfunction (Ernst et al., 2003; Johansen, Aase, Meyer, & Sagvolden, 2002). This circuit encompasses the DLPFC, the temporal cortex, and the ACC as well as the mesolimbic system, including both the amygdala and hippocampus (Swartz, 1999). Altered reward and motivational processing in ADHD is thought to result from disruption of or altered pathways in this circuitry (Johansen et al., 2002). The pursuit of immediate reward is a particularly salient feature in ADHD, due perhaps to ineffective top-down control of the ventral striatum by the orbital PFC. In addition to top-down control deficits, hypoactivation in the ventral striatum during reward anticipation may underlie the propensity toward reward-seeking behaviors, impulsivity, and hyperactivity in ADHD as a compensatory mechanism (Scheres, Milham, Knutson, & Castellanos, 2007). From a life course perspective, ADHD symptoms may remit, in part, as a result of the progressive white matter myelination of prefrontal regions through adolescence, and of continued synaptic pruning, both of which increase efficiency of neural communication and top-down executive control (Durston & Casey, 2006).

Schizophrenia

Given this chapter's focus on attention, the genesis of the term schizophrenia is instructive. Bleuler created the term from the Greek roots schizen ("split") and phren- ("mind") to highlight the disconnect between higher-order thought processes and sensory perception that is characteristic of the disorder. Schizophrenia typically manifests in late adolescence and early adulthood, when higher-order, executive abilities mediated by the PFC reach maturation. As described in chapter 8, the etiology of schizophrenia is complex and determined by the interplay of genetic vulnerabilities and environmental risk factors. While highly heritable, with some estimates of its overall heritability as high as 70% (Jones & Cannon, 1998; Kendler, 1988) (see also table 8-6), schizophrenia is a disorder of multifactorial inheritance. Most likely, several genes interact to elevate biological risk for schizophrenia. Genetic evidence for the role of the environment in the etiology of schizophrenia comes from the observation that in monozygotic twins, who share 100% of their genes, sometimes one twin is affected but the other twin is not; the review of 10 studies in chapter 8 suggests that when one identical twin has been so diagnosed, the second twin has between a 41%–79% chance of developing the disorder, depending on the particular study (see also Cardno & Gottesman, 2000) . Additional potential, and difficult to evaluate, predisposing environmental agents may include prenatal complications (Dalman, Allebeck, Cullberg, Grunewald, & Koster, 1999), maternal exposures to stress (King, Laplante, & Joober, 2005), influenza (A. S. Brown et al., 2004), taxoplasma (A. S. Brown et al., 2005), and lower socioeconomic status (Fox, 1990) in vulnerable individuals.

Evidence from behavioral and neuroimaging studies further demonstrates that early (Cervellione, Burdick, Cottone, Rhinewine, & Kumra, 2007; Frangou, Hadjulis, & Vourdas, 2008; Zanelli et al., 2010), perhaps prodromal features (Cannon et al., 2006; Jahshan, Heaton, Golshan, & Cadenhead, 2010) of schizophrenia include deficits in executive function. This executive function deficit during adolescent and early adult development and the associated transitions to functional independence either may unmask or trigger vulnerability, as when making decisions about living arrangements, career, and relationships (Eaton & Harrison, 2001). The detection and diagnosis of schizophrenia illustrate how development of a mental disorder often involves an interaction between diathesis (predisposition) and stress arising from environmental and social expectations. A variety of cross-sectional neuroimaging studies comparing brain images of controls and of individuals with schizophrenia have observed differences in DLPFC structure and function at both early and later stages of the disorder (Barch et al., 2001; Berman, Illowsky, & Weinberger, 1988; Davatzikos et al., 2005; Frangou, 2010; Weinberger, Berman, Suddath, & Torrey, 1992). In addition, older adults with schizophrenia show larger deficits in executive function relative to controls than do younger cases (Fucetola et al., 2000). To date, however, no prospective data have disclosed whether individuals with schizophrenia are at increased risk for accelerated declines in executive function with age.

The deficits in executive function and other cognitive functions in schizophrenia co-occur with psychiatric symptomatology such as disturbances of thought (delusions) and perception (visual or auditory hallucinations). These disturbances have been theorized to reflect deficits in inhibitory executive functions and to give rise to mood disturbances and withdrawal (Green, 1996; Liddle, 1987; Mueser & McGurk, 2004). Other cognitive disruptions in schizophrenia include alterations in attention, motivation, and affect, all governed in part by the ACC (Devinsky, Morrell, & Vogt, 1995) within the cortical–limbic network (Benes, 1993; Benes, Turtle, Khan, & Farol, 1994). Altered inhibitory function is thought to reflect deficits in both prefrontal and ACC activity with increasing cognitive demand (Blasi et al., 2009). These alterations in functional neural networks may represent part of a developmental cascade in which one developmental deficit gives rise to another, ultimately leading to the cognitive symptomatology observed in schizophrenia.

The hypothalamic-pituitary-adrenal (HPA) axis is an important limbic neural network that matures more rapidly than the prefrontal cortical network. Like the PFC, the HPA axis is a pathway involved in reacting to real and perceived environmental threats; its dysregulation increases vulnerability to schizophrenia. (For a review, see Walker, Mittal, & Tessner, 2008.) Evidence for HPA dysregulation among adolescents with schizophrenia (Muck-Seler et al., 2004; Walsh, Spelman, Sharifi, & Thakore, 2005) has been found in the form of reduced hippocampal volume (Geuze, Vermetten, & Bremner, 2005; Steen, Mull, McClure, Hamer, & Lieberman, 2006) and altered dopamine in mesolimbic circuits (Marinelli, Rudick, Hu, & White, 2006). During adolescence, marked increases in cortisol, the stress hormone regulated by the HPA axis, have been linked to the development of schizophrenia (Walker, Walder, & Reynolds, 2001). The excitatory pathways in the HPA are influenced by limbic structures responsible for emotional processing such as the amygdala and hippocampus, which in turn are upregulated and downregulated by the cognitive control of emotions through the PFC (Ochsner et al., 2004).

From the standpoint of biological vulnerability, many genes have been implicated in schizophrenia (Kirov, O'Donovan, & Owen, 2005); they act primarily on glutamatergic neurotransmission. (For a review, see Lisman et al., 2008.) The vulnerability–stress model of schizophrenia suggests that a confluence of latent and developmental environmental exposures with dopaminergic dysfunction not only affecting executive function in the PFC but also leading to autonomic hyperactivity in the HPA axis and limbic structures (Nuechterlein et al., 1994).

Depression

In early adulthood and midlife, feelings of anhedonia, fatigue, and loss of motivation are crippling symptoms of depressive disorders. The lifetime prevalence of depression, which is often accompanied by functional disability, is estimated at between 2% and 15% (Üstün,

Ayuso-Mateos, Chatterji, Mathers, & Murray, 2004). This range is consistent with the 1-year prevalence rate of 5.3% reported in the review of 42 studies in chapter 1. Depression occurs more frequently in females than in males. This gender disparity begins around the age of 13, coinciding with the earlier development of the hypothalamic-pituitary-gonadal system in girls than boys (Angold & Costello, 2006). Rates become more uniform across genders by age 55 (Bebbington, 1996; Bebbington et al., 1998). The median age of onset of major depressive disorder has been estimated to be 30 years (Kessler, Chiu, Demler, Merikangas, & Walters, 2005), occurring concurrently with independence and seminal developmental milestones such as establishing a career, home, marriage, and family. In older adults, the prevalence of depression is significantly less than in younger adults (Jorm, 2000; Kessler et al., 2005), and as reported in chapter 6, incidence rates decline sharply after age 65. Early or cumulative life course stressors may trigger depressive episodes in genetically and environmentally at-risk individuals by altering prefrontal networks and mesolimbic dopamine networks. (For a review, see Cabib & Puglisi-Allegra, 1996.)

Individuals with depressive disorders often have a predisposition to focus on negative rather than positive aspects of experiences, exemplified by negative attention and recall biases (Clark & Beck, 1999) that may make them more cognitively vulnerable when exposed to stressors (Abela & Hankin, 2008). From a neurocognitive perspective, individuals with depression generally exhibit limited top-down executive control and excessive bottom-up (detail-oriented) processing of events and information, which may restrict their ability to regulate and put negative biases in context (Beck, 2008). A general pattern of brain activation observed in patients with depression includes hypoactivity in frontal regions and hyperactivity in limbic regions such as the amygdala (Siegle, Steinhauer, Thase, Stenger, & Carter, 2002; Siegle, Thompson, Carter, Steinhauer, & Thase, 2007) and insula (Mayberg et al., 1999). Disruption of the prefrontal–limbic circuit results in mood dysregulation as a result of the limited top-down prefrontal control over limbic emotional processing centers. For example, in individuals without depression, reappraisal of negative stimuli involves activation of the left ventromedial PFC with downregulation of the amygdala, whereas those with depression exhibit bilateral PFC recruitment and excitation of the amygdala, suggesting an inability to effectively modulate emotions despite enhanced PFC activity (Johnstone, van Reekum, Urry, Kalin, & Davidson, 2007). Patients with depression also have been found to have decreased brain volume, regional cerebral blood flow, and metabolism in regions of the subgenual PFC (Drevets et al., 1997). In mid- to late life, those with depression display decreased prefrontal volume (Coffey et al., 1993; Krishnan et al., 1992) compared with those without depressive disorders. In late life, depression is associated with white matter microstructural changes within the DLPFC that may disrupt connectivity with limbic structures responsible for emotion (Taylor et al., 2004). Moreover, older adults with depression exhibit executive dysfunction (Lockwood, Alexopoulos, & van Gorp, 2002), which may have an adverse effect on treatment response and adherence (Alexopoulos et al., 2000; Mohlman, 2005). As a result, cognitive behavioral therapies often implement strategies to bolster executive cognitive skills (Mohlman et al., 2010). The growing understanding of the role of the PFC in dysfunctional modulation of emotional systems has substantial implications both for cognitive-based interventions that build on executive skills and for pharmacotherapies that target deficits in executive function and associated networks.

Generalized Anxiety Disorder

Generalized anxiety disorder (GAD) is characterized by chronic, excessive, and uncontrollable worry that occurs most days and persists for at least six months (APA, 2000). It also must be accompanied by at least three other symptoms, such as difficulty concentrating, severe insomnia, irritability, muscle tension, restlessness, and fatigue. Ultimately, lifetime symptoms are associated with missed work (Olfson et al., 1997), hypertension (Barger &

Sydeman, 2005; B. Kennedy & Schwab, 1997), and increased risk for coronary heart disease (Kubzansky et al., 1997). Comorbidity with depression is estimated at 12% in individuals between the ages of 11 and 32 years (Moffitt et al., 2007).

The onset of GAD generally occurs between the late teens and late 20s, with significantly less frequency after age 35 (Barlow, Blanchard, Vermilyea, Vermilyea, & DiNardo, 1986; Rogers et al., 1999). Like other major mental disorders, GAD is considered a chronic disorder; symptoms may remit and recur for decades (Kessler & Wittchen, 2002) and become exacerbated during periods of stress (APA, 2000). Epidemiologic studies estimate the lifetime prevalence of GAD in the United States at between 4% and 7% of the population (Blazer, Hughes, George, Swartz, & Boyer, 1991; Kessler, DuPont, Berglund, & Wittchen, 1999; Wittchen, Zhao, Kessler, & Eaton, 1994). It is twice as prevalent in women as in men (Robins & Regier, 1991).

Generalized anxiety disorder is characterized by a reliance on worry as an emotional regulation strategy. Worry may be provoked by negative perceptions of ambiguous information (Dugas, Buhr, & Ladouceur, 2004; Dugas, Gosselin, & Ladouceur, 2001; Ladouceur et al., 1999), automatic encoding and retrieval of threatening information (MacLeod & Rutherford, 2004), or poor understanding of or negative response to aversive emotions (Mennin, Heimberg, Turk, & Fresco, 2005); alternatively, it may be perceived as a problem solving strategy (Wells, 1999, 2004). The possible triggers of GAD are integrated into one of the most influential models on this topic: the avoidance theory of worry (Borkovec, Alcaine, & Behar, 2004; Borkovec & Inz, 1990; Borkovec, Ray, & Stober, 1998).

Like behavioral avoidance, worry is a mechanism by which the unpleasant, anxious arousal provoked by aversive stimuli may be mitigated; as a result, worry becomes a learned and maintained behavior (Mowrer, 1947). Unlike behavioral avoidance, worry is initiated as a cognitive avoidance strategy when a threat is perceived and cannot be circumvented. Physiological consequences of worry include low vagal tone and reduced heart rate variability, which diminish the flexibility of parasympathetic HPA response to changing environmental demands (Lyonfields, Borkovec, & Thayer, 1995; Thayer, Friedman, & Borkovec, 1996; Thayer & Lane, 2000, 2002).

As noted above, the PFC exerts cognitive control through downregulation of activity in limbic structures responsible for emotional processing, such as the amygdala (Ochsner et al., 2004) and insula (Goldin, McRae, Ramel, & Gross, 2008). Electroencephalography indicates that prefrontal areas are involved actively during worry and anxious arousal (W. R. Carter, Johnson, & Borkovec, 1986; Heller, Nitschke, Etienne, & Miller, 1997; Hofmann et al., 2005; Nitschke & Heller, 2002). Moreover, induction of worry in individuals who otherwise are not worried is associated with similar increased activity in the medial orbital frontal gyrus and decreased activity in the amygdala and insula (Hoehn-Saric, Lee, McLeod, & Wong, 2005). In a pharmacological treatment study in generalized anxiety disorder, decreases in activity of prefrontal and thalamostriatal regions were observed following treatment using a similar worry induction paradigm (Hoehn-Saric, Schlund, & Wong, 2004). These prefrontal regions mediate inhibitory control, a process positively related to the severity of worry (Price & Mohlman, 2007) and to medial orbitofrontal volume (Mohlman et al., 2009). In all, worry appears to activate prefrontal resources to overexpress executive inhibitory control over limbic structures that are implicated in fear processing and autonomic arousal.

Neurodegenerative Disorders

Huntington's disease (HD), Parkinson's disease (PD), and Alzheimer's disease (AD) are all progressive neurologic disorders. Huntington's disease, an autosomal dominant disorder with 100% penetrance, is characterized genetically by an unstable expanded trinucleotide CAG repeat coding for glutamine. It leads to degeneration of the caudate nucleus in the striatum and results in the insidious development of involuntary movements (chorea), impaired voluntary movement, and prominent executive dysfunction beginning in an individual's late 40s and early 50s. Parkinson's disease was first described in 1817 by James Parkinson, who

identified a group of patients with a shaking palsy (resting tremor), and involves degeneration of the putamen in the striatum. The etiology of the disease is attributed to unknown interactions among genetic vulnerabilities and environmental factors such as head injury and toxin exposure. The prevalence of PD rises markedly with age, from 1% of the population over age 55 in the United States to 3% over age 70. The most common age-related neurodegenerative disorder is AD, characterized by a gradual deterioration in memory, language, and other cognitive functions as well as by changes in behavior and impairments in activities of daily living. After age 65 years, the prevalence and incidence of AD increase exponentially with age, doubling every five years with advancing age (Jorm & Jolley, 1998; C. Qiu, De Ronchi, & Fratiglioni, 2007; Ziegler-Graham, Brookmeyer, Johnson, & Arrighi, 2008). In 2006, the worldwide prevalence of AD was 26.6 million cases, a figure expected to rise fourfold over the next 50 years (Brookmeyer, Johnson, Ziegler-Graham, & Arrighi, 2007). The causes of AD are not well understood, but many risk factors have been identified, among them genes (described in chapter 8), vascular factors (e.g., hypertension, diabetes, and obesity), diet and nutritional factors, and psychosocial and lifestyle factors (e.g., social networks, leisure activities, and physical activities). (For reviews, see C. Qiu et al., 2007; Studenski et al., 2006.)

Regardless of age, executive processes are defective in both HD (Aron et al., 2003; Lawrence & Jette, 1996; Sprengelmeyer, Lange, & Homberg, 1995) and PD (Cools, Barker, Sahakian, & Robbins, 2001; Gauntlett-Gilbert, Roberts, & Brown, 1999; Lees & Smith, 1983; Pollux, 2004). These deficits appear to result from degeneration of frontostriatal circuits linking the PFC to the caudate and putamen (R. G. Brown & Marsden, 1990; Gotham, Brown, & Marsden, 1988) delineated by Cummings (1993). In HD, small changes in set-shifting demands (one of the three components of executive function noted above) lead to costly errors and increased reaction time when a prepotent, or highly practiced, motor response must be inhibited (Aron et al., 2003). These impairments are thought to reflect diminished inhibitory control. Like individuals with HD, those with PD display deficits in set shifting (Cools et al., 2001; Lees & Smith, 1983). However, in contrast to HD patients, PD patients experience set-shifting costs only when the shifts are unpredictable and require inhibition of distractors (Cools et al., 2001), possibly as a result of diminished prefrontal control over motor behavior (Aron et al., 2003). Some studies suggesting that these deficits occur only in the absence of external cues, requiring patients to rely on internal strategies (Brown & Marsden, 1988) offer insights into potential intervention strategies to buffer and exercise these attentional abilities. (For a review, see Ogden, 2005.)

UTILITY OF BIOMARKERS IN MENTAL DISORDERS

For each of the mental disorders summarized above, functional and structural neuroimaging have been essential to establish and specify the PFC networks implicated in disease-related cognitive, emotional, and functional deficits. However, these methods have yet to have been translated into early detection, diagnosis, and treatment in the same way that biomarkers have been applied to aid in the diagnosis of other diseases such as diabetes and cardiovascular disease. These biomarkers often are linked directly to the pathophysiology and mechanism of a disease. In the case of mental disorders, however, clinicians rely mainly on symptom expression; biomarkers are used far less routinely to aid in diagnosis of underlying pathology. The current diagnostic system for mental disorders (the nosology articulated in the fourth edition of the *Diagnostic and Statistical Manual of Mental Disorders* [APA, 2000]) has been criticized as insufficient with regard to etiology despite high reliability in diagnosis (McHugh & Slavney, 1998). Thanks to new technologies including neuroimaging, genetic analytical techniques, and both neurochemical and neuropathologic methodologies, biomarkers increasingly are proving valuable to the understanding of some mental disorders, particularly those progressive neuropathologic disorders in which

biological changes can be tracked along with symptom progression. These biomarkers can help improve accuracy of diagnoses, explain pathogenesis and pathophysiology, and predict prognosis. They also can function as intermediate indices of treatment effects in the evaluation of novel therapies. We discuss each contribution in turn.

Biomarkers Can Help Improve Diagnostic Accuracy

The first contribution of biomarkers is to help improve the accuracy of diagnoses of mental disorders. A symptom-based diagnostic system for mental disorders in the absence of measures of pathophysiology can give rise to a greater likelihood of misclassifications or delayed classifications. Biomarkers may serve as useful adjuncts to improve the classification of mental disorders, especially in the early course of a disease. For example, neurodegenerative dementias such as HD, PD, and AD are chronic disorders with insidious onset and long preclinical periods. The memory symptoms of individuals in the early or prodromal stages of AD are not sufficient to affect daily function and thus do not meet current criteria for its diagnosis. As a result, several biomarkers have been proposed for incorporation into AD diagnostic criteria to improve both sensitivity and specificity of diagnosis. Among the candidate biomarkers are magnetic resonance imaging measures of hippocampal atrophy (Desikan et al., 2008; Kerchner et al., 2010), lumbar measures of cerebrospinal fluid to detect low levels of $A\beta_{42}$ and increased levels of tau protein, and positron emission tomography imaging to measure in vivo amyloid plaque burden (Dubois et al., 2007). Biomarkers also may be used to differentiate between unipolar depression and bipolar disorder, specifically following a first depressive episode and prior to a first episode of mania (Phillips & Vieta, 2007). Further, biomarkers may help predict onset of a mental disorder in people either with elevated familial risk or prodromal symptoms. For example, individuals with prodromal AD who show structural alterations in the medial temporal cortex may be more likely to develop psychotic symptoms (Pantelis et al., 2003).

Biomarkers and Mental Disorder Pathophysiology

Biomarkers also may help unravel the etiologic factors and pathophysiology of mental disorders. Many neurochemical, electrophysiological, and neuroimaging biomarkers have been found to be associated with mental disorders. These biomarkers can be considered endophenotypes—intermediate phenotypes (Gottesman & Gould, 2003). Endophenotypes may represent the intermediate steps on the pathophysiological pathways from genotype to phenotype (observable symptoms) and are supposed to have simpler genetic architectures than the disease syndrome itself. In the search for candidate genes in mental disorders, phenotypic heterogeneity may contribute in part to small effect sizes and the failure to replicate most findings (Burmeister, McInnis, & Zollner, 2008).

However, when one combines endophenotypes with functional polymorphisms or other genetic variants, they both increase the likelihood of identifying the underlying causes of mental disorders and facilitate understanding of the pathogenesis. This method, for example, has provided insight into the role in schizophrenia of the dopamine system, in which dysregulation may serve as a mechanism through which working memory is affected (Diaz-Asper et al., 2008). Deficits in sensorimotor gating represent another widely studied, schizophrenia-related neurophysiological biomarker (Adler et al., 1982; Braff & Geyer, 1990). Such deficits provide a biologically plausible pathway to account for well-characterized difficulties in filtering information from multiple sensory inputs (Grillon, Courchesne, Ameli, Geyer, & Braff, 1990). In addition, use of this neurophysiological biomarker has resulted in identification of a potential susceptibility locus on chromosome 15 (R. Freedman et al., 1997).

It is difficult to establish animal models for mental disorders, especially those affecting insight and involving subjective psychological experiences, such as schizophrenia. Identification of endophenotypes permits mental disorders to be modeled in animals, since they can be objectively measured in parallel in humans and animals. Once an animal model of mental disorders is established, it can help guide the search for underlying mechanisms of onset and progression and can serve to provide intermediate outcomes in the identification of novel pharmacologic agents and therapies. For example, prepulse inhibition, by serving as a measurable behavioral outcome in mouse models of schizophrenia, has facilitated investigation of the genetic bases of sensorimotor gating and advanced knowledge about the pathophysiology and neurobiology of schizophrenia in humans (Geyer, McIlwain, & Paylor, 2002; Swerdlow & Geyer, 1998).

Biomarkers in Clinical Practice

Biomarkers may play an important role in clinical practice in providing information about the prognosis of mental disorders. For example, in early AD, positive amyloid imaging, low levels of $A\beta_{42,}$ and increased levels of tau protein in cerebrospinal fluid represent good predictors of conversion from a preclinical memory disorder with mild cognitive impairment to AD (Jack et al., 2010). In addition, objective, reliable outcome measures offer advantages over subjective measures such as self-reported improvement in symptoms, which are sometimes unreliable, particularly in individuals experiencing cognitive declines. The use of biomarkers as outcome measures may confer an advantage in identifying intermediate treatment effects that target mechanism(s) of the disease. For example, neuroimaging has demonstrated that phobia is associated with hyperactivation in the insula and ACC and that successful cognitive behavioral therapy attenuates activity in these regions (Straube, Glauer, Dilger, Mentzel, & Miltner, 2006). In addition to monitoring effect of behavioral treatments, genetic biomarkers may also be used to predict drug responses (Nnadi & Malhotra, 2007).

Biomarkers and New Therapeutic Developments

Finally, an improved understanding of pathophysiology is important to developing effective therapies. Biomarkers with known neurochemical bases can be used to identify novel targets for treatment and develop animal models on which new compounds can be tested. For the treatment of schizophrenia, new compounds have been developed to target altered glutamate neurotransmission (Patil et al., 2007). The elevated activity observed in the auditory cortex of schizophrenia patients during hallucinations has served as a target for intervention in the use of transcranial magnetic stimulation on the temporal lobe to attenuate hallucinations (Jandl et al., 2006). Biomarkers also may aid in development of drugs for the treatment of a variety of mental disorders. For example, past clinical trials of disease-modifying agents for AD have been unsuccessful, perhaps as a result of insufficiently sensitive measures to detect effects coupled with a failure to identify targeted populations entering a critical window for treatment effects (Fleisher, Donohue, Chen, Brewer, & Alsen, 2009). To increase the power of such trials, it has been proposed that clinical trials of disease-modifying agents be enriched with biomarkers to identify individuals at greatest risk for progression to AD.

INTERVENTIONS FOR EXECUTIVE DYSFUNCTION ACROSS THE LIFE COURSE

This chapter has outlined several mental disorders across the life course that share a common deficit in executive functions; it also has described the neural pathways that support this complex set of behaviors that are important to social interaction and independent functioning. Identifying these overlapping pathways affords the opportunity to find common solutions. These findings collectively argue for the design and implementation of efficacious and effective cognitive health programs to promote the development (in ADHD, depression, and schizophrenia) and maintenance (in GAD, HD, and PD) of executive functions and their supporting prefrontal substrates. The findings further suggest that therapies and rehabilitation strategies used to improve planning and problem solving in one disorder may be applicable to other disorders

with deficits in executive function, regardless of their underlying etiologies.

Among adolescents, the goal is to remediate developmental delays and deficits (as well as environmental barriers) during the critical arc of brain–behavior development. In later life, the goal is to mitigate rates of decline that may be exacerbated by normal aging. At both ends of the life course, individuals may be especially vulnerable to environmental stressors during identifiable windows of development, particularly when prefrontal circuits do not effectively differentiate between and inhibit excitatory pathways in the amygdala and HPA axis to evaluate the emotional salience and threat of objects or events.

Successful intervention appears possible. What follows provides evidence for the continued plasticity of the prefrontal circuits in individuals at elevated risk for executive dysfunction and dementia when they are placed in enriched environments that exercise multiple components of executive function.

It is clear from the literature that executive functions and the neural pathways that support them are important to social interaction and independent functioning across a range of mental disorders. These findings collectively argue for the design and implementation of effective cognitive and functional health programs to promote the development and maintenance of executive functions and their supporting prefrontal brain circuits. In children, the goal can extend beyond remediating developmental delays. Programs focused on cognitive health also can capitalize on what is known about brain development in enriched environments, such as aiding and encouraging children to read, an important vehicle to learning during the critical early years of brain–behavior development. Similarly, in later life, the goal is not only to mitigate cognitive decline and dementia risk but also to enrich the lives of others. At both ends of the age spectrum, individuals remain social organisms. The malleable pathways through which environmental deprivation adversely affects mental health and development in both childhood and later life remain the same pathways through which cognitive, mental, and functional health can be enriched.

Experience Corps, an intergenerational, community-based model of health promotion for retired adults age 60 and older makes older adults the agents of social health promotion to improve both academic and behavioral outcomes among children. The Experience Corps program was initially designed and implemented in a national demonstration by Linda Fried and Marc Freedman (M. Freedman & Fried, 1999). It was refined further and evaluated in a pilot randomized trial in Baltimore, Maryland, in 1999–2001, through a research–community partnership with Sylvia McGill and the Greater Homewood Community Corporation. (For more details, see Rebok et al., 2011.) Structures within this program were designed to enhance the number of older-adult volunteers in elementary schools by requiring both a high bolus of volunteer service (15 hours a week) and social support and networks through team training and team service. Many volunteers live near the schools they serve and get physical exercise by walking to and from, as well as within, the schools. Cognitive activities for the older-adult volunteers include training in roles that required flexibility, problem solving, and other executive functions while supporting children's literacy, math skill development, and motivation to read; assisting in school libraries; and promoting conflict resolution.

A short-term randomized controlled pilot study of the Experience Corps volunteer intervention both targeted and was found to substantially improve executive functions among African American, community-dwelling older adults with poor executive function at baseline (Carlson et al., 2008). These promising short-term findings suggest that this type of high-impact intervention may help ameliorate, perhaps even reverse, executive deficits. A six-month pilot neuroimaging study examined whether the Experience Corps intervention affects the PFC pathways that regulate executive function. Program-specific improvements in executive function were once again observed, accompanied by increased functional activity in regions of the PFC and in the ACC (Carlson, Erickson, et al., 2009). Thus at-risk individuals exhibited measurable brain plasticity in direct response to environmental

enrichment, providing initial evidence of this program's potential to reverse cognitive and corresponding neural deficits. In summary, those individuals at greatest risk for deficits in executive functions showed substantial and clinically meaningful improvements in these and other functions as a result of participating in this intervention over a short interval— suggesting that those with the most to lose have the most to gain from environmental enrichment (Carlson et al., 2008; Carlson, Erickson, et al., 2009).

These findings offer initial evidence that older adults at high risk for executive dysfunction maintain great potential for brain plasticity and cognitive resilience. The high bolus of enrichment offered by Experience Corps led within a short time to gains in brain regions vulnerable to aging. Through a larger randomized trial of Experience Corps in Baltimore that incorporates neuroimaging and other measures of physiologic dysregulation in the study of memory and physical function, it will be increasingly possible to discern whether programs such as this can help buffer and boost PFC and hippocampal regions important to executive and memory function and to regulation of responses to emotional and perceived threats in the environment. Although the extent and limits of brain plasticity in response to increased environmental enrichment remain unknown, the work stands as a springboard to a new generation of interventions that target top-down executive strategies to help rewire or reverse dysfunctional networks.

SUMMARY AND CONCLUSIONS

This chapter has presented an overview of a number of mental disorders over the life course that are characterized by deficits in executive function and associated prefrontal–striatal brain networks. These deficits often emerge during critical windows during the PFC's long developmental trajectory. While the etiologies underlying these executive deficits differ, all appear in some way to disrupt those frontostriatal circuits (Cropley, Fujita, Innis, & Nathan, 2006; Tisserand & Jolles,

2003). Disruptions may occur in part because of cell loss (Raz, Rodrigue, Head, Kennedy, & Acker, 2004), white matter axonal damage (Gunning-Dixon & Raz, 2003), and dopamine deficiencies (Volkow et al., 1998). Nonetheless, promising research in persons at risk for executive dysfunction indicates that plastic adaptations can be induced in these complex pathways to reverse or buffer against executive dysfunction.

Each of the mental disorders discussed has a long, potentially progressive course involving executive deficits that may become exacerbated with age, placing individuals at elevated risk for late-life disability. Given the lifelong chronicity of these mental disorders and the associated need for pharmacologic and behavioral management and for health care resources, their combined prevalence in the population leads to an aggregate public health care burden affecting individuals, families, and the larger society (Rubenstein, Chrischilles, & Voelker, 1997; Schenkman, Wei Zhu, Cutson, & Whetten-Goldstein, 2001). Targeting these disorders in the aggregate using large-scale programs to promote and augment executive functions may help individuals sustain functional independence and reduce the burden on public health care systems. The work summarized here reinforces the utility of neurobiological tools, including peripheral biomarkers and brain imaging, in measuring the impact of these emerging intervention designs on underlying prefrontal–striatal networks. With the worldwide aging of the population and the accompanying potential exacerbation of executive deficits, a need exists to develop large-scale disease-modifying treatments that intervene on the pathobiological processes involved in the progression of cognitive and mental decline and of neuropathologic diseases.

REFERENCES

Abela, J., & Hankin, B. L. (2008). Cognitive vulnerability to depression in children and adolescents: A developmental psychopathology perspective. In J. Abela (Ed.), *Handbook of depression in children and adolescents* (pp. 35–78). New York, NY: Guilford.

Adleman, N. E., Menon, V., Blasey, C. M., White, C. D., Warsofsky, I. S., Glover, G. H., & Reiss, A. L. (2002). A developmental fMRI study of the Stroop color-word task. *Neuroimage, 16*(1), 61–75.

Adler, L. E., Pachtman, E., Franks, R. D., Pecevich, M., Waldo, M. C., & Freedman, R. (1982). Neurophysiological evidence for a defect in neuronal mechanisms involved in sensory gating in schizophrenia. *Biological Psychiatry 17*(6), 639–654.

Alexopoulos, G. S., Meyers, B. S., Young, R. C., Kalayam, B., Kakuma, T., Gabrielle, M.,... Hull, J. (2000). Executive dysfunction and long-term outcomes of geriatric depression. *Archives of General Psychiatry, 57*(3), 285–290.

American Psychiatric Association. (2000). *Diagnostic and statistical manual of mental disorders* (4th ed., text rev.). Washington, DC: Author.

Angold, A., & Costello, E. J. (2006). Puberty and depression. *Child and Adolescent Psychiatry Clinics of North America, 15*(4), 919–937.

Aron, A. R., Watkins, L., Sahakian, B. J., Monsell, S., Barker, R. A., & Robbins, T. W. (2003). Task-set switching deficits in early-stage Huntington's disease: Implications for basal ganglia function. *Journal of Cognitive Neuroscience, 15*(5), 629–642.

Baddeley A. D., Bressi, S., Della Sala, S., Logie, R., & Spinnler, H. (1991). The decline of working memory in Alzheimer's disease: A longitudinal study. *Brain, 114*(Pt. 6), 2521–2542.

Baddeley, A., Logie, R., Bressi, S., Della Sala, S., & Spinnier, H. (1986). Dementia and working memory. *Quarterly Journal of Experimental Psychology A, 38*(4), 603–618.

Banich, M. T., Milham, M. P., Atchley, R., Cohen, N. J., Webb, A., Wszalek, T.,... Magin, R. (2000). fMRI studies of Stroop tasks reveal unique roles of anterior and posterior brain systems in attentional selection. *Journal of Cognitive Neuroscience, 12*(6), 988–1000.

Banich, M. T., Milham, M. P., Jacobson, B. L., Webb, A., Wszalek, T., Cohen, N. J., & Kramer, A. F. (2001). Attentional selection and the processing of task-irrelevant information: Insights from fMRI examinations of the Stroop task. *Progress in Brain Research, 134,* 459–470.

Barch, D.M., Carter, C.S., Braver, T.S., Sabb, F. W., MacDonald, A., 3rd, Noll, D. C., & Cohen, J. D. (2001). Selective deficits in prefrontal cortex function in medication-naive patients with schizophrenia. *Archives of General Psychiatry, 58*(3), 280–288.

Barger, S., & Sydeman, S. J. (2005). Does generalized anxiety disorder predict coronary heart disease risk factors independently of major depressive disorder? *Journal of Affective Disorders, 88*(1), 87–91.

Barkley, R. (1997). Behavioral inhibition, sustained attention, and executive functions: Constructing a unifying theory of ADHD. *Psychological Bulletin, 121*, 65–94.

Barkley, R. (1998). How should attention deficit disorder be described? *Harvard Mental Health Letter, 14*, 8.

Barlow, D., Blanchard, E. B., Vermilyea, J. A., Vermilyea, B. B., & DiNardo, P. A. (1986). Generalized anxiety and generalized anxiety disorder: Description and reconceptualization. *American Journal of Psychiatry, 143*(1), 40–44.

Bebbington, P. (1996). The origins of sex differences in depressive disorder: Bridging the gap. *International Review of Psychiatry, 8*, 295–332.

Bebbington, P. E., Dunn, G., Jenkins, R., Lewis, G., Brugha, T., Farrell, M., & Meltzer, H. (1998). The influence of age and sex on the prevalence of depressive conditions: Report from the National Survey of Psychiatric Morbidity. *Psychological Medicine, 28*(1), 9–19.

Beck, A. (2008). The evolution of the cognitive model of depression and its neurobiological correlates. *American Journal of Psychiatry, 165*(8), 969–977.

Benes, F. M. (1993). Neurobiological investigations in cingulate cortex of schizophrenic brain. *Schizophrenia Bulletin, 19*(3), 537–549.

Benes, F. M., Turtle, M., Khan, Y., & Farol, P. (1994). Myelination of a key relay zone in the hippocampal formation occurs in the human brain during childhood, adolescence, and adulthood. *Archives of General Psychiatry, 51*(6), 477–484.

Berman, K. F., Illowsky, B. P., & Weinberger, D. R. (1988). Physiological dysfunction of dorsolateral prefrontal cortex in schizophrenia. IV. Further evidence for regional and behavioral specificity. *Archives of General Psychiatry, 45*(7), 616–622.

Biederman, J., Mick, E., & Faraone, S. V. (2000). Age-dependent decline of symptoms of attention deficit hyperactivity disorder: Impact of remission definition and symptom type. *American Journal of Psychiatry, 157*(5), 816–818.

Blasi, G., Taurisano, P., Papazacharias, A., Caforio, G., Romano, R., Lobianco, L.,...Bertolino, A. (2009). Nonlinear response of the anterior cingulate and prefrontal cortex in schizophrenia as a function of variable attentional control. *Cerebral Cortex, 20*(4), 837–845.

Blazer, D. G., Hughes, D., George, L. K., Swartz, M., & Boyer, R. (1991). Generalized anxiety disorder. In L. N. Rogers & D. A. Regier (Eds.). *Psychiatric disorders in America: The Epidemiologic Catchment Area study* (pp. 180–203). New York, NY: Free Press.

Bleuler, M. (1963). Conception of schizophrenia within the last fifty years and today [abridged]. *Proceedings of the Royal Society of Medicine, 56*(10), 945–952.

Borkovec, T. D., Alcaine, O. M., & Behar, E. (2004). Avoidance theory of worry and generalized anxiety disorder. In R. G. Heimberg, C. L. Turk, & D. S. Mennin (Eds.), *Generalized anxiety disorder: Advances in research and practice* (pp. 77–108). New York, NY: Guilford.

Borkovec, T. D., & Inz, J. (1990). The nature of worry in generalized anxiety disorder: A predominance of thought activity. *Behaviour Research and Therapy, 28*(2), 153–158.

Borkovec, T. D., Ray, W. J., & Stober, J. (1998). Worry: A cognitive phenomenon intimately linked to affective, physiological, and interpersonal behavioral processes. *Cognitive Therapy and Research, 22*(6), 561–576.

Botvinick, M., Nystrom, L. E., Fissell, K., Carter, C. S., & Cohen J. D. (1999). Conflict monitoring versus selection-for-action in anterior cingulate cortex. *Nature, 402*(6758), 179–181.

Boyle, P. A., Malloy, P. F., Salloway, S., Cahn-Weiner, D. A., Cohen, R., & Cummings, J. L. (2003). Executive dysfunction and apathy predict functional impairment in Alzheimer disease. *American Journal of Geriatric Psychiatry, 11*(2), 214–221.

Braff, D. L., & Geyer, M. A. (1990). Sensorimotor gating and schizophrenia: Human and animal model studies. *Archives of General Psychiatry, 47*(2), 181–188.

Brookmeyer, R., Johnson, E., Ziegler-Graham, K., & Arrighi, H. M. (2007). Forecasting the global burden of Alzheimer's disease. *Alzheimer's and Dementia, 3*(3), 186–191.

Brown, A. S., Begg, M. D., Gravenstein, S., Schaefer, C. A., Wyatt, R. J., Bresnahan, M.,...Susser, E. S. (2004). Serologic evidence of prenatal influenza in the etiology of schizophrenia. *Archives of General Psychiatry, 61*(8), 774–780.

Brown, R. G., & Marsden, C. D. (1988). Internal versus external cues and the control of attention in Parkinson's disease. *Brain, 111*(Pt 2), 323–345.

Brown, A. S., Schaefer, C. A., Quesenberry, C. P., Jr., Liu, L., Babulas, V. P., & Susser, E. S. (2005). Maternal exposure to toxoplasmosis and risk of schizophrenia in adult offspring. *American Journal of Psychiatry, 162*(4), 767–773.

Buckner, R. L. (2004). Memory and executive function in aging and Alzheimer's disease: Multiple factors that cause decline and reserve factors that compensate. *Neuron, 44*(1), 195–208.

Bunge, S. A., Dudukovic, N. M., Thomason, M. E., Vaidya, C. J., & Gabrieli, J. D. (2002). Immature frontal lobe contributions to cognitive control in children: Evidence from fMRI. *Neuron, 33*(2), 301–311.

Burmeister, M., McInnis, M. G., & Zollner, S. (2008). Psychiatric genetics: Progress amid controversy. *Nature Reviews Genetics, 9*(7), 527–540.

Bush, G., Luu, P., & Posner, M. I. (2000). Cognitive and emotional influences in anterior cingulate cortex. *Trends in Cognitive Sciences, 4*(6), 215–222.

Bush, G., Valera, E., & Seidman, L. (2005). Functional neuroimaging of attention-deficit/hyperactivity disorder: A review and suggested future directions. *Biological Psychiatry, 57*(11), 1273–1284.

Bush, G., Whalen, P. J., Shin, L. M., & Rauch, S. L. (2006). The counting Stroop: A cognitive interference task. *Nature Protocols, 1*(1), 230–233.

Cabib, S., & Puglisi-Allegra, S. (1996). Different effects of repeated stressful experiences on mesocortical and mesolimbic dopamine metabolism. *Neuroscience, 73*(2), 375–380.

Cahn, D. A., Sullivan, E. V., Shear, P. K., Pfefferbaum, A., Heit, G., & Silverberg, G. (1998). Differential contributions of cognitive and motor component processes to physical and instrumental activities of daily living in Parkinson's disease. *Archives of Clinical Neuropsychology, 13*(7), 575–583.

Cahn-Weiner, D. A., Boyle, P. A., & Malloy, P. F. (2002). Tests of executive function predict instrumental activities of daily living in community-dwelling older individuals. *Applied Neuropsychology, 9*(3), 187–191.

Cahn-Weiner, D. A., Farias, S. T., Julian, L., Harvey, D. J., Kramer, J. H., Reed, B. R.,...Chui, H. (2007). Cognitive and neuroimaging predictors of instrumental activities of daily living. *Journal of the International Neuropsychological Society, 13*(5), 747–757.

Cahn-Weiner, D. A., Ready, R. E., & Malloy, P. F. (2003). Neuropsychological predictors of everyday memory and everyday functioning in patients with mild Alzheimer's disease. *Journal of Geriatric Psychiatry and Neurology, 16*(2), 84–89.

Cannon, M., Moffitt, T. E., Caspi, A., Murray, R. M., Harrington, H., & Poulton, R. (2006). Neuropsychological performance at the age of 13 years and adult schizophreniform disorder: Prospective birth cohort study. *British Journal of Psychiatry, 189*, 463–464.

Cardno, A. G., & Gottesman, I. I. (2000). Twin studies of schizophrenia: from bow-and-arrow concordances to star wars Mx and functional genomics. *American Journal of Medical Genetics, 97*(1), 12–17.

Carlson, M. C., Erickson, K. I., Kramer, A. F., Voss, M. W., Bolea, N., Mielke, M.,...Fried, L. P. (2009). Evidence for neurocognitive plasticity in at-risk older adults: The Experience Corps program. *Journals of Gerontology, Series A: Biological Sciences and Medical Sciences, 64*(12), 1275–1282.

Carlson, M. C., Saczynski, J. S., Rebok, G. W., Seeman, T., Glass, T. A., McGill, S.,...Fried, L. P. (2008). Exploring the effects of an "everyday" activity program on executive function and memory in older adults: Experience Corps. *Gerontologist, 48*(6), 793–801.

Carlson, M. C., Xue, Q. L., Zhou, J., & Fried, L. P. (2009). Executive decline and dysfunction precedes declines in memory: The Women's Health and Aging Study II. *Journals of Gerontology, Series A: Biological Science and Medical Sciences, 64*(1), 110–117.

Carter, C. S., Mintun, M., & Cohen, J. D. (1995). Interference and facilitation effects during selective attention: An $H_2^{15}O$ PET study of Stroop task performance. *Neuroimage, 2*(4), 264–272.

Carter, W. R., Johnson, M. C., & Borkovec, T. D. (1986). Worry: An electrocortical analysis. *Advances in Behaviour Research & Therapy, 8*(4), 193–204.

Casey, B. J., Castellanos, F. X., Giedd, J. N., Marsh, W. L., Hamburger, S. D., Schubert, A. B.,...Rapoport, J. L. (1997). Implication of right frontostriatal circuitry in response inhibition and attention-deficit/hyperactivity disorder. *Journal of the American Academy of Child and Adolescent Psychiatry, 36*(3), 374–383.

Casey, B. J., Getz, S., & Galvan, A. (2008). The adolescent brain. *Developmental Review, 28*(1), 62–77.

Casey, B. J., Giedd, J. N., & Thomas, K. M. (2000). Structural and functional brain development and its relation to cognitive development. *Biological Psychology, 54*(1–3), 241–257.

Casey, B. J., Thomas, K. M., Davidson, M. C., Kunz, K., & Franzen, P. L. (2002). Dissociating striatal and hippocampal function developmentally with a stimulus–response compatibility task. *Journal of Neuroscience, 22*(19), 8647–8652.

Castellanos, F. X., Giedd, J. N., Berquin, P. C., Walter, J. M., Sharp, W., Tran, T., ... Rapoport, J. L. (2001). Quantitative brain magnetic resonance imaging in girls with attention-deficit/hyperactivity disorder. *Archives of General Psychiatry, 58*(3), 289–295.

Castellanos, F. X., Giedd, J. N., Marsh, W. L., Hamburger, S. D., Vaituzis, A. C., Dickstein, D. P., ... Rapoport, J. L. (1996). Quantitative brain magnetic resonance imaging in attention-deficit hyperactivity disorder. *Archives of General Psychiatry, 53*(7), 607–616.

Castellanos, F. X., Lee, P. P., Sharp, W., Jeffries, N. O., Greenstein, D. K., & Clasen, L. S. (2002). Developmental trajectories of brain volume abnormalities in children and adolescents with attention-deficit hyperactivity disorder. *Journal of the American Medical Association, 288*(14), 1740–1748.

Cervellione, K. L., Burdick, K. E., Cottone, J. G., Rhinewine, J. P., & Kumra, S. (2007). Neurocognitive deficits in adolescents with schizophrenia: Longitudinal stability and predictive utility for short-term functional outcome. *Journal of the American Academy of Child and Adolescent Psychiatry, 46*(7), 867–878.

Clark, D., & Beck, A. (1999). *Scientific foundations of cognitive theory and therapy of depression.* New York, NY: John Wiley & Sons.

Coffey, C., Wilkinson, W. E., Weiner, R. D., Parashos, I. A., Djang, W. T., Webb, M. C., ... Spritzer, C. E. (1993). Quantitative cerebral anatomy in depression: A controlled magnetic resonance imaging study. *Archives of General Psychiatry, 50*(1), 7–16.

Cools, R., Barker, R. A., Sahakian, B. J., & Robbins, T. W. (2001). Enhanced or impaired cognitive function in Parkinson's disease as a function of dopaminergic medication and task demands. *Cerebral Cortex, 11*(12), 1136–1143.

Cropley, V. L., Fujita, M., Innis, R. B., & Nathan, P. J. (2006). Molecular imaging of the dopaminergic system and its association with human cognitive function. *Biological Psychiatry, 59*(10), 898–907.

Cummings, J. L. (1993). Frontal–subcortical circuits and human behavior. *Archives of Neurology, 50*(8), 873–880.

Dalman, C., Allebeck, P., Cullberg, J., Grunewald, C., & Koster, M. (1999). Obstetric complications and the risk of schizophrenia: A longitudinal study of a national birth cohort. *Archives of General Psychiatry, 56*(3), 234–240.

Davatzikos, C., Shen, D., Gur, R. C., Wu, X., Liu, D., Fan, Y., ... Gur, R. E. (2005). Whole-brain morphometric study of schizophrenia revealing a spatially complex set of focal abnormalities. *Archives of General Psychiatry, 62*(11), 1218–1227.

Desikan, R. S., Fischl, B., Cabral, H. J., Kemper, T. L., Guttmann, C. R., Blacker, D., ... Killiany, R. J. (2008). MRI measures of temporoparietal regions show differential rates of atrophy during prodromal AD. *Neurology, 71*(11), 819–825.

D'Esposito, M., Detre, J. A., Alsop, D. C., Shin, R. K., Atlas, S., & Grossman, M. (1995). The neural basis of the central executive system of working memory. *Nature, 378*(6554), 279–281.

Devinsky, O., Morrell, M. J., & Vogt, B. A. (1995). Contributions of anterior cingulate cortex to behaviour. *Brain, 118*(Pt. 1), 279–306.

Diamond, A. (2002). Normal development of prefrontal cortex from birth to young adulthood: Cognitive functions, anatomy, and biochemistry. In D. T. Stuss & R. T. Knight (Eds.), *Principals of frontal lobe function* (pp. 466–503). New York, NY: Oxford University Press.

Diaz-Asper, C. M., Goldberg, T. E., Kolachana, B. S., Straub, R. E., Egan, M. F., & Weinberger, D. R. (2008). Genetic variation in catechol-O-methyltransferase: Effects on working memory in schizophrenic patients, their siblings, and healthy controls. *Biological Psychiatry, 63*(1), 72–79.

Drevets, W. C., Price, J. L., Simpson, J. R., Jr., Todd, R. D., Reich, T., Vannier, M., & Raichle, M. E. (1997). Subgenual prefrontal cortex abnormalities in mood disorders. *Nature, 386*(6627), 824–827.

Drewe, E. A. (1975). Go–no go learning after frontal lobe lesions in humans. *Cortex, 11*(1), 8–16.

Dubois, B., Feldman, H. H., Jacova, C., Dekosky, S. T., Barberger-Gateau, P., Cummings, J., ... Scheltens, P. (2007). Research criteria for the diagnosis of Alzheimer's disease: Revising the NINCDS-ADRDA criteria. *Lancet Neurology, 6*(8), 734–746.

Dugas, M., Buhr, K., & Ladouceur, R. (2004). The role of intolerance of uncertainty in etiology and maintenance of generalized anxiety disorder. In R. G. Heimberg, C. L. Turk, & D. S. Mennin (Eds.), *Generalized anxiety disorder: Advances in research and practice* (pp.143–163). New York, NY: Guilford.

Dugas, M. J., Gosselin, P., & Ladouceur, R. (2001). Intolerance of uncertainty and worry: Investigating specificity in a nonclinical sample. *Cognitive Therapy and Research, 25*(5), 551–558.

Durston, S. (2003). A review of the biological bases of ADHD: What have we learned from imaging studies? *Mental Retardation and Developmental Disabilities Research Review, 9*(3), 184–195.

Durston, S., & Casey, B. J. (2006). What have we learned about cognitive development from neuroimaging? *Neuropsychologia, 44*(11), 2149–2157.

Eaton, W. W., & Harrison, G. (2001). Life chances, life planning, and schizophrenia: A review and interpretation of research on social deprivation. *International Journal of Mental Health, 30,* 58–81.

Ernst, M., Kimes, A. S., London, E. D., Matochik, A. K., Eldreth, D., Tata, S.,... Bolla, K. (2003). Neural substrates of decision making in adults with attention deficit hyperactivity disorder. *American Journal of Psychiatry, 160*(6), 1061–1070.

Fleisher, A. S., Donohue, M., Chen, K., Brewer, J. B., & Alsen, P. S. (2009). Applications of neuroimaging to disease-modification trials in Alzheimer's disease. *Cognitive and Behavioral Neurology, 21*(1), 29–136.

Fox, J. W. (1990). Social class, mental illness, and social mobility: The social selection-drift hypothesis for serious mental illness. *Journal of Health and Social Behavior, 31*(4), 344–353.

Frangou, S. (2010). Cognitive function in early onset schizophrenia: A selective review. *Frontiers in Human Neuroscience, 3,* 79.

Frangou, S., Hadjulis, M., & Vourdas, A. (2008). The Maudsley early onset schizophrenia study: Cognitive function over a 4-year follow-up period. *Schizophrenia Bulletin, 34*(1), 52–59.

Freedman, M., & Fried, L. (1999). *Launching Experience Corps: Findings from a two-year pilot project mobilizing older Americans to help inner-city elementary schools.* Oakland, CA: Civic Ventures.

Freedman, R., Coon, H., Myles-Worsley, M., Orr-Ortreger, A., Olincy, A., Davis, A.,... Byerleys, W. (1997). Linkage of a neurophysiological deficit in schizophrenia to a chromosome 15 locus. *Proceedings of the National Academy of Sciences of the United States of America, 94*(2), 587–592.

Fucetola, R., Seidman, L. J., Kremen, W. S., Faraone, S. V., Goldstein, J. M., & Tsuang, M. T. (2000). Age and neuropsychologic function in schizophrenia: A decline in executive abilities beyond that observed in healthy volunteers. *Biological Psychiatry, 48*(2), 137–146.

Fuster, J. M. (1989). *The prefrontal cortex: Anatomy, physiology, and neuropsychology of the frontal lobe* (2nd ed.). New York, NY: Raven Press.

Garavan, H., Ross, T. J., & Stein, E. A. (1999). Right hemispheric dominance of inhibitory control: An event-related functional MRI study. *Proceedings of the National Academy of Sciences of the United States of America, 96*(14), 8301–8306.

Garon, N., Bryson, S. E., & Smith, I. M. (2008). Executive function in preschoolers: A review using an integrative framework. *Psychological Bulletin, 134*(1), 31–60.

Gatzke-Kopp, L. M., & Beauchaine, T. P. (2007). Direct and passive prenatal nicotine exposure and the development of externalizing psychopathology. *Child Psychiatry and Human Development, 38*(4), 255–269.

Gauntlett-Gilbert, J., Roberts, R. C., & Brown, V. J. (1999). Mechanisms underlying attentional set-shifting in Parkinson's disease. *Neuropsychologia, 37*(5), 605–616.

Geuze, E., Vermetten, E., & Bremner, J. D. (2005). MR-based in vivo hippocampal volumetrics: 2. Findings in neuropsychiatric disorders. *Molecular Psychiatry, 10*(2), 160–184.

Geyer, M. A., McIlwain, K. L., & Paylor, R. (2002). Mouse genetic models for prepulse inhibition: An early review. *Molecular Psychiatry, 7*(10), 1039–1053.

Giedd, J. N., Blumenthal, J., Jeffries, N. O., Castellanos, F. X., Liu, H., Zijdenbos, A.,... Rapoport, J. L. (1999). Brain development during childhood and adolescence: A longitudinal MRI study. *Nature Neuroscience, 2*(10), 861–863.

Gogtay, N., Giedd, J. N., Lusk, L., Hayashi, K. M., Greenstein, D., Vaituzis, A. C.,... Thompson, P. M. (2004). Dynamic mapping of human cortical development during childhood through early adulthood. *Proceedings of the National Academy of Sciences of the United States of America, 101*(21), 8174–8179.

Goldin, P. R., McRae, K., Ramel, W., & Gross, J. J. (2008). The neural bases of emotion regulation: Reappraisal and suppression of negative emotion. *Biological Psychiatry, 63*(6), 577–586.

Gotham, A. M., Brown, R. G., & Marsden, C. D. (1988). "Frontal" cognitive function in patients with Parkinson's disease "on" and "off" levodopa. *Brain, 111*(Pt. 2), 299–321.

Gottesman, I. I., & Gould, T. D. (2003). The endophenotype concept in psychiatry: etymology and strategic intentions. *American Journal of Psychiatry 160*(4), 636–645.

Green, M. F. (1996). What are the functional consequences of neurocognitive deficits in schizophrenia? *American Journal of Psychiatry, 153*(3), 321–330.

Grillon, C., Courchesne, E., Ameli, R., Geyer, M. A., & Braff, D. L. (1990). Increased distractibility in schizophrenic patients: Electrophysiologic and behavioral evidence. *Archives of General Psychiatry, 47*(2), 171–179.

Gunning-Dixon, F. M., & Raz, N. (2003). Neuro-anatomical correlates of selected executive functions in middle-aged and older adults: A prospective MRI study. *Neuropsychologia, 41*(14), 1929–1941.

Hazeltine, E., Bunge, S. A., Scanlon, M. D., & Gabrieli, J. D. (2003). Material-dependent and material-independent selection processes in the frontal and parietal lobes: An event-related fMRI investigation of response competition. *Neuropsychologia, 41*(9), 1208–1217.

Hazeltine, E., Poldrack, R., & Gabrieli, J. D. (2000). Neural activation during response competition. *Journal of Cognitive Neuroscience, 12*(Suppl. 2), 118–129.

Heller, W., Nitschke, J. B., Etienne, M. A., & Miller, G. A. (1997). Patterns of regional brain activity differentiate types of anxiety. *Journal of Abnormal Psychology, 106*(3), 376–385.

Hoehn-Saric, R., Lee, J. S., McLeod, D. R., & Wong, D. F. (2005). Effect of worry on regional cerebral blood flow in nonanxious subjects. *Psychiatry Research, 140*(3), 259–269.

Hoehn-Saric, R., Schlund, M. W., & Wong, S. H. (2004). Effects of citalopram on worry and brain activation in patients with generalized anxiety disorder. *Psychiatry Research: Neuroimaging, 131*(1), 11–21.

Hofmann, S. G., Moscovitch, D., Litz, B., Kim, H.-J., Davis, L., & Pizzagalli, D. (2005). The worried mind: Autonomic and prefrontal activation during worrying. *Emotion, 5*(4), 464–475.

Jack, C. R., Jr., Knopman, D. S., Jagust, W. J., Shaw, L. M., Alsen, P. S., Weiner, M. W., ... Trojanowski, J. Q. (2010). Hypothetical model of dynamic biomarkers of the Alzheimer's pathological cascade. *Lancet Neurology, 9*(1), 119–128.

Jahshan, C., Heaton, R. K., Golshan, S., & Cadenhead, K. S. (2010). Course of neurocognitive deficits in the prodrome and first episode of schizophrenia. *Neuropsychology, 24*(1), 109–120.

Jandl, M., Steyer, J., Weber, M., Linden, D. E., Rothmeier, J., Maurer, K., & Kaschka, W. P. (2006). Treating auditory hallucinations by transcranial magnetic stimulation: A randomized controlled cross-over trial. *Neuropsychobiology, 53*(2), 63–69.

Jernigan, T. L., Archibald, S. L., Berhow, M. T., Sowell, E. R., Foster, D. S., & Hesselink, J. R. (1991). Cerebral structure on MRI, part I: Localization of age-related changes. *Biological Psychiatry, 29*(1), 55–67.

Johansen, E. B., Aase, H., Meyer, A., & Sagvolden, T. (2002). Attention-deficit/hyperactivity disorder (ADHD) behaviour explained by dysfunctioning reinforcement and extinction processes. *Behavioural Brain Research 130*(1–2), 37–45.

Johnstone, T., van Reekum, C. M., Urry, H. L., Kalin, N. H., & Davidson, R. J. (2007). Failure to regulate: Counterproductive recruitment of top-down prefrontal–subcortical circuitry in major depression. *Journal of Neuroscience, 27*(33), 8877–8884.

Jorm, A. (2000). Does old age reduce the risk of anxiety or depression? A review of epidemiological studies across the adult life span. *Psychological Medicine, 30*(1), 11–22.

Jones, P., & Cannon, M. (1998). The new epidemiology of schizophrenia. *Psychiatric Clinics of North America, 21*(1), 1–25.

Jorm, A. F., & Jolley, D. (1998). The incidence of dementia: A meta-analysis. *Neurology, 51*(3), 728–733.

Kendler, K. S. (1988). The genetics of schizophrenia. In M. T. Tsuang & J. C. Simpson (Eds.), *Handbook of schizophrenia* (Vol. 3, pp. 437–462). Amsterdam: Elsevier Science.

Kennedy, B., & Schwab, J. J. (1997). Utilization of medical specialists by anxiety disorder patients. *Psychosomatics, 38*(2), 109–112.

Kennedy, K. M., Erickson, K. I., Rodrigue, K. M., Voss, M. W., Colcombe, S. J., Kramer, A. F., ... Raz, N. (2009). Age-related differences in regional brain volumes: A comparison of optimized voxel-based morphometry to manual volumetry. *Neurobiology of Aging, 30*(10), 1657–1676.

Kerchner, G. A., Hess, C. P., Hammond-Rosenbluth, K. E., Xu, D., Rabinovici, G. D., Kelley, D. A., ... Miller, B. L. (2010). Hippocampal CA1 apical neuropil atrophy in mild Alzheimer disease visualized with 7-T MRI. *Neurology, 75*(15), 1381–1387.

Kessler, R. C., Chiu, W. T., Demler, O., Merikangas, K. R., & Walters, E. E. (2005). Prevalence, severity, and comorbidity of 12-month DSM-IV disorders in the National Comorbidity Survey Replication. *Archives of General Psychiatry, 62*(6), 617–627.

Kessler, R. C., DuPont, R. L., Berglund, P., & Wittchen, H. U. (1999). Impairment in pure and comorbid generalized anxiety disorder and major depression at 12 months in two national surveys. *American Journal of Psychiatry, 156*(12), 1915–1923.

Kessler, R. C., & Wittchen, H. U. (2002). Patterns and correlates of generalized anxiety disorder in community samples. *Journal of Clinical Psychiatry, 63*(Suppl. 8), 4–10.

King, S., Laplante, D., & Joober, R. (2005). Understanding putative risk factors for schizophrenia: Retrospective and prospective studies. *Journal of Psychiatry and Neuroscience, 30*(5), 342–348.

Kirov, G., O'Donovan, M. C., & Owen, M. J. (2005). Finding schizophrenia genes. *Journal of Clinical Investigation, 115*(6), 1440–1448.

Kramer, A. F., & Atchley, P. (2000). Age-related effects in the marking of old objects in visual search. *Psychology and Aging, 15*(2), 286–296.

Krishnan, K. R. R., McDonald, W. M., Escalona, P. R., Doraiswamy, P. M., Na, C., Husain, M. M.,... Nemeroff, C. B. (1992). Magnetic resonance imaging of the caudate nuclei in depression. *Archives of General Psychiatry, 49*(7), 553–558.

Kubzansky, L. D., Kawachi, I., Spiro, A., Weiss, S. T., Vokonas, P. S., & Sparrow, D. (1997). Is worrying bad for your heart? A prospective study of worry and coronary heart disease in the Normative Aging study. *Circulation, 95*(4), 818–824.

Ladouceur, R., Dugas, M. J., Freeston, M. H., Rheaume, J., Blais, F., Boisvert, J. M.,... Thibodeau, N. (1999). Specificity of generalized anxiety disorder symptoms and processes. *Behavior Therapy, 30*, 191–207.

Lambert, N. M., & Hartsough, C. S. (1998). Prospective study of tobacco smoking and substance dependencies among samples of ADHD and non-ADHD participants. *Journal of Learning Disabilities, 31*(6), 533–544.

Lawrence, R. H., & Jette, A. M. (1996). Disentangling the disablement process. *Journals of Gerontology, Series B: Psychological Sciences and Social Sciences, 51*(4), s173–s182.

Lees, A. J., & Smith, E. (1983). Cognitive deficits in the early stages of Parkinson's disease. *Brain, 106*(Pt. 2), 257–270.

Liddle, P. F. (1987). Schizophrenic syndromes, cognitive performance and neurological dysfunction. *Psychological Medicine, 17*(1), 49–57.

Lisman, J. E., Coyle, J. T., Green, R. W., Javitt, D. C., Benes, F. M., Heckers, S., & Grace, A. A. (2008). Circuit-based framework for understanding neurotransmitter and risk gene interactions in schizophrenia. *Trends in Neuroscience, 31*(5), 234–242.

Lockwood, K. A., Alexopoulos, G. S., & van Gorp, W. G. (2002). Executive dysfunction in geriatric depression. *American Journal of Psychiatry, 159*(7), 1119–1126.

Lyonfields, J., Borkovec, T. D., & Thayer, J. F. (1995). Vagal tone in generalized anxiety disorder and the effects of aversive imagery and worrisome thinking. *Behavior Therapy, 26*, 457–466.

MacDonald, A. W., 3rd, Cohen, J. D., Stenger, V. A., & Carter, C. S. (2000). Dissociating the role of the dorsolateral prefrontal and anterior cingulate cortex in cognitive control. *Science, 288*(5472), 1835–1838.

MacLeod, C., & Rutherford, E. (2004). Information-processing approaches: Assessing the selective functioning of attention, interpretation, and retrieval. In R. G. Heimberg, C. L. Turk, & D. S. Mennin (Eds.), *Generalized anxiety disorder: Advances in research and practice* (pp. 109–142). New York, NY: Guilford.

Madden, D. J. (2000). Neuroimaging of memory: Introduction. *Microscopy Research and Technique, 51*(1), 1–5.

Madden, D. J., Whiting, W. L., Huettel, S. A., White, L. E., McFall, J. R., & Provenzale, J. M. (2004). Diffusion tensor imaging of adult age differences in cerebral white matter: Relation to response time. *Neuroimage, 2*(3), 1174–1181.

Marinelli, M., Rudick, C. N., Hu, X. T., & White, F. J. (2006). Excitability of dopamine neurons: Modulation and physiological consequences. *CNS & Neurological Disorders—Drug Targets, 5*(1), 79–97.

Mayberg, H. S., Liotti, M., Brannan, S. K., McGinnis, S., Mahurin, R. K., Jerabek, P. A.,... Fox, P. T. (1999). Reciprocal limbic–cortical function and negative mood: Converging PET findings in depression and normal sadness. *American Journal of Psychiatry, 156*(5), 675–682.

McHugh, P. R., & Slavney, P. R. (1998). *The perspectives of psychiatry* (2nd ed.). Baltimore, MD: Johns Hopkins University Press.

Mennin, D. S., Heimberg, R. G., Turk, C. L., & Fresco, D. M. (2005). Preliminary evidence for an emotion dysregulation model of generalized anxiety disorder. *Behavior Research and Therapy, 43*(10), 1281–1310.

Meyer, D. E., & Kleras, D. E. (1997). A computational theory of executive control processes and multiple-task performance: Basic mechanisms. *Psychological Review, 104*(1), 3–65.

Milham, M. P., Erickson, K. I., Banich, M. T., Kramer, A. F., Webb, A., Wszalek, T., & Cohen, N. J. (2002). Attentional control in the aging brain: Insights from an fMRI study of the Stroop task. *Brain and Cognition, 49*(3), 277–296.

Moffitt, T., Harrington, H. L., Caspi, A., Kim-Cohen, J., Goldberg, D., Gregory, A. M., & Poulton, R. (2007). Depression and generalized anxiety disorder cumulative and sequential comorbidity in a birth cohort followed prospectively to age 32 years. *Archives of General Psychiatry, 64*(6), 651–660.

Mohlman, J. (2005). Does executive dysfunction affect treatment outcome in late-life mood and anxiety disorders? *Geriatric Psychiatry and Neurology, 18*(2), 97–108.

Mohlman, J., Price, R., Eldreth, D. A., Chazin, D., Glover, D., & Kates, W. R. (2009). The relation of worry to prefrontal cortex volume in late life generalized anxiety disorder. *Psychiatry Research, 173*(2), 121–127.

Mohlman. J., Reel, D. H., Chazin, D., Ong, D., Georgescu, B., Tiu, J., & Dobkin, R. D. (2010). A novel approach to treating anxiety and enhancing executive skills in an older adult with Parkinson's disease. *Clinical Case Studies, 9*(1), 74–90.

Mowrer, O. (1947). On the dual nature of learning: A re-interpretation of "conditioning" and "problem-solving." *Harvard Educational Review*, 102–148.

Muck-Seler, D., Pivac, N., Mustapic, M., Crncevic, J., Jakovlevic, M., & Sagud, M. (2004). Platelet serotonin and plasma prolactin and cortisol in healthy, depressed and schizophrenic women. *Psychiatry Research, 127*(3), 217–226.

Mueser, K. T., & McGurk, S. R. (2004). Schizophrenia. *Lancet, 363*(9426), 2063–2072.

Nieuwenhuis, S., Ridderinkhof, K. R., de Jong, R., Kok, A., & van der Molen, M. W. (2000). Inhibitory inefficiency and failures of intention activation: Age-related decline in the control of saccadic eye movements. *Psychology and Aging, 15*(4), 635–647.

Nitschke, J. B., & Heller, W. (2002). The neuropsychology of anxiety disorders: Affect, cognition and neural circuitry. In H. D'Haenen, J. A. den Boer, H. Westenberg, & P. Willner (Eds.), *Textbook of biological psychiatry* (pp. 975–988). London, UK: Wiley.

Nnadi, C. U., & Malhotra, A. K. (2007). Individualizing antipsychotic drug therapy in schizophrenia: The promise of pharmacogenetics. *Current Psychiatry Reports, 9*(4), 313–318.

Norman, W., & Shallice, T. (1986). Attention to action. In R. J. Davidson, G. E. Schwartz, & D. Shapiro (Eds.), *Consciousness and self regulation: Advances in research and theory* (Vol. 4, pp. 1–18). New York, NY: Plenum.

Nuechterlein, K. H., Dawson, M. E., Ventura, J., Gitlin, M., Subotnik, K. L., Snyder, K. S.,... Bartzokis, G. (1994). The vulnerability/stress model of schizophrenic relapse: A longitudinal study. *Acta Psychiatrica Scandinavica, 382*(Suppl.), 58–64.

Ochsner, K. N., Ray, R. D., Cooper, J. C., Robertson, E. R., Chopra, S., Gabrieli, J. D., Gross, J. J. (2004). For better or for worse: Neural systems supporting the cognitive down- and up-regulation of negative emotion. *Neuroimage, 23*(2), 483–499.

Ogden, J. A. (2005). *Fractured minds: A case-study approach to clinical neuropsychology* (2nd ed.). New York, NY: Oxford University Press.

Olfson, M., Fireman, B., Weissman, M. M., Leon, A. C., Sheehan, D. V., Kathol, R. G.,... Farber, L. (1997). Mental disorders and disability among patients in a primary care group practice. *American Journal of Psychiatry, 154*(12), 1734–1740.

Olincy, A., Ross, R. G., Young, D. A., & Freedman, R. (1997). Age diminishes performance on an antisaccade eye movement task. *Neurobiology of Aging, 18*(5), 483–489.

Pantelis, C., Velakoulis, D., McGorry, P. D., Wood, S. J., Suckling, J., Phillips, L. J.,... McGuire, K. P. (2003). Neuroanatomical abnormalities before and after onset of psychosis: A cross-sectional and longitudinal MRI comparison. *Lancet, 361*(9354), 281–288.

Pardo, J. V., Pardo, P., Janer, K. W., & Raichle, M. E. (1990). The anterior cingulate cortex mediates processing selection in the Stroop attentional conflict paradigm. *Proceedings of the National Academy of Sciences of the United States of America, 87*(1), 256–259.

Patil, S. T., Zhang, L., Martenyi, F., Lowe, S. L., Jackson, K. A., Andreev, B. V.,... Schoepp, D. D. (2007). Activation of mGlu2/3 receptors as a new approach to treat schizophrenia: A randomized phase 2 clinical trial. *Nature Medicine, 13*(9), 1102–1107.

Paus, T., Zijdenbos, A., Worsley, K., Collins, D. L., Blumenthal, J., Giedd, J. N.,... Evans, A. C. (1999). Structural maturation of neural pathways in children and adolescents: In vivo study. *Science, 283*(5409), 1908–1911.

Phillips, M. L., & Vieta, E. (2007). Identifying functional neuroimaging biomarkers of bipolar disorder: Toward DSM-V. *Schizophrenia Bulletin, 33*(4), 893–904.

Polanczyk, G., deLima, M. S., Horta, B. L., Biederman, J., & Rohde, L. A. (2007). The worldwide prevalence of ADHD: A systematic review and metaregression analysis. *American Journal of Psychiatry, 164*(6), 942–948.

Pollux, P. M. (2004). Advance preparation of set-switches in Parkinson's disease. *Neuropsychologia, 42*(7), 912–919.

Price, R. B., & Mohlman, J. (2007). Inhibitory control and symptom severity in late life generalized anxiety disorder. *Behaviour Research & Therapy, 45*(11), 2628–2639.

Qiu, A., Crocetti, D., Adler, M., Mahone, E. M., Denckla, M. B., Miller, M. I., & Mostofsky, S. H. (2009). Basal ganglia volume and shape in children with attention deficit hyperactivity disorder. *American Journal of Psychiatry, 166*(1), 74–82.

Qiu, C., De Ronchi, D., & Fratiglioni, L. (2007). The epidemiology of the dementias: An update. *Current Opinions in Psychiatry, 20*(4), 380–385.

Rafal, R., Gershberg, F., Egly, R., Ivry, R., Kingstone, A., & Ro, T. (1996). Response channel activation and the lateral prefrontal cortex. *Neuropsychologia, 34*(12), 1197–1202.

Raz, N. (2000). Aging of the brain and its impact on cognitive performance: Integration of structural and functional findings. In F. I. M. Craik & T. A. Salthouse (Eds.), *Handbook of aging and cognition* (pp. 1–90). Hillsdale, NJ: Lawrence Erlbaum.

Raz, N., Rodrigue, K. M., Head, D., Kennedy, A. M., & Acker, J. D. (2004). Differential aging of the medial temporal lobe: A study of a five-year change. *Neurology, 62*(3), 433–438.

Rebok, G. W. Carlson, M. C., Barron, J. S., Frick, K. D., McGill, S., Parisi, J., ... Fried, L. P. (2011). Experience Corps®: A civic engagement–based public health intervention in the public schools. In P. E. Hartman-Stein & A. La Rue (Eds.), *Enhancing cognitive fitness in adults: A guide to the use and development of community-based programs* (pp. 469–487). New York, NY: Springer.

Resnick, S. M., Pham, D. L., Kraut, M. A., Zonderman, A. B., & Davatzikos, C. (2003). Longitudinal magnetic resonance imaging studies of older adults: A shrinking brain. *Journal of Neuroscience, 23*(8), 3295–3301.

Robins, L., & Regier, D. A. (Eds.). (1991). *Psychiatric disorders in America: The Epidemiologic Catchment Area study.* New York, NY: Free Press.

Rogers, M., Warshaw, M. G., Goisman, R. M., Goldenberg, I., Rodriguez-Villa, F., Mallya, G., ... Keller, M. B. (1999). Comparing primary and secondary generalized anxiety disorder in a long-term naturalistic study of anxiety disorders. *Depression and Anxiety, 10*(1), 1–7.

Rosenthal, D. (1963). *The Genain quadruplets: A case study and theoretical analysis of heredity and environment in schizophrenia.* New York, NY: Basic Books.

Royall, D. R., Palmer, R., Chiodo, L. K., & Polk, M. J. (2004). Declining executive control in normal aging predicts change in functional status: The Freedom House study. *Journal of the American Geriatrics Society, 52*(3), 346–352.

Royall, D. R., Palmer, R., Chiodo, L. K., & Polk, M. J. (2005). Executive control mediates memory's association with change in instrumental activities of daily living: The Freedom House study. *Journal of the American Geriatrics Society, 53*(1), 11–17.

Rubenstein, L. M., Chrischilles, E. A., & Voelker, M. D. (1997). The impact of Parkinson's disease on health status, health expenditures, and productivity: Estimates from the National Medical Expenditure Survey. *Pharmacoeconomics, 12*(4), 486–498.

Rubia, K., Overmeyer, S., Taylor, E., Brammer, M., Williams, S. C., Simmons, A., ... Bullmore, E. T. (2000). Functional frontalisation with age: Mapping neurodevelopmental trajectories with fMRI. *Neuroscience and Biobehavioral Reviews, 24*(1), 13–19.

Rubia, K., Smith, A. B., Brammer, M. J., & Taylor, E. (2003). Right inferior prefrontal cortex mediates response inhibition while mesial prefrontal cortex is responsible for error detection. *Neuroimage, 20*(1), 351–358.

Rubia, K., Smith, A. B., Taylor, E., & Brammer, M. (2007). Linear age-correlated functional development of right inferior fronto-striato-cerebellar networks during response inhibition and anterior cingulate during error-related processes. *Human Brain Mapping, 28*(11), 1163–1177.

Satterfield, J. H., & Schell, A. (1997). A prospective study of hyperactive boys with conduct problems and normal boys: Adolescent and adult criminality. *Journal of the American Academy of Child and Adolescent Psychiatry, 36*(12), 1726–1735.

Schenkman, M., Wei Zhu, C., Cutson, T. M., & Whetten-Goldstein, K. (2001). Longitudinal evaluation of economic and physical impact of Parkinson's disease. *Parkinsonism and Related Disorders, 8*(1), 41–50.

Scheres, A., Milham, M. P., Knutson, B., & Castellanos, F. X. (2007). Ventral striatal hyporesponsiveness during reward anticipation in attention-deficit/ hyperactivity disorder. *Biological Psychiatry, 61*(5), 720–724.

Schulz, K. P., Tang, C. Y., Fan, J., Marks, D. J., Newcorn, J. H., Cheung, A. M., & Halperin, J. M. (2005). Differential prefrontal cortex activation during inhibitory control in adolescents with and without childhood attention-deficit/ hyperactivity disorder. *Neuropsychology, 19*(3), 390–402.

Shallice, T. (1994). Multiple levels of control processes. In C. Umilta & M. Moscovich (Eds.), *Attention and performance XV* (pp. 395–420). Cambridge, MA: MIT Press.

Shaw, P., Eckstrand, K., Sharp, W., Blumenthal, J., Lerch, J. P., Greenstein, D., ... Rapoport, J. L. (2007). Attention-deficit/hyperactivity disorder is characterized by a delay in cortical maturation. *Proceedings of the National Academy of*

Sciences of the United States of America, 104(49), 19649–19654.

Siegle, G. J., Steinhauer, S. R., Thase, M. E., Stenger, V. A., & Carter, C. S. (2002). Can't shake that feeling: Event-related fMRI assessment of sustained amygdala activity in response to emotional information in depressed individuals. *Biological Psychiatry, 51*(9), 693–707.

Siegle, G. J., Thompson, W., Carter, C. S., Steinhauer, S. R., & Thase, M. E. (2007). Increased amygdala and decreased dorsolateral prefrontal BOLD responses in unipolar depression: Related and independent features. *Biological Psychiatry, 61*(2), 198–209.

Smith, E. E., & Jonides, J. (1999). Storage and executive processes in the frontal lobes. *Science, 283*(5408), 1657–1661.

Sowell, E. R., Thompson, P. M., Tessner, K. D., & Toga, A. W. (2001). Mapping continued brain growth and gray matter density reduction in dorsal frontal cortex: Inverse relationships during postadolescent brain maturation. *Journal of Neuroscience, 21*(22), 8819–8829.

Sprengelmeyer, R., Lange, H., & Homberg, V. (1995). The pattern of attentional deficits in Huntington's disease. *Brain, 118*(Pt. 1), 145–152.

Steen, R. G., Mull, C., McClure, R., Hamer, R. M., & Lieberman, J. A. (2006). Brain volume in first-episode schizophrenia: Systematic review and meta-analysis of magnetic resonance imaging studies. *British Journal of Psychiatry, 188*, 510–518.

Straube, T., Glauer, M., Dilger, S., Mentzel, H. J., & Miltner, W. H. (2006). Effects of cognitive–behavioral therapy on brain activation in specific phobia. *Neuroimage, 29*(1), 125–135.

Studenski, S., Carlson, M. C., Fillit, H., Greenough, W. T., Kramer, A., & Rebok, G. W. (2006). From bedside to bench: Does mental and physical activity promote cognitive vitality in late life? *Science of Aging Knowledge Environment, 10*, pe21.

Swartz, J. (1999). Dopamine projections and frontal systems function. In B. L. Miller & J. L. Cummings (Eds.), *The human frontal lobes: Functions and disorders* (pp. 159–173). New York, NY: Guilford.

Swerdlow, N. R., & Geyer, M. A. (1998). Using an animal model of deficient sensorimotor gating to study the pathophysiology and new treatments of schizophrenia. *Schizophrenia Bulletin, 24*(2), 285–301.

Tamm, L., Menon, V., & Reiss, A. L. (2002) Maturation of brain function associated with response inhibition. *Journal of the American Academy of Child and Adolescent Psychiatry, 41*(10), 1231–1238.

Taylor, W. D., MacFall, J. R., Payne, M. E., McQuoid, D. R., Provenzale, J. M., Steffens, D. C., & Krishnan, K. R. R. (2004). Late-life depression and microstructural abnormalities in dorsolateral prefrontal cortex white matter. *American Journal of Psychiatry, 161*(7), 1293–1296.

Thayer, J., Friedman, B. H., & Borkovec, T. D. (1996). Autonomic characteristics of generalized anxiety disorder and worry. *Biological Psychiatry, 39*(4), 255–266.

Thayer, J. F., & Lane, R. D. (2000). A model of neurovisceral integration in emotion regulation and dysregulation. *Journal of Affective Disorders, 61*(3), 201–216.

Thayer, J. F., & Lane, R. D. (2002). Perseverative thinking and health: Neurovisceral concomitants. *Psychology and Health, 17*(5), 685–695.

Tisserand, D. J., & Jolles, J. (2003). On the involvement of prefrontal networks in cognitive ageing. *Cortex, 39*(4–5), 1107–1128.

Üstün, T. B. Ayuso-Mateos, J., Chatterji, S., Mathers, C., & Murray, C. J. (2004). Global burden of depressive disorders in the year 2000. *British Journal of Psychiatry, 184*, 386–392.

Vaidya, C. J., Austin, G., Kirkorian, G., Ridlehuber, H. W., Desmond, J. E, Glover, G. H., & Gabrieli, J. D. (1998). Selective effects of methylphenidate in attention deficit hyperactivity disorder: A functional magnetic resonance study. *Proceedings of the National Academy of Sciences of the United States of America, 95*(24), 14494–14499.

Volkow, N. D., Gur, R. C., Wang, G. J., Fowler, J. S., Moberg, P. J., Ding, Y. S.,...Logan, J. (1998). Association between decline in brain dopamine activity with age and cognitive and motor impairment in healthy individuals. *American Journal of Psychiatry, 155*(3), 344–349.

Walker, E., Mittal, V., & Tessner, K. (2008). Stress and the hypothalamic pituitary adrenal axis in the developmental course of schizophrenia. *Annual Review of Clinical Psychology, 4*, 189–216.

Walker, E. F., Walder, D. J., & Reynolds, F. (2001). Developmental changes in cortisol secretion in normal and at-risk youth. *Developmental Psychopathology, 13*(3), 721–732.

Walsh, P., Spelman, L., Sharifi, N., & Thakore, J. H. (2005). Male patients with paranoid schizophrenia have greater ACTH and cortisol secretion in response to metoclopramide-induced

AVP release. *Psychoneuroendocrinology, 30*(5), 431–437.

Weinberger, D. R., Berman, K. F., Suddath, R., & Torrey, E. F. (1992). Evidence of dysfunction of a prefrontal–limbic network in schizophrenia: A magnetic resonance imaging and regional cerebral blood flow study of discordant monozygotic twins. *American Journal of Psychiatry, 149*(7), 890–897.

Wells, A. (1999). A cognitive model of generalized anxiety disorder. *Behaviour Modification, 23*(4), 526–555.

Wells, A. (2004). A cognitive model of GAD: Metacognitions and pathological worry. In R. G. Heimberg, C. L. Turk, & D. S. Mennin (Eds.), *Generalized anxiety disorder: Advances in research and practice* (pp. 164–186). New York, NY: Guilford.

West, R. L. (1996). An application of prefrontal cortex function theory to cognitive aging. *Psychological Bulletin, 120*(2), 272–292.

Wittchen, H. U., Zhao, S., Kessler, R. C., & Eaton, W. W. (1994). DSM-III-R generalized anxiety disorder in the National Comorbidity Survey. *Archives of General Psychiatry, 51*(5), 355–364

Zanelli, J., Reichenberg, A., Morgan, K., Fearon, P., Kravariti, E., Dazzan, P., . . . Murray, R. M. (2010). Specific and generalized neuropsychological deficits: A comparison of patients with various first-episode psychosis presentations. *American Journal of Psychiatry, 167*(1), 78–85.

Ziegler-Graham, K., Brookmeyer, R., Johnson, E., & Arrighi, H. M. (2008). Worldwide variation in the doubling time of Alzheimer's disease incidence rates. *Alzheimer's and Dementia, 4*(5), 316–323.

10

Models of Stress and Adapting to Risk: A Life Course, Developmental Perspective

CATHERINE P. BRADSHAW

GEORGE W. REBOK

BENJAMIN ZABLOTSKY

LAREINA N. LAFLAIR

TAMAR MENDELSON

WILLIAM W. EATON

Key Points

- Stress often plays a critical role in the development of mental health and mental and behavioral disorders

- The life course perspective helps in understanding the link between stress and mental health problems, because it shows the importance of both human development and the social context as each evolves over the course of life

- Biological, social, and psychological factors all influence the perception of stress and its link with mental and behavioral disorders

- Stress can be measured in several ways, including self-report checklists, interviews, and physiological assessments

- Stress has been linked with several physical health problems, including hypertension, coronary heart disease, and cancer, as well as dysregulation of physiological systems like the hypothalamic-pituitary-adrenal axis

- The diathesis–stress model provides a conceptual framework for understanding the influence of stress on the etiology of mental and behavioral disorders
- The concept of resilience is helpful in understanding why not all individuals exposed to risk will develop mental and behavioral disorders

INTRODUCTION

The ability to adapt to stress and adversity is a central component of human development over the life course. Although a certain amount of stress is normal and necessary for survival, too much stress can trigger or exacerbate a range of mental problems of varying severity. Stress has been defined in many ways (S. Cohen, Kessler, & Gordon, 1995). For the purposes of this chapter, stress is conceptualized as major or minor life events that disrupt biological and behavioral mechanisms that maintain stability of an individual's physiology, emotion, and cognition (Lazarus & Folkman, 1984; Luthar & Zigler, 1991; Monroe & Simons, 1991). Because stress appears to have important physiological, psychological, and social consequences, it is a common focus of public mental health research. A number of theories have been proposed to link the experience of stress with mental health problems across the life course. These theories have directed attention to the role of biological, genetic, and social factors that may influence the experience or perception of stress or may modulate responses to stress. Thus understanding and characterizing stress and its mental health consequences are critical subjects in the field of public mental health.

This chapter explores the role of stress in the conduct of both public mental health research and practice. It begins with a discussion of the leading definitions and theories of stress proposed in relation to the experience of mental problems, followed by an examination of the multiple perspectives related to the measurement and study of stress. Given the ubiquitous nature of stress and its association with developmental challenges, this review is couched within a broader life course perspective. This perspective highlights the significance of both human development and the social context in examining the link between stress and mental health problems. We identify a range of developmental stressors spanning different life stages and describe their effects on mental health and adjustment problems.

PERSPECTIVES ON STRESS

Despite long-standing interest in stress within the scientific community, debates about its definition, measurement, and utility as a concept persist (S. Cohen et al., 1995; Kopp et al., 2010; Pollock, 1988; Vingerhoets & Marcelissen, 1988). In his classic description of stress, Hans Selye (1956) proposed that stressors are events that strain an individual's adaptive capability, giving rise to disruption of routine or habitual functioning. Other proposed definitions of stress share this notion of a threat to a balanced system of functioning (e.g., Chrousos & Gold, 1992; Hinkle, 1987; McEwen, 2000). Stress thus is commonly agreed to represent an interference with a system's physiological and psychological homeostasis (Ingram & Luxton, 2005). However, theories of stress differ in a number of ways, including the extent to which they emphasize physiological and psychological processes and the extent to which they highlight subjective appraisals of the stressor.

Historical Perspectives on Stress

The concept of stress and its role in mental problems dates to the work of Freud in the early 1900s (J. P. Wilson, 1994). While working with Josef Breuer on the disorder now called posttraumatic stress disorder (PTSD), Freud initially endorsed a posttraumatic seduction theory approach to describe responses to trauma (Breuer &

Freud, 1895). However, he later supported a model based on anxiety resulting from intrapsychic threats or conflicts. While much of Freud's career focused on anxiety and the unconscious rather than on external stressors, his writings reflect an awareness of the potential significance of perceived threats and conflicts as sources of stress. While not commonly invoked in contemporary public mental health research, the psychoanalytic perspective laid the groundwork for subsequent psychological research on personality and mental health factors; it also highlighted the significance of early childhood experiences for the onset of subsequent adjustment problems. Despite the popular use of the term stress in the 19th and early 20th centuries, the concept was rarely discussed in the mental health literature prior to the end of World War II, when increased concern arose about symptoms of PTSD displayed by combat veterans. Since that time, the concept of stress has gained widespread popularity in relation to mental and physical disorders (Pollock, 1988; Vingerhoets & Marcelissen, 1988).

In the behavioral sciences, the notion of stress initially was adapted from concepts in engineering and physics (Pollock, 1988; Sapolsky, 2004). In its nascence, stress research had a predominantly physiological emphasis. Walter Cannon's work in the 1920s identified the impact of emotional arousal on the physiological responses of an organism, highlighting the role of the sympathetic nervous system (Cannon, 1929; Vingerhoets & Marcelissen, 1988). A pioneer in stress research, Selye proposed the general adaptation syndrome model to describe the process by which chronic exposure to stress stimuli increased the risk for disease. According to Selye (1956), the stress response occurs in three successive stages: alarm reaction, resistance, and exhaustion. Subsequent research has focused on the biological aspects of the stress response and how chronic exposure to stressful conditions exerts wear and tear on the body's response system, in turn increasing the risk for both physical and mental health problems

(McEwen, 1998). In this line of research, stress most often is considered the reaction process, whereas the stressors are environmental stimuli (Hankin, Abela, Auerbach, McWhinnie, & Skitch, 2005).

Other research, focused on the role of psychological processes, has explored the extent to which the appraisal of an event as stressful could influence the physiological response. Lazarus and Folkman (1984) elaborated the transactional nature of the stress process, describing it as a dynamic interplay between environmental events and an individual's appraisal of those events. They proposed that stress occurs when an individual perceives the demands of a situation to exceed his or her resources and capacity to cope with those demands.[1] Stress appraisal is an internalized process; its assessment relies on individual subjective reports (Lazarus & Folkman, 1984). Other theories also have incorporated appraisal as a critical factor in shaping emotional and physiological outcomes (e.g., Leventhal, 1984; Leventhal & Scherer, 1987).

Rather than focus on subjective appraisal, other researchers have emphasized "objective" environmental circumstances that contribute to stress (e.g., Holmes & Rahe, 1967). Adopting a stimulus-based approach, Grant and colleagues (2003) defined stress as "environmental events or chronic conditions that objectively threaten...physical and/or psychological health or wellbeing" (p. 449). Those circumstances include discrete negative or adverse life events, such as the death of a loved one, divorce, or a natural disaster, as well as chronic exposure to adversity, such as living in a violent neighborhood or battling a chronic physical illness. Even positively valenced life events—such as marriage or a job promotion—could create a level of stress that demands adaptive changes to the existing biological and psychological systems (Brown & Harris, 1989; Dohrenwend & Shrout, 1985).

----

1. Coping is the process by which individuals respond to a stressor, either by attempting to modify a stressful situation (problem-focused coping) or by managing their internal emotional reactions (emotion-focused coping).

Characteristics of Stress

SITUATIONAL AND DEVELOPMENTAL STRESSORS

Stress often results from change, from the process of adapting to change, and from developmental challenges. Even small changes in rapid succession can lead to stress and susceptibility to physical and mental health problems (Selye, 1956). Stressors can be described as either situational or developmental (maturational). Situational stressors result from unanticipated or unplanned events that threaten an individual's homeostasis or equilibrium, such as family illness, separation or divorce, unemployment, relocation, natural or man-made disasters, and the birth of a child with a physical, behavioral, or neurological impairment. Developmental or maturational stressors, part of normal growth and development, occur as an individual or a family as a whole moves from one developmental stage to another. Developmental stressors also may be associated with the achievement of developmental tasks, such as weaning, toilet training, establishing a sexual identity, school success or failure, choosing a career, and retirement. Family developmental stressors include adapting to a new family member, childbearing, and family relocation. Whether developmental stressors result from individual or family development, generally the family as a whole is affected.

DIMENSIONS OF STRESS

A number of dimensions of stress are thought to influence its effect on adjustment. The positive or negative aspect of the event—its valence—may influence the extent to which it results in distress. Most researchers concur that negative events tend to be more stressful than positive events (Dohrenwend, 1998). An event's predictability also may influence the level of experienced stress. The death of a chronically ill grandparent, for example, may be less stressful than the unexpected death of a spouse in a car accident. Another potential factor influencing the stress response is the extent to which an individual feels a lack of

control when faced with adversity—a sense of fatefulness (Dohrenwend, 2000; Dohrenwend, Raphael, Schwartz, Stueve, & Skodol,1993; Pearlin & Schooler, 1978). Other factors likely to moderate the impact of life events include their centrality (i.e., importance) to identity and functioning and their magnitude (i.e., severity) (Dohrenwend, 2000).

TYPES OF STRESSORS

The National Scientific Council on the Developing Child (2005) recommended conceptualizing stress as toxic, tolerable, or positive. Toxic stress, illustrated throughout the preceding section, is a consequence of strong or frequent activation of the body's stress system that may be sustained over a long period, potentially leading to dysregulation of the body's physiological response patterns. Such toxic stress is thought to produce long-term changes in brain functioning and sensitivity to environmental stimuli. Tolerable stress occurs in small doses and with lower frequency; compared with toxic stress, it is relatively short-lived. If tolerable stress is well managed and occurs in a supportive environment, it can be beneficial for an individual. Finally, positive stress most often arises from short-lived stressors that are expected in an individual's life course and that carry no negative connotations. Such positive stress includes that experienced in preparing for an exam, in meeting new people, and in the early stages of a romantic relationship. All serve as opportunities to grow without constant or frequent activation of the body's physiological response to stress (see below for information on the hypothalamic-pituitary-adrenal [HPA] system).

HASSLES VERSUS STRESSORS

Other researchers have distinguished between the day-to-day experience of minor stressors and severe, relatively rare life events (Pearlin & Skaff, 1995). Everyday adversities can be further subdivided into chronic stressors and daily hassles (Serido, Almeida, & Wethington, 2004). Chronic stressors are ongoing events or concerns, such as fear of losing one's job or disagreements with one's neighbors. These persistent difficulties often are associated with factors such as being overworked or balancing competing demands of multiple social roles (e.g., being a parent and a wife as well as an employee). In contrast, daily hassles are relatively minor frustrating and distressing experiences resulting from everyday transactions with the environment, such as traffic congestion, minor arguments, and unexpected deadlines (Turner, Wheaton, & Lloyd, 1995). While seemingly minor, daily hassles have been found to adversely affect health and well-being (DeLongis, Folkman, & Lazarus, 1988; Eckenrode, 1984; Pett & Johnson, 2005). Stress researchers also have examined the extent to which pervasive factors related to the social structure may produce stress. Thus, for example, stress is theorized to result from prejudice, discrimination, and structural inequities that can place certain individuals and groups in a disadvantaged status (Clark, Anderson, Clark, & Williams, 1999; I. L. Meyer, 2003).

ACUTE STRESS EXPOSURE

Awareness of the significant impact of acute stress exposure on mental health and illnesses such as PTSD has been growing since World War II. As described in chapter 1, symptoms of PTSD include recurrent memories or flashbacks of trauma, avoidance of reminders of the trauma, increased arousal or hyperarousal, and a diminished range of emotional expression. (See also the fourth edition of the *Diagnostic and Statistical Manual of Mental Disorders* [American Psychiatric Association , 1994].) While the lifetime prevalence of PTSD in the general population is approximately 3–4% (with a range of 1–9%), it is considerably higher among individuals exposed to war. For example, studies of Vietnam veterans suggest that the prevalence in this population was approximately 15% (Kulka, 1990), while the prevalence among Gulf War veterans was 10% (Kang, Natelson, Mahan, Lee, & Murphy, 2003). In early studies of Iraq War veterans, the prevalence of combat-related PTSD was approximately 12%, and another 4% had other mental problems (Hoge et al., 2004). Some evidence suggests a dose–response effect, a linear association between the number of firefights in which a soldier engaged and the risk for combat-related PTSD (Hoge et al., 2004).

Because it was long thought that children were either immune to stress or resilient in the face of stressors, much of the early work on acute stress responses and PTSD focused on adults. Building on her father's work, Anna Freud and her colleague Dorothy Burlingham (1943) investigated the emotional health status of children who had lost a parent during World War II or who had been abandoned and were living at the Hampstead War Nursery in London. Their work documented the children's responses to war and highlighted the significance of caring adults who were physically and emotionally available to support the children. It also appeared that the children looked to the adults around them to gauge their responses to the stress of war. Decades later, Lenore Terr (1990) documented the significant short- and long-term effects of a traumatic experience endured by a group of children from Chowchilla, California: being kidnapped and buried underground in a van for over 12 hours. Her qualitative research drew national attention to the importance of providing traumatized children with psychiatric care and dramatically debunked the myth that children were immune to serious psychological effects of traumatic events. Some of her research suggests that young children may be even more vulnerable than adults to experiencing adjustment problems in response to trauma (Terr, 1990).

More recent empirical studies have examined the short- and long-term effects on both children and adults of natural and man-made disasters such as Hurricane Katrina in the Gulf Coast area (Burton et al., 2009; P. S. Wang et al., 2007) and the September 11, 2001, attacks on the World Trade Center (Comer et al., 2010; Hoven et al., 2005; Schlenger et al., 2002). Immediately following the 9/11 attacks, the prevalence of PTSD was substantially higher among New York City's adult residents than in the rest of the country; the probability of PTSD was linked to direct exposure to the event (Schlenger et al., 2002). High proportions of New York City public school children were found to be suffering from PTSD and other anxiety disorders (including childhood depression) six months after exposure to the 9/11 attacks. Similarly, postdisaster mental health effects, particularly mood and anxiety disorders, have been reported among survivors of Hurricane Katrina. However, few of those individuals received adequate care following the disaster (P. S. Wang et al., 2007). Older adults appeared especially vulnerable to the effects of Katrina, as evidenced by high rates of morbidity and increased rates of emergency room visits and hospitalizations (Burton et al., 2009). (For further discussion of research on crisis-related acute trauma, see chapter 11.)

Physiological Mechanisms Involved in the Stress Responses

The specific physiological mechanisms involved in the stress response are a topic of growing interest. One particular brain chemistry circuit that has received considerable attention is the HPA axis, which is activated in response to a perceived threat (Evans, 2003; Gunnar & Donzella, 2002; Gunnar, Talge, & Herrera, 2009). The HPA axis involves the hypothalamus, the pituitary gland, and the adrenal gland, which act in concert to produce the stress hormone cortisol (see figure 10-1). When the system is activated by a stressor, the paraventricular nucleus of the hypothalamus releases corticotropin-releasing factor (CRF), which in turn activates the anterior pituitary gland to release adrenocorticotropic hormone. This triggers the adrenal gland, which is situated on top of the kidney, to release androgens and to produce cortisol. Cortisol, a glucocorticoid and a corticosteroid hormone, is released into the bloodstream, activating the sympathetic nervous system and preparing the body for a fight-or-flight response. Immediate physiological changes resulting from the effects of cortisol include pupil dilation and increased heart rate, blood pressure, and breathing rate (Gunnar & Donzella, 2002). Secondary functions such as digestion are inhibited to provide more energy for the

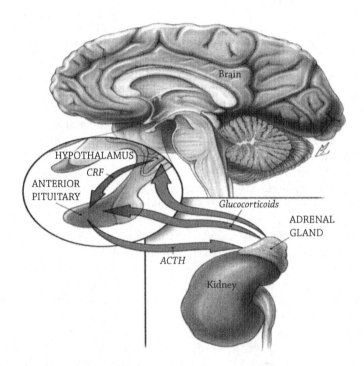

Figure 10-1   **Hypothalamic-Pituitary-Adrenal Axis And Stress Reactivity**
ACTH = adrenocorticotropic hormone; CRF = corticotropin-releasing factor.

Source: Reproduced with permission from Niehoff, 2002.

fight-or-flight response. Because the HPA axis is a highly regulated system, increased levels of circulating cortisol inhibit the release of CRF by the hypothalamus through a stepwise process that effectively halts release of additional, potentially excessive cortisol.

While acute activation of the HPA axis is adaptive and plays an important role in mobilizing a response to stress, chronic activation of the system can give rise to hippocampal damage, including reductions in dendritic branching (arborization) and neurogenesis (Watanabe, Gould, & McEwen, 1992). Because the hippocampus plays a role in inhibiting the hypothalamus from releasing CRF, continuous HPA activation can lead to dysregulation of the HPA axis altogether. Moreover, chronic activation of the sympathetic nervous system can lead to a compromised immune system (Littrell, 2008), changing an adaptive process into a maladaptive one (Perry, 1997; Perry, Pollard, Blakley, Baker, & Vigilante, 1995). Several mental disorders have been associated with both a dysregulated physiological stress response and a reduction in hippocampal volume, among them depressive illness (Sheline, Wang, Gado, Csernansky, & Vannier, 1996), and anxiety disorders (U. Meyer, van Kampen, Isovich, Flugge, & Fuchs, 2001), including PTSD (Bremner et al., 1995).

Allostasis is the term used to describe a complex, "dynamic, highly interactive set of multiple physiological systems of equilibrium maintenance" (Evans, 2003, p. 924; also see McEwen, 1998). Allostasis represents the body's attempt to balance itself in response to an encountered stressor or series of stressors, resulting in the ongoing adjustment of its typical operating range or set points (Evans, 2003). This maintenance process increases a body's allostatic load, the cumulative negative effects of—or the price the body pays for—adapting to psychosocial challenges and adverse environmental stimuli (Seeman, Singer, Rowe, Horowitz, & McEwen, 1997). The chronic wear and tear on body and brain from mobilizing resources to respond to stress results in adverse effects on the body, in what often is described as the "scarring" model. In some instances, downregulation of the system

is necessary to maintain internal stability. As Evans (2003) wrote:

> Allostatic load is not simply a consequence of environmental demands. Rather, it is a complex, dynamic system of physiological changes in multiple systems created by responses to environmental demands that are modulated by prior experience with stressors, genetic predisposition and lifestyle choices. (p. 925)

Physiological signs of the consequences of this downregulation include elevated blood pressure, cortisol, epinephrine, and norepinephrine; hyperactivity; and poor recovery from acute demand. Common indicators of allostatic load are found in the body's neurophysiological systems, notably measures of heart rate and arousal, cortisol functioning, and blood pressure (McEwen, 1998).

One elegant example of the association between risk exposure and allostatic load comes from a study of rural children by Evans (2003). Expanding on Rutter's (1986, 1987) theory of cumulative risk, Evans examined the association between a set of environmental and socioemotional risk factors (e.g. crowding, noise level, violence exposure, single parenthood) and indicators of allostatic load. He documented an association between cumulative risk exposure and a number of physiological changes, including alterations in self-regulatory behavior, learned helplessness, cardiovascular functioning, neuroendocrine functioning, body mass index, and a composite index of total allostatic load. This work also highlights the potential psychological and physiological impact the developmental timing of stress exposure can have on adjustment, both in the short term and across the life course.

Measuring Stress

While symptoms of PTSD are commonly assessed in clinical and epidemiologic studies, researchers often are interested in quantifying exposure to life events using methods that can capture objective characteristics of the exposure rather than subjective responses to it (see, e.g., Brown & Harris, 1989; Dohrenwend &

Shrout, 1985). Self-report measures of life events are the methods most widely used to ascertain stress levels (Kopp et al., 2010; Turner et al., 1995). Checklists of stressful life events (typically amassed through self-reports or interviews) vary in content, scope, and specificity of events and experiences. Life event scales in use today are fairly consistent in their approach to measuring stressful life events, including such factors as work-, family-, relationship-, neighborhood-, and race-related issues.

The conceptualization or definition of stress chosen by researchers can have significant bearing on both the content of the measure and the manner in which the instrument is administered. For example, consistent with an objective perspective on stress, checklists generally assess the cumulative number of positive and negative events experienced within a specific time frame (e.g., a 1-year period). Items most often are weighted according to severity. This approach assumes that participants perceive events similarly without regard to individual demographics (Turner et al., 1995). Holmes and Rahe's (1967) Social Readjustment Rating Scale (SRRS) is one of the life event checklists most commonly used in measuring potentially stressful events. The SRSS elaborates on the Schedule of Recent Experiences (Hawkins, Davies, & Holmes, 1957) and defines stress as the cumulative change or adjustment resulting from responses to both positive and negative environmental events. When developing the weights for the SRSS, life events were objectively weighted by a randomly selected panel of judges who rated the amount of adjustment deemed appropriate for each experience. Modifications to the SRSS to reflect age-specific stressors have made the instrument more developmentally appropriate for participants of different ages, from children and adolescents to older adults (Hankin et al., 2005).

Interview measures of life events are an alternative to the self-report checklist. In some cases, researchers may read checklist items aloud to participants and use probes or structured interview questions to inquire about particular reported events. Interview approaches often can provide a richer description of specific events and additional contextual information about the stress experienced. Not surprisingly, these approaches also place greater emphasis on participants' appraisal of events than do self-report checklists (Rudolph et al., 2000). Research studies also use other tools, such as daily event records and diaries, to pinpoint the timing of stress, thus helping to link exposure to particular stressors with specific behavioral or psychological problems (e.g., linking work-related stress with substance use).

Although interviews and checklists are used broadly by researchers and can be efficiently administered, both approaches are vulnerable to measurement error, recall bias, and social desirability bias. Self-report measures of stress may not readily measure objective threat, may exclude the period of the event, and may not distinguish whether the stressors are independent of an individual's behavior (Hankin et al., 2005).

As a result of the limitations of self-report measures, interest is growing in exploring physiological measures of stress, such as salivary cortisol levels. Released by the HPA axis, cortisol is reactive to stress; further, chronically high cortisol levels predict poor health outcomes such as insulin resistance and other risk factors for diabetes and cardiovascular disease (Wolkowitz, Epel, & Reus, 2001). Cortisol levels can be assessed from blood, urine, or saliva samples. Concentrations of easy-to-collect salivary hormones are considered reliable and valid measures of the concentrations of hormones in the blood (Kirschbaum & Hellhammer, 1994). Cortisol sampling can assess various aspects of HPA activity, including basal cortisol levels, diurnal variation, and response to acute stressors (Nicolson, 2008).

Because recurrent cardiovascular arousal has been posited as a stress-related pathway that may increase risk for disease, researchers also often rely on this phenomenon when assessing the effects of stress (Brunner et al., 2002; Schneiderman, 1987). Blood pressure, for example, provides a broad assessment of cardiac arousal. Other indices of cardiovascular function provide more nuanced information about the nature of the arousal and the relative involvement of the sympathetic and parasympathetic systems. For instance, the high-frequency power component of heart rate variability (HF-HRV) is an index of parasympathetic control (Berntson et al., 1997); reduced HF-HRV has been linked to increased cardiovascular disease and mortality (Liao et al., 1997; Thayer & Lane, 2007). Impedance cardiography, another measure of cardiovascular response, isolates two distinct arousal components: cardiac output (the amount of blood pumped by the heart) and total peripheral resistance (vasoconstriction of blood vessels). Chronic levels of increased total peripheral resistance are associated with vascular hypertrophy, hypertension, and other untoward cardiovascular outcomes (McFetridge & Sherwood, 1999). Adverse cardiac responses such as increases in total peripheral resistance relative to cardiac output can be induced by threat-related stress (i.e., demands in excess of perceived resources) (Blascovich & Mendes, 2000). Based on established guidelines, these cardiovascular measures can be assessed noninvasively with the use of special analytic software to obtain relevant measures from signals recorded by spot electrodes (Sherwood et al., 1990).

FROM STRESS TO DISTRESS

While the definitions and measures of stress may have varied over time, the links among stress and physical and mental problems, as well as more general social adjustment problems, have long been recognized. Strong evidence shows that stressful life events can disrupt daily functioning and can degrade the quality of life to the point of disorder. These effects appear to vary both by developmental level and by the presence of other vulnerabilities.

Link Between Stress and Mental Disorders

A growing body of research documents a link between adverse life events and a variety of mental problems (Eaton, 1978; Jordanova et al., 2007; Surtees et al., 1986). Both cross-sectional and longitudinal studies of adverse life events have shown an association with mental disorders (Kessler, 1997; Paykel, 1994; Surtees et al., 1986). Research has found that

most episodes of depression, perhaps as many as 50%, are preceded by a major life event (Brown & Harris, 1978; Nazroo, 2001). The psychological toll claimed by stress also is seen in its role in the etiology of other mental disorders such as PTSD and anxiety.

Consistent with the definition of stress developed by Lazarus and Folkman (1984), compelling evidence exists for an association between subjectively appraised stressors and mental disorders such as depression (Surtees et al., 1986). In fact, among the most consistent depression research findings are that stressful life events, including both major and minor stressors, often precede the onset of depression and that an accumulation of stressors can have a graded relationship with the severity of the resulting depressive disorder (Lewinsohn, Hoberman, & Rosenbaum, 1988). Severe life events—physical assault, death of a close relative, unemployment, marital problems, divorce, or termination of romantic relationship—have been found to be associated with more severe depression. The greatest risk for onset appears to occur within one month of the stressor event (Kendler et al., 1995; Lewinsohn et al., 1988).

Not surprisingly, stress has been linked with lower overall productivity; it further can contribute to distal adverse outcomes such as poor academic or work performance, risk of accidents and injuries, and low socioeconomic status (Giaconia et al., 1995; Swaen, van Amelsvoort, Bültmann, Slangen, & Kant, 2004). Stress also can affect social relationships, such as by disrupting the social environment and social interactions in ways that in turn can create a vulnerability to further psychological and physiological distress or can exacerbate the effects of the existing stress (Joiner, 2000).

Link Between Stress and Physical Health

The health-related outcomes of stress are both numerous and far-reaching. For example, stress appears to contribute to poor physical health (Jemmott & Locke, 1984), including complications such as upper respiratory problems, allergies, hypertension, coronary heart disease, and cancer (Chen & Miller, 2007; Chida, Hamer, Wardle, & Steptoe, 2008; Figueredo, 2009; Smith & Nicholson, 2001; Turner Cobb & Steptoe, 1998). In addition, stress can produce deleterious physiological effects by dysregulating physiological systems like the HPA axis (Nemeroff et al., 2006; Sapolsky, 1999), as well as by disrupting patterns of sleeping and eating. Numerous studies have linked high stress levels to a range of other physical health problems, among them chronic fatigue, heart disease, headaches, muscle tension, upset stomach, dizziness, and obesity.

Because multiple regulatory systems in the body interact in a nonlinear fashion, stress can promote disease through both direct and indirect physiological pathways (Kamarck & Jennings, 1991; Kubzansky & Kawachi, 2000). For instance, cardiovascular responses to stress include patterns of increased vascular resistance that have adverse health effects (Tomaka, Blascovich, Kelsey, & Leitten, 1993). Research also suggests that stress may impair the autonomic nervous system, particularly the parasympathetic (vagal) branch, associated with restorative functions. Lower vagal tone has been linked to anxiety, depression, and hostility (Demaree & Everhart, 2004; Kawachi, Sparrow, Vokonas, & Weiss, 1995; Porges, 2003; Thayer, Friedman, & Borkovec, 1996) and further is associated with increased risk for morbidity and mortality from cardiovascular disease (Thayer & Lane, 2007). Other work has linked stress and associated distress with catecholamine secretion or dysregulation of the HPA axis and secondary metabolic disturbances (Stansfeld, Fuhrer, Shipley, & Marmot, 2002). Not surprisingly, research has sought to discern physiological mechanisms that might mediate the influence of stress on both physical and psychological well-being. Such physiological factors also may modulate responsiveness to environmental stress. These pathways are considered in greater detail below.

Cause or Consequence of Stress?

Because life events thought to cause stress actually may be undetected consequences of a physical or mental illness (Thoits, 1981), additional research must be conducted to tease apart the relationships between stress and health. Further, research to date typically has not controlled for preexisting mental problems, despite the fact that a history of psychopathology may influence future mental health outcomes. For example, an Australian longitudinal study of 1,947 adolescents with preexisting depressive and anxiety symptoms found early adverse life events to be associated with an eightfold increased risk for subsequent adverse life events, which in turn were predictive of subsequent major depressive disorder (Patton, Coffey, Posterino, Carlin, & Bowes, 2003).

THEORIES OF STRESS AND ADAPTATION

Why do some people exposed to stress develop mental problems while others do not? Empirical evidence suggests that prior experience, coping skills, and personal and social coping resources (including the availability of social support) can mitigate the impact of adverse life events and help reduce the risk for mental problems (Eaton, 1978). While the study of the biological mechanisms and potential modifiers underlying stress and stress reactions can help in better understanding potential causes of mental problems, numerous environmental stressors also play a critical role in stress response processes. Bronfenbrenner's ecological systems theory (1979) illustrates the multiple internal and external systems or levels that influence development and adjustment to risk, and delineates the transactional processes occurring across the ecological system (see figure 10-2). Bronfenbrenner characterized a set of nested levels of influence, each with a significant influence on development across the life course (Bronfenbrenner & Morris, 1998). For example, individuals can experience both risk and protection at the individual level through factors such as genetics, intelligence, and temperament. The next level of influence is within the microsystem, which includes a combination of family and peer relationships. However, exposure to the greater exosystem—the surrounding social

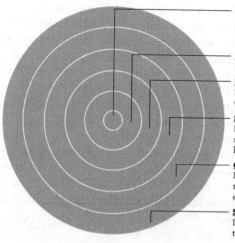

Individual Factors
Includes individual traits (e.g., race, sexual orientation, learning and other disabilities, religion, ethnicity, gender). Also includes any biological, genetic and psychological strengths and challenges or issues.

Family
Includes influences due to family life, structure, and relationship dynamics.

Peer Relationships
Includes influences of interpersonal relationships and group dynamics with peers.

School and Work
Includes the effects of all aspects of the school or work environment, such as policies and implementation, climate, available resources, leadership style and commitment, and involvement.

Community and Culture
Includes influences of the community (e.g., services and resources, support networks), the cultural context including factors (e.g., race, religion), and experience of inclusion or exclusion.

Society
Includes state and societal policies, practices and dominant social norms that affect an individual's opportunities.

Figure 10-2   **Bronfenbrenner's Ecological Systems Theory.**

Source: From Mishna, 2012. Reproduced with permission from Oxford University Press.

environment—also affects individuals within the microsystem. The final level of influence, the macrosystem, is composed of the underlying values and customs of the larger environment and can include policies and national events (Bronfenbrenner & Morris, 1998).

Factors at each level have the potential to exert a direct or indirect influence on the risk for mental problems. Some factors, such as a supportive home environment, can buffer risks from other ecological systems, such as exposure to violence in the community (Zielinski & Bradshaw, 2006). A number of theories have been posited that describe the process by which stress increases the risk for mental health disorders. Several of the leading theories are considered below, drawing on the ecological model and providing examples of specific disorders across the life course.

Diathesis–Stress Models

The effect of stress on mental health is best characterized by the diathesis–stress (or vulnerability–stress) model (see figure 10-3). Initially developed to delineate the etiology of schizophrenia (Bleuler, 1963; Rosenthal, 1963), the model has evolved to include other disorders with dynamic interactions with the environment (McKeever & Huff, 2003; Monroe

& Simons, 1991; Zubin & Spring, 1977). The diathesis–stress model provides a conceptual framework for exploring the influence of stress on the etiology of mental disorders.

Models of the diathesis–stress type are dependent on the relationship between a biological vulnerability (the diathesis) and an environmental influence (the stressor). The combination of these two factors contributes to the likelihood that an individual will develop

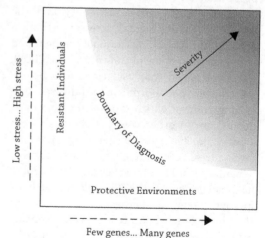

Figure 10-3   **Diathesis–Stress Model.**

Source: © Johns Hopkins University.

a mental disorder. Several diathesis–stress models have been developed, each apportioning different relative weights to the two factors. The most basic are threshold models, in which the combination of factors becomes significant if their sum (additive model) or product (multiplicative model) crosses an arbitrary, predesignated threshold. These models place no greater emphasis on either vulnerability or stressor, since a large stressor may be enough for the threshold to be crossed with minimal input from a biological vulnerability. Similarly, in the presence of a biological vulnerability, such as a genetic abnormality, only a small (or even no) environmental stressor may be needed for the threshold to be crossed and the disorder to manifest. Thus without regard to the relative weight of the two factors, if the threshold is crossed, the individual will manifest the disorder; if it is not crossed, the disorder will not become manifest. The most notable threshold model was proposed by Zubin and Spring (1977) to explain the etiology of schizophrenia. Zubin and Spring believed every individual to have a minimal biological vulnerability for the symptoms of schizophrenia. According to their model, the determining factor in the onset of schizophrenic symptoms is that the individual's environment has sufficient detrimental influences to push an individual over the threshold for the disease. The ipsative model, a variant of the additive model, posits that an inverse relationship can exist between a biological vulnerability and the impact of environmental stressors (Hankin et al., 2005). A working example can be found in the research of Caspi and colleagues (2003), who determined that variations of a neurotransmitter polymorphism minimized the tipping point at which stress led to manifest depression. In other words, individuals with a particular biological vulnerability required fewer adverse events to evidence symptoms of a mental disorder. McKeever and Huff (2003) have suggested that PTSD follows such an ipsative model of diathesis–stress, positing that the disorder shows an inverse relationship between stress and vulnerability to disorder (e.g., increased stress lowers the threshold for psychopathology). Traumatic stress and PTSD are discussed in greater detail in chapter 11.

The risk–resilience continuum model is an extension of the ipsative model in which the presence of previous environmental stressors increases the threshold for disorder expression (Ingram & Price, 2001). Betancourt and Khan (2008) have explored the extent to which children from countries at war are able to develop mental resiliency as a result of managing to live with a constant level of trauma. They caution, however, that adverse mental health outcomes are equally or even more likely, in which case the kindling model, in which environmental stressors decrease the threshold at which a disorder arises, may be more applicable (Post, 1992).

Genetic Susceptibility and Environmental Risk

Much of the recent work on diathesis–stress models has examined genetic vulnerabilities for mental problems within the context of environmental risks. A review of the literature by Belsky and Pluess (2009), for example, provides a framework for evaluating the evidence in favor of differential susceptibility. They highlight the importance of considering a range of phenotypic, endophenotypic, genetic, and emotional markers for mental disorders within the diathesis–stress paradigm. They also emphasize the importance of the gene–environment interaction perspective in future mental health research.

When the environment and an individual's innate trait interact, they form genotype–environment associations (Plomin, DeFries, & Loehlin, 1977) that may help explain the process through which genetic factors interact with or, in some cases, are correlated with environmental experiences. Three common genotype–environment relationships—passive, reactive, and active—most often are considered in research on mental disorders. Passive correlations depend on a shared genetic and environmental condition, such as a family unit in which parents share genes and environment with their children. Parents shape the household based on their own genetic code; parental personality traits can be passed on to their children as a consequence of modeling. Thus Kelley and Fals-Stewart (2004) determined that children of drug-abusing parents were more likely to develop mental disorders, including substance abuse, than were children of parents who did not abuse substances.

Reactive genotype–environment relationships occur when the environment must be modified to accommodate an individual's innate traits, as when parenting is adjusted to accommodate a child's behaviors associated with attention deficit hyperactivity disorder (ADHD). Similarly, based on the same child's behavior, his or her peers may need to reshape their relationships, potentially resulting in a decrement in the quality of the child's friendships (Normand, Schneider, & Robaey, 2007). Finally, active relationships (also called evocative associations) occur when an individual's innate traits lead him or her to seek out different environments. Extroverted individuals who seek out new scenarios that challenge them socially may be the best examples of this relationship. Similarly, academically focused individuals may continue to challenge themselves by attending graduate school after college.

A growing body of literature is examining the interplay of susceptibility factors and environmental predictors, with a particular focus on genetic polymorphisms associated with psychopathology (Rutter, 2008). Much of the research on biological risk factors for stress has focused on neurotransmitters associated with mental disorders. These factors are explored as potential mediators or moderators of the stress response. A series of studies by Caspi and colleagues (2002, 2003) have investigated the interaction between particular genetic vulnerabilities and environmental stressors. One such study found a significant link between a serotonin polymorphism (the long vs. short alleles of the 5-HTT gene) and adverse psychiatric outcomes (i.e. depression and suicidality) following an adverse life event (Caspi et al., 2003). Caspi and colleagues (2002) also found that when an individual had experienced childhood maltreatment, the presence of the monoamine oxidase A (MAOA) gene polymorphism was associated with a decreased threshold for aggressive behaviors.

Since those groundbreaking studies, several others examining the relationship between MAOA and childhood maltreatment or adversity have generally concluded that mental disorders, including ADHD, are significantly more frequent among individuals who possess the short MAOA allele and who also have faced or are facing adversity (Kim-Cohen et al., 2006). Similarly, a broad array of researchers (e.g., Caspi et al., 2003; Zalsman et al., 2006) have linked another serotonin polymorphism (5-HTTLPR) and stressful life events with depressive symptoms. However, a meta-analysis by Risch and others (2009) failed to confirm this association when pooling 14 separate studies investigating this particular gene–environment interaction. More recently, Cicchetti, Rogosch, Sturge-Apple, and Toth (2010) explored whether genetic variation in the serotonin transporter polymorphism (5-HTTLPR) moderated the association between child maltreatment and suicidal ideation among school-age children. Higher suicidal ideation was found among children who had been maltreated than among those who had not; there also was an interaction between the maltreatment and the genetic polymorphism. Similarly, in a longitudinal study of stressful life events among adults, Kendler and colleagues (1995) found that while most participants did not develop major depressive disorder, the risk for depression was 2.4 times greater in those at high genetic vulnerability than among those at low genetic risk. Animal models (using female rhesus macaques) have provided additional evidence for the association between increased life stressors and neurotransmitters, showing that lower levels of cortisol and a major serotonin metabolite in the cerebrospinal fluid (5-HIAA) are linked to increased aggression (Westergaard et al., 2003). Together, these findings highlight the need to consider both genetic and environmental factors when exploring risks for mental disorders (Rutter, 2008).

Social–Cognitive Risk Factors

As noted earlier, a considerable body of research on gene–environment interactions has examined childhood risk factors such as maltreatment. A number of studies have documented an association between physical abuse as a form of child maltreatment and a range of mental problems. The majority of the research in this area has examined vulnerable personality traits such as high levels of fearfulness, impulsivity, and shyness and a propensity toward anger. These features, when combined with parental factors (e.g., parental power assertions and parenting quality and effectiveness), are associated with psychological distress, including but not limited to externalizing and internalizing behavior problems.

The strength of the attachment between parent and child arguably is one of the most important and telling predictors of both current and future life stress. John Bowlby's (1969, 1973) seminal work illustrates the need for children to have an attachment figure who provides a secure base from which the child can explore the world while receiving consistent and sensitive care. The absence of such a relationship leads to adverse life events, as illustrated in countless animal and human scenarios. One of the earlier explorations was the seminal work by Harry Harlow examining the effects that deprivation of a maternal figure has on the behavior and social–emotional well-being of young rhesus monkeys (Harlow & Harlow, 1969). The studies highlighted the significant impact of early attachment experiences on both adjustment and response to stress. This work has been extended in other animal studies to explore physiological systems involved in this process as well as gene–environment interactions that may increase the vulnerability of some individuals to stress associated with neglect or abuse (Belay et al., 2011; Rutter, 2008; Suomi, 2006). Several of the findings have been replicated in human populations, for example, in studies of orphaned children in developing countries (Gunnar, Bruce, & Grotevant, 2000) and insecurely attached children of young mothers (Chisholm, 1998).

Child maltreatment has been one of the more heavily researched factors that have been linked to adverse life events and the inability to form secure attachments (Bradshaw & Garbarino, 2004; Cicchetti, 1989; Dodge, Bates, & Pettit, 1990). The absence of secure attachments in turn has been associated with affect dysregulation and impairment of interpersonal functioning, including depression and behavioral problems (Cicchetti, 2002; Cicchetti & Lynch, 1995). In contrast, a secure attachment confers mental health benefits and promotes both stability across the life span and healthy adult relationships (Cicchetti, Rogosch, Lynch, & Holt, 1993; Collins & Read, 1990; Waters, Merrick, Treboux, Crowell, & Albersheim, 2000).

Low socioeconomic status (SES) is a common stressor that has been broadly explored in the literature. Hollingshead and Redlich (1958) found psychopathology was more prevalent in children from low-SES families than in those from high-SES families. Indeed, as many as a quarter of impoverished youth have social and emotional difficulties (Keenan, Shaw, Walsh, Delliquadri, & Giovannelli, 1997). Because SES is a composite variable, it cannot be summarized readily as a single risk factor; instead, it can be best expressed as a combination of risk factors such as limited resources, potential adverse events, parental psychopathology, and lower levels of educational attainment (Hollingshead, 1965). Theorists have long speculated that the effects of social status operate above and beyond material aspects of social position such as access to resources (Wilkinson, 1997). Indeed, subjective perceptions of social status have been found to predict health outcomes even after controlling for material aspects of status (Adler, Epel, Castellazzo, & Ickovics, 2000; Ostrove, Adler, Kuppermann, & Washington, 2000). Perceived lower social status is hypothesized to exert its negative effects through stress pathways (Adler, 2009). Consistent with an ecological perspective, SES and other risk factors operate not only at the level of the individual and family but also at the community level. For example, community-wide low SES may lead to domestic crowding as well as overcrowded schools. In many instances, as risk factors cumulate and the number of lower SES families grouped together increases, the potential for stressful life events is likely to rise. The groundbreaking research of William Julius Wilson (1991, 1997) highlights the significant untoward impact of concentrated disadvantage on a range of outcomes, including mental health, education, and employment.

Models of Risk, Protection, and Resiliency

Many researchers argue that not all stress is bad; rather, it can play a potentially important adaptive role in human development. In the right context, both positive and tolerable stress contribute to resilience. In fact, such circumstances may give rise to stress inoculation, through which an individual becomes immune to particular stressors after having tolerated the effects of similar stressors. The diathesis–stress model is applicable in these instances; examples are found, in particular, in research from war-torn parts of the world. A curious example comes from the work of Alvarez and Hunt (2005), who identified increased resilience to PTSD among longtime firefighters. It has been conjectured that the community feel of the firefighters' workplace provides protective effects, buffering against adverse life events and acute stressful situations otherwise associated with the job. Werner (1995) identified individual characteristics that may protect against stressful environments, such as effective problem-solving and communication skills, positive self-esteem, a high level of autonomy, and both social and academic competence. Other researchers distinguish between protective effects (which arise only in the face of risk) and promotive effects (which occur without regard to contextual risk) (Stouthamer-Loeber, Loeber, Wei, Rarrington, & Wikstroem, 2002).

The concept of resilience is relevant to any discussion of risk and protective factors. Resilience is the relative capacity for healthy adaptation to adversities over the life course (Simeon et al., 2007). As an important subject for both research and clinical investigation, biopsychosocial substrates of resilience are becoming better elucidated (Charney, 2004). A number of factors have been implicated in healthy adaptation: temperament, childhood trauma, attachment style, baseline and stress-related cortisol measures, and cognitive performance under stress.

Studies have defined and measured resilience in a variety of ways, including by assessing overall psychosocial functioning or measuring hardiness and coping skills (Connor & Zhang, 2006). Critically, the absence of major psychopathology in and of itself is not an adequate indicator of resilience. Nevertheless, developing a comprehensive understanding of resilience across the life span is important for mental health promotion, as resilience has been vastly understudied compared with disease and vulnerability.

The majority of research on resilience has focused on ascertaining why some people overcome significant life adversity while others succumb to difficult life events. Traditionally, such research, focused on children and adolescents, has sought to identify individuals who succeed despite the risk. Few studies have considered how young, middle-aged, and older adults might achieve such resilience in the first place (Hildon, Smith, Netuveli, & Blane, 2008; Rowe & Kahn, 2000). Rutter (2006) posits that because "resilience in relation to childhood adversities may stem from positive adult experiences, a life span trajectory approach is needed" (p. 1).

The term resilient can describe individuals with relatively good psychological outcomes despite risk experiences that would be expected to bring about serious adverse sequelae. Yet resilience is not simply an expression of social competence (Masten, 2006) or positive mental health. While important concepts, both refer to something different from resilience. At its core, resilience is an interactive process that yields a relatively positive psychological outcome despite serious risk experiences. As suggested by the diathesis–stress model, while most individuals are likely to be somewhat resilient (Tolan, 1996), the level of resilience may well differ among individuals (Fergus & Zimmerman, 2005).

The act of coping with adversity or adverse events is related to the resilience process (Compas, Connor-Smith, & Jaser, 2004). Coping skills enable an individual to adapt in the face of a life challenge or stress (Rutter, 2006). The coping process is likely to involve physiological adaptation, psychological habituation, a sense of efficacy, the acquisition of effective coping strategies, and a cognitive redefinition of the experience. As Rutter (2006) notes,

> the notion of resilience focuses attention on coping mechanisms, mental sets,

and the operation of personal agency. In other words, it requires a move from a focus on external risks to a focus on *how* these external risks are dealt with by the individual. (p. 4)

Critically, however, both the capacity to cope and resilience have limits; if exposed to enough stress, an individual may be unable to bounce back.

Researchers agree that in both health and development, gains and growth exist in fine balance with deterioration and loss, a balance that involves interactions between protective and risk factors (Baltes & Graf, 1996; Breslow, 1999). Luthar and Cicchetti (2000) concluded that research on resilience "should target protective and vulnerability forces at multiple levels of influence" (p. 878). In fact, a relatively recent shift toward promotion of assets and strengths has occurred in the field of mental disorder prevention, since such efforts may

both buffer individuals from the harmful effects of stress and foster successful coping (O'Connell, Boat, & Warner, 2009). (For several examples of the application of these theoretical approaches to stress, see chapter 17.)

A LIFE COURSE PERSPECTIVE ON ADAPTING TO STRESS

It behooves social science researchers to adopt a life course, developmental perspective when attempting to understand the dynamic interaction between stressors and the development of psychopathology. The life course, social field model (see figure 10-4) is a commonly cited developmental model that has guided public mental health research (Kellam, Branch, Agrawal, & Ensminger, 1975; Kellam & Rebok, 1992). For example, early in life, children may face developmental challenges and problems

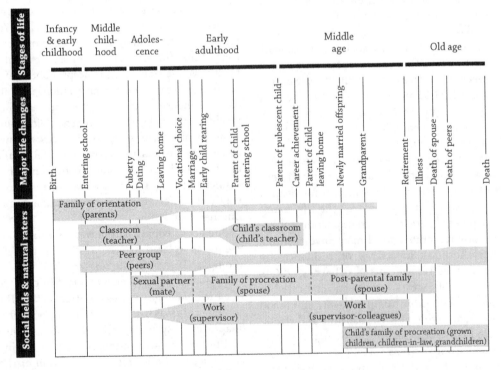

Figure 10-4   **Life Course Social Field Model.**

Source: Adapted from Kellam, S. G., Branch, J. D., Agrawal, K. C., & Ensminger, M. E. (1975). *Mental health and going to school: The Woodlawn program of assessment, early intervention and intervention and evaluation.* Chicago, IL: University of Chicago.. © Johns Hopkins University.

from traumatic life events (e.g., death of a parent) and major chronic stressors (e.g., poverty) to more normative difficulties (e.g., peer relations problems) and daily hassles (e.g., conflict with siblings) (Skinner & Zimmer-Gembeck, 2007). During adolescence and young adulthood, forming a sense of self—an identity—and forging romantic relationships emerge as key developmentally salient challenges. Youth experience increased stress with growing role responsibilities and demands associated with the transition to adulthood. Other challenges and stresses arise throughout adulthood. Individuals have to negotiate marriage and family, employment and retirement, acute and chronic illness, and even death, along with the developmental stress associated with these life events.

The frequency and types of stressors experienced across the life course undergo developmental changes as well. For example, the absolute number of uncontrollable life events begins to increase around age 13; along the same trajectory, levels of negative emotions are rising, leading to the potential development of depressive symptoms in early and midadolescence (Ge, Lorenz, Conger, Elder, & Simons, 1994; Larson, Moneta, Maryse, & Wilson, 2002).

Consistent with ecological systems theory, as children grow and respond to their environments, they are shaped and guided by their interactions with individuals within their communities (including the previously discussed genotype–environment relationships). The majority of children will follow a typical trajectory with age-appropriate events, including developmental (e.g., taking first steps and speaking first words) and social milestones (e.g., first day of school and first romantic relationship). A child who does not reach these milestones is at risk of falling into a maladaptive trajectory. Further, when social milestones occur earlier than expected (e.g., early marriage and early pregnancy), the negotiating process that occurs during all transitions becomes more stressful than normal.

Adolescents must confront and manage stressful physiological changes concurrent with exposure to new, demanding social situations as they adapt to growing independence and responsibility. Unsurprisingly, given differences in both development and social behavior between boys and girls, not all adolescents are exposed to the same environmental and biological stresses. The coping mechanisms manifested in young men and women have the potential to differ externally and internally, with young men more likely to display aggressive behaviors, perhaps as a consequence of their life course development and exposure to deviant and violent behavior (Loeber & Stouthamer-Loeber, 1998). These differences underscore the need to better understand the disparate gender-related effects of stress and resilience.

Finally, by adopting a life span perspective, underlying problems that arise throughout an individual's development can be better recognized. Behavior disorders are prime examples, given the recognized evolution from ADHD to conduct disorder to antisocial personality disorder (Burke, Loeber, Lahey, & Rathouz, 2005; Monuteaux, Faraone, Michelle Gross, & Biederman, 2007). Rutter (1989) introduced the term *heterotypic continuity* to describe this continuation of an underlying problem as a constant in different yet similar disorders over the life span. On the other hand, *homotypic continuity* results when the same psychopathologic trait continues to manifest in the same way over the life course. Merikangas and colleagues (2003) provided an example of this phenomenon in their longitudinal study of a community-based cohort with stable depression and anxiety over the course of 15 years.

The following sections examine how individuals adapt to different developmental challenges and stressors at different life stages, starting with family, peer, and school relationships in childhood and early adolescence, proceeding to romantic and marital relationships in later adolescence and young adulthood, and ending with the social contexts of work and retirement as potential stressors during the adult and aging years.

Family Relations

As important as the developmental period in which certain stressors may occur is the ecological context within which they arise: the family structure and dynamic, including early childhood attachments and related consequences. Attachment theory, as proposed by Bowlby (1969, 1973) and by Ainsworth, Blehar, Waters, and Wall (1978), has had a profound impact on the understanding of human development and behavior, particularly with respect to normative processes of child development. Researchers have invoked attachment theory as a way to understand the development and course of non-normative and maladaptive behavior, including poor self-regulation, peer functioning, and romantic functioning (Davila, Ramsay, Stroud, & Steinberg, 2005; Hazan & Shaver, 1987).

A child may face a number of stressors in the course of development. Within the family, research has focused on stressors such as marital conflict and divorce (Davies & Cumming, 1994; Ge, Natsuaki, & Conger, 2006), domestic violence between parents (Ireland & Smith, 2009), death of a parent (Tennant, 1988; Tyrka, Wier, Price, Ross, & Carpenter, 2008), and child maltreatment, including neglect and both physical and sexual abuse (Arnow, 2004). Ge and colleagues (2006), for example, conducted an 11-year longitudinal study of depressive symptoms of children in divorced and nondivorced families in the rural Midwest. Children who experienced parental divorce by age 15 showed a greater increase in depressive symptoms than children from nondivorced families. The stressful life events experienced by the children shortly after the divorce mediated the divorce's impact on depressive symptoms. Overall, females experienced a greater number of depressive symptoms in adolescence and young adulthood than did males.

Intelligence also has been examined within the context of family risk environment. Sameroff, Seifer, Baldwin, and Baldwin's (1993) seminal study of children ages 4–13 documented the association between IQ and cumulative risk factors (e.g., stressful life events, poor maternal mental health, low family social support, and low family SES). The researchers reported a that linear accumulation of risk—not any specific patterns of risk—affected developmental outcomes, underscoring the importance of acknowledging the cumulative effects of the risk environment.

Research, including genetic epidemiology studies, has confirmed that childhood maltreatment is associated with elevated risk for a wide range of behavioral symptoms, including maladaptive personality traits (Kendler et al., 2000). In a study of suicidal ideation among more than a thousand 8-year-old children identified as maltreated or at risk for maltreatment, Thompson and colleagues (2005) found that almost 10% reported suicidal ideation. The severity of abuse, chronicity of maltreatment, and presence of multiple types of maltreatment were associated with such ideation. Children who have been maltreated, as well as those exposed to community or domestic violence, are at increased risk for suicidal ideation (Cicchetti et al., 2010; Lambert, Copeland-Linder, & Ialongo, 2008; Thompson et al., 2005). Leitenberg, Gibson, and Novy (2004) found that individuals with extensive histories of child abuse relied more than others on disengagement coping (wishful thinking, problem avoidance, social withdrawal, and self-criticism). However, engagement coping (problem solving, cognitive restructuring, obtaining social support, and expressing emotions), did not show a corresponding decrease with increased exposure to childhood stressors or abuse. Thus some individuals with significantly adverse or abusive childhood histories may rely, in the face of subsequent stressors, on maladaptive coping strategies rather than more socially acceptable strategies.

Physical abuse is one of the clearest examples of an objective stressor that acts as a risk factor for negative behaviors. Physical abuse within the first five years of life has repeatedly been found to be a strong and consistent predictor of later youth violence and aggression (Cicchetti, Toth, & Maughan, 2000; Coie & Dodge, 1998; Hankin et al., 2005). Childhood abuse or maltreatment, including certain forms of dysfunction within the child's immediate family environment, also strongly predicts poor adult behavioral and physical health outcomes. Children who experience abuse, neglect, or other family dysfunction are more likely to have internalizing and externalizing behavior problems, have other types of mental disorders, have more physical symptoms, and engage in more risk-taking behaviors than children who have not been abused (Arnow, 2004). Moreover, studies indicate at least a twofold increased risk of adult revictimization among those who have experienced childhood physical or sexual abuse or have been child witnesses to violence (Wyatt, Guthrie, & Notgrass, 1992).

The more severe the abuse, the stronger the association with poor outcomes in adulthood. Further, the effects of adverse childhood events on mental health outcomes may well be cumulative. Cumulative risk is salient to traumatic stress studies, as the accumulation of events over time may be more toxic to physical and mental life than any individual event appraised in isolation (Rutter, 1987, 2006). The dose–response relationship or graded relationship between adverse childhood events and negative outcomes has been empirically substantiated (Anda et al., 2006; Felitti et al., 1998; Lu, Mueser, Rosenberg, & Jankowski, 2008). For example, Anda and associates (2006) reported a dose–response relationship between the number of adverse childhood events experienced and an increased risk of mental health problems and somatic disturbances, including substance abuse, memory problems, hypersexuality, and aggression. The findings are entirely consistent with the theory that the sum of risks has greater impact than any individual risk (Rutter, 1987, 2006).

The finding that child maltreatment in the form of physical abuse strongly predicts later behavior problems such as conduct disorder, aggression, and delinquency could reflect:

- the direct effect of physical abuse
- the indirect effect of genetic risk factors passed from parent to child that increase the likelihood of both abusive experiences and engagement in antisocial behavior (i.e., a gene–environment correlation)
- a combination of both effects (Hankin et al., 2005).

In a study testing these competing hypotheses, Jaffee, Caspi, Moffitt, and Taylor (2004) found that independent of known genetic risk, physical abuse is an environmentally mediated process directly involved in causally contributing to youths' behavioral problems. As

discussed previously, Cicchetti and colleagues (2010) reported a gene–environment interaction for suicidal ideation, but not depression. More work is needed to determine with greater confidence how vulnerability and protective factors combine with life experiences to lead to the development of a maladaptive personality (Hankin et al., 2005).

Despite the negative outcomes associated with child maltreatment, numerous studies have shown great heterogeneity in the effects of maltreatment (see Zielinski & Bradshaw, 2006). For example, while depression, substance use, aggression, criminal behavior, and sexual problems are more prevalent among adults who have been abused as children than among those who have not been maltreated, nearly one fourth of abused children evidence no long-term symptoms (McGloin & Widom, 2001). This heterogeneity in outcomes has been attributed to a variety of factors, including the type, onset, chronicity, and severity of the abuse, as well as the characteristics of the perpetrator(s). Characteristics of the child (e.g., sex, age, mental health status, and temperament) are also important factors in later outcomes.

The question of how ecological and contextual variables may influence the developmental consequences of child maltreatment is of growing interest (Zielinski & Bradshaw, 2006), particularly since the vast majority of studies in this area focus exclusively on a child's immediate family environment. A pressing need exists to broaden current research to include the effects that peer groups, schools, and neighborhoods have on children who have been maltreated.

Peer and School Relationships

From midchildhood through adolescence, the peer group emerges as a developmentally salient social phenomenon that influences children's attitudes and behaviors (Rubin, Bukowski, & Parker, 2006). Research suggests that in many cases, children who have difficulty in peer relationships (e.g., being victimized or bullied by peers at school or not having a close friend) may be at increased risk for behavioral and emotional disorders, substance abuse, and delinquency (Deater-Deckard, 2001; La Greca & Harrison, 2005; Woodward & Ferguson, 1999). Being a victim of negative peer experiences has been associated, for example, with the development of depression, particularly in girls. This greater vulnerability among girls has been linked to socialization experiences that give rise to passivity and a lack of assertiveness (Keenan et al., 2010). Further, children with low-quality or unstable friendships are more likely to experience academic problems (Ladd, Kochenderfer, & Coleman, 1996), to be bullied (Hodges, Boivin, Vitaro, & Bukowski, 1999), and to feel lonely (Parker & Seal, 1996) than are children with solid friendships.

Children with developmental disorders appear to be particularly vulnerable to peer rejection. Researchers have established that children with ADHD often are rejected by their peers (e.g., Normand et al., 2007). While the data clearly show these children are often excluded from close friendships, reasons underlying the inability to maintain existing friendships are not entirely clear. Comorbid oppositional defiant disorder or conduct disorder may aggravate their difficulties, contributing to observed deficits in social functioning. Researchers also have studied the impact of other mental disorders on peer relations. Chen, Cohen, Johnson, and Kasen (2009), who investigated adolescent mental disorders and peer relationships, found that mental disorders in adolescence did not predict the frequency of peer conflict during early adulthood. However, adolescent depression, disruptive disorders, and substance abuse did predict increased peer conflict during adolescence, without regard to the frequency of contact. In contrast, youth with anxiety disorders reported less peer conflict than those without these disorders, a finding that might be the product of conflict avoidance by highly anxious adolescents.

To what degree might other developmental contexts, such as the family, mitigate the effects of negative peer relations? In a sample of 1,023 adolescents, Sentse, Lindenberg, Omvlee, Ormel, and Veenstra (2010) found that when analyzing parent and peer effects simultaneously, both the protective effects of parental acceptance and the adverse impact of peer rejection were diminished. In contrast, the protective effect of peer acceptance and the risk effect of parental rejection remained strong. Thus peer acceptance buffered parental rejection, but parental acceptance did not buffer peer rejection, suggesting that the parent and peer contexts are independent of each other.

In a review of research on the impact of peer relationships on the development of psychopathology in childhood and adolescence, Deater-Deckard (2001) addressed the long-term negative effects of peer rejection and victimization, noting that much research remains to be done from a life span perspective on the long-term impact of adverse peer experiences. Some promising areas for inquiry include the heterogeneity of life course developmental processes, gender-based norms, multilevel modeling across different developmental contexts, and the utility of gene–environment process models (Deater-Deckard, 2001).

Romantic Relationships

From a developmental perspective, romantic relationships are widely considered to be a hallmark feature of adolescence. Yet relatively little is known about whether and how the duration or depth of adolescent romantic relationships may affect long-term development and well-being (Collins, Welsh, & Furman, 2009). Depending on their duration, nature, and quality, adolescent romantic relationships have been associated both with social competence and with risk for adjustment problems (Furman, Low, & Ho, 2009; Furman & Shomaker, 2008). Furman and colleagues (2009) reported that greater amounts of romantic experience among 10th-grade students were associated with higher levels of social acceptance and of both friendship and romantic competence. At the same time, however, increased romantic experience was associated with more substance use, delinquent behavior, and genital sexual behaviors. Multiple poor-quality relationships of short duration have been found to be associated with increased depressive symptoms (Joyner & Udry, 2000) and with problem behaviors between partners

(Zimmer-Gembeck, Siebenbruner, & Collins, 2001). Further, adolescent relationships leading to early marriage consistently have been associated with early divorce and high levels of marital dissatisfaction (Karney & Bradbury, 1995).

Gender differences appear to be salient in the mental health effects of romantic relationships. In a study using two waves of data from the National Longitudinal Study of Adolescent Health (N = 8,181), Joyner and Udry (2000) found that that males and females who became romantically involved between interviews experienced a larger increase in depression than their counterparts who did not. However, females experienced a more significant increase in depression than males in response to romantic involvement. Simon and Barrett (2010), studying gender differences in the mental health consequences of romantic relationships of young adults, discovered that current involvements and recent breakups were more closely associated with the mental health of women than men. Conversely, support and strain in an ongoing relationship were more closely associated with well-being among men than among women. These findings underscore why the particular period in the life course and the experiences of specific age cohorts are important in theorizing about gender differences in the effects of romantic relationships on mental health.

One particularly influential theory, attachment theory, can help unravel the role of romantic relationships across the life span. While the cognitive and emotional requisites of mature romantic relationships rarely appear before late adolescence, the developmental process begins much earlier, with a redistribution of attachment functions (e.g., proximity seeking) and reliance on individuals other than parents for unconditional acceptance (Collins et al., 2009). While early attachment theory work focused on the parent–child relationship, the models have been extended to describe attachments across the life course. Bowlby's (1969, 1973) theory of how attachments between parent and child affect later development has been applied to close relationships in adulthood and development. Hazan and Shaver (1994) posited that attachment theory could be used to understand the nature and developmental course of adult romantic relationships and that adult romantic relationships were comparable to attachment relationships earlier in life and similarly affect intra- and interpersonal functioning. Research supporting this notion has found that adult attachment security in romantic relationships is positively associated with various aspects of functioning in romantic relationships (Davila et al., 2005). Conversely, attachment insecurity has been linked with relationship dysfunction, adjustment problems, and mental problems, including personality disorders (Van Uzendoom, Schuengel, & Bakersman-Krannenburg, 1999).

Marriage

Marriage is perhaps the most important relationship for many adults. Marital happiness can have beneficial effects on mental health, yet the quality of marital relationships increasingly is recognized as an important stressor with potentially deleterious health consequences, such as depression (e.g., Beach & O'Leary, 1993). Robles and Kiecolt-Glaser (2003) reviewed both earlier studies suggesting that unhappy marriages are associated with greater morbidity and mortality and other, more recent studies on the impact of marital functioning on the health of the cardiovascular, endocrine, and immune systems. They found that negative, hostile behavior during marital conflict and discussions was associated not only with elevated cardiovascular activity but also with alterations in stress-related hormones and immune function dysregulation.

Building on this work, Barnett, Steptoe, and Gareis (2005) estimated the relationship between the quality of one's marital role and three indicators of psychobiological stress—self-reported stress, cortisol levels, and ambulatory blood pressure (ABP). They found that without regard to gender, marital role concerns (but not marital role rewards) were related to all three stress indicators. Participants with more significant marital concerns reported greater stress throughout the day, showed an attenuated cortisol increase after waking and a flatter cortisol slope over the day, and had elevated ambulatory diastolic blood pressure over the middle of the workday, with a similar trend in systolic pressure. These results suggest that in addition to the carryover of work stress into domestic life that has been evident for many years, domestic strain exerts an influence on biological function over the working day and evening. While previous research suggested that depressed immune functioning may act as a mechanism that links troubled marriages to potentially adverse health outcomes, Barnett and colleagues (2005) found a potential second mechanism: poorer stress-related biological response.

Recent studies illustrate how the physiological changes associated with marital functioning in the studies just described may have implications for long-term health outcomes. In their examination of ABP among married and single men and women, Holt-Lunstad, Birmingham, and Jones (2008) found that both marital status and marital quality affect morbidity. Married individuals had greater satisfaction with life and lower blood pressure than single individuals; high marital quality was associated with lower ABP, lower stress and depression, and higher satisfaction with life than found among unmarried individuals. Compared with individuals in low-quality marriages, however, single individuals had lower ABP, suggesting that they fare better than their unhappily married counterparts. The presence of a supportive network did not moderate (i.e., buffer) the adverse effects of being single or unhappily married. These results highlight the complex nature of the influence of social relationships on long-term health and may help clarify the physiological pathways through which such associations are created.

The developmental consequences of marriage for an individual do not occur in isolation; they are closely interrelated with those of other individuals, foremost among them marital partners. Using 35-year longitudinal data on 178 married couples from the Seattle Longitudinal Study, Hoppmann, Gerstorf, Willis, and Schaie (2011) found spousal similarities not only in level of happiness but also in fluctuations in happiness over time. Consistent with a life course perspective,

these findings complement earlier research on age-related changes in individual well-being by pointing to the value of exploring the marriage as the unit of analysis.

Work

Generally, paid employment has been found to benefit psychological well-being; in contrast, various forms of nonemployment, including unemployment, adversely affect mental health (Matthews, Hertzman, Ostry, & Power, 1998; Thomas, Benzeval, & Stansfeld, 2005). Transitions from paid employment to either unemployment or long-term sick leave are associated with increased psychological distress for both men and women (Thomas et al., 2005). Among women, similar psychological distress is associated with leaving the workplace for maternity leave or with staying home to look after the family. Conversely, transitions from those roles to formal employment led to improved mental health, most significantly within the first six months. Unemployment also has been found to be associated with physiological stress (F. Cohen et al., 2007). Cohen and colleagues (2007) examined the effects of unemployment and reemployment on natural killer cell cytotoxicity (NKCC), higher levels of which are associated with better immune function. As they had hypothesized, people who were persistently unemployed had significantly lower NKCC levels than a matched group of employed people; NKCC levels increased significantly after the unemployed participants became reemployed.

It is also important to consider gender when examining the long-term effects of employment and unemployment (Mossakowski, 2009). While layoffs may have deleterious consequences for women's physical and mental health, the large-scale engagement of women in the workforce has enhanced women's overall self-rated health, owing largely to greater educational attainment. Increased female employment, however, has created its own set of stressors, resulting in greater gender equality in the adoption of risky behaviors such as binge drinking and smoking. This rise in women's health risks may be tempered by a concurrent reported increase in women's assertiveness and overall empowerment (Wood & Eagly, 2002).

Older adults may be particularly vulnerable to involuntary displacement from the workforce, particularly because of their increased vulnerability to various health-related problems. Given the additional distress associated with loss of income and possible loss of medical insurance coverage, work displacement has the potential to exacerbate those problems for older adults (Mandal & Roe, 2008). Not only do older adults suffer longer periods of involuntary unemployment than younger individuals, but also their skills may not be transferable to new positions, resulting in a substantial loss of earnings. Millions of older Americans cope with physical limitations, cognitive changes, and various losses commonly associated with aging, such as bereavement. Job loss simply adds to the growing number of stresses faced by individuals as they age.

Retirement

Although retirement is one of the most important transitions in late adult life (Theriault, 1994; M. Wang, Henkens, & van Solinge, 2011), knowledge about its effects on mental health is fragmentary at best (Kim & Moen, 2002). For many older adults, retirement is a life event marking passage into later stages of life. As such, it has important social and economic implications that extend well beyond the individual. Increasingly, retirement is a gradual rather than an abrupt transition, involving changes in patterns, hours, and types of work. Whether quick or protracted, retirement is not merely an objective point of transition; rather, it is marked by developmental and social–psychological significance that may affect physical and psychological well-being (Moen, 2001). For some individuals, retirement may signal a break from job-related stressors, such as high work demands and low latitude for decision making; as a result, it may lead to greater autonomy and personal fulfillment. Others, however, may experience retirement as the loss of a valued occupational role, the loss of a social network of coworkers, and a diminished sense of personal identity, each

of which can give rise to reduced psychological well-being (Kim & Moen, 2002).

Empirical evidence on the physical and psychological consequences of retirement has been inconsistent. Christ and colleagues (2007) reported that workers age 65 and above report better mental health status than nonworkers in the same age range. Those researchers also found that white-collar workers have lower levels of depression than service sector workers. In a longitudinal study of short- and long-term effects of retirement, Kim and Moen (2002) found that whereas men experience a morale boost as they enter retirement, they show more depressive symptoms after being retired for a longer period. Women did not demonstrate a similar pattern. The short-term improvements in mental health status among the newly retired may reflect the "honeymoon" phase proposed by Atchley (1976). Immediately following retirement, individuals may experience a boost in energy, health, and life satisfaction as they pursue desired plans that may have been postponed and experiment with new roles and activities. Consistent with this perspective, several studies report that greater autonomy leads retirees to have better mental health and lower stress levels (Drentea, 2002; Matthews et al., 1998; Midanik, Soghikian, Ransom, & Tekawa, 1995). Mandal and Roe (2008) reported that reentering the workforce following involuntary job loss is also psychologically beneficial to retirees and that after retirement, women generally exhibit better psychological well-being than men.

From a life course perspective, retirement should be seen both as a process (with differences in well-being between the newly retired and those who have been continuously retired over a longer period) and as a life event occurring in particular contexts (Kim & Moen, 2002). The impact of retirement on mental health may depend on prior levels of psychological well-being and stress experiences. For example, individuals with depressive symptoms before retirement may be vulnerable to even more such symptoms as well as other mental problems as they transition into retirement. Retirees reporting earlier stressful work environments report higher levels of alcohol consumption in retirement than do retirees reporting less stressful earlier work environments (Richman, Zlatoper, Zackula Ehmke, & Rospenda, 2006). On the other hand, individuals reporting that workplace demands interfered with family life in late midlife experienced fewer depressive symptoms after retirement (Coursolle, Sweeney, Raymo, & Ho, 2010).

Thus, depending on preretirement life and work experience, retirement may come more as a relief than as a stressor. These findings underscore the importance of context and the potential of residual effects of workplace stress during retirement. Marital context also appears to play an important role in retirement well-being. Using data from the Health and Retirement Survey, Szinovacz and Davey (2004) found that having a retired spouse exerts a beneficial influence on both recently retired and longer retired men. In contrast, retired women show beneficial effects of a spouse's employment arise, but only when very recently retired. Taken together, all of the above findings about effects of retirement underscore the complexity of the retirement adaptation process and the need for a life course approach to mitigating stress and reducing its potentially adverse mental health effects.

CONCLUSION AND FUTURE DIRECTIONS

While the association between adverse life events and mental health problems has been the subject of considerable empirical inquiry, it remains unclear whether adverse life events actually cause later adverse life events or mental disorders like depression. At the physiological level, chronic stress may have detrimental effects, leading to both a reduced hippocampal volume and a compromised immune system. To understand stress at an ecological level, it is necessary to transition from an individual stress activation model to a more holistic model that incorporates life events and experiences. Although any life event may activate the HPA axis, the context of the activating stressor is of great importance and can be understood by applying diathesis–stress models. While risk and protective factors have the potential to be both biological and environmental, they also

may reflect the interplay of both factors—this line of research is worthy of further inquiry.

One promising area of investigation is the degree to which early-life stressors may set the stage for stressors later in life (Grant & McMahon, 2005). For example, abuse in childhood may give rise additional stressors and distress in adolescence and adulthood. Thus stressors experienced in childhood may predict both maladaptive coping strategies and psychopathology that in turn set the stage for still other stressful experiences later in life (Gibb, 2002; Magnus, Diener, Fujita, & Payot, 1993; Monroe & Simons, 1991).

The relationship between varying types of psychopathology and stressors experienced at various points in development is another promising area of inquiry. As the brain develops, capacities for particular types of cognitive mediation develop concurrently, providing the mediational link between stressors and emerging manifestations of particular types of disorder (Mash & Barkeley, 2003). The ways in which development constrains or fosters potential mediating cognitive abilities, the degree to which stressors might operate within a developmental context to facilitate or inhibit the development of particular cognitive processes, and the degree to which developmental influences on cognitive mediation might explain developmental variation in the manifestation of psychopathology represent interrelated and promising avenues for research.

Resilience is another topic that merits continued investigation. To grasp resilience in its full complexity, one must adopt a multiple-levels-of-analysis approach that encompasses the biological, psychological, and environmental context domains. Although it is impractical for most investigators to include all levels of analysis in a single experimental design, the growing movement toward collaborative interdisciplinary research within the disciplines of neuroscience and developmental psychopathology offers optimism that a multiple-levels approach will become increasingly prevalent. The adoption of such a perspective will result in a more sophisticated and comprehensive portrayal of resilience that will not only advance scientific knowledge of this phenomenon but also inform efforts to translate research on positive adaptation in the face of adversity into interventions to promote resilient functioning.

REFERENCES

Adler, N. E. (2009). Health disparities through a psychological lens. *American Psychologist, 64*(8), 663–672.

Adler, N. E., Epel, E. S., Castellazzo, G., & Ickovics, J. R. (2000). Relationship of subjective and objective social status with psychological and physiological functioning: Preliminary data in healthy white women. *Journal of Health Psychology, 19*(6), 586–592.

Ainsworth, M. D., Blehar, M. C., Waters, E., & Wall, S. (1978). *Patterns of attachment: A psychological study of the strange situation.* Hillsdale, NJ: Lawrence Erlbaum.

Alvarez, J., & Hunt., M. (2005). Risk and resilience in canine search and rescue handlers after 9/11. *Journal of Traumatic Stress, 18*(5), 497–505.

American Psychiatric Association. (1994). *Diagnostic and statistical manual of mental disorders* (4th ed.). Washington, DC: Author.

Anda, R. F., Felitti, V. J., Bremner, J. D., Walker, J. D., Whitfield, C., Perry, B. D., & Giles, W. H. (2006). The enduring effects of abuse and related adverse experiences in childhood: A convergence of evidence from neurobiology and epidemiology. *European Archives of Psychiatry and Clinical Neuroscience, 256*(3), 174–186.

Arnow, B. A. (2004). Relationships between childhood maltreatment, adult health and psychiatric outcomes, and medical utilization. *Journal of Clinical Psychiatry, 65*(Suppl. 12), 10–15.

Atchley, R. (1976). Selected social and psychological differences between men and women in later life. *Journal of Gerontology, 31*(2), 204–211.

Baltes, P. B., & Graf, P. (1996). Psychological aspects of aging: Facts and frontiers. In D. Magnusson (Ed.), *Life span development of individuals: Behavioral, neurobiological, and psychosocial perspectives* (pp. 427–460). Cambridge, UK: Cambridge University Press.

Barnett, R. C., Steptoe, A., & Gareis, K. C. (2005). Marital-role quality and stress-related psychobiological indicators. *Annals of Behavioral Medicine, 30*(1), 36–43.

Beach, S. R., & O'Leary, D. K. (1993). Marital discord and dysphoria: For whom does the marital relationship predict depressive symptomatology? *Journal of Social and Personal Relationships, 10,* 405–420.

Belay, H., Burton, C. L., Lovic, V., Meaney, M. J., Sokolowski, M., & Fleming, A. S. (2011). Early adversity and serotonin transporter genotype interact with hippocampal glucocorticoid receptor mRNA expression, corticosterone, and behavior in adult male rats. *Behavioral Neuroscience, 125*(2), 150–160.

Belsky, J., & Pluess, M. (2009). Beyond diathesis stress: Differential susceptibility to environmental influences. *Psychological Bulletin, 135*(6), 885–908.

Berntson, G. G., Bigger, J. T., Eckberg, D. L., Grossman, P., Kaufmann, P. G., Malik, M, . . . Van Der Molen, M. W. (1997). Heart rate variability: Origins, methods, and interpretive caveats. *Psychophysiology, 34*(6), 623–648.

Betancourt, T. S., & Khan, K. T. (2008). The mental health of children affected by armed conflict: Protective processes and pathways to resilience. *International Review of Psychiatry, 20*(3), 317–328.

Blascovich, J., & Mendes, W. B. (2000). Challenge and threat appraisals: The role of affective cues. In J. Forgas (Ed.), *Feeling and thinking: The role of affect in social cognition* (pp. 59–82). Cambridge, UK: Cambridge University Press.

Bleuler, M. (1963). Conception of schizophrenia within the last fifty years and today. *Proceedings of the Royal Society of Medicine, 56,* 945–952.

Bowlby, J. (1969). *Attachment and loss, Vol.1: Attachment.* New York, NY: Basic Books.

Bowlby, J. (1973). *Attachment and loss, Vol. 2: Separation, anxiety and anger.* New York, NY: Basic Books.

Bradshaw, C. P., & Garbarino, J. (2004). Social cognition as a mediator of the influence of family and community violence on adolescent development: Implications for intervention. *Annals of the New York Academy of Sciences, 1036,* 85–105.

Bremner, J. D., Randall, P., Scott, T. M., Bronen, R. A., Seibyl, J. P., Southwick, S. M., . . . Innis, R. B. (1995). MRI-based measurement of hippocampal volume in patients with combat-related posttraumatic stress disorder. *American Journal of Psychiatry, 152*(7), 973–981.

Breslow, L. (1999). From disease prevention to health promotion. *Journal of the American Medical Association, 281*(11), 1030–1033.

Breuer, J. & Freud, S. (1895). *Studies on hysteria* (standard ed., Vol 2). London: Hogarth Press, 1955.

Bronfenbrenner, U. (1979). *The ecology of human development: Experiments by nature and design.* Cambridge, MA: Harvard University Press.

Bronfenbrenner, U., & Morris, P. (1998). The ecology of developmental processes. In W. Damon (Ed.), *Handbook of child psychology* (Vol. 1, pp. 993–1028). New York, NY: John Wiley & Sons.

Brown, G. W., & Harris, T. O. (1978). *The social origins of depression: A study of psychiatric disorder in women*. London, UK: Tavistock.

Brown, G. W., & Harris, T. O. (1989). Depression. In G. W. Brown and T. O. Harris (Eds.), *Life events and illness* (pp. 49–93). New York, NY: Guilford.

Brunner, E. J., Hemingway, H., Walker, B. R., Page, M., Clarke, P., Juneia, M.,...Marmot, M. G. (2002). Adrenocortical, autonomic, and inflammatory causes of the metabolic syndrome: Nested case–control study. *Circulation, 106*(21), 2659–2665.

Burke, J. D., Loeber, R., Lahey, B. B., & Rathouz, P. J. (2005). Developmental transitions among affective and behavioral disorders in adolescent boys. *Journal of Child Psychology and Psychiatry, 46*(11), 1200–1210.

Burton, L. C., Skinner, E. A., Uscher-Pines, L., Lieberman, R., Leff, B., Clark, R.,...Weiner, J. P. (2009). Health of Medicare Advantage plan enrollees at 1 year after Hurricane Katrina. *American Journal of Managed Care, 15*(1), 13–22.

Cannon, W. B. (1929). *Bodily changes in pain, hunger, fear, and rage* (2nd ed.). New York, NY: D. Appleton.

Caspi, A., McClay, J., Moffitt, T. E., Mill, J., Martin, J., Craig, I. W.,...Poulton, R. (2002). Role of genotype in the cycle of violence in maltreated children. *Science, 297*(5582), 851–854.

Caspi, A., Sugden, K., Moffitt, T. E., Taylor, A., Craig, I. W., Harrington, H.,...Poulton, R. (2003). Influence of life stress on depression: Moderation by a polymorphism in the *5-HTT* gene. *Science, 301*(5631), 386–389.

Charney, D. S. (2004). Psychobiological mechanisms of resilience and vulnerability: Implications for successful adaptation to extreme stress. *American Journal of Psychiatry, 161*(2), 195–216.

Chen, E., & Miller, G. E. (2007). Stress and inflammation in exacerbations of asthma. *Brain, Behavior, and Immunity, 21*(8), 993–999.

Chen, H., Cohen, P., Johnson, J. G., & Kasen, S. (2009). Psychiatric disorders during adolescence and relationships with peers from age 17 to 27. *Social Psychiatry and Psychiatric Epidemiology, 44*(3), 223–230.

Chida, Y., Hamer, M., Wardle, J., & Steptoe, A. (2008). Do stress-related psychosocial factors contribute to cancer incidence and survival? *Nature Clinical Practice Oncology, 5*(8), 466–475.

Chisholm, K. (1998). A three year follow-up of attachment and indiscriminate friendliness in children adopted from Romanian orphanages. *Child Development, 69*(4), 1092–1106.

Christ, S., Lee, D., Flemings, L., LeBlanc, W., Arheart, K., Chung-Bridges, K.,...McCollister, K. (2007). Employment and occupation effects on depressive symptoms in older Americans: Does working past age 65 protect against depression? *Journals of Gerontology, Series B: Social Sciences, 6*(6), s399–s403.

Chrousos, G. P., & Gold, P. W. (1992). The concepts of stress systems disorders: Overview of physical and behavioral homeostasis. *Journal of the American Medical Association, 267*(9), 1244–1252.

Cicchetti, D. (1989). How research on child maltreatment has informed the study of child development. In D. Cicchetti & V. Carlson (Eds.), *Child maltreatment* (pp. 377–431). Cambridge, UK: Cambridge University Press.

Cicchetti, D. (2002). The impact of social experience on neurobiological systems: Illustrations from a constructivist view of child maltreatment. *Cognitive Development, 17*, 1407–1428.

Cicchetti, D., & Lynch, M. (1995). Failures in the expectable environment and their impact on individual development: The case of child maltreatment. In D. Cicchetti & D. J. Cohen (Eds.), *Developmental psychopathology* (Vol. 2, pp. 32–71). New York, NY: Wiley.

Cicchetti, D., Rogosch, F. A., Lynch, M., & Holt, K. D. (1993). Resilience in maltreated children: Processes leading to adaptive outcome. *Developmental Psychopathology, 5*, 629–648.

Cicchetti, D., Rogosch, F. A., Sturge-Apple, M., & Toth, S. L. (2010). Interaction of child maltreatment and *5-HTT* polymorphisms: Suicidal ideation among children from low-SES backgrounds. *Journal of Pediatric Psychology, 35*(5), 536–546.

Cicchetti, D., Toth, S. L., & Maughan, A. (2000). An ecological-transactional model of child maltreatment. In A. Sameroff, M. Lewis, & S. M. Miller (Eds.), *Handbook of developmental psychopathology* (3rd ed.). New York, NY: Plenum.

Clark, R., Anderson, N. B., Clark, V. R., & Williams, D. R. (1999). Racism as a stressor for African Americans: A biopsychosocial model. *American Psychologist, 54*(10), 805–816.

Cohen, F., Kemeny, M. E., Zegans, L. S., Johnson, P., Kearney, K. A., & Stites, D. P. (2007). Immune function declines with unemployment and recovers after stressor termination. *Psychosomatic Medicine, 69*(3), 225–234.

Cohen, S., Kessler, R. C., & Gordon, L. U. (1995). *Measuring stress.* New York, NY: Oxford University Press.

Coie, J. D., & Dodge, K. A. (1998). Aggression and antisocial behavior. In W. Damon (Series Ed.) & N. Eisenberg (Vol. Ed.), *Handbook of child psychology: Vol. 3. Social, emotional, and personality development* (5th ed., pp. 770–862). New York, NY: Wiley.

Collins, N. L., & Read, S. J. (1990). Adult attachment, working models, and relationship quality in dating couples. *Journal of Personality and Social Psychology, 58*(4), 644–663.

Collins, W. A., Welsh, D. P., & Furman, W. (2009). Adolescent romantic relationships. *Annual Review of Psychology, 60*, 631–652.

Comer, J. S., Fan, B., Duarte, C. S., Wu, P., Musa, G. J., Mandell, D. J., ... Hoven, C. W. (2010). Attack-related life disruption and child psychopathology in New York City public schoolchildren 6-months post-9/11. *Journal of Clinical Child and Adolescent Psychology, 39*(4), 460–469.

Compas, B. E., Connor-Smith, J., & Jaser, S. S. (2004). Temperament, stress reactivity and coping: Implications for depression in childhood and adolescence. *Journal of Clinical Child and Adolescent Psychology, 33*(1), 21–31.

Connor, K. M., & Zhang, W. (2006). Resilience: Determinants, measurement and treatment responsiveness. *CNS Spectrums, 11*(10, Suppl. 12), 5–12.

Coursolle, K. M., Sweeney, M. M., Raymo, J. M., & Ho, J. H. (2010). The association between retirement and emotional wellbeing: Does prior work–family conflict matter? *Journals of Gerontology, Series B: Psychological and Social Sciences, 69*(5), 609–620.

Davies, P. T., & Cummings, E. M. (1994). Maternal conflict and child adjustment: An emotional security hypothesis. *Psychological Bulletin, 116*(3), 387–411.

Davila, J., Ramsay, M., Stroud, C. B., & Steinberg, S. J. (2005). Attachment as vulnerability to the development of psychopathology. In B. L. Hankin & J. R. Z. Abela (Eds.), *Development of psychopathology: A vulnerability–stress perspective* (pp. 215–242). Thousand Oaks, CA: Sage.

Deater-Deckard, K. (2001). Annotation: Recent research examining the role of peer relationships in the development of psychopathology. *Journal of Child Psychology and Psychiatry, 42*(5), 565–579.

DeLongis, A., Folkman, S., & Lazarus, R. S. (1988). The impact of daily stress on health and mood: Psychological and social resources as mediators. *Journal of Personality and Social Psychology, 54*(3), 486–495.

Demaree, H. A., & Everhart, D. E. (2004). Reduced parasympathetic activity and decreased sympathovagal flexibility during negative emotional processing. *Personality and Individual Differences, 36*, 457–469.

Dodge, K. A., Bates, J. E., & Pettit, G. S. (1990). Mechanisms in the cycle of violence. *Science, 250*(4988), 1678–1683.

Dohrenwend, B. P. (1998). *Adversity, stress and psychopathology.* London, UK: Oxford University Press.

Dohrenwend, B. P. (2000). The role of adversity and stress in psychopathology: Some evidence and its implications for theory and research. *Journal of Health and Social Behavior, 41*(1), 1–19.

Dohrenwend, B. P., Raphael, K. G., Schwartz, S., Stueve, A., & Skodol, A. (1993). The Structured Event Probe and Narrative Rating method for measuring stressful life events. In L. Goldberger & S. Breznitz (Eds.), *Handbook of stress: Theoretical and clinical aspects* (pp. 174–199). New York, NY: Free Press.

Dohrenwend, B. P., & Shrout, P. (1985). "Hassles" in the conceptualization and measurement of life stress variables. *American Psychologist, 40*, 780–785.

Drentea, P. (2002). Retirement and mental health. *Journal of Aging and Health, 14*(2), 167–194.

Eaton, W. W. (1978). Life events, social supports and psychiatric symptoms: A re-analysis of the New Haven data. *Journal of Health and Social Behavior, 19*(2), 230–234.

Eckenrode, J. (1984). Impact of chronic and acute stressors on daily reports of mood. *Journal of Personality and Social Psychology, 46*(4), 907–918.

Evans, G. W. (2003). A multimethodological analysis of cumulative risk and allostatic load among rural children. *Developmental Psychology, 39*(5), 924–933.

Felitti, V. J., Anda, R. F., Nordenberg, D., Williamson, D. F., Spitz, A. M., Koss, M. P., & Marks, J. S. (1998). Relationship of child abuse and household dysfunction to many of the leading causes of death in adults. *American Journal of Preventive Medicine, 14*(4), 245–258.

Fergus, S., & Zimmerman, M. A. (2005). Adolescent resilience: A framework for understanding healthy development in the face of risk. *Annual Review of Public Health, 26*, 399–419.

Figueredo, V. (2009). The time has come for physicians to take notice: The impact of psychosocial stressors on the heart. *American Journal of Medicine, 122*(8), 704–712.

Freud, A., & Burlingham, D. (1943). *War and children*. New York, NY: International Universities Press.

Furman, W., Low, S., & Ho, M. J. (2009). Romantic experience and psychosocial adjustment in middle adolescence. *Journal of Clinical Child and Adolescent Psychology, 38*(1), 75–90.

Furman, W., & Shomaker, L. B. (2008). Patterns of interaction in adolescent romantic relationships: Distinct features and links to other close relationships. *Journal of Adolescence, 31*(6), 771–788.

Ge, X., Lorenz, F. O., Conger, R. D., Elder, G. H., & Simons, R. L. (1994). Trajectories of stressful life events and the emergence of gender differences in adolescent depressive symptoms. *Developmental Psychology, 30*(4), 467–483.

Ge, X., Natsuaki, M. N., & Conger, R. D. (2006). Trajectories of depressive symptoms and stressful life events among male and female adolescents in divorced and non-divorced families. *Developmental Psychopathology, 18*(1), 253–273.

Giaconia, R. M., Reinherz, H. Z., Silverman, A. B., Bilge, P., Frost, A. K., & Cohen, E. (1995). Traumas and posttraumatic stress disorder in a community population of older adolescents. *Journal of the American Academy of Child and Adolescent Psychiatry, 34*(10), 1369–1380.

Gibb, B. E. (2002). Childhood malnutrition and negative cognitive styles: A quantitative and qualitative review. *Clinical Psychology Review, 22*(2), 223–246.

Grant, K. E., Compas, B. E., Stuhlmacher, A. F., Thurm, A. E., McMahon, S. D., & Halpert, J. A. (2003). Stressors and child and adolescent psychopathology: Moving from markers to mechanisms of risk. *Psychological Bulletin, 129*(3), 447–466.

Grant, K. E., & McMahon, S. D. (2005). Conceptualizing the role of stressors in the development of psychopathology. In B. L. Hankin & J. R. Z. Abela (Eds.), *Development of psychopathology: A vulnerability–stress perspective* (pp. 3–31). Thousand Oaks, CA: Sage.

Gunnar, M. R., Bruce, J., & Grotevant, H. D. (2000). International adoption of institutionally reared children: Research and policy. *Development and Psychopathology, 12*(4), 677–693.

Gunnar, M. R., & Donzella, B. (2002). Social regulation of the cortisol levels in early human development. *Psychoneuroendocrinology, 27*(1–2), 199–220.

Gunnar, M. R., Talge, N. M., & Herrera, A. (2009). Stressor paradigms in developmental studies: What does and does not work to produce mean increases in salivary cortisol. *Psychoneuroendocrinology, 34*(7), 953–967.

Hankin, B. L., Abela, J. R. Z., Auerbach, R. P., McWhinnie, C. M., & Skitch, S. A. (2005). Development of behavioral problems over the life course. In B. L. Hankin & J. R. Z. Abela (Eds.), *Development of psychopathology: A vulnerability–stress perspective* (pp. 385–416). Thousand Oaks, CA: Sage.

Harlow, H. F., & Harlow, M. K. (1969). Effects of various mother–infant relationships on rhesus monkey behaviours. In B. M. Foss (Ed.), *Determinants of infant behavior, 4* (pp. 15–36). London, UK: Methuen.

Hawkins, N. G., Davies, R., & Holmes, T. H. (1957). Evidence of psychosocial factors in the development of pulmonary tuberculosis. *American Review of Tuberculosis, 75*(5), 768–780.

Hazan, C., & Shaver, P. R. (1987). Romantic love conceptualized as an attachment process. *Journal of Personality and Social Psychology, 52*(3), 511–524.

Hazan, C., & Shaver, P. R. (1994). Attachment as an organizational framework for research on close relationships. *Psychological Inquiry, 5*(1), 1–22.

Hildon, Z., Smith, G., Netuveli, G., & Blane, D. (2008). Understanding adversity and resilience at older ages. *Sociology of Health and Illness, 30*(5), 726–740.

Hinkle, L. E. (1987). Stress and disease: The concept after 50 years. *Social Science and Medicine, 25*(6), 561–566.

Hodges, E. V. E., Boivin, M., Vitaro, F., & Bukowski, W. M. (1999). The power of friendship: Protection against an escalating cycle of peer victimization. *Developmental Psychology, 35*(1), 94–101.

Hoge, C. W., Castro, C. A., Messer, S. C., McGurk, D., Cotting, D. I., & Koffman, R. L. (2004). Combat duty in Iraq and Afghanistan, mental health problems, and barriers to care. *New England Journal of Medicine, 351*(1), 13–22.

Hollingshead, A. B. (1965). *Two-factor index of social position*. Unpublished report, Yale University, New Haven, CT.

Hollingshead, A. B., & Redlich, F. C. (1958). *Social class and mental illness: Community study*. Hoboken, NJ: John Wiley & Sons.

Holmes, T. H., & Rahe, R. H. (1967). The Social Readjustment Rating Scale. *Journal of Psychosomatic Research, 11*(2), 213–218.

Holt-Lunstad, J., Birmingham, W., & Jones, B. Q. (2008). Is there something unique about marriage? The relative impact of marital status, relationship quality, and network social support on ambulatory blood pressure and mental health. *Annals of Behavioral Medicine, 35*(2), 239–244.

Hoppmann, C. A., Gerstorf, D., Willis, S. L., & Schaie, K. W. (2011). Spousal interrelations in happiness in the Seattle Longitudinal Study. *Developmental Psychology, 47*(1), 1–8.

Hoven, C. W., Duarte, C. S., Lucas, C. P., Wu, P., Mandell, D. J., Goodwin, R. D.,...Susser, E. (2005). Psychopathology among New York City public school children 6 months after September 11. *Archives of General Psychiatry, 62*(5), 545–552.

Ingram, R. E., & Luxton, D. D. (2005). Vulnerability-stress models. In B. L. Hankin & J. R. Z. Abela (Eds.), *Development of psychopathology: A vulnerability-stress perspective* (pp. 32–46). Thousand Oaks, CA: Sage.

Ingram, R. E., & Price, J. M. (Eds.). (2001). *Vulnerability to psychopathology: Risk across the lifespan.* New York, NY: Guilford.

Ireland, T. O., & Smith, C. A. (2009). Living in partner-violent families: Developmental links to antisocial behavior and relationship violence. *Journal of Youth and Adolescence, 38*(3), 323–339.

Jaffee, S. R., Caspi, A., Moffitt, T. E., & Taylor, A. (2004). Physical maltreatment victim to antisocial child: Evidence of an environmentally mediated process. *Journal of Abnormal Psychology, 113*(1), 44–55.

Jemmott, J. B., & Locke, S. E. (1984). Psychosocial factors, immunologic mediation and human susceptibility to infectious diseases: How much do we know? *Psychological Bulletin, 95*(1), 78–108.

Joiner, T. E. (2000). Depression's vicious scree: Self-propagatory and erosive factors in depression chronicity. *Clinical Psychology: Science and Practice, 7*, 203–218.

Jordanova, V., Stewart, R., Goldberg, D., Bebbington, P. E., Brugha, T., Singleton, N.,...Meltzer, H. (2007). Age variation in life events and their relationship with common mental disorder in a national survey population. *Social Psychiatry and Psychiatric Epidemiology, 42*(8), 611–616.

Joyner, K., & Udry, R. J. (2000). You don't bring me anything but down: Adolescent romance and depression. *Journal of Health and Social Behavior, 41*(4), 369–391.

Kamarck, T., & Jennings, J. R. (1991). Biobehavioral factors in sudden cardiac death. *Psychological Bulletin, 109*(1), 42–75.

Kang, H. K., Natelson, B. H., Mahan, C. M., Lee, K. Y., & Murphy, F. M. (2003). Post-traumatic stress disorder and chronic fatigue syndrome-like illness among Gulf War veterans: A population-based study of 30,000 veterans. *American Journal of Epidemiology, 157*(2), 141–148.

Karney, B. R., & Bradbury, I. N. (1995). The longitudinal course of marital quality and stability: A review of theory, method and research. *Psychological Bulletin, 118*(1), 3–34.

Kawachi, I., Sparrow, D., Vokonas, P. S., & Weiss, S. T. (1995). Decreased heart rate variability in men with phobic anxiety (data from the Normative Aging Study). *American Journal of Cardiology, 75*(14), 882–885.

Keenan, K., Hipwell, A., Feng, X., Rischall, M., Henneberger, A., & Klosterman, S. (2010). Lack of assertion, peer victimization and risk for depression in girls: Testing a diathesis–stress model. *Journal of Adolescent Health, 47*(5), 526–528.

Keenan, K., Shaw, D. S., Walsh, B., Delliquadri, E., & Giovannelli, J. (1997). DSM-III-R disorders in preschool children from very low-income families. *Journal of American Academy of Child and Adolescent Psychiatry, 36*(5), 620–627.

Kellam, S. G., Branch, J. D., Agrawal, K. C., & Ensminger, M. E. (1975). *Mental health and going to school: The Woodlawn program of assessment, early intervention and intervention and evaluation.* Chicago, IL: University of Chicago.

Kellam, S. G., & Rebok, G. W. (1992). Building developmental and etiological theory through epidemiologically based preventive intervention trials. In J. McCord & R. E. Tremblay (Eds.), *Preventing antisocial behavior: Interventions from birth through adolescence* (pp. 162–195). New York, NY: Guilford.

Kelley, M. L., & Fals-Stewart, W. (2004). Psychiatric disorders of children living with drug-abusing, alcohol-abusing, and non-substance-abusing fathers. *Journal of the American Academy of Child and Adolescent Psychiatry, 43*(5), 621–628.

Kendler, K. S., Bulik, C. M., Silberg, J., Hettema, J. M., Myers, J., & Prescott, C. A. (2000). Childhood sexual abuse and adult psychiatric and substance use disorders in women: An epidemiological and co-twin control analysis. *Archives of General Psychiatry, 57*(10), 953–959.

Kendler, K. S., Kessler, R. C., Walters, E. E., MacLean, C., Neale, M. C., Heath, A. C., & Eaves, L. J. (1995). Stressful life events, genetic liability, and onset of an episode of major depression in women. *American Journal of Psychiatry, 152*(6), 833–842.

Kessler, R. C. (1997). The effects of stressful life events on depression. *Annual Review of Psychology, 48*, 191–214.

Kim, J., & Moen, P. (2002). Retirement transitions, gender, and psychological wellbeing. *Journals of Gerontology, Series A: Psychological Science and Social Sciences, 57*(3), 212–222.

Kim-Cohen, J., Caspi, A., Taylor, A., Williams, B., Newcombe, R., Craig, I. W., & Moffitt, T. E. (2006). MAOA, maltreatment, and gene–environment interaction predicting children's mental health: New evidence and a meta-analysis. *Molecular Psychiatry, 11*(10), 903–913.

Kirschbaum, C., & Hellhammer, D. H. (1994). Salivary cortisol in psychoneuroendocrine research: Recent developments and applications. *Psychoneuroendocrinology, 19*(4), 313–333.

Kopp, M. S., Konkolÿ Thege, B., Balog, P., Stauder, A., Salavecz, G., Rózsa, S.,…Ádám, S. (2010). Measures of stress in epidemiological research. *Journal of Psychosomatic Research, 69*(2), 211–225.

Kubzansky, L. D., & Kawachi, I. (2000). Going to the heart of the matter: Do negative emotions cause coronary heart disease? *Journal of Psychosomatic Research, 48*(4–5), 323–337.

Kulka, R. A. (1990). *Trauma and the Vietnam War generation: Report of findings from the National Vietnam Veterans Readjustment study.* New York, NY: Brunner/Mazel.

Ladd, G. W., Kochenderfer, B. J., & Coleman, C. (1996). Friendship quality as a predictor of young children's early school adjustment. *Child Development, 67*(3), 1103–1118.

La Greca, A. M., & Harrison, H. M. (2005). Adolescent peer relations, friendships, and romantic relationships: Do they predict social anxiety and depression? *Journal of Clinical Child and Adolescent Psychology, 34*(1), 49–61.

Lambert, S. F., Copeland-Linder, N., & Ialongo, N. S. (2008). Longitudinal associations between community violence exposure and suicidality. *Journal of Adolescent Health, 43*(4), 380–386.

Larson, R. W., Moneta, G., Maryse, H., & Wilson, S. (2002). Continuity, stability and change in daily emotional experience across adolescence. *Child Development, 73*(4), 1151–1165.

Lazarus, R. S., & Folkman, S. (1984). *Stress, appraisal, and coping.* New York, NY: Springer.

Leitenberg, H., Gibson, L. E., & Novy, P. L. (2004). Individual differences among undergraduate women in methods of coping with stressful events: The impact of cumulative childhood stressors and abuse. *Child Abuse and Neglect, 28*(2), 181–192.

Leventhal, H. (1984). A perceptual motor theory of emotion. In: K. R. Scherer & P. Ekman (Eds.), *Approaches to emotion* (pp. 271–291). Hillsdale, NJ: Lawrence Erlbaum.

Leventhal, H., & Scherer, K. (1987). The relationship of emotion to cognition: A functional approach to semantic controversy. *Cognition & Emotion, 1,* 3–28.

Lewinsohn, P. M., Hoberman, H. M., & Rosenbaum, M. (1988). A prospective study of risk factors for unipolar depression. *Journal of Abnormal Psychology, 97*(3), 251–264.

Liao, D., Cai, J., Rosamond, W. D., Barnes, R. W., Hutchinson, R. G., Whitsel, E. A.,…Heiss, G. (1997). Cardiac autonomic function and incident coronary heart disease: A population-based case-cohort study. The ARIC Study. *American Journal of Epidemiology, 145*(8), 696–706.

Littrell, J. (2008). The mind–body connection: Not just a theory anymore. *Social Work in Health Care, 46*(4), 17–37.

Loeber, R., & Stoudhamer-Loeber, M. (1998). Development of juvenile aggression and violence: Some common misconceptions and controversies. *American Psychologist, 53*(2), 242–259.

Lu, W., Mueser, K. T., Rosenberg, S. D., & Jankowski, M. K. (2008). Correlates of adverse childhood experiences among adults with severe mood disorders. *Psychiatric Services, 59*(9), 1018–1026.

Luthar, S. S., & Cicchetti, D. (2000). The construct of resilience: Implications for intervention and social policy. *Developmental Psychopathology, 12*(4), 857–885.

Luthar, S. S., & Zigler, E. (1991). Vulnerability and competence: A review of research on resilience in childhood. *American Journal of Orthopsychiatry, 61*(1), 6–22.

Magnus, K., Diener, E., Fujita, F., & Payot, W. (1993). Extraversion and neuroticism as predictors of objective life events: A longitudinal analysis. *Journal of Personality and Social Psychology, 65*(5), 1046–1053.

Mandal, B., & Roe, B. (2008). Job loss, retirement and the mental health of older Americans. *Journal of Mental Health Policy Economics, 11*(4),167–176.

Mash, E. J., & Barkley, R. A. (2003). *Child psychopathology* (2nd ed.). New York, NY: Guilford.

Masten, A. S. (2006). Developmental psychopathology: Pathways to the future. *International Journal of Behavioral Development, 30*(1), 47–54.

Matthews, S., Hertzman, C., Ostry, A., & Power, C. (1998). Gender, work roles and psychosocial work characteristics as determinants of health. *Social Science and Medicine, 46*(11), 1417–1424.

McEwen, B. S. (1998). Stress, adaptation, and disease: Allostasis and allostatic load. *Annals of the New York Academy of Sciences, 840,* 33–44.

McEwen, B. (2000). Definitions and concepts of stress. In Fink, G. (Ed.), *Encyclopedia of stress* (Vol. 3, pp. 508–509). San Diego, CA: Academic Press.

McFetridge, J., & Sherwood, A. (1999). Impedance cardiography for noninvasive measurements of cardiovascular hemodynamics. *Nursing Research, 48*(2), 109–113.

McGloin, J. M., & Widom, C. S. (2001). Resilience among abused and neglected children grown up. *Development and Psychopathology, 13*(4), 1021–1038.

McKeever, V. M., & Huff, M. E. (2003). A diathesis–stress model of posttraumatic stress disorder: Ecological, biological, and residual stress pathways. *Review of General Psychology, 7*(3), 237–250.

Merikangas, K. R., Zhang, H., Avenevoli, S., Acharyya, S., Neuenschwander, M., & Angst, J. (2003). Longitudinal trajectories of depression and anxiety in a prospective community study. *Archives of General Psychiatry, 60*(10), 993–1000.

Meyer, I. L. (2003). Prejudice, social stress and mental health in lesbian, gay and bisexual populations: Conceptual issues and research evidence. *Psychological Bulletin, 129*(5), 674–697.

Meyer, U., van Kampen, M., Isovich, E., Flugge, G., & Fuchs, E. (2001). Chronic psychosocial stress regulates the expression of both GR and MR mRNA in the hippocampal formation of tree shrews. *Hippocampus, 11*(3), 329–336.

Midanik, J., Soghikian, K., Ransom, L., & Tekawa, I. (1995). The effect of retirement on mental and health behaviors: The Kaiser Permanente Retirement study. *Journals of Gerontology, Series B: Psychological Sciences and Social Sciences, 50*(1), 859–861.

Mishna, F. (2012). *Bullying: a guide to research, intervention, and prevention.* New York, NY: Oxford University Press.

Moen, P. (2001). The gendered life course. In L. K. George and R. H. Binstock (Eds.), *Handbook of aging and social sciences* (5th ed., pp. 179–196). San Diego, CA: Academic Press.

Monroe, S. M., & Simons, A. D. (1991). Diathesis-stress theories in the context of life-stress research: Implications for the depressive disorders. *Psychological Bulletin, 110*(3), 406–425.

Monuteaux, M. C., Faraone, S. V., Michelle Gross, L., & Biederman, J. (2007). Predictors, clinical characteristics and outcome of conduct disorder in girls with attention-deficit/hyperactivity disorder: A longitudinal study. *Psychological Medicine, 37*(12), 1731–1741.

Mossakowski, K. N. (2009). The influence of past unemployment duration on symptoms of depression among young women and men in the United States. *American Journal of Public Health, 99*(10), 1826–1832.

National Scientific Council on the Developing Child. (2005). *Excessive stress disrupts the architecture of the developing brain* (NSCDC Working Paper No. 3). Waltham, MA: Brandeis University.

Nazroo, J. Y. (2001, March 1). Exploring gender difference in depression. *Psychiatric Times, 18*(3). Retrieved from http://www.psychiatrictimes.com/depression/content/article/10168/1158326?pageNumber=3

Nemeroff, C. B., Bremner, J. D., Foa, E. B., Mayberg, H. S., North, C. S., & Stein, M. B. (2006). Posttraumatic stress disorder: A state-of-the-science review. *Journal of Psychiatric Research, 40*(1), 1–21.

Nicolson, N. A. (2008). Measurement of cortisol. In L. J. Leucken & L. C. Gallo (Eds.), *Handbook of physiological research methods in health psychology* (pp. 37–74). Thousand Oaks, CA: Sage.

Niehoff, D. (2002). *The biology of violence (how understanding the brain, behavior, and environment can break the vicious circle of aggression).* New York, NY: Free Press.

Normand, S., Schneider, B. H., & Robaey, P. (2007). Attention-deficit/hyperactivity disorder and the challenges of close friendship. *Journal of the Canadian Academy of Child and Adolescent Psychiatry, 16*(2), 67–73.

O'Connell, M. E., Boat, T., & Warner, K. E. (2009). *Preventing mental, emotional, and behavioral disorders among young people: Progress and possibilities.* Washington, DC: National Academies Press.

Ostrove, J. M., Adler, N. E., Kuppermann, M., & Washington, A. E. (2000). Objective and subjective assessments of socioeconomic status and their relationship to self-rated health in an ethnically diverse sample of pregnant women. *Journal of Health Psychology, 19*(6), 613–618.

Parker, J. G., & Seal, J. (1996). Forming, losing, renewing and replacing friendships: Applying temporal parameters to the assessment of children's friendship experiences. *Child Development, 67*, 2248–2268.

Patton, G. C., Coffey, C., Posterino, M., Carlin, J. B., & Bowes, G. (2003). Life events and early onset depression: Cause or consequence? *Psychological Medicine, 33*(7), 1203–1210.

Paykel, E. S. (1994). Life events, social support and depression. *Acta Psychiatrica Scandinavica, 377*(Suppl.), 750–758.

Pearlin, L. I., & Schooler, C. (1978). The structure of coping. *Journal of Health and Social Behavior, 19*(1), 2–21.

Pearlin, L. I., & Skaff, M. M. (1995). Stressors and adaptation in late life. In M. Gatz (Ed.), *Emerging issues in mental health and aging* (pp. 97–123). Washington, DC: American Psychological Association.

Perry, B. (1997). Incubated in terror: Neuro-developmental factors in the "cycle of violence." In J. D. Osofsky (Ed.), *Children in a violent society* (pp. 124–149). New York, NY: Guilford.

Perry, B. D., Pollard, R. A., Blakley, T. L., Baker, W. L., & Vigilante, D. (1995). Childhood trauma, the neurobiology of adaptation, and "use-dependent" development of the brain: How "states" become "traits." *Infant Mental Health Journal, 16*(4), 271–291.

Pett, M. A., & Johnson, M. J. M. (2005). Development and psychometric evaluation of the revised University Student Hassles Scale. *Educational and Psychological Measurement, 65*(6), 984–1010.

Plomin, R., DeFries, J. C., & Loehlin, J. C. (1977). Genotype–environment interaction and correlation in the analysis of human behavior. *Psychological Bulletin, 84*(2), 309–322.

Pollock, K. (1988). On the nature of social stress: Production of a modern mythology. *Social Science and Medicine, 26*(3), 381–392.

Porges, S. W. (2003). The polyvagal theory: Phylogenetic contributions to social behavior. *Physiology and Behavior, 79*(3), 503–513.

Post, R. M. (1992). Transduction of psychosocial stress into the neurobiology of recurrent affective disorder. *American Journal of Psychiatry, 149*(8), 999–1010.

Richman, J. A., Zlatoper, K. W., Zackula Ehmke, J. L., & Rospenda, K. M. (2006). Retirement and drinking outcomes: Lingering effects of workplace stress? *Addictive Behaviors, 31*(5), 767–776.

Risch, N., Herrell, R., Lehner, T., Liang, K.-Y., Eaves, L., Hoh, J., ... Merikangas, K. R. (2009). Interaction between the serotonin transporter gene (*5-HTTLPR*), stressful life events, and risk of depression: A meta-analysis. *Journal of the American Medical Association, 301*(23), 2462–2471.

Robles, T. F., & Kiecolt-Glaser, J. K. (2003). The physiology of marriage: Pathways to health. *Physiological Behavior, 79*(3), 409–416.

Rosenthal, D. (1963). A suggested conceptual framework. In D. Rosenthal (Ed.), *The Genian quadruplets* (pp. 505–516). New York, NY: Basic Books.

Rowe, J. W., & Kahn, R. L. (2000). Successful aging and disease prevention. *Advances in Renal Replacement Therapy, 7*(1), 70–77.

Rubin, K. H., Bukowski, W. M., & Parker, J. G. (2006). Peer interactions, relationships and groups. In W. Damon, R. M. Lerner, & N. Eisenberg (Eds.), *Handbook of child psychology: Vol. 3. Social, emotional, and personality development* (6th ed., pp. 571–645). New York, NY: Wiley.

Rudolph, K. D., Hammen, C., Burge, D., Lindberg, N., Herzberg, D., & Daley, S. E. (2000). Toward an interpersonal life-stress model of depression: The developmental context of stress generation. *Development and Psychopathology, 12*(2), 215–234.

Rutter, M. (1986). Meyerian psychobiology, personality development and the role of life experiences. *American Journal of Psychiatry, 143*(9), 1077–1087.

Rutter, M. (1987). Psychological resilience and protective mechanisms. *American Journal of Orthopsychiatry, 57,* 598–611.

Rutter, M. (1989). Pathways from childhood to adult life. *Journal of Child Psychology and Psychiatry, 30*(1), 23–51.

Rutter, M. (2006). Implications of resilience concepts for scientific understanding. *Annals of the New York Academy of Sciences, 1094,* 1–12.

Rutter, M. (2008). Biological implications of gene–environment interaction. *Journal of Abnormal Child Psychology, 36*(7), 969–975.

Sameroff, A. J., Seifer, R., Baldwin, A., & Baldwin, C. (1993). Stability of intelligence from preschool to adolescence: The influence of social and family risk factors. *Child Development, 64*(1), 80–97.

Sapolsky, R. M. (1999). Glucocorticoids, stress, and their adverse neurological effects: Relevance to aging. *Experimental Gerontology, 34*(6), 721–732.

Sapolsky, R. M. (2004). *Why zebras don't get ulcers: The acclaimed guide to stress, stress-related diseases and coping* (3rd ed.). New York, NY: Henry Holt.

Schlenger, W. E., Caddell, J. M., Ebert, L., Jordan, B. K., Rourke, K. M., Wilson, D., ... Kulka, R. A. (2002). Psychological reactions to terrorist attacks: Findings from the National Study of Americans' Reactions to September 11. *Journal of the American Medical Association, 288*(5), 581–588.

Schneiderman, N. (1987). Psychophysiologic factors in atherogenesis and coronary artery disease. *Circulation, 76*(1, Pt. 2), 141–147.

Seeman, T. E., Singer, B., Rowe, J. W., Horowitz, R., & McEwen, B. S. (1997). The price of adaptation—allostatic load and its health consequences: McArthur Studies of Successful Aging. *Archives of Internal Medicine, 157*(11), 2259–2268.

Selye, H. (1956). *The stress of life.* New York, NY: McGraw-Hill.

Sentse, M., Lindenberg, S., Omvlee, A., Ormel, J., & Veenstra, R. (2010). Rejection and acceptance across contexts: Parents and peers as risks and buffers for early adolescent psychopathology: The TRAILS study. *Journal of Abnormal Child Psychology, 38*(1), 119–130.

Serido, J., Almeida, D. M., & Wethington, E. (2004). Chronic stressors and daily hassles: Unique and interactive relationships with psychological distress. *Journal of Health and Social Behavior, 45*(1), 17–33.

Sheline, Y. I., Wang, P. W., Gado, M. H., Csernansky, J. G., & Vannier, M. W. (1996). Hippocampal atrophy in recurrent major depression. *Proceedings of the National Academy of Sciences of the United States of America, 93*(9), 3908–3913.

Sherwood, A., Allen, M. T., Fahrenberg, J., Kelsey, R. M., Lovallo, W. R., & van Doornen, L. J. (1990). Methodological guidelines for impedance cardiography. *Psychophysiology, 27*(1), 1–23.

Simeon, D., Yehuda, R., Cunhill, R., Knutelska, M., Putnam, F. W., & Smith, L. M. (2007). Factors associated with resilience in healthy adults. *Psychoendocrinology, 32*(8–10), 1149–1152.

Simon, R. W., & Barrett, A. E. (2010). Nonmarital romantic relationships and mental health in early adulthood: Does the association differ for women and men? *Journal of Health and Social Behavior, 51*(2), 168–182.

Skinner, E. A., & Zimmer-Gembeck, M. J. (2007). The development of coping. *Annual Review of Psychology, 58*, 119–144.

Smith, A., & Nicholson, K. (2001). Psychosocial factors, respiratory viruses and exacerbation of asthma. *Psychoneuroendocrinology, 26*(4), 411–420.

Stansfeld, S. A., Fuhrer, R., Shipley, M. J., & Marmot, M. G. (2002). Psychological distress as a risk factor for coronary heart disease in the Whitehall II study. *International Journal of Epidemiology, 31*(1), 248–255.

Stouthamer-Loeber, M., Loeber, R., Wei, E., Rarrington, D. P., & Wikstroem, P. (2002). Risk and promotive effects in the explanation of persistent serious delinquency in boys. *Journal of Consulting and Clinical Psychology, 70*(1), 111–123.

Suomi, S. J. (2006). Risk, resilience, and gene × environment interactions in rhesus monkeys. *Annals of the New York Academy of Sciences, 1094*, 52–62.

Surtees, P. G., Miller, P. M., Ingham, J. G., Kreitman, N. B., Rennie, D., & Sashidharan, S. P. (1986). Life events and the onset of affective disorder: A longitudinal general population study. *Journal of Affective Disorders, 10*(1), 37–50.

Swaen, G. M., van Amelsvoort, L. P., Bültmann, U., Slangen, J. J., & Kant, I. J. (2004). Psychosocial work characteristics as risk factors for being injured in an occupational accident. *Journal of Occupational and Environmental Medicine, 46*(6), 521–527.

Szinovacz, M. E., & Davey, A. (2004). Honeymoons and joint lunches: Effects of retirement and spouse's employment on depressive symptoms. *Journals of Gerontology, Series B: Psychological Sciences and Social Sciences, 59*(5), 233–245.

Tennant, C. (1988). Parental loss in childhood: Its effect in adult life. *Archives of General Psychiatry, 45*(11), 1045–1050.

Terr, L. (1990). *Too scared to cry: Psychic trauma in childhood.* New York, NY: Basic Books.

Thayer, J. F., Friedman, B. H., & Borkovec, T. D. (1996). Autonomic characteristics of generalized anxiety disorder and worry. *Biological Psychiatry, 39*(4), 255–266.

Thayer, J. F., & Lane, R. D. (2007). The role of vagal function in the risk for cardiovascular disease and mortality. *Biological Psychology, 74*(2), 224–242.

Theriault, J. (1994). Retirement as a psychosocial transition: Process of adaptation to change. *International Journal of Aging and Human Development, 38*(2), 153–170.

Thoits, P. (1981). Undesirable life events and psychophysiological distress: A problem of operational confounding. *American Sociological Review, 46*(1), 97–109.

Thomas, C., Benzeval, M., & Stansfeld, S. A. (2005). Employment transitions and mental health: An analysis from the British Household Panel survey. *Journal of Epidemiology and Community Health, 59*(3), 243–249.

Thompson, R., Briggs, E., English, D. J., Dubowitz, H., Lee, L. C., Brody, K., ... Hunter, W. M. (2005). Suicidal ideation among 8-year olds who are maltreated and at risk: Findings from the LONGSCAN studies. *Child Maltreatment, 10*(1), 26–36.

Tolan, P. (1996). How resilient is the concept of resilience? *Community Psychologist, 29*(4), 12–15.

Tomaka, J., Blascovich, J., Kelsey, R. M., & Leitten, C. L. (1993). Subjective, physiological, and behavioral effects of threat and challenge appraisal. *Journal of Personality and Social Psychology, 65*(2), 248–260.

Turner, R. J., Wheaton, B., & Lloyd, D. A. (1995). The epidemiology of social stress. *American Sociological Review, 60*(1), 104–125.

Turner Cobb, J. M., & Steptoe, A. (1998). Psychosocial influences on upper respiratory infectious illness in children. *Journal of Psychosomatic Research, 45*(4), 319–330.

Tyrka, A. R., Wier, L., Price, L. H., Ross, N. S., & Carpenter, L. L. (2008). Childhood parental loss and adult psychopathology: Effects of loss characteristics and contextual factors. *Journal of Psychiatry and Medicine, 38*(3), 329–344.

Van IJzendoom, M. H., Schuengel, C., & Bakersman-Krannenburg, M. J. (1999). Disorganized attachment in early childhood: Meta-analysis of precursors, concomitants, and sequelae. *Development and Psychopathology, 11*(2), 225–249.

Vingerhoets, A. J. J. M., & Marcelissen, F. H. G. (1988). Stress research: Its present status and issues for future developments. *Social Science and Medicine, 26*(3), 279–291.

Wang, M., Henkens, K., & van Solinge, H. (2011). Retirement adjustment: A review of theoretical and empirical advances. *American Psychologist, 66*(3), 204–213.

Wang, P. S., Gruber, M. J., Schoenbaum, M., Speier, A. H., Wells, K. B., & Kessler, R. C. (2007). Mental health service use among Hurricane Katrina survivors in the eight months after the disaster. *Psychiatric Services, 58*(11), 403–411.

Watanabe, Y., Gould, E., & McEwen, B. S. (1992). Stress induces atrophy of apical dendrites of hippocampus CA3 pyramidal neurons. *Brain Research, 588*(2), 341–344.

Waters, E., Merrick, S., Treboux, D., Crowell, J., & Albersheim, L. (2000). Attachment security in infancy and early adulthood: A twenty-year longitudinal study. *Child Development, 71*(3), 684–689.

Werner, E. E. (1995). Resilience in development. *Current Directions in Psychological Science, 4*(3), 81–85.

Westergaard, G. C., Suomi, S. J., Chavanne, T. J., Houser, L., Hurley, A., Cleveland, A., . . . Higley, J. D. (2003). Physiological correlates of aggression and impulsivity in free-ranging female primates. *Neuropsychopharmacology, 28*(6), 1045–1055.

Wilkinson, R. G. (1997). Socioeconomic determinants of health. Health inequalities: Relative or absolute material standards? *British Medical Journal, 314*(7080), 591–595.

Wilson, J. P. (1994). The historical evolution of PTSD diagnostic criteria: From Freud to DSM-IV. *Journal of Trauma and Stress, 7*(4), 681–698.

Wilson, W. J. (1991). Public policy research and "the truly disadvantaged." In C. Jencks & P. E. Peterson (Eds.), *The urban underclass* (pp. 460–481). Washington, DC: Brookings Institute.

Wilson, W. J. (1997). *When work disappears: The world of the new urban poor.* New York, NY: Random House.

Wolkowitz, O. M., Epel, E. S., & Reus, V. I. (2001). Stress hormone–related psychopathology: Pathophysiological and treatment implications. *World Journal of Biological Psychiatry, 2*(3), 115–143.

Wood, W., & Eagly, A. H. (2002). A cross-cultural analysis of the behavior of women and men: Implications for the origins of sex differences. *Psychological Bulletin, 128*(5), 699–727.

Woodward, L. J., & Ferguson, D. M. (1999). Childhood peer relationship problems and psychosocial adjustment in late adolescence. *Journal of Abnormal Child Psychology, 27*(1), 85–102.

Wyatt, G. E., Guthrie, D., & Notgrass, C. M. (1992). Differential effects of women's child sexual abuse and subsequent sexual revictimization. *Journal of Consulting and Clinical Psychology, 60*(2), 167–173.

Zalsman, G., Huang, Y.-Y., Oquendo, M. A., Burke, A. K., Hu, X.-z., Brent, D. A., . . . Mann, J. J. (2006). Association of a triallelic serotonin transporter gene promoter region (*5-HTTLPR*) polymorphism with stressful life events and severity of depression. *American Journal of Psychiatry, 163*(9), 1588–1593.

Zielinski, D. S., & Bradshaw, C. P. (2006). Ecological influences on the sequelae of child maltreatment: A review of the literature. *Child Maltreatment, 11*(1), 49–62.

Zimmer-Gembeck, M. J., Siebenbruner, J., & Collins, W. A. (2001). Diverse aspects of dating: Associations with psychosocial functioning from early to middle adolescence. *Journal of Adolescence, 24*(3), 313–336.

Zubin, J., & Spring, B. (1977). Vulnerability: A new view of schizophrenia. *Journal of Abnormal Psychology, 86*(2), 103–126.

11

Adapting to Acute Crisis

CARLA L. STORR

MELISSA AZUR

JUDITH K. BASS

HOLLY C. WILCOX

Key Points

- Most people experience some form of crisis or trauma in their lifetime, and some proportion will experience a mental syndrome or disorder as a result

- Abnormal reactions to crisis events arising from a wide variety of situations show similar patterns

- Survivors of crises may experience anxiety disorders, mood changes, and behavioral changes

- Mental health reactions are determined the type and severity of the crisis event, individual-level factors, and access to care after the event

- Providers of care often fail to recognize abnormal emotional responses to a crisis, because individuals more readily seek help for pain and physical ailments attributed to the crisis

- Psychological first aid is an evidence-based intervention used to aid people in the immediate aftermath of disasters, community violence, and other traumatic events

- Common treatments include cognitive behavior therapy and group counseling, but more work is needed in prevention

INTRODUCTION

To many people, a crisis is an unexpected tragedy with the potential to change lives irrevocably. Some crises are the product of large-scale events, such as natural or man-made disasters, life-threatening accidents, or other cataclysmic events. Others arise from more personal predicaments: divorce, terminal illness, sexual identity conflicts, and other emotional, interpersonal, or individual issues. While any of these life events can induce stress and distress, this chapter's focus is on the mental health issues associated with crises that arise at the community or societal level, ranging from acts of terrorism to the impact of war on soldiers and civilians, and from the ravages of earthquakes and tornadoes to the very fear of an impending crisis itself. Unfortunately, crises are all too common around the world, affecting the mental and physical health of individuals, families, communities, and even entire societies. The public health impact of such crises cannot be overestimated. Crises exponentially increase the risk for mental health problems and amplify the factors that compromise the capacity to cope.

Each year, an estimated 6–7% of the US population is exposed to disaster or trauma, ranging from motor vehicle accidents and crime to natural and human-caused disasters (Norris, 1988). The need to understand the range of potential reactions to crises is a public health imperative. At the individual level, these reactions can give rise to changes in behavior, physical well-being, psychological health, thinking patterns, and social interactions. At the family, community, and societal levels, disruption of social relations, physical relocation, and dissolution of infrastructure may lower the capacity to cope.

Reactions also may differ based on the nature of the crisis and on the characteristics of individuals affected by it. For example, individuals with direct exposure to a crisis are more likely to develop emotional distress than other groups. Concentric circles of exposure spread out from the epicenter to include bystanders witnessing the event, first responders and rescue workers, and family and friends of victims. It is also important to consider variation in who is at risk for suffering the effects of crises, since an individual's physical and psychological vulnerabilities, personal resources, and social connections can act as risk factors for or protective factors against adverse reactions. Understanding responses to crises can help in creating prevention and intervention strategies that mitigate both the immediate and long-term mental health repercussions of crises.

NORMAL, COMMON REACTIONS TO CRISES

Not all reactions to crises interfere with the ability to cope or are indicative of a more significant mental health problem. After a crisis, many people say they feel as if they are on a roller coaster or are going crazy when in fact they are experiencing normal reactions to a very distressing event. Symptoms and reaction times differ among individuals; moreover, the same person may feel and react differently to similar experiences arising at different times. Most people who live through a crisis or cope with the aftermath of a disaster experience only transitory symptoms. For some, the process of recovering from a crisis may even facilitate health and a reorientation of values and goals (Tedeschi, Park, & Calhoun, 1998).

When faced with a crisis, the human body activates the automatic fight-or-flight response—a response of long-ago ancestors to either physically protect themselves or escape a dangerous situation. Through a combination of neural and hormonal signals, the brain's hypothalamus prompts the body's adrenal glands to release a surge of hormones, the most abundant of which are adrenaline and cortisol. Adrenaline increases blood pressure and heart rate and sends glucose (sugar) to the muscles to help speed escape. Once the immediate danger subsides, the body begins to release cortisol to help shut down the stress response. Table 11-1 displays a range of physical, cognitive, and emotional symptoms that commonly arise during and shortly after a disaster or crisis. They are considered normal because they are time limited and resolve relatively rapidly.

The first emotional reactions to a crisis may be fear and disbelief (A. R. Roberts, 2000);

Table 11-1. Common Reactions Experienced During a Crisis

PHYSICAL SYMPTOMS	COGNITIVE SYMPTOMS	EMOTIONAL SYMPTOMS
Nausea	Confusion	Anger
Sweating	Hypervigilance	Fear or horror
Shock	Need to appoint blame	Excitement
Fast breathing	Poor problem solving	Disbelief
Pounding heart	Poor memory	Feeling overwhelmed
Shaking	Disorientation	Panic
Weakness		Irritability
Fainting		Outbursts

cognitive processes may be so hampered that reactions are based purely on instinct. This stage most commonly lasts up to 72 hours after the triggering event, though reactions may persist longer or may vary in intensity for some time. Other strong emotions may begin to appear from 24 hours to several weeks later, as a person struggles to manage crisis-related stress and upset using existing coping skills. (See box 11-1.) Finally, after an extended period of emotional and physical arousal, most people experience exhaustion. Intense fear, anger, confusion, and guilt may alternate with denial and avoidance of anything connected to the event. Anger is a natural by-product, providing a sense of control, if only in a limited way.

PATHOLOGIC OR UNHEALTHY REACTIONS TO CRISES

While the majority of trauma-exposed individuals recover within the first few weeks or

---

Box 11-1. Common Reactions Experienced Days Following a Traumatic Event

Fear and anxiety about danger to self or loved ones, being alone, being in other frightening situations, or a similar event happening again

Avoidance of situations or thoughts that remind one of the traumatic event

Being easily startled by loud noises or sudden movements

Flashbacks or mentally reexperiencing the event

Little interest in usual activities, including loss of appetite

Sadness or feelings of loss or aloneness

Shock or disbelief at what has happened; feeling numb, unreal, isolated, or detached from other people

Cognitive problems; trouble concentrating or remembering things

Preoccupation with thinking about the trauma

Guilt and self-doubt for not having acted in some other way during the trauma or for being better off than others; feeling responsible for another person's death or injury

Anger or irritability at what has happened, at the senselessness of it all, or at what caused the event to happen; often asking, "Why me?"

months after a crisis, a substantial minority continue to experience symptoms of distress and discomfort related to the traumatic experience. For those individuals, behavioral problems most often arise within a year or two following the trauma; the onset of posttraumatic stress disorder (PTSD), however, may be delayed even longer (Andrews, Brewin, Philpott, & Stewart, 2007; Smid, Mooren, van der Mast, Gersons, & Kleber, 2009). The duration of symptoms also may vary, based on factors associated with the individual, the trauma, and the type and quality of treatment received. Thus research has found, for example, that the duration of a PTSD episode may be longer for females than males (Breslau, Kessler, et al., 1998). For some individuals, symptoms that resolve may recur when they are confronted with reminders of the event; new life events or trauma may reactivate or exacerbate symptoms. In this way, mental health problems associated with traumatic events are similar to other chronic medical problems characterized by periods of relapse and remission.

A number of the mental disorders and other behavior problems common among survivors of crises or disasters are described below. They include a range of anxiety disorders as well as both mood and behavior changes.

Anxiety Disorders

Under certain circumstances, anxiety is beneficial. When an individual is faced with an unfamiliar challenge, anxiety spurs that person to prepare for the upcoming event and may even ready the body for action to flee impending danger. However, when the level of anxiety is out of proportion to the threat and when fears become overwhelming and interfere with daily living, an individual may be suffering from an anxiety disorder (see box 11-2).

GENERALIZED ANXIETY DISORDER

General anxiety disorder (GAD) is characterized by chronic, exaggerated worry and tension, even when little or nothing has provoked it. The unrealistic distress about everyday things characteristic of the disorder extends beyond normal anxieties that people experience every day. For individuals with GAD, the very thought of getting through the day may produce anxiety. What feel like crises and disasters are ongoing occurrences, arising in relationship to issues of money, health, family, and work. Diagnostic significance is reached when a person spends at least six months worrying excessively about everyday problems (American Psychiatric Association [APA], 1994). Compared with other individuals, those who report experiencing a life-threatening event, an injury or severe illness, or a death in the family have been found to experience an increased prevalence of GAD (Muhsen, Lipsitz, Garty-Sandalon, Gross, & Green, 2008).

POSTTRAUMATIC STRESS DISORDER

Posttraumatic stress disorder constitutes an excessive reaction to a deeply shocking and disturbing experience. Characterized by intense fear, helplessness, or horror, the disorder arises most often after experiencing,

---

Box 11-2. Symptoms Characteristic of Anxiety Disorders

Irrational feelings of fear, dread, or being in danger

Tension

Worry

Helplessness or a sense of uncontrollability

Physical symptoms such as agitation, trembling, nausea, hot or cold flashes, dizziness, shortness of breath, or frequent urination

witnessing, or confronting an event involving a serious injury or a threat to the physical integrity of others. A diagnosis of PTSD is based on an assessment of symptoms, their duration of a month or longer, and significant distress or impairment (APA, 1994). Some research has shown the impact of PTSD on workplace absenteeism and inefficiency to be comparable to work-related impairment associated with major depressive disorder (Kessler & Frank, 1997). Thus, for example, an individual with an affective disorder such as major depression or an anxiety disorder on average has more than five times the number of lost or reduced work days as an employee with no mental disorder (11 vs. 2 lost work days per 100 workers and 66 vs. 11 reduced work days per 100 workers, respectively).

Both clinicians and researchers have found that a PTSD diagnosis often does not capture the severe psychological harm that results from chronic, prolonged, and repeated trauma (Bryant, 2010). In long-term trauma, such as childhood physical and sexual abuse, hostage situations, and kidnappings, a victim generally is held physically or emotionally under the control of a perpetrator. Symptoms of such prolonged trauma may be diagnosed mistakenly as a personality disorder (Allen, Huntoon, & Evans, 1999). Thus while five clinically meaningful personality clusters (alienated, withdrawn, aggressive, suffering, and adaptive) have been found among traumatized women, the same clusters do not regularly emerge among other individuals with PTSD (S. Taylor, Asmundson, & Carleton, 2006). People with this type of complex PTSD usually meet PTSD criteria but also may require additional, special treatment considerations.

In mid- to high-income countries, only a small proportion of individuals exposed to a traumatic event meet criteria for PTSD. The lifetime cumulative incidence and 12-month prevalence of PTSD in such countries range from 1.3% to 12.2% and from undetectable to 3.5%, respectively (Breslau, 2009). While less is known about the general prevalence of PTSD in lower income countries, it is substantially higher in countries in which war and disease are endemic. Community population surveys in four postconflict settings found the lifetime

cumulative rate of PTSD to range from 16% to 37% (de Jong et al., 2001).

Studies of at-risk populations demonstrate higher rates of PTSD than are found in general population samples. Following disasters, the prevalence of PTSD is approximately 30–40% among direct victims, 10–20% among rescue workers, and 5–10% in the general population (Galea, Nandi, & Vlahov, 2005).

ACUTE STRESS DISORDER

Acute stress disorder (ASD) is characterized by the development of PTSD-like symptoms immediately after exposure to an extreme traumatic stressor (APA, 1994). Severe anxiety and both dissociative and other symptoms usually begin within a month of the trauma and persist from a minimum of two days to as many as four weeks. (If symptoms persist for more than a month, however, a diagnosis of PTSD is made.)

Ongoing research seeks to understand how many people with ASD go on to develop PTSD (Creamer, O'Donnell, & Pattison, 2004). Prospective studies that followed people after several kinds of traumas have found that between 30% and 80% of those diagnosed with ASD subsequently develop PTSD; the proportion of those with diagnosed PTSD who report previous ASD ranges from 10% to 60% (Bryant, Creamer, O'Donnell, Silove, & McFarlane, 2008).

The prevalence of ASD in the general population is not known. In a population exposed to a serious traumatic stressor, however, prevalence is dependent on the degree of exposure and the extent and persistence of the trauma. Higher rates of ASD have been reported following human-caused trauma than following trauma resulting from natural disaster (Bryant, 2000). Rates ranging from approximately 5% to 30% have been reported in individuals exposed to violent crime, admitted to the hospital following traumatic injury, or informed they have cancer (Brewin, Andrews, Rose, & Kirk, 1999; Bryant et al., 2008; Kangas, Henry, & Bryant, 2007).

Mood Disorders

Changes in mood are common throughout life; over time, most people experience both ups (happiness) and downs (sadness). However, following a crisis, some ups and downs exceed the norm. They do not resolve readily over time; they interfere with daily functioning (see box 11-3).

MAJOR DEPRESSIVE DISORDER

Depressive illness, among the most frequent psychiatric sequelae of loss and traumatic injuries (Bryant et al., 2010), is characterized by long-lasting feelings of sadness and a loss of interest in activities that used to be enjoyable or fun. Unlike transient sadness, major depressive disorder is a persistent problem that changes sleep patterns, appetite, and the way one thinks about things and oneself (APA, 1994).

In almost 50% of cases of individuals exposed to traumatic events, major depressive disorder has been found to co-occur with PTSD (Kessler, Sonnega, Bromet, Hughes, & Nelson, 1995). The similarity of symptoms, coupled with common causation and sequential occurrence, help explain the overlap between the disorders. Nonetheless, some individuals develop depression or PTSD alone in response to trauma (O'Donnell, Creamer, & Pattison, 2004; Shalev et al., 1998).

TRAUMATIC AND COMPLICATED GRIEF

Grief is a universal and very painful personal response that can dominate one's emotions for months. Traumatic grief may occur following the death of a significant person in one's life—bereavement—or as the result of another type of loss (e.g., loss of a limb, loss of a job, or loss of status). The experience may be sudden and unexpected, or it may be anticipated. Traumatic losses, however they arise, often are overwhelming and may complicate the grieving process.

In traumatic grief due to the death of a significant person, symptoms interfere with the ability to experience the typical bereavement process. The combination of trauma and grief symptoms is so severe that any thoughts or reminders, even happy ones, of the person who has died can lead to frightening images, memories, or thoughts of that death (Horowitz et al., 1997). Grief-stricken individuals may find it difficult to move on with their lives. In children, traumatic grief also may interfere with everyday activities, from schoolwork to socializing with friends. Clinical concern is triggered when symptoms persist with significant intensity for longer than two months.

Long-term grief reactions appear to be common following crises. Complicated grief has been found in 46% of family members as long as six months after the death of a loved one in an intensive care unit (Anderson, Arnold, Angus, & Bryce, 2008). Three years following the attacks of September 11, 2001, 43% of bereaved adults continued to screen as positive for complicated grief (Neria et al., 2007).

Box 11-3. Symptoms Characteristic of Mood Disorders

Feeling sad or blue

Decreased interest or activities that used to be pleasurable

Grief

Fatigue

Gastrointestinal problems (indigestion, constipation, or diarrhea)

Headache

Backache

Anxiety, apathy, or anger

Behavior Changes

ALCOHOL AND DRUG USE DISORDERS

Substance use disorders (including both abuse and dependence on alcohol or drugs) often go hand in hand with trauma and other personal stressors, such as issues related to conflict or intimacy in relationships) (Chilcoat & Breslau, 1998; Kessler et al., 1995). Many people self-medicate with drugs or alcohol in an effort to cope with upsetting events, to numb themselves, and to try to manage difficult thoughts, feelings, and memories related to traumatic experiences (Leeise, Pagura, Sareen, & Bolton, 2010). While such behavior may appear to offer a quick solution, it actually may lead to more significant problems. In fact, heavy drinking or drug use may complicate treatment of co-occurring anxiety and mood disorders by interfering with both psychotherapeutic and pharmacologic treatments.

Estimates from a prospective study that followed people for a decade found that neither PTSD nor trauma exposure increased the incidence of alcohol disorders (Breslau, Davis, & Schultz, 2003). The same study further revealed that drug disorders were four times more likely to emerge among people with PTSD than among those without the disorder.

TOBACCO SMOKING

The literature suggests that smoking rates are significantly higher among persons exposed to a traumatic event than among the general population (Feldner, Babson, & Zvolensky, 2007; Fu et al., 2007). Exposure to a traumatic event appears to be associated with increased smoking (including onset, frequency, and nicotine dependence); the increase is most significant among individuals with PTSD. The relationships may be bidirectional, since nicotine may help reduce affective symptoms; withdrawal may exacerbate symptoms of hyperarousal (Feldner, Babson, Zvolensky, et al., 2007). Anxiety disorders have been found to hinder tobacco cessation efforts, since they heighten the risk for relapse (Zvolensky, Bernstein, Marshall, & Feldner, 2006).

In the US general population, the rate of cigarette smoking is 22%. However, approximately 45% of persons with current PTSD are also current smokers; 70% of them smoke more than a pack (20 cigarettes) per day (Feldner, Babson, & Zvolensky, 2007). A prospective study that followed people for 10 years found that nicotine dependence developed in an estimated 10% of persons with no trauma history, 20% of those with a traumatic exposure but no PTSD, and 32% of those with PTSD (diagnosis of which requires exposure to a traumatic event) (Breslau et al., 2003).

DISRUPTIVE BEHAVIORS AND FUNCTIONAL IMPAIRMENT

Reactions to a traumatic event may include uncontrollable feelings of anger or sadness that result in attention problems, aggression, and impulsive behavior. Anger normally is a natural, healthy emotion that provides increased energy to persist in the face of obstacles and helps people manage life's adversities. However, intense anger may give rise to aggressive behavior that can harm intimate relationships, friendships, and employment. Such feelings also may affect individuals' feelings about themselves and their roles in society. Individuals with PTSD show greater anger, hostility, and aggression scores than those without the disorder (Lasko, Gurvits, Kuhne, Orr, & Pitman, 1994; Orth & Wieland, 2006).

Some individuals engage in behaviors designed to deflect blame or responsibility onto others. Other signs of coping behavior failures include regular temper tantrums, resentment, bullying and threatening others, destroying property, and strong defiance of authority figures. If these behaviors become part of a long-term conduct pattern together, they may be diagnostic of a disruptive behavior disorder. Functional impairment from disorders such as these that arise following a severe trauma can result in academic failure, teen pregnancy, involvement with the criminal justice system, marital problems, and unemployment.

In the wake of a traumatic event, children in particular may experience behavior changes. Among children living in the Gaza Strip, 37% were found to have conduct problems; 23%, hyperactivity problems; and 60%, peer relationship problems (Thabet, Abu Tawahina, El Sarraj, & Vostanis, 2008). In the United States, childhood trauma exposure has been associated with widespread impairment at age 18, including higher rates of overall behavioral-emotional problems, interpersonal problems, and academic failure (Giaconia et al., 1995).

SUICIDE

Suicide is a fatal, self-inflicted destructive act with an explicit or inferred intent to die. A complex event, suicide rarely is attributable to a single traumatic event. A combination of both risk and protective processes interact to increase or decrease an individual's potential for suicide. (Box 11-4 lists symptoms that indicate that a person may be suicidal.) Early traumatic experiences such as sexual, emotional, or physical abuse have a high attributable risk for suicidal behaviors, including thoughts (ideation) and actions (both attempts and completions) (Brent, Baugher, Bridge, Chen, & Chiappetta, 1999; Brown, Cohen, Johnson, & Smailes, 1999; Fergusson, Horwood, & Lynskey, 1996). Studies have shown that life events interact with genetic vulnerability to increase one's risk for suicide attempts (Caspi et al., 2003; Gibb, McGeary, Beevers, & Miller, 2006; Roy, Hu, Janal, & Goldman, 2007). Often, adolescent suicide attempts are precipitated by stressful events such as family or discipline problems, public humiliation, run-ins with the law, or the threat or recent experience of separation from a loved one (Shaffer, 1974; Shafii, Steltz-Lenarsky, Derrick, Beckner, & Whittinghill, 1988). A crisis or traumatic event can act as a precipitant for suicidal behaviors among more vulnerable individuals, such as those with a history of mood disorder, impulsivity, or aggression (Mann, Waternaux, Haas, & Malone, 1999).

A history of trauma exposure appears to increase the risk for suicide. As many as 75–85% of people with suicidal behaviors have such a trauma history (Belik, Cox, Stein, Asmundson, & Sareen, 2007). Research also suggests that suicide attempts are associated not only with a past trauma but also with a diagnosis of PTSD. In a large community sample of young adults followed since first grade, 10% of the participants with PTSD subsequently attempted suicide, compared with 5% or less among those participants without PTSD (Wilcox, Storr, & Breslau, 2009). Further, among individuals who experienced assaultive violence, a diagnosis of PTSD raised the risk for suicide more than threefold. In contrast, suicide risk was not significantly increased among those with PTSD who had experienced nonassaultive violence (Wilcox et al., 2009).

NONSUICIDAL SELF-INJURY

Nonsuicidal self-injury (NSSI) is the socially unsanctioned practice of deliberately and directly injuring oneself, as in the practice of cutting (see box 11-5). Although self-harm is neither well understood nor extensively studied, commonly cited risk factors for this behavior are known to include such stressful experiences as family conflict and sexual or physical abuse (Boudewyn & Liem, 1995; Bureau et al., 2009; Turell & Armsworth, 2000). NSSI also has been reported as a way in

---

Box 11-4. Several Symptoms That Might Signal a Suicidal Person

Expressions of hopelessness and helplessness

Current suicidal ideation

Previous suicide attempts

History of depressive disorder or another psychiatric disorder

History of impulsive or aggressive behavior

Box 11-5. Common Self-Injurious Behaviors

Cutting

Branding or burning

Hitting (with an object), bone breaking, punching, or head banging

Drinking harmful chemicals

---

which individuals with PTSD attempt to control or reduce symptom severity (Weierich & Nock, 2008). Linehan (1993) postulated that early-childhood environments characterized by abuse, neglect, and stifled emotional expression give rise to poor interpersonal and emotion regulation skills that in turn lead to later, maladaptive coping behaviors, such as NSSI. While appearing as a diagnostic criterion for borderline personality disorder in the fourth edition of the *Diagnostic and Statistical Manual of Mental Disorders* (DSM-IV) (APA, 1994), NSSI also is seen frequently in young people with developmental disabilities, eating disorders, and mood, anxiety, and substance use disorders. Studies of adolescents and young adults estimate that lifetime self-injury prevalence ranges from 12% to 38%, with many engaging in self-inflicted physical injury as a means of coping with an overwhelming situation or emotion (Whitlock, 2010).

Comorbidity

Psychiatric comorbidity is the simultaneous or serial presence of two or more diagnosable mental disorders in an individual within a specific period. A number of studies document high rates of psychiatric comorbidity following traumatic crises. The correlation estimates found in table 11-2 (below) display the disorders that most often co-occur within one year following exposure to a trauma-inducing crisis (Kessler, Chiu, Demler, Merikangas, & Walters, 2005).

Up to 80% of individuals with PTSD are estimated to have at least one co-occurring mental disorder. The co-occurrence of affective disorders can present in 26–65% of PTSD cases, anxiety disorders in 30–60% of cases, personality disorders in 40–60% of cases, and alcoholism or drug abuse in over half of cases (60–80%) (Brady, Kileen, Brewerton, & Lucerini, 2000; Breslau, Davis, Andreski, Federman, & Anthony 1998; Creamer, Burgess, & McFarlane, 2001; Kulka et al., 1990). Depressive disorders are the most common; occurring in nearly all cases of PTSD (as high as 70%) (Kessler, DuPont, Berglund, & Wittchen, 1999).

The heightened impairment and suffering resulting from comorbidity commensurately

Table 11-2. Comorbidity of Mental Disorders Following Trauma

TETRACHLORIC CORRELATIONS OF PSYCHIATRIC DISORDERS IN THE PAST 12 MONTHS

	GAD	PTSD	AD	DD
MDD	0.62	0.50	0.37	0.40
GAD		0.44	0.31	0.35
PTSD			0.34	0.25
AD				0.71

GAD = generalized anxiety disorder; PTSD = posttraumatic stress disorder; AD = alcohol dependence; DD = drug dependence; MDD = major depressive disorder.

Source: Data from Kessler et al., 2005.

increase the burden of mental disorders at the individual and public health levels. The combination of multiple severe symptoms, greater functional disability, longer illness duration, and less social competence may give rise to both higher service use and increased risky health behaviors (Bakken, Landheim, & Vaglum, 2007; de Graaf, Bijl, Ten Have, Beekman, & Vollebergh, 2004; Rauch et al., 2008; Renouf, Kovacs, & Mukerji, 1997). Given the extensive overlap of symptoms among the disorders, many clinicians who readily identify and treat symptoms of anxiety or depression may not recognize PTSD (Samson, Bensen, Beck, Price, & Nimmer, 1999; Zimmerman & Mattia, 1999).

A prior history of a mental disorder may be a risk factor or marker for developing a second disorder after experiencing trauma. The pre-existing disorder either could predispose an individual to exposure to a traumatic event or could amplify the risk for developing the second disorder following a trauma. Biological processes also may be at work. Adaptations in brain chemistry associated with chronic stress may predispose or unmask a vulnerability to psychiatric disorders, substance use disorders, or both (Brady & Sinha, 2005).

Physical Reactions

The emotional response to trauma can have adverse effects on physical health as well as on cognitive and behavioral well-being. People with PTSD present a particularly good case model. Such individuals, for example, are likely to seek medical help for musculoskeletal, gastrointestinal, cardiovascular, pelvic, and neurologic complaints as well as for pulmonary disease, hypertension, and peptic ulcer (Boscarino, 1997; Davidson, Hughes, Blazer, & George, 1991; Samson et al., 1999; Schnurr & Jankowski, 1999; Spitzer et al., 2009). Norman and colleagues (2006) suggest that the expression of of trauma-related experiences may vary by gender. Unfortunately, without regard to gender issues, PTSD is poorly recognized in both general medical and psychiatric clinical practice (Davidson et al., 1991; Samson et al., 1999). As a result, individuals may be treated for general physical complaints that actually

are symptomatic of PTSD. This same type of problem arises with other co-occurring physical and mental disorders.

Several mechanisms have been proffered to explain the co-occurrence of mental and physical conditions following a traumatic experience. At its simplest, the trauma may be a causal factor in both a physical illness or injury and subsequent pathologic emotional responses. A somewhat circular relationship between the physical and mental may arise. In such an instance, called mutual maintenance, pain acts as a reminder of the trauma, triggering efforts to avoid situations that might lead to further pain and recalled trauma (Asmundson, Coons, Taylor, & Katz, 2002). For example, the association of PTSD with chronic pain has been hypothesized to be related to mutual maintenance (McWilliams, Cox, & Enns, 2003).

Alternatively, a life-threatening illness may precipitate an emotional disorder in reaction to the illness. Many studies, for example, have found that individuals recovering from heart attacks, stroke, cancer. or severe accidents can develop diagnosable depressive illness related in part to the perceived or actual loss of independence, altered body image, or changes in self-efficacy (Noyes et al., 1990). Individuals with life-threatening conditions who also are depressed report a greater number of physical symptoms and use more medical treatment than such individuals who are not depressed (Strik, Lousberg, Cheriex, & Honig, 2004). Thus co-occurring disorders may well have public health and health economic implications.

Third, abnormalities in the hypothalamic-pituitary-adrenal (HPA) axis seen in mental disorders such as PTSD may give rise to increased physical complications (Yehuda et al., 1995). These and other neurochemical changes may produce a vulnerability to hypertension and atherosclerotic heart disease; they also may precipitate abnormalities in thyroid and other hormone functions, heightening susceptibility to infections and immunologic disorders.

Finally, given the high rates of trauma-induced comorbid mental disorders, the physical disorder actually may be related to multiple co-occurring mental disorders. The physical health effects of PTSD, for example, may be attributed in part to comorbid depressive and anxiety disorders.

Genetic and Physiological Changes

Stressful situations mobilize numerous brain regions, including the amygdala, hippocampus, and prefrontal cortex. Research suggests that exposure to chronic stress may have deleterious consequences on brain functioning. For example, long-term dysregulation of specific neurochemical and neuropeptide systems in the brain appears to be involved in the development of both clinical depression and anxiety disorders (Neumeister, Henry, & Krystal, 2007; Reagan, Grillo, & Piroli, 2008). Several neurotransmitter and neuroendocrine systems appear to be involved in the stress response (Southwick et al., 2007).

The HPA axis, a major part of the neuroendocrine system, maintains homeostasis in times of increased stress. Stressful experiences during critical periods of brain development in the formative years shape not only the ways individuals interpret threatening experiences but also the length and strength of stress responses to a threat. Moreover, the experience of stress during these key periods of brain development may permanently change the response of the HPA axis to stress, increasing vulnerability to psychopathology in response to excessive or chronic stress (Gunnar & Donzella, 2002; Gunnar & Quevedo, 2007; Heim & Nemeroff, 2001; Nemeroff, 2004).

The HPA axis also appears to be influenced by other early life experiences (Francis & Meaney, 1999; Weaver, Grant, & Meaney, 2002). The strongest evidence comes from preclinical animal studies in which the offspring of rats who engage in high licking and grooming of their young exhibit both better regulation of the HPA axis and reduced anxiety in later adulthood. These effects clearly are not genetic, since they also can be produced in rat pups cross-fostered from low- to high-licking-and-grooming mothers (Francis & Meaney, 1999). Pharmacologic intervention, however, can alter the findings. When centrally infused with methionine, offspring of low-licking-and-grooming mothers displayed reversal of the effects of maternal behavior on subsequent anxious behavior, HPA axis regulation, and glucocorticoid receptor methylation (Weaver et al., 2005).

Genetics may play a role in the relative vulnerability of trauma victims to developing subsequent PTSD (Broekman, Olff, & Boer, 2007; Segman, Shalev, & Gelernter, 2007). PTSD also may be related to preexisting structural brain abnormalities. For example, both smaller hippocampal volume and abnormalities in the septum pellucidum have been linked to a higher susceptibility to PTSD and other anxiety disorders (Gilbertson et al., 2002; Gross & Hen, 2004; May, Chen, Gilbertson, Shenton, & Pitman, 2004; Talbot, 2004).

TRAUMA AND MENTAL HEALTH: HISTORY AND EPIDEMIOLOGY

The notion that stress could contribute to the development and expression of mental disorders existed long before formal nosologic classifications such as the DSM were created (Yehuda & McFarlane, 1995). Early classifications used terms such as gross stress reaction and transient situational disturbances to describe acute distress experienced after war or other catastrophes. Individuals with attenuated symptoms were thought to be suffering from neuroses. In the 1970s, research disclosed that long-term responses to interpersonal trauma such as the child abuse syndrome, the rape trauma syndrome, and the battered woman syndrome were similar to those found in returning war veterans. However, the diagnostic system at the time had no way to classify such chronic conditions that may arise in previously healthy individuals following exposure to a traumatic event. It was not until the 1980s, with publication of the third edition of the DSM (APA, 1980), that PTSD became part of the nosology and that inquiry into the mental responses to trauma became an integral part of contemporary basic, clinical, and epidemiologic research.

The very definition of a traumatic event, and the scope of events subsumed in that definition, has evolved over time (Friedman, Resick, & Keane, 2007; Monson, Friedman, & La Bash, 2007; Rechtman, 2004; van der Kolk, 2007).

Initially a traumatic experience was defined as an overwhelming and disturbing unusual experience. However, the DSM-IV definition, still in use, broadens the concept of trauma to encompass all events with potential clinical significance (APA, 1994). At the same time, however, the definition requires:

• a direct experience of the trauma (i.e., witnessing or being confronted with an event involving actual or threatened death or serious injury or a threat to the physical integrity of oneself or others)
• a response of intense fear, helplessness, or horror.

By some estimates, the DSM-IV's broadened definition increased the number of diagnostically relevant traumatic events in the general population from 68% to 90% (Breslau & Kessler, 2001). Current studies often use lists of specific types of events to assess traumatic exposure (e.g., Elhai, Gray, Kashdan, & Franklin, 2005). Diagnostic assessment of PTSD involves an exploration of the relationship between described symptoms and a specific qualifying traumatic event. Increased prevalence rates for both PTSD and other acute emotional reactions to trauma also result from the subjective, emotional components of the DSM-IV's diagnostic criterion for PTSD (Creamer, McFarlane, & Burgess, 2005).

For the foregoing reasons, estimates of the prevalence of exposure to traumatic events vary by stressor (event) criteria and other methodological differences, such as how exposure to the traumatic event was assessed. In high-resource nations such as the United States, estimates suggest that at least 50% of the population will experience one traumatic event in their lifetimes; many experience more than one such event. Yet only a fraction of those exposed to trauma develop PTSD.

In war-torn and low-resource countries, the prevalence of crises is high. The consequences of conflict, including forced relocation and violence (often in the context of war and terrorism), may give rise to prevalence rates of PTSD much greater than that found in the United States (de Jong et al., 2001; Murthy, 2007). (See table 11-3.)

In addition to differences in the definition and assessment of trauma exposure, other methodological differences among studies must be kept in mind in efforts to assess the epidemiology of responses to disasters and other traumatic events. Sampling and design issues are among the most important (Galea, Maxwell, & Norris, 2008; Kessler, Keane, Ursano, Mokdad, & Zaslavsky, 2008; Wittchen, Gloster, Beesdo, Schönfeld, & Peronigg, 2009). Outcome measure comparability (e.g., the difference between assessments based on stress symptoms and on diagnostic criteria) is also important. Assessments using stress symptoms, for example, tend to overestimate PTSD prevalence (Boals & Hathaway, 2009; Terhakopian, Sinaii, Engel, Schnurr, & Hoge, 2008). Other important factors include the timing of the assessment (affecting whether the study addresses short- or long-term consequences) and event factors (e.g., type of trauma, proximity to and role in the event), and potential societal or cultural implications.

TYPES OF TRAUMATIC EVENTS

Although the classification of traumatic events is not straightforward, this section provides a few classification examples, grouped by the scope of the experience and by the "cause." For purposes of this description, individual traumatic experiences are distinguished from traumatic events, such as disaster and war, that involve large groups of people, often entire communities. While reaction to traumas resulting from a wide variety of situations show surprisingly similar patterns, much of the history and research on traumatic stress has focused on specific traumas or specific population samples, such as combat duty military and disaster victims. Less is known about trauma-specific consequences in the general population or about the conditional risk of mental problems among trauma victims in general populations.

Individual Traumatic Events

VIOLENCE

Exposure to violence has been associated with a number of mental health problems, including

Table 11-3. Exposure to Traumatic Events and PTSD Prevalence in Selected Large Community or General Population Samples

COUNTRY	SOURCE	PREVALENCE OF TRAUMA EXPOSURE[a] (%)	PREVALENCE OF PTSD (%)	
			LIFETIME	12 MONTH OR RECENT
GENERAL TYPES OF EVENTS				
United States	Kessler et al., 1995	50–60	7.8	
	Breslau Kessler, et al., 1998	90	12.2	
Canada	Van Ameringen, Mancini, Patterson, & Boyle, 2008	76	9.2	
Mexico	Norris et al., 2003	77	11.2	
Chile	Zlotnick et al., 2006	40	4.4	
Australia	Rosenman, 2002	57		1.5
	Creamer et al., 2001	50–65		1.3
New Zealand	Kazantzis et al., 2009	61		
Israel	Bleich, Gelkopf, Melamed, & Solomon, 2006	36 ?[b]	9.0[b]	
Germany	Perkonigg, Kessler, Storz, & Wittchen, 2000	17	1.3	0.7
Switzerland	Hepp et al., 2006	28		0
Netherlands	De Vries & Olff, 2009	81	7.4	
Sweden	Frans, Rimmo, Aberg, & Fredrikson, 2005	81	5.6	
Europe (six countries)	Darves-Bornoz et al., 2008	64		1.1

(continued)

Table 11-3. (Continued)

COUNTRY	SOURCE	PREVALENCE OF TRAUMA EXPOSURE[a] (%)	PREVALENCE OF PTSD (%)	
			LIFETIME	12 MONTH OR RECENT
WAR-ORIENTED EVENTS				
Afghanistan	Cardozo et al., 2004	62 (>3 events)		42.1[b]
	Scholte et al., 2004	67		20.4[b]
Lebanon	Karam et al., 2006	55	3.4	
Rwanda	Pham, Weinstein & Longman 2004	75	24.8b	
Sudan	B. Roberts, Damundu, Lomoro, & Sondorp, 2009	92		36.2[b]
Kosovo	Lopes Cardozo, Vergara, Agani, & Gotway, 2000	66	17.1[b]	
Algeria	de Jong et al., 2001	92	37.4	
Cambodia	de Jong et al., 2001	74	28.4	
Ethiopia	de Jong et al., 2001	78	15.8	
Gaza Strip	de Jong et al., 2001	59	17.8	

[a]Types of events varied and often no cumulative percentage for exposure to any event was reported; therefore used highest estimate from a single event.
[b]Symptom assessment versus structured clinical interview.

suicide, substance misuse, depression, and PTSD (Caetano & Cunradi, 2003; Lambert, Copeland-Linder, & Ialongo, 2008; Rutherford, Zwi, Grove, & Butchart, 2007). Epidemiologic surveys in the US general population have shown that 15%–24% of individuals exposed to violence will develop PTSD (Breslau, Kessler, et al., 1998). Rates of PTSD among victims of crime range between 19% and 75% (Kilpatrick & Resnick, 1993). Experiences of assaultive violence, such as rape and other sexual assault, torture, kidnapping, and unwilling captivity, are among the traumatic events most likely to lead to mental disorders. PTSD develops in about half of those who experience assaultive violence, compared with only 2% of individuals who have learned that a close relative experienced such violence (Breslau, Kessler, et al., 1998).

The impact of being exposed to violence or abuse varies by age and developmental stage. Because it affects the chain of development, early, more prolonged exposure may give rise to significant problems. Childhood maltreatment and abuse have been shown to interfere with a young person's ability to regulate emotions, which in turn may lead to extreme or out-of-control emotions such as anger and rage (Chemtob, Novaco, Hamada, Gross, & Smith, 1997), substance abuse and dependence (Anda et al., 2006), and various forms of self-injury later in life, among them self-starving, cutting, and suicide attempts (van der Kolk, Perry, & Herman, 1991).

Children and adolescents living in homes with domestic violence (now also called intimate partner violence) are at increased risk for emotional and behavioral problems (Holt, Buckley, & Whelan, 2008). Estimates suggest that in the United States, 9% of adolescents have witnessed parental violence, and 38% have witnessed community violence (Zinzow et al., 2009). Both forms of witnessed violence are associated with double the likelihood of PTSD and major depressive disorder compared with peers who have not witnessed such violence (Zinzow et al., 2009).

ACCIDENTS AND ACUTE INJURY

Behavioral complications of physical injury are an increasing public health concern,

particularly now that advances in trauma care have increased the number of individuals surviving traumatic injury. Each year in the United States, approximately 2.5 million individuals experience an injury requiring admission to an acute care facility (Bonnie, Fulco, & Liverman, 1999). Survivors of severe physical injury experience psychiatric sequelae similar to those found among survivors of other types of trauma. A few studies have reported the prevalence of acute stress disorder at 12% to 16% among individuals with physical injuries (Bryant & Harvey, 1998; Harvey & Bryant, 1999a, 1999b; Mellman, David, Bustamante, Fins, & Esposito, 2001). Battle-injured soldiers and individuals who have been seriously injured or burned are at particularly high risk for developing PTSD and depression (Grieger et al., 2006; Laugharne, van de Watt, & Jance, 2011; O'Donnell, Creamer, Bryant, Schnyder, & Shalev, 2003; Van Loey & Van Son, 2003). The US National Study on the Costs and Outcomes of Trauma estimated the prevalences of PTSD and depression a year after being hospitalized for an injury at 20% and 7%, respectively (Zatzick et al., 2008).

The experiences of war veterans and civilians wounded in combat areas tell a similar story about the interconnectedness of physical and mental disorders. Explosive munitions place soldiers at risk for loss of a limb during combat missions. Further, both peacekeepers and residents in strife-torn areas are at risk of amputation and other life-threatening injury from as many as 90 to 110 million unexploded, unmarked antipersonnel land mines (Aboutanos & Baker, 1997). A limited number of studies have explored mental health outcomes of amputations. Two studies following war veterans over an extended period found that 32–52% of amputees needed mental health care to treat PTSD, depression, and impulse control difficulties (Dougherty, 2003; Ebrahimzadeh, Fattahi, & Nejad, 2006).

ILLNESS

Emotional distress is common among patients with chronic disorders or potentially fatal illnesses, such as cancer (Kross, Gries, & Curtis, 2008; Mehnert & Koch, 2007). Similar distress is found among families of individuals who die from or even survive a critical acute illness (Kross et al., 2008). While the DSM-IV (APA, 1994) considers a diagnosed life-threatening illness as a form of trauma, questions remain about whether stress and fears of intensive, often invasive medical procedures and treatments also may be traumatic stressors. Analyses of studies of intensive care unit survivors found clinically significant depressive symptoms among an average of 28% of patients and clinically significant PTSD symptoms among an average of 22% of patients (Davydow, Gifford, Desai, Bienvenu, & Needham, 2009; Davydow, Gifford, Desai, Needham, & Bienvenu, 2008).

CONFLICT AND WAR: MILITARY PERSONNEL

Service in the military increases not only the likelihood of witnessing injury and death but also the potential of captivity or life-threatening situations. In comparison with both civilian populations and peers with no combat exposure, combat veterans and soldiers have a higher prevalence of PTSD, suicide, aggressive behavior, and excessive use of alcohol or drugs (see table 11-4). An individual's exposure to war zone stress has been found to vary with the nature of the conflict and the demands of each deployment (Hoge et al., 2004; Kang, Natelson, Mahan, Lee, & Murphy, 2003; Richardson, Frueh, & Acierno, 2010; Sareen et al., 2007; Schlenger et al.,1992). Prisoners of war have the highest risk of PTSD; high rates persist even 40 years following release (Goldstein, van Kammen, Shelly, Miller, & van Kammen, 1987; Kluznick, Speed, VanValkenburg, & Magraw, 1986).

Similarly, the psychological effects of peacekeeping vary based on the demands of the mission, which can range from benign observation or humanitarian operations to more dangerous work to maintain cease-fires or engage civilian combatants. The majority of peacekeepers cope well with the stress of their service and do not exhibit psychological distress. Nonetheless, some do experience PTSD and other forms of psychological distress, such as depression and alcoholism (see table 11-4).

Between April 2004 and October 2007, children in 19 countries and territories were actively involved in armed conflict as members of government forces or nonstate armed groups (Coalition to Stop the Use of Child Soldiers, 2008). Child soldiers may be used to lay mines, gather intelligence, and act as guards, helpers, and sex partners. Studies document an extremely high degree of trauma exposure and symptoms of posttraumatic stress among these children and youth (Somasundaram, 2002). (See table 11-4.)

CONFLICT AND WAR: CITIZENS AND REFUGEES

During times of war, civilians may experience many violent events (armed conflict, the impact of bombs and land mines, mutilation, and other atrocities). Less evident, nonviolent events such as inadequate food, fuel, or housing also inflict trauma on the civilian population. Studies have documented a host of war-related mental health problems among civilian populations exposed to the traumas of war and torture (Johnson & Thompson, 2008; Steel et al., 2009). For example, more than 15 years after the 1980–1988 war between Iraq and Iran, individuals in a town exposed to chemical weapons and other high-intensity warfare experienced anxiety, depression, and PTSD at rates markedly higher than those in a town that experienced low-intensity warfare (respectively, 65% vs. 18%, 41% vs. 6%, and 33% vs. 2%) (Hashemian et al., 2006).

Unsurprisingly, PTSD is more common among concentration camp survivors than individuals not interned during wartime (Kuch & Cox, 1992). Moreover, long-term consequences of psychiatric problems have also been found among Holocaust survivors (Eaton, Sigal, & Weinfeld, 1982; Trappler, Cohen, & Tulloo, 2007).

Like concentration camp survivors, refugees frequently experience multiple war-related traumatic events (Marshall, Schell, Elliott, Berthold, & Chun, 2005; Onyut et al., 2009; Sabin, Lopes Cardozo, Nackerud, Kaiser, & Varese, 2003). Studies of adult refugees have found prevalence rates from 4% to 86% for PTSD and from 5% to 31% for depression

Table 11-4. Examples of Psychopathology in War

EXPOSURE CIRCUMSTANCE	SOURCE	PSYCHOPATHOLOGY POST DEPLOYMENT
ADULT COMBAT OPERATIONS		
Vietnam War	Dohrenwend et al., 2006	19% lifetime war-related PTSD, 9% PTSD a decade later
	O'Toole et al., 1996	19% PTSD, 6% MDD, 8% GAD, 43% AUD
Persian Gulf War (Desert Storm)	Wolfe, Erickson, Sharkansky, King, & King, 1999	3% PTSD immediately following war, 8% PTSD 2 years after war
	Kang et al., 2003	23% PTSD (4% nondeployed, 10% deployed but no combat)
1982 Lebanon war	Z. Solomon & Mikulincer, 2006	PTSD with CSR: 1 year 54%, 2 years 47%, 3 years 38%, 20 years 27%
		PTSD, no CSR: 1 year 12%, 2 years 7%, 3 years 6%, 20 years 7%
Afghanistan	Hoge et al., 2004	Army: 6% PTSD, 7% depression, 7% anxiety, 18% alcohol misuse
Iraq	Hoge et al., 2004	Army: 13% PTSD, 8% depression, 8% anxiety, 21% alcohol misuse
		Marine: 12% PTSD, 7% depression, 7% anxiety, 29% alcohol misuse
Active Canadian military	Sareen et al., 2007	12 month: 2% PTSD, 7% MDD, 2% GAD, 5% AUD, 4% suicidal ideation
PRISONERS OF WAR/HOSTAGES		
Bataan & Corregidor, 1941	Goldstein et al., 1987	50% PTSD 40 years later
World War II	Kluznick et al., 1986	67% PTSD, 24% MDD, 55% GAD, 27% AUD 40 years later
	Kang, Bullman, & Taylor, 2006	Pacific theater: 22% PTSD, European theater: 17% PTSD

Table 11-4. (Continued)

EXPOSURE CIRCUMSTANCE	SOURCE	PSYCHOPATHOLOGY POST DEPLOYMENT
Yom Kippur War	Ohry et al., 1994	13% PTSD (vs. 3% in combat control) 18 years later
PEACEKEEPING OPERATIONS		
Somalia	Litz, Orsillo, Friedman, Ehrlich, & Batres, 1997; Gray, Bolton, & Litz, 2004	8% PTSD 5 months after return
United Nations Interim Forces, Lebanon, 1978–1991	Thoresen & Mehlum, 2008; Mehlum & Weisaeth, 2002	5% PTSD, 6% suicide 7 years after service
UK Armed Forces (various operations)	Greenberg et al., 2008	4% PTSD
CHILD SOLDIERS		
Germany	Kuwert, Spitzer, Rosenthal, & Freyberger, 2008	5% PTSD since war, 2% current PTSD approximately 50 years later
Nepal	Kohrt et al, 2008	55% PTSD, 53% depression, 46% anxiety
Uganda	Derluyn, Broekaert, Schuyten, & De Temmerman, 2004	97% had clinical level of PTSD symptoms

PTSD = posttraumatic stress disorder; MDD = major depressive disorder; GAD = generalized anxiety disorder; AUD = alcohol use disorder; CSR = chronic stress reaction.

(Hollifield et al., 2009). An estimated 11% of refugee children meet criteria for PTSD (Fazel, Wheeler, & Danesh, 2005). In general, and not surprisingly, displaced persons express significantly more distress than people who have not been displaced, even when the latter have experienced considerable war stress. Studies also have found that mental health effects on trauma-exposed refugees persist years after permanent resettlement in host countries (Marshall, Schell, Elliott, Berthold, & Chun, 2005; Steel et al., 2009).

Mass Traumatic Events/Disasters

Disasters are mass traumatic events with broad adverse effects on people and their environments. In addition to causing both morbidity and mortality, major disasters often result in evacuation and even permanent relocation, with significant disruption to health care services and systems for both patients and staff (Weisler, Barbee, & Townsend, 2006). Natural disasters occur throughout the world, often as a result of extreme weather (e.g., a tornado or cyclone) or a geologic event (e.g., a volcano or earthquake). Disasters also can be caused by humans: Some are accidental, such as forest fires; others are caused with the goal of inflicting trauma and instilling fear, such as school shootings, bombings, and terror attacks.

A disaster's genesis may affect how individuals and communities respond to the trauma both physically and emotionally. Without regard to the cause, for every disaster victim with a physical injury, many more are likely to have significant mental health needs. A meta-analysis of 39 disaster studies estimated that a disaster yields a 17% increase in the rate of psychopathology (Rubonis & Bickman, 1991). Other studies have found that the prevalence of PTSD following natural disasters (5–60% in the first one to two years) is generally lower than that after man-made disasters (25%–75% in the first year) (Galea et al., 2005).

Disasters also can have a profound impact on first responders and rescue workers (Benedek, Fullerton, & Ursano, 2007; Bills et al., 2008; Briggs et al., 2010; Galea et al., 2005; Laugharn et al., 2011). Public safety and health care workers may experience adverse emotional consequences from exposure to the traumatic event, from working with disrupted systems and stressed populations, and from taking on additional workload and demands, all while worrying about their own families.

MASS VIOLENCE/TERRORISM

Terrorism is the use of force or violence against persons or property for the express purpose of generating fear and other adverse psychological effects in the target population. It includes assassinations, kidnappings, hijackings, bomb threats and bombings, computer-based cyber attacks, and the use of chemical, biological, nuclear, and radiologic weapons. Critically, these acts include not only the actual violence but also the threat of such violence. Terrorists may gain publicity for their cause by using threats to instill fear in the public or by trying to convince citizens that their government is powerless against the terror threat.

Several research reviews on the consequences of terrorism demonstrate elevated dis-tress, particularly PTSD, in the weeks following a terrorist attack (DiMaggio & Galea, 2006; Galea et al., 2005; Gidron, 2002; Laugharne, Janca, & Widiger, 2007). (See table 11-5.)

INDUSTRIAL ACCIDENTS

Other types of man-made disaster are the results of failed technology, such as engineering failures, transport disasters, or environmental disasters, as evidenced in recent history by the *Exxon Valdez* tanker and Gulf oil well spills, the toxic waste at Love Canal, the collapse of old bridges and dams in the Northeast and Midwest of the United States, and the chemical leak in Bhopal, India. The aftermath of such accidents can affect victims for many years, in part from the direct physical danger but also in part from the fragmentation of the community at large. Table 11-6 summarizes the findings of studies evaluating the mental health outcomes of several types of industrial disaster.

NATURAL DISASTERS

Mother Nature is a force of destruction like no other. Worldwide, over 300 disasters occur

Table 11-5. Examples of Psychopathology Following Terrorist Attacks

TERRORIST EVENT	SOURCE	SAMPLE	TIME POST EVENT	PREVALENCE		
				PTSD	DEPRESSION	OTHER PSYCHOPATHOLOGY
BOMBINGS						
Oklahoma City, 1995	North et al., 2004	Survivors	6 months	32%		45% psychological disorder
			17 months	31%		
	Shariat, Mallonee, Kruger, Farmer, & North, 1999	Survivors	18–36 months		27%	28% anxiety
Nairobi, Kenya, 1998	Njenga, Nicholls, Nyamai, Kigamwa, & Davidson, 2004	Nonrandom residents	1–3 months	24%		
NYC and Pentagon, Sept 11, 2001	Galea et al., 2002	NYC residents	4–6 weeks	8%	10%	
	Schlenger et al., 2002	NYC residents	1–2 months	11%		
		DC residents	1–2 months	3%		
		US population	1–2 months	4%		
	Grieger, Fullerton, & Ursano, 2003, 2004	Pentagon employees	7 months	14%		13% increased alcohol use
	Grieger et al., 2005	Pentagon employees	1 year	23%	4%	
		Pentagon employees	2 years	14%	7%	
	Vlahov et al., 2004	NYC residents	6–9 months			10% smoking, 18% alcohol, 3% marijuana use increase
Madrid, 2004	Miquel-Tobal et al., 2006	Residents	1–3 months	2%	8%	
	Gabriel et al., 2007	Injured in attack	5–12 weeks	44%	32%	13% GAD

	Conejo-Galindo et al., 2008	Residents	5–12 weeks	12%	8%	9% GAD
		Police officers	5–12 weeks	1%	1%	0.7% GAD
		Hospitalized	1 month	36%	29%	12% suicide, 12% GAD
		Survivors	6 months	34%	23%	16% suicide, 11% GAD
			12 months	29%	29%	14% suicide, 12% GAD

SHOOTINGS

Killeen, TX, 1991	North, McCutcheon, Spitznagel, & Smith, 2002	Survivors	1 month	26%	10%
			1 year	14%	10%
			3 years	18%	10%
Clayton Courthouse, 1992	S. D. Johnson, North & Smith, 2002	Survivors	6–8 weeks	5%	4%
			1 year	3%	3%
			3 years	3%	3%

OTHER

Tokyo subway, chemical attack, 1995	Ohtani et al., 2004	Survivors	5 years	17%	
Israel, second intifada, 2000–2004	Bleich et al., 2006	General population	19 months	9%	59%
			44 months	9%	30%

PTSD = posttraumatic stress disorder; NYC = New York City; DC = Washington, DC; GAD = generalized anxiety disorder.

Table 11-6. Examples of Psychopathology Following Industrial Disasters

EVENT TYPE	SOURCE	SAMPLE[a]	TIME POST EVENT	PSYCHOPATHOLOGY
NUCLEAR DISASTERS				
Pennsylvania: Three Mile Island, 1979	Dew & Bromet,1993	Survivors	10 years	Increased rates of GAD and depression
Kyiv: Chernobyl, 1986	Havenaar et al., 1996	Population	6 years	36% any psychiatric diagnosis
	Bromet, Gluzman, Schwartz, & Goldgaber, 2002	Survivors	11 years	18% PTSD (10% controls)
OIL SPILLS				
Alaska: Exxon Valdez, 1989	Palinkas, Russell, Downs, & Petterson, 1992	Population	1 year	43% one or more disorder (23% nonexposed)
	Palinkas, Petterson, Russell, & Downs, 1993	Population	1 year	20% GAD, 9% PTSD, 17% depression (CESD > 16)
Taean, Korea: Hebei Spirit, 2007	Song et al., 2009	Survivors	8 weeks	78% depression (CESD > 16), 18% suicidal impulses
EXPLOSIONS				
Rome, Italy: gas leak, 2001	Raja, Onofri, Azzoni, Borzellino, & Melchiorre, 2008	Survivors	20 months	37% PTSD, 7% GAD
Toulouse, France: chemical factory, 2001	Rivière et al., 2008	Population	18 months	19% & 8% PTSD (residents in immediate and peripheral areas, respectively)
Enschede, Netherlands: fireworks depot, 2000	Soeteman et al., 2007	Survivors	1 year	Increase of psychological and musculoskeletal problems
	Yzermans et al., 2005	Survivors	2.5 years	Increase of psychological problems, unexplained physical symptoms, and gastrointestinal problems
STRUCTURAL FAILURES				
West Virginia: Buffalo Creek dam collapse, 1972	Green et al., 1990	Survivors	2 years	44% PTSD adults, 32% PTSD children
			14 years	28% PTSD, 30% other psychopathology
South Wales: Aberfan coal slag heap collapse, 1966	Gleser, Green, & Winget, 1981	Survivors	2 years	70% MDD, 60% GAD, 44% increase in smoking
	Morgan, Scourfield, Williams, Jasper, & Lewis, 2003	Survivors	33 years	29% PTSD

GAD: generalized anxiety disorder; PTSD = posttraumatic stress disorder; CESD = [definel; MDD = major depressive disorder. CESD: Center for Epidemiologic Studies Depression Scale

[a]Survivor samples were selected because exposed; population samples were selected from community or households.

each year. (See table 11-7.) Natural hazards result in hundreds or thousands of deaths and cost billions of dollars by disrupting commerce, destroying communities and critical infrastructure, and decimating livelihoods as well as lives. The level of destruction depends on the intensity of the event, the population density at the event's epicenter, and the degree of preparedness, such as warning systems and physical protections.

A comprehensive review and analysis of worldwide natural hazards was compiled as part of the International Strategy for Disaster Reduction (United Nations International Strategy for Disaster Reduction Secretariat, 2009). Many of the 10 worst natural disasters have occurred in Asia (Udomratn, 2008). Earthquakes and earthquake-induced ocean floor movements often generate tsunamis that leave a wide path of death and destruction, as seen in the 2011 tsunami in Japan.

While natural disasters in the United States may appear to occur at random, some regions are more prone to certain types of natural disasters than others. Hurricanes, for example, strike more often in the Southeast and Mid-Atlantic regions (Bourque, Siegel, Kano, & Wood, 2006). Tornadoes tend to frequent the center of the nation, most notably in what has come to be known as Tornado Alley, and the West Coast experiences the greatest number of earthquakes and wildfires.

While studies assessing long-term mental health outcomes following earthquakes are readily found in the literature, far less is known about the emotional and behavioral consequences of other natural disasters, such as fires and drought. Table 11-8 summarizes a range of studies examining the mental health impact of geophysical and hydrometeorological natural disasters.

EMERGING EPIDEMICS AND BIOTERRORISM

The recent occurrence of highly infectious viruses and influenzas (e.g., H1N1) has rekindled interest in the psychological impact of disease outbreaks and what might occur in the wake of a bioterrorism attack. As public health officials and clinicians work to manage an outbreak's threat, public uncertainty is heightened by the novelty of the infectious agent and the unpredictability of the disease's course. Individuals who contract the illness may be confronted with compulsory isolation and experimental treatments. They must face the immediate threat not only to their own life and health but potentially also to those of family and friends. Because health care workers and other first responders are at risk for contracting a potentially lethal disease, they face added anxiety and stress.

A review of 10 observational studies found high prevalences of clinically significant symptoms of depression (17% to 43%), PTSD (21% to 35%), and nonspecific

Table 11-7. Disaster Occurrences, Mortality, and Morbidity

YEAR	NUMBER	DEATHS	AFFECTED (MILLIONS)
2000	413	8,686	173
2001	379	30,981	199
2002	422	12,657	660
2003	360	109,991	255
2004	355	241,647	162
2005	434	89,162	160
2006	401	23,502	122
2007	416	16,871	211
2008	321	235,816	212

Source: http://www.unisdr.org/eng/media-room/press-release/2009/pr-2009-
-01-disaster-figures-2008.pdf

Table 11-8. Examples of Psychopathology Following Natural Disasters

TYPE OF DISASTER	SOURCE	SAMPLE[a]	TIME POST EVENT	PREVALENCE[†]		
				PTSD	DEPRESSION	OTHER PSYCHOPATHOLOGY
EARTHQUAKES						
Chi Chi, Taiwan, 1999 (7.3 on Richter scale)	Chou et al., 2007	Survivors	6 months	8%	12%	4% suicide, 2% DAD
			2 years	10%	7%	6% suicide, 2% DAD
			3 years	4%	6%	6% suicide, 5% DAD
Marmara, Turkey, 1999 (7.4 on Richter scale)	Onder, Tural, Aker, Kiliç, & Erdoğan, 2006	Population	36 months	19%	19%	
			3 years	12%	10%	
VOLCANOES & LAND/MUDSLIDES						
Mt. Unzen, Japan, 1991	Ohta et al., 2003	Survivors	6/44 months			66%/46% distress
Sarno, Italy, 1998	Catapano et al., 2001	Population	1 year	28%		
Tezuitlan, Mexico, 1999	Norris, Murphy, Baker, & Perilla, 2004	Population	6 months	31%	4%	
FIRES						
California, October 2003	Marshall et al., 2007	Survivors	3 months	24%	33%	
Australian bushfire, 1983	McFarlane & Van Hooff, 2009	Survivors	20 years	2%		

TSNAMI

Aech and North Sumatra, 2004	van Griensven et al., 2006	Population, displaced	3/9 months	12%/7%	30%/17%	37%/25% anxiety
		Population, not displaced	3/9 months	7%/2%	20%/14%	30%/26% anxiety

HURRICANES

Mitch, Nicaragua, 1998	Caldera, Palma, Penayo, & Kullgren, 2001	Primary care patients	6 months	6%		10% suicide
Katrina, Gulf Coast US, 2005	Office of Applied Studies, 2008	Population, displaced	1 year	19%		26% distress, 12% SUD
		Population, not displaced	1 year	6%		9% distress, 8% SUD
	Kessler, Galea, et al., 2008	Population	5–8 months	15%		3% suicidal ideation
			17–20 months	21%		6% suicidal ideation

PTSD = posttraumatic stress disorder; DAD = drug abuse/dependence; SUD = substance use disorder.
aSurvivors exhibited nonprobability in selection; population samples were selected at random from community or households.

anxiety (23% to 48%) among patients surviving acute respiratory distress syndrome (ARD) (Davydow, Desai, Needham, & Bienvenu, 2008). In a retrospective study of ARD in patients at a Hong Kong hospital, the cumulative incidence of a DSM-IV mental disorder was 59%; up to one third of patients continued to experience the mental disorder some 30 months following their ARD treatment (Mak, Chu, Pan, Yiu, & Chan, 2009). At 30-month follow up, PTSD was found to be twice as prevalent among health care workers, who represented 30% of the study sample, as among the rest of the sample. Psychological distress also has been found to be more common among residents of equine influenza–infected areas (34%) than in the general population (12%) (M. R. Taylor, Agho, Stevens, & Raphael, 2008).

WHO IS AT RISK?

Not everyone exposed to a traumatic event develops a mental disorder such as depression or PTSD. Wide variation has been found not only in the symptoms and disorders experienced and their timing (immediate or delayed) but also, critically, in who is most likely to have an adverse mental health response to a crisis. Emotional and behavioral reactions to crises are determined in part by individual factors such as current and past mental health status, capacity for self-care, and availability of social and emotional support. Reactions also are affected by event-specific factors (type and severity of the crisis) and by post-disaster access to care and services (Bonanno, Galea, Bucciarelli, & Vlahov, 2007; Bonanno & Mancini, 2008; Walsh, 2007). Further, a growing body of evidence suggests that risk factors for ongoing, chronic PTSD may not be the same as the factors that place a person at risk for PTSD. What follows is a discussion of some of the factors that either increase or decrease the risk for mental disorders following trauma.

Gender

Men tend to have a greater likelihood of exposure to traumatic events and to experience different types of trauma than women (Breslau, Kessler et al., 1998; Kessler et al., 1995). For example, whereas lifetime experience of rape is higher among women, being threatened with a weapon is more common among men (Kessler et al., 1995). In contrast to the findings regarding rates of exposure, general population studies have found significantly higher lifetime PTSD prevalence in women, about double that seen in men (Breslau, Kessler et al., 1998; Kessler et al., 1995). Some researchers posit that the difference is attributable to the greater likelihood for women to experience more severe trauma than men (e.g., rape and sexual assault) and to the generally higher prevalence of a history of depression or other mood disorders in women (Breslau, Davis, Andreski, Peterson, & Schultz,1997; Bromet, Sonnega, & Kessler, 1998).

Women's roles and status in society are linked to their vulnerability during and after disasters, making a woman more likely than a man to die or suffer long-term consequences from a disaster (Raphael, Taylor, & McAndrew, 2008). Women may be burdened with additional mental stress while they maintain household responsibilities and care for children under difficult, even life-threatening circumstances. While girls and women draw support from their cultural connections and identity, they also may feel the weight of cultural pressures to be strong, to remain silent about personal issues, and to refrain from discussing problems outside the family.

Age and Experience

The risk of experiencing a traumatic event is greatest between the ages of 15 and 24 years; thereafter the risk declines consistently with age (Breslau, 2009; Breslau, Kessler et al., 1998; Bromet et al., 1998; Norris, 1992). However, the literature provides little definitive information on the relationship between age and the risk for PTSD (see Breslau, Chilcoat, Kessler, & Davis, 1999; Brewin, Andrews, & Valentine, 2000; Cherniack, 2008; Kessler et al., 1995). Older adults may be less likely to develop trauma-related emotional disorders, possibly because they have had more experience coping with painful or stressful events. At the same time, however, frail, elderly individuals with posttraumatic experiences often exhibit grave impairment in the ability to conduct the affairs of daily life. Even more critically, they often do not receive optimal treatment for PTSD, despite frequent visits to health care providers for somatic complaints and conditions (van Zelst, deBeurs, Beekman, van Dyck, & Deeg, 2006). It is difficult for health care workers, families, and even the elderly themselves to distinguish between problems related to aging and those linked to mental illness.

Race and Ethnicity

In the United States, racial and ethnic differences also have been noted in the prevalence of exposure to traumatic events and in the development of PTSD. Higher rates of exposure to violence have been noted among African Americans, American Indians, and Alaska Natives than in members of other population groups (Jenkins & Bell, 1997; US Department of Health and Human Services, 2001). Recent immigrants to the United States may be at risk for PTSD from preimmigration exposure to war-related trauma (Farias, 1994).

Previous History of Trauma and Psychiatric History

People who inappropriately feel responsible for a traumatic event, who regard the event as punishment for personal wrongdoing, or who generally have negative or pessimistic worldviews are more likely to develop a pathologic reaction to a traumatic event than are those with more positive life views who do not personalize the trauma. Past exposure to trauma may increase the likelihood of an adverse mental reaction to subsequent trauma (Breslau et al., 1999), though some research suggests that prior trauma actually may inoculate individuals against later trauma (Norris & Murrell, 1988).

A past history of mental illness, most notably depression, has been found to be a potent risk factor for PTSD (Breslau, Davis et al., 1998). Following a disaster or other traumatic event, people with chronic mental illnesses are particularly vulnerable to PTSD and suicidal behaviors, including both attempts and completions. While little research has been

undertaken in this challenging area, experiences from Hurricane Katrina suggest that in times of crisis, people with the most serious mental disorders may lack access to their medications and to needed mental health care, with potentially adverse results (Wang et al., 2008).

A family history of psychopathology also may be a risk factor for PTSD among trauma-exposed individuals (Breslau, Davis, Andreski, & Peterson, 1991; Bromet et al., 1998; Davidson, Swartz, Storck, Krishnan, & Hammett, 1985). Twin studies indicate that certain inherited abnormalities in both brain hormone levels and brain structure may increase a person's susceptibility to stress disorders following exposure to trauma (Afifi, Asmundson, Taylor, & Jang, 2010).

Social Support

People with a network of close friends and relatives are less likely to develop adverse emotional reactions to a traumatic event than individuals with less social support (Brewin et al., 2000; Moscardino, Scrimin, Capello, & Altoè, 2010; S. Solomon & Smith, 1994). In much the same way that relationships can act as a protective factor against PTSD and other adverse reactions to trauma, supportive environments, too, promote healthier prognoses (Ozer and Weinstein, 2004). Such networks of understanding can both help mitigate the trauma and improve the chance of recovery. Although providing emotional support sometimes means listening repeatedly to the story of an individual's trauma, sharing emotions about the event can help an emotionally traumatized person feel less alone.

Exposure Type and Severity

The impact of a trauma is measured by its cause, scope, and duration. Natural disasters (floods, earthquakes, hurricanes, etc.) or accidents (airplane crashes, workplace explosions, etc.) actually are less traumatic for most people than are human acts of intentional cruelty or terrorism. Terrorist-inflicted trauma appears to produce particularly high rates of both PTSD and ASD in survivors and bystanders.

Studies show a modest association between event severity (sometimes referred to as life threat experience) and PTSD (Brewin et al., 2000; Ozer, Best, Lipsey, & Weiss, 2003).

Proximity to and Duration of Exposure

A number of studies have found evidence for a dose–response relationship between proximity to a traumatic event and pathologic reactions such as PTSD. Prevalence of mental disorders is consistently higher among persons closer to the epicenter of a traumatic event than among those further away (Hashemian et al., 2006; van Griensven et al., 2006). Similarly, subsequent emotional health and pathology may be influenced by the roles individuals performed during and immediately following the traumatic event (first responder, health professional, etc.). Most studies have focused on the mental health effects on the victims of the traumatic event; more recently, studies have also explored the emotional impact on individuals involved in rescue efforts (Benedek et al., 2007; Bills et al., 2008). Some studies have assessed effects on more than one group after the same traumatic event, facilitating direct comparisons of the effect of level of exposure on mental status (Gabriel et al., 2007; Schlenger et al., 2002).

Presence of Other Stressors

Cumulative exposure to stressors appears to worsen the prognosis for both PTSD and depression (Breslau & Davis, 1987; Catani, Jacob, Schauer, Kohila, & Neuner, 2008). Broader environmental and social factors (e.g., torture and starvation in refugee camps, limited resources, and physical displacement) may interact with personal factors to shape an individual's mental health response to traumatic events (Steel et al., 2009).

PREVENTION AND INTERVENTION STRATEGIES

With the growth of knowledge about the mental health implications of traumatic experiences, increased attention has turned to the prevention and treatment of adverse emotional responses to trauma. While a review of all crisis-focused interventions and treatments is beyond the scope of this chapter, the following section provides a selective review of interventions and treatments found to be of help both in the immediate aftermath of a traumatic event and in the weeks following. (See box 11-6 for links to other resources and sources of information.)

Psychological First Aid

Psychological first aid (PFA) is an evidence-informed intervention to support and assist people in the immediate aftermath of disasters, community violence, or other traumatic events. Often compared to physical first aid, PFA incorporates principles of crisis intervention to help "reduce the initial distress caused by traumatic events, and to foster short and long-term adaptive functioning" (Brymer et al., 2006, p. 6). PFA provides information, offers support, facilitates access to necessary resources, and identifies individuals who may need formal help for an emotional problem (Everly & Flynn, 2006).

While a number of PFA models are being used, they tend to follow a similar process (Brymer et al., 2006; Everly & Flynn, 2006). Once engaged, an individual's immediate needs are assessed, among them physical safety, medical care needs, and emotional health. As noted earlier in this chapter, a traumatic event may give rise to a wide range of normal and abnormal responses. While some individuals experience mild distress, others may have severe reactions that interfere with their ability to function, ranging from increased risk-taking behavior to disorientation and from physical shocklike reactions to feeling emotionally overwhelmed (Brymer et al., 2006).

Stabilization, one of the core components of PFA, is introduced early in the course of the intervention to help orient individuals who may be experiencing the most severe immediate reactions to the event. Another key component of PFA is assessing the immediate needs of a victim of a traumatic event; further needs are then identified. This activity most often is undertaken in a private, safe location where the individual can talk about the trauma experience. Individuals who do not want to share their experience are not pressured into discussing the event. PFA providers do more than provide an ear and support; they also can help educate about common physical and emotional reactions to traumatic events and about coping mechanisms, as well as provide information about available resources. Perhaps most important, PFA helps trauma survivors develop a mental health plan of action that may link them to local resources and supports, help identify personal support systems, and refer to sources of further treatment for a potential emotional problem as needed.

With adaptations for developmental level and cultural practices, PFA can be a valuable tool after a mass trauma for use among individuals of all ages, cultures, and ethnicities (Brymer et al., 2006). Ideally, disaster mental health teams are briefed on the cultural norms of the affected populations. In the absence of such information, however, the disaster mental health team either can gather information from community leaders or can observe and take cues from how people interact. Finally,

while PFA has become standard practice following disasters and other large-scale traumatic events, the practice would benefit from further, ongoing, and rigorous evaluation of its effectiveness.

PFA and other immediate services can help people define a "new normal" and better understand their emotional response to the traumatic event. As noted earlier in this chapter, the good news is that the vast majority of individuals exposed to these kinds of traumatic crises will not need formal mental health services. However, also without question, in the weeks following a traumatic event, some children, women, and men of all ages will develop symptoms indicative of a need for treatment. The following section describes a number of trauma-informed treatment programs that have been used successfully in the United States and abroad.

Trauma-Focused Cognitive Behavior Therapy

An evidence-based practice, trauma-focused cognitive behavior therapy (TF-CBT), is designed to address symptoms of PTSD, depression, and behavioral problems in children who have been exposed to trauma (Cohen and Mannarino, 2008). A short-term psychotherapy, TF-CBT is grounded in cognitive behavioral, attachment, family, and humanistic theories (Child Sexual Abuse Task Force, Research & Practice Core, 2004). Both children and their parents or caregivers are engaged in the 12- to 16-week treatment. Core components covered in TF-CBT include:

• educates children and caregivers about common responses to trauma
• teaches stress management and relaxation techniques, parenting skills, and affective modulation
• explains the relationships among thoughts, feelings, and behaviors
• engages the child in a trauma narrative designed to help him or her process the event and master reminders
• facilitates communication in joint parent–child sessions
• addresses safety issues and other individual child and family emotional needs (Child Sexual Abuse Task Force, Research & Practice Core, 2004).

Randomized TF-CBT trials suggest that it can help reduce symptoms of PTSD and, in some cases, those of depression and anxiety among children who have been sexually abused (Cohen, Deblinger, Mannarino, & Steer, 2004; Cohen & Mannarino, 1996; Deblinger, Mannarino, Cohen, & Steer, 2006), are disaster survivors (CATS Consortium & Hoagwood, 2007), have been exposed to violence (Smith et al., 2007), or have been in car accidents (Smith et al., 2007). Children in those studies experienced greater improvement in symptomatology than others who either received treatment as usual or were wait-listed. Research by Stein and colleagues (2003) suggests that TF-CBT can be modified successfully for use in school settings to reduce PTSD even without traditional parental involvement. In that study, three months following the intervention, children who participated in TF-CBT had lower PTSD and depression scores than were found among wait-listed

controls. The use of TF-CBT administered in a school environment may help overcome barriers to treatment that otherwise might inhibit families from seeking care. While the use of TF-CBT with children has a solid research base, further investigation can help elucidate both the optimal number of sessions and the intervention elements essential to positive outcomes (Cohen, 2003).

Training resources for TF-CBT have been translated into a host of different languages and include guidelines on how best to integrate a family's culture and values into the treatment and setting (Child Sexual Abuse Task Force, Research & Practice Core, 2004). While studies of the core components of TF-CBT offer support for its use across multiple cultures (Cox et al., 2007; Layne et al., 2001), rigorous evaluation of the cross-cultural use of TF-CBT has yet to be undertaken, suggesting the need for additional research.

Exposure Therapy

Exposure therapy enables individuals who have been exposed to severe trauma to relive their frightening memories in a safe, structured environment until the fear and anxiety associated with the memory diminish (Rothbaum, Hodges, Ready, Graap, & Alarcon, 2001). The process is undertaken over multiple sessions, during which the intensity and duration of exposure to the memory increases until it no longer results in avoidant behavior. Numerous studies have evaluated the effectiveness of exposure therapy for individuals diagnosed with PTSD. For example, in a controlled study, Neuner and colleagues (2008) found that among war-affected refugees from Rwanda and Somalia, posttrauma symptoms diminished with either exposure therapy or general trauma counseling. Another study exploring the benefits of exposure therapy among refugees found that the therapy reduced symptoms not only of PTSD but also of both anxiety and depressive disorders (Paunovic & Ost, 2001). Exposure therapy also has been used and evaluated with military veterans and sexual assault survivors. Based on a literature review, Rothbaum and colleagues (2001) concluded that research supports exposure therapy as an effective means of reducing PTSD in each of these traumatized populations.

A new approach to exposure therapy, made possible by technological advances in virtual reality (VR), has received increasing research and clinical interest. Goggles, headphones, joysticks, and other gaming equipment are used along with computers to simulate the traumatic event (Wood et al., 2009). For example, VR technology can simulate the sounds of helicopters flying overhead or the sensation of driving a Humvee. Other technology monitors physiological responses such as heart rate and respiration during the therapeutic VR experience. In a sense, VR provides a full immersion in the traumatic event within the safety of the therapeutic environment, creating an interactive traumatic environment that doesn't rely solely on an individual's detailed recollections of the event (Wood et al., 2009). Case studies and preliminary results from VR-assisted exposure therapy suggest it may well be a promising approach to treating PTSD in military personnel (Gamito et al., 2009; McLay, McBrien, Wiederhold, & Wiederhold, 2010; Wood et al., 2009). Additional rigorous research in this area is warranted.

Mixed Interventions and Non-Trauma-Focused Interventions

Researchers also have developed interventions that incorporate treatments and activities designed to promote positive development and decrease the likelihood of developing mental disorders following trauma exposure. For example, Tol and colleagues (2008) studied a school-based psychosocial program for youth affected by political violence in rural Indonesia. This secondary prevention program focused on youth already exhibiting some behavioral difficulties but not yet meeting diagnostic criteria for a mental disorder. It combined cognitive behavioral techniques, such as psychoeducation, safety building, and relaxation, with creative activities that allowed the children to express their distress through art and movement. The randomized, controlled design found that this type of intervention helped promote psychosocial well-being, such as maintaining hope in the face of challenges.

In an extension of their early work on trauma-focused CBT in schools, Layne and colleagues (2008) developed a three-tiered program of:

- psychoeducation for students exposed to trauma and experiencing distress
- combined psychoeducation and trauma- or grief-focused CBT for students experiencing trauma-related distress
- referral to mental health services for students with significant mental health issues.

The first two program tiers were the subject of a randomized, controlled trial with war-affected Bosnian adolescents. Both program elements were found to lower symptomatology for depression and PTSD, to help the youth manage their grief in more appropriate, productive ways, and to improve their social relationships.

Not all trauma-related programs focus on treating symptoms, however. In the United States, Weine and colleagues (2008) investigated a family group approach for trauma-affected Bosnians who had been relocated to Chicago, Illinois. They found that that a multi-family group approach to care increased access to mental health services. Further, Gould, Greenberg, and Hetherton (2007) implemented a stigma reduction program among military personnel in the United Kingdom and found that psychoeducation and training could improve attitudes toward PTSD, stress, and seeking help, important factors associated with prevention and early intervention for anxiety disorders such as PTSD.

Interpersonal Psychotherapy

In addition to symptoms of mental problems resulting from having experienced traumatic events, people also may experience depression and anxiety associated with life in the aftermath of trauma. Thus treatment should not be limited to PTSD; assessment and intervention for depression and anxiety may also be warranted for trauma-affected populations. One such treatment is interpersonal psychotherapy (IPT), a manualized, brief treatment focused on the connection between mental health and interpersonal relationships (Weissman,

Markowitz, & Klerman, 2000). The treatment involves:

- educating clients about their mental disorders, how the disorders may impair relationships, and how relationships can trigger symptoms of disorders
- identifying problematic relationships
- intervening with clients in the areas of grief, role disputes, role transitions, and interpersonal deficits, as appropriate to the individual (Campanini et al., 2010).

IPT initially was developed to treat depression; subsequently, it has been adapted both to treat other disorders and to be used in a group format (Wilfley et al., 1993). Studies have explored the effectiveness of group IPT in treating depression in victims of trauma. Bolton and colleagues (2007) examined the benefits of using group IPT to treat depression and anxiety among war-affected adolescents in northern Uganda. They found that the intervention, in the hands of local counselors, helped reduce the severity of the crisis- and trauma-related symptoms experienced by these youth. Group IPT has more recently been modified to treat depression among individuals with comorbid PTSD. While further research is warranted, studies suggest that group IPT also may be effective in reducing symptoms of PTSD as well as depression symptoms in individuals who have experienced childhood abuse and interpersonal violence (Bleiberg & Markowitz, 2005; Campanini et al., 2010; Krupnick et al., 2008; Robertson, Rushton, Batrim, Moore, & Morris, 2007), as well among military veterans (Ray & Webster, 2010; Robertson et al., 2007).

CONCLUSIONS AND RECOMMENDATIONS

During their lifetimes, human beings inevitably will experience some type of crisis or traumatic event. Some events, such as natural disasters and accidents, cannot be avoided altogether. The only way to reduce or eliminate the frequency and severity of man-made traumas is through concerted social change locally, nationally, and worldwide. Acute crises happen; individual and community preparation

and response can help mitigate their physical and emotional toll. Unfortunately, today, while local and federal crisis management provide an immediate emergency response, they often neglect to plan for or respond to long-term crisis sequelae.

On a positive note, however, research has advanced knowledge about human responses to highly stressful or traumatic experiences. It is known that many responses to the same traumatic event are possible and that while some individuals suffer few or no emotional ill effects, others cannot forget their traumatic experiences and develop serious emotional sequelae. Moreover, just as the experience of a trauma is quite personal, so, too, is the healing process. Both the availability of resources and the recognition that services can help may determine when and how real healing occurs for individuals and for communities.

REFERENCES

Aboutanos, M. B., & Baker, S. P. (1997). Wartime civilian injuries: Epidemiology and intervention strategies. *Journal of Trauma, 43*(4), 719–726.

Afifi, T. O., Asmundson, G. J., Taylor, S., & Jang, K. L. (2010). The role of genes and environment on trauma exposure and posttraumatic stress disorder symptoms: A review of twin studies. *Clinical Psychological Review, 30*(1), 101–112.

Allen, J. G., Huntoon, J., & Evans, R. B. (1999). Complexities in complex posttraumatic stress disorder in inpatient women: Evidence from cluster analysis of MCMI-III personality disorder scales. *Journal of Personality Assessment, 73*(3), 449–471.

American Psychiatric Association. (1980). *Diagnostic and statistical manual of mental disorders* (3rd ed.). Washington, DC: Author.

American Psychiatric Association. (1994). *Diagnostic and statistical manual of mental disorders* (4th ed.). Washington, DC: Author.

Anda, R. F., Felitti, V. J., Bremner, J. D., Walker, J. D., Whitfield, C., Perry, B. D.,…Giles, W. H. (2006). The enduring effects of abuse and related adverse experiences in childhood: A convergence of evidence from neurobiology and epidemiology. *European Archives of Psychiatry and Clinical Neuroscience, 256*(3), 174–186.

Anderson, W. G., Arnold, R. M., Angus, D. C., & Bryce, C. L. (2008). Posttraumatic stress and complicated grief in family members of patients in the intensive care unit. *Journal of General Internal Medicine, 23*(11), 1871–1876.

Andrews, B., Brewin, C. R., Philpott, R., & Stewart, L. (2007). Delayed-onset posttraumatic stress disorder: A systematic review of the evidence. *American Journal of Psychiatry, 164*(9), 1319–1326.

Asmundson, G. J. G., Coons, M. J., Taylor, S., & Katz, J. (2002). PTSD and the experience of pain: Research and clinical implications of shared vulnerability and mutual maintenance models. *Canadian Journal of Psychiatry, 47*(10), 930–937.

Bakken, K., Landheim, A. S., & Vaglum, P. (2007). Axis I and II disorders as long-term predictors of mental distress: A 6-year prospective follow-up of substance-dependent patients. *BMC Psychiatry, 7*, 29–41.

Belik, S. L., Cox, B. J., Stein, M. B., Asmundson, G. J., & Sareen, J. (2007). Traumatic events and suicidal behavior: Results from a national mental health survey. *Journal of Nervous and Mental Disease, 195*(4), 342–349.

Benedek, D. M., Fullerton, C., & Ursano, R. J. (2007). First responders: Mental health consequences of natural and human-made disasters for public health and public safety workers. *Annual Review of Public Health, 28*, 55–68.

Bills, C. B., Levy, N. A., Sharma, V., Charney, D. S., Herbert, R., Moline, J., & Katz, C. L. (2008). Mental health of workers and volunteers responding to events of 9/11: Review of the literature. *Mount Sinai Journal of Medicine, 75*(2), 115–127.

Bleiberg, K. L., & Markowitz, J. C. (2005). A pilot study of interpersonal psychotherapy for posttraumatic stress disorder. *American Journal of Psychiatry, 162*(1), 181–183.

Bleich, A., Gelkopf, M., Melamed, Y., & Solomon, Z. (2006). Mental health and resiliency following 44 months of terrorism: A survey of an Israeli national representative sample. *BMC Medicine, 4*, 21–32.

Boals, A., & Hathaway, L. M. (2009). The importance of the DSM-IV E and F criteria in self-report assessments of PTSD. *Journal of Anxiety Disorders, 24*(1), 161–166.

Bolton, P., Bass, J., Betancourt, T., Speelman, L., Onyango, G., Clougherty, K., ... Verdeli, H. (2007). Interventions for depression symptoms among adolescent survivors of war and displacement in Northern Uganda: A randomized controlled trial. *Journal of the American Medical Association, 298*(5), 519–527.

Bonanno, G. A., Galea, S., Bucciarelli, A., & Vlahov, D. (2007). What predicts psychological resilience after disaster? The role of demographics, resources and life stress. *Journal of Consulting and Clinical Psychology, 75*(5), 671–682.

Bonanno, G. A., & Mancini, A. D. (2008). The human capacity to thrive in the face of potential trauma. *Pediatrics, 121*(2), 369–375.

Bonnie, R. J., Fulco, C. E., & Liverman, C. T. (Eds.). (1999). *Reducing the burden of injury: Advancing prevention and treatment*. Washington, DC: National Academies Press.

Boscarino, J. A. (1997). Diseases among men 20 years after exposure to severe stress: Implications for clinical research and medical care. *Psychosomatic Medicine, 59*(6), 605–614.

Boudewyn, A. C., & Liem, J. H. (1995). Childhood sexual abuse as a precursor to depression and self-destructive behavior in adulthood. *Journal of Traumatic Stress, 8*(3), 445–459.

Bourque, L. B., Siegel, J. M., Kano, M., & Wood, M. M. (2006). Weathering the storm: The impact of hurricanes on physical and mental health. *Annals of the American Academy of Political and Social Science, 604*, 129–151.

Brady, K. T., Killeen, T. K., Brewerton, T., & Lucerini, S. (2000). Comorbidity of psychiatric disorders and posttraumatic stress disorder. *Journal of Clinical Psychiatry, 61*(Suppl. 7), 22–32.

Brady, K. T., & Sinha, S. (2005). Co-occurring mental and substance use disorders: The neurobiological effects of chronic stress. *American Journal of Psychiatry, 162*(8), 1483–1493.

Brent, D. A., Baugher, M., Bridge, J., Chen, T., & Chiappetta, L. (1999). Age- and sex-related risk factors for adolescent suicide. *Journal of the American Academy of Child and Adolescent Psychiatry, 38*(12), 1497–1505.

Breslau, N. (2009). The epidemiology of trauma, PTSD, and other post-trauma disorders. *Trauma, Violence & Abuse, 10*(3), 198–210.

Breslau, N., Chilcoat, H. D., Kessler, R. C., & Davis, G. C. (1999). Previous exposure to trauma and PTSD effects of subsequent trauma: Results from the Detroit Area Survey of Trauma. *American Journal of Psychiatry, 156*(6), 902–907.

Breslau, N., & Davis, G. C. (1987). Posttraumatic stress disorder: The etiologic specificity of wartime stressors. *American Journal of Psychiatry, 144*(5), 578–583.

Breslau, N., Davis, G. C., Andreski, P., Federman, B., & Anthony, J. C. (1998). Epidemiological findings on posttraumatic stress disorder and comorbid disorders in the general population. In B. P. Dohrenwend (Ed.), *Adversity, stress, and psychopathology* (pp. 319–328). London, UK: Oxford University Press.

Breslau, N., Davis, G. C., Andreski, P., & Peterson, E. (1991). Traumatic events and posttraumatic stress disorder in an urban population of young adults. *Archives of General Psychiatry, 48*(3), 216–222.

Breslau, N., Davis, G. C., Andreski, P., Peterson, E. L., & Schultz, L. R. (1997). Sex differences in posttraumatic stress disorder. *Archives of General Psychiatry, 54*(11), 1044–1048.

Breslau, N., Davis, G. C., & Schultz, L. R. (2003). Posttraumatic stress disorder and the incidence of nicotine, alcohol, and other drug disorders in persons who have experienced trauma. *Archives of General Psychiatry, 60*(3), 289–294.

Breslau, N., & Kessler, R. (2001). The stressor criterion in DSM-IV posttraumatic stress disorder: An epidemiological investigation. *Biological Psychiatry, 50*(9), 699–704.

Breslau, N., Kessler, R. C., Chilcoat, H. D., Schultz, L. R., Davis, G. C., & Andreski, P. (1998). Trauma and posttraumatic stress disorder in the community: The 1996 Detroit Area Survey of Trauma. *Archives of General Psychiatry, 55*(7), 626–632.

Brewin, C. R., Andrews, B., Rose, S., & Kirk, M. (1999). Acute stress disorder and posttraumatic stress disorder in victims of violent crime. *American Journal of Psychiatry, 156*(3), 360–366.

Brewin, C. R., Andrews, B., & Valentine, J. D. (2000). Meta-analysis of risk factors for posttraumatic stress disorder in trauma-exposed adults. *Journal of Consulting and Clinical Psychology, 68*(5), 748–766.

Briggs, Q. M., Fullerton, C. S., Reeves, J. J., Grieger, T. A., Reissman, D., & Ursano, R. J. (2010). Acute stress disorder, depression, and tobacco use in disaster workers following 9/11. *American Journal of Orthopsychiatry, 80*(4), 586–592.

Broekman, B. F., Olff, M., & Boer, F. (2007). The genetic background to PTSD. *Neuroscience and Biobehavioral Reviews, 31*(3), 348–362.

Bromet, E. J., Gluzman, S., Schwartz, J. E., & Goldgaber, D. (2002). Somatic symptoms in women 11 years after the Chornobyl accident: Prevalence and risk factors. *Environmental Health Perspectives, 110*(Suppl. 4), 625–629.

Bromet, E., Sonnega, A., & Kessler, R. C. (1998). Risk factors for DSM-III-R posttraumatic stress disorder: Findings from the National Comorbidity Survey. *American Journal of Epidemiology, 147*(4), 353–361.

Brown, J., Cohen, P., Johnson, J. G., & Smailes, E. M. (1999). Childhood abuse and neglect: Specificity of effects on adolescent and young adult depression and suicidality. *Journal of the American Academy of Child and Adolescent Psychiatry, 38*(12), 1490–1496.

Bryant, R. A. (2000). Acute stress disorder. *PTSD Research Quarterly, 11*(2), 1–7.

Bryant, R. A. (2010). The complexity of complex PTSD. *American Journal of Psychiatry, 167*(8), 879–881.

Bryant, R. A., Creamer, M., O'Donnell, M. L., Silove, D., & McFarlane, A. C. (2008). A multisite study of the capacity of acute stress disorder diagnosis to predict posttraumatic stress disorder. *Journal of Clinical Psychiatry, 69*(6), 923–929.

Bryant, R. A., & Harvey, A. G. (1998). Relationship between acute stress disorder and posttraumatic stress disorder following mild traumatic brain injury. *American Journal of Psychiatry, 155*(5), 625–629.

Bryant, R. A., O'Donnell, M. L., Creamer, M., McFarlane, A. C., Clark, C. R., & Silove, D. (2010). The psychiatric sequelae of traumatic injury. *American Journal of Psychiatry, 67*(3), 312–320.

Brymer, M., Jacobs, A., Layne, C., Pynoos, R., Ruzek, J., Steinberg, A.,...Watson, P. (2006). *Psychological first aid: Field operations guide* (2nd ed.). Rockville, MD: Substance Abuse and Mental Health Services Administration, US Department of Health and Human Services.

Bureau, J. F., Martin, J., Freynet, N., Poirier, A. A., Lafontaine, M. F., & Cloutier, P. (2009). Perceived dimensions of parenting and non-suicidal self-injury in young adults. *Journal of Youth and Adolescence, 39*(5), 484–494.

Caetano, R., & Cunradi, C. (2003). Intimate partner violence and depression among Whites, Blacks, and Hispanics. *Annals of Epidemiology, 13*(10), 661–665.

Caldera, T., Palma, L., Penayo, U., & Kullgren, G. (2001). Psychological impact of the hurricane Mitch in Nicaragua in a 1-year perspective. *Social Psychiatry and Psychiatric Epidemiology, 36*(3), 108–114.

Campanini, R. F., Schoedl, A. F., Pupo, M. C., Costa, A. C., Krupnick, J. L., & Mello, M. F. (2010). Efficacy of interpersonal therapy-group format adapted to post-traumatic stress disorder: An open-label add-on trial. *Depression and Anxiety, 27*(1), 72–77.

Cardozo, B. L., Bilukha, O. O., Crawford, C. A., Shaikh, I., Wolfe, M. I., Gerber, M. L., & Anderson, M. (2004). Mental health, social functioning and disability in postwar Afghanistan. *Journal of the American Medical Association, 292*(5), 575–584.

Caspi, A., Sugden, K., Moffitt, T. E., Taylor, A., Craig, I. W., Harrington, H.,...Poulton, R. (2003). Influence of life stress on depression:

Moderation by a polymorphism in the 5-HTT gene. *Science, 301*(5631), 386–389.

Catani, C., Jacob, N, Schauer, E., Kohila, M., & Neuner, F. (2008). Family violence, war, and natural disasters: A study of the effect of extreme stress on children's mental health in Sri Lanka. *BMC Psychiatry, 8,* 33.

Catapano, F., Malafronte, R., Lepre, F., Cozzolino, P., Arnone, R., Lorenzo, E,...Maj, M. (2001). Psychological consequences of the 1998 landslide in Sarno, Italy: A community study. *Acta Psychiatrica Scandinavica, 104*(6), 438–442.

CATS Consortium & Hoagwood, K. (2007). Implementing CBT for traumatized children and adolescents after September 11: Lessons learned from the Child and Adolescent Trauma Treatments and Services (CATS) project. *Journal of Clinical Child and Adolescent Psychology, 36*(4), 581–592.

Chemtob, C. M., Novaco, R. W., Hamada, R. S., Gross, D. M., & Smith, G. (1997). Anger regulation deficits in combat-related posttraumatic stress disorder. *Journal of Traumatic Stress, 10*(1), 17–35.

Cherniack, E. P. (2008). The impact of natural disasters on the elderly. *American Journal of Disaster Medicine, 3*(3), 133–139.

Chilcoat, H. D., & Breslau, N. (1998). Investigations of causal pathways between PTSD and drug use disorders. *Addictive Behaviors, 23*(6), 827–840.

Child Sexual Abuse Task Force, Research & Practice Core. (2004). *How to implement trauma-focused cognitive behavioral therapy.* Durham, NC: National Center for Child Traumatic Stress.

Chou, F. H., Wu, H. C., Chou, P., Su, C. Y., Tsai, K. Y., Chao, S. S.,...Ou-Yang, W. C. (2007). Epidemiologic psychiatric studies on post-disaster impact among Chi-Chi earthquake survivors in Yu-Chi, Taiwan. *Psychiatry and Clinical Neurosciences, 61*(4), 370–378.

Coalition to Stop the Use of Child Soldiers. (2008). *Child soldiers, global report 2008.* London, UK: Bell and Bain.

Cohen, J. A. (2003). Treating acute posttraumatic reactions in children and adolescents. *Biological Psychiatry, 53*(9), 827–833.

Cohen, J. A., Deblinger, E., Mannarino, A. P., & Steer, R. (2004). A multi-site, randomized controlled trial for children with abuse-related PTSD symptoms. *Journal of the American Academy of Child and Adolescent Psychiatry, 43*(4), 393.

Cohen, J. A., & Mannarino, A. P. (1996). A treatment outcome study for sexually abused preschool children: Initial findings. *Journal of the American Academy of Child and Adolescent Psychiatry, 35*(1), 42–50.

Cohen, J. A., & Mannarino, A. P. (2008). Disseminating and implementing trauma-focused CBT in community settings. *Trauma, Violence & Abuse, 9*(4), 214–226.

Conejo-Galindo, J., Medina, O., Fraguas, D., Terán, S., Sainz-Cortón, E., & Arango, C. (2008). Psychopathological sequelae of the 11 March terrorist attacks in Madrid: An epidemiological study of victims treated in a hospital. *European Archives of Psychiatry and Clinical Neurosciences, 258*(1), 28–34.

Cox, J., Davies, D. R., Burlingame, G. M., Campbell, J. E., Layne, C. M., & Katzenbach, R. J. (2007). Effectiveness of a trauma/grief-focused group intervention: A qualitative study with war-exposed Bosnian adolescents. *International Journal of Group Psychotherapy, 57*(3), 319–345.

Creamer, M., Burgess, P., & McFarlane, A. C. (2001). Post-traumatic stress disorder: Findings from the Australian National Survey of Mental Health and Well-Being. *Psychological Medicine, 31*(7), 1237–1247.

Creamer, M., McFarlane, A. C., & Burgess, P. (2005). Psychopathology following trauma: The role of subjective experience. *Journal of Affective Disorders, 86*(2–3), 175–182.

Creamer, M., O'Donnell, M. L., & Pattison, P. (2004). The relationship between acute stress disorder and posttraumatic stress disorder in severely injured trauma survivors. *Behavior, Research and Therapy, 42*(3), 315–328.

Darves-Bornoz, J. M., Alonso, J., de Girolamo, G., de Graaf, R., Haro, J. M., Kovess-Masfety, V.,...Gasquet, I. (2008). Main traumatic events in Europe: PTSD in the European Study of the Epidemiology of Mental Disorders survey. *Journal of Traumatic Stress, 21*(5), 455–462.

Davidson, J. R. T., Hughes, D., Blazer, D. G., & George, L. K. (1991). Post-traumatic stress disorder in the community: An epidemiological study. *Psychological Medicine, 3,* 713–721.

Davidson, J., Swartz, M., Storck, M., Krishnan, R. R., & Hammett, E. (1985). A diagnostic and family study of posttraumatic stress disorder. *American Journal of Psychiatry, 142*(1), 90–93.

Davydow, D. S., Desai, S. V., Needham, D. M., & Bienvenu, O. J. (2008). Psychiatric morbidity in survivors of the acute respiratory distress syndrome: A systematic review. *Psychosomatic Medicine, 70*(4), 512–519.

Davydow, D. S., Gifford, J. M., Desai, S. V., Bienvenu, O. J., & Needham, D. M. (2009). Depression in general intensive care unit survivors: A systematic review. *Intensive Care Medicine, 35*(5), 796–809.

Davydow, D. S., Gifford, J. M., Desai, S. V., Needham, D. M., & Bienvenu, O. J. (2008). Posttraumatic stress disorder in general intensive care unit survivors: A systematic review. *General Hospital Psychiatry, 30*(5), 421–434.

Deblinger, E., Mannarino, A. P., Cohen, J. A., & Steer, R. A. (2006). A follow-up study of a multisite, randomized, controlled trial for children with sexual abuse–related PTSD symptoms. *Journal of the American Academy of Child and Adolescent Psychiatry, 45*(12), 1474–1484.

de Graaf, R., Bijl, R. V., Ten Have, M., Beekman, A. T., & Vollebergh, W. A. (2004). Pathways to comorbidity: The transition of pure mood, anxiety and substance use disorders into comorbid conditions in a longitudinal population-based study. *Journal of Affective Disorders, 82*(3), 461–467.

de Jong, J. T., Komproe, I. H., Van, O. M., El, M. M., Araya, M., Khaled, N., ... Somasundaram, D. (2001). Lifetime events and posttraumatic stress disorder in 4 postconflict settings. *Journal of the American Medical Association, 286*(5), 555–562.

Derluyn, I., Broekaert, E., Schuyten, G., & De Temmerman, E. (2004). Post-traumatic stress in former Ugandan child soldiers. *Lancet, 363*(9412), 861–863.

de Vries, G. J., & Olff, M. (2009). The lifetime prevalence of traumatic events and posttraumatic stress disorder in the Netherlands. *Journal of Traumatic Stress, 22*(4), 259–267.

Dew, M. A., & Bromet, E. J. (1993). Predictors of temporal patterns of psychiatric distress during 10 years following the nuclear accident at Three Mile Island. *Social Psychiatry and Psychiatric Epidemiology, 28*(2), 49–55.

DiMaggio, C., & Galea, S. (2006). The behavioral consequences of terrorism: A meta-analysis. *Academic Emergency Medicine, 13*(5), 559–566.

Dohrenwend, B. P., Turner, J. B., Turse, N. A., Adams, B. G., Koenen, K. C., & Marshall, R. (2006). The psychological risks of Vietnam for U.S. veterans: A revisit with new data. *Science, 313*(5789), 979–982.

Dougherty, P. J. (2003). Long-term follow-up of unilateral transfemoral amputees from the Vietnam war. *Journal of Trauma, 54*(4), 718–723.

Eaton, W. W., Sigal, J. J., & Weinfeld, M. (1982). Impairment in Holocaust survivors after 33 years: Data from an unbiased community sample. *American Journal of Psychiatry, 139*(6), 773–777.

Ebrahimzadeh, M. H., Fattahi, A. S., & Nejad, A. B. (2006). Long-term follow-up of Iranian veteran upper extremity amputees from the Iran–Iraq war (1980–1988). *Trauma, 61*(4), 886–888.

Elhai, J. D., Gray, M. J., Kashdan, T. B., & Franklin, C. L. (2005). Which instruments are most commonly used to assess traumatic event exposure and posttraumatic effects? A survey of traumatic stress professionals. *Journal of Traumatic Stress, 18*(5), 541–545.

Everly, G. S., Jr., & Flynn, B. W. (2006). Principles and practical procedures for acute psychological first aid training for personnel without mental health experience. *International Journal of Emergency Mental Health, 8*(2), 93–100.

Farias, P. (1994). Central and South American refugees: Some mental health challenges. In A. J. Marsella, T. Bornemann, S. Ekblad, & J. Orley (Eds.), *Amidst peril and pain: The mental health and well-being of the world's refugees* (pp. 101–113). Washington, DC: American Psychological Association.

Fazel, M., Wheeler, J., & Danesh, J. (2005). Prevalence of serious mental disorder in 7000 refugees resettled in Western countries: A systematic review. *Lancet, 365*(9467), 1309–1314.

Feldner, M. T., Babson, K. A., & Zvolensky, M. J. (2007). Smoking, traumatic event exposure, and post-traumatic stress: A critical review of the empirical literature. *Clinical Psychology Review, 27*(1), 14–45.

Feldner, M., Babson, K., Zvolensky, M. J., Vujanovic, A. A., Lewis, S. F., Gibson, L. E., ... Bernstein, A. (2007). Posttraumatic stress symptoms and smoking to reduce negative affect: An investigation of trauma-exposed daily smokers. *Addictive Behaviors, 32*(2), 214–227.

Fergusson, D. M., Horwood, L. J., & Lynskey, M. T. (1996). Childhood sexual abuse and psychiatric disorder in young adulthood: II. Psychiatric outcomes of childhood sexual abuse. *Journal of the American Academy of Child and Adolescent Psychiatry, 35*(10), 1365–1374.

Francis, D. D., & Meaney, M. J. (1999). Maternal care and the development of stress responses. *Current Opinion in Neurobiology, 9*(1), 128–134.

Frans, O., Rimmo, P. A., Aberg, L., & Fredrikson, M. (2005). Trauma exposure and post-traumatic stress disorder in the general population. *Acta Psychiatrica Scandinavica, 111*(4), 291–299.

Friedman, M. J., Resick, P. A., & Keane, T. M. (2007). PTSD: Twenty-five years of progress and challenges. In M. J. Friedman, T. M. Keane, & P. A. Resick (Eds.), *Handbook of PTSD: Science and practice* (pp. 3–18). New York, NY: Guilford.

Fu, S. S., McFall, M., Saxon, A. J., Beckham, J. C., Carmody, T. P., Baker, D. G., & Joseph, A. M. (2007). Post-traumatic stress disorder and smoking: A systematic review. *Nicotine and Tobacco Research, 9*(11), 1071–1084.

Gabriel, R., Ferrando, L., Cortón, E. S., Mingote, C., García-Camba, E., Liria, A. F., & Galea, S. (2007). Psychopathological consequences after a terrorist attack: An epidemiological study among victims, the general population, and police officers. *European Psychiatry, 22*(6), 339–346.

Galea, S., Ahern, J., Resnick, H., Kilpatrick, D., Bucuvalas, M., Gold, J, & Vlahov, D. (2002). Psychological sequelae of September 11 terrorist attacks in New York City. *New England Journal of Medicine, 346*(13), 982–987.

Galea, S., Maxwell, A. R., & Norris, F. (2008). Sampling and design challenges in studying the mental health consequences of disasters. *International Journal of Methods in Psychiatric Research, 17*(Suppl. 2), s21–s28.

Galea, S., Nandi, A., & Vlahov, D. (2005). The epidemiology of post-traumatic stress disorder after disasters. *Epidemiologic Reviews, 27,* 78–91.

Gamito, P., Oliveira, J., Morais, D., Oliveira, S., Durate, N., Saraiva, T., . . . Rosa, P. (2009). Virtual reality therapy controlled study for war veterans with PTSD: Preliminary results. *Studies of Health Technology and Informatics, 144,* 269–272.

Giaconia, R. M., Reinherz, H. Z., Silverman, A. B., Pakiz, B., Frost, A. K., & Cohen, E. (1995). Traumas and posttraumatic stress disorder in a community population of older adolescents. *Journal of the American Academy of Child and Adolescent Psychiatry, 34*(10), 1369–1380.

Gibb, B. E., McGeary, J. E., Beevers, C. G., & Miller, I. W. (2006). Serotonin transporter (*5-HTTLPR*) genotype, childhood abuse and suicide attempts in adult psychiatric inpatients. *Suicide and Life-Threatening Behavior, 36*(6), 687–693.

Gidron, Y. (2002). Posttraumatic stress disorder after terrorist attacks: A review. *Journal of Nervous and Mental Disease, 190*(2), 118–121.

Gilbertson, M. W., Shenton, M. E., Ciszewski, A., Kasai, K., Lasko, N. B., Orr, S. P., & Pitman R. K. (2002). Smaller hippocampal volume predicts pathologic vulnerability to psychological trauma. *Nature Neuroscience, 5*(11), 1242–1247.

Gleser, G., Green, B., & Winget, C. (1981). *Prolonged psychological effects of disaster: A study of Buffalo Creek.* New York, NY: Academic Press.

Goldstein, G., van Kammen, W., Shelly, C., Miller, D. J., & van Kammen, D. P. (1987). Survivors of imprisonment in the Pacific theater during World War II. *American Journal of Psychiatry, 144*(9), 1210–1213.

Gould, M., Greenberg, N., & Hetherton, J. (2007). Stigma and the military: Evaluation of a PTSD psychoeducational program. *Journal of Trauma and Stress, 20*(4), 505–512.

Gray, M. J., Bolton, E. E., & Litz, B. T. (2004). A longitudinal analysis of PTSD symptom course: Delayed-onset PTSD in Somalia peacekeepers. *Journal of Consulting and Clinical Psychology, 72*(5), 909–913.

Green, B. L., Lindy, J. D., Grace, M. C., Gleser, G. C., Leonard, A. C., Korol, M., & Winget, C. (1990). Buffalo Creek survivors in the second decade: Stability of stress symptoms. *American Journal of Orthopsychiatry, 60*(1), 43–54.

Greenberg, N., Iversen, A., Hull, L., Bland, D., & Wessely, S. (2008). Getting a peace of the action: Measures of post traumatic stress in UK military peacekeepers. *Journal of Royal Society of Medicine, 101*(2), 78–84.

Grieger, T. A., Cozza, S. J., Ursano, R. J., Hoge, C., Martinez, P. E., Engel, C. C., & Wain, H. J. (2006). Posttraumatic stress disorder and depression in battle-injured soldiers. *American Journal of Psychiatry, 163*(10), 1777–1783.

Grieger, T. A., Fullerton, C. S., & Ursano, R. J. (2003). Posttraumatic stress disorder, alcohol use, and perceived safety after the terrorist attack on the Pentagon. *Psychiatric Services, 54,* 1380–1382.

Grieger, T. A., Fullerton, C. S., & Ursano, R. J. (2004). Posttraumatic stress disorder, depression, and perceived safety 13 months following the terrorist attack on the Pentagon. *Psychiatric Services, 55,* 1061–1063.

Grieger, T. A., Waldrep, D. A., Lovasz, M. M., & Ursano, R. J. (2005). Follow-up of Pentagon employees 2 years after the terrorist attack of September 11, 2001. *Psychiatric Services, 56*(11), 1374–1378.

Gross, C., & Hen, R. (2004). Genetic and environmental factors interact to influence anxiety. *Neurotoxicity Research, 6*(6), 493–501.

Gunnar, M. R., & Donzella, B. (2002). Social regulation of the cortisol levels in early human development. *Psychoneuroendocrinology, 27*(1–2), 199–220.

Gunnar, M. R., & Quevedo, K. M. (2007). Early care experiences and HPA axis regulation in children: A mechanism for later trauma vulnerability. *Progress in Brain Research, 167,* 137–149.

Harvey, A. G., & Bryant, R. A. (1999a). Acute stress disorder across trauma populations. *Journal of Nervous and Mental Disease, 187*(7), 443–446.

Harvey, A. G., & Bryant, R. A. (1999b). Predictors of acute stress following motor vehicle accidents. *Journal of Traumatic Stress, 12*(3), 519–525.

Hashemian, F., Khoshnood, K., Desai, M. M., Falahati, F., Kasl, S., & Southwick, S. (2006).

Anxiety, depression and posttraumatic stress in Iranian survivors of chemical warfare. *Journal of the American Medical Association, 296*(5), 560–566.

Havenaar, J. M., Van den Brink, W., Van den Bout, J., Kasyanenko, A. P., Poelijoe, N. W., Wholfarth, T., & Meijler-Iljina, L. I. (1996). Mental health problems in the Gomel region (Belarus): An analysis of risk factors in an area affected by the Chernobyl disaster. *Psychological Medicine, 26*(4), 845–855.

Heim, C., & Nemeroff, C. B. (2001). The role of childhood trauma in the neurobiology of mood and anxiety disorders: Preclinical and clinical studies. *Biological Psychiatry, 49*(12), 1023–1039.

Hepp, U., Gamma, A., Milos, G., Eich, D., Ajdacic-Gross, V., Rössler, W.,…Schnyder, U. (2006). Prevalence of exposure to potentially traumatic events and PTSD: The Zurich Cohort Study. *European Archives of Psychiatry and Clinical Neuroscience, 256*(3), 151–158.

Hoge, C. W., Castro, C. A, Messer, S. C., McGurk, D., Cotting, D. I., & Koffman, R. L. (2004). Combat duty in Iraq and Afghanistan, mental health problems and barriers to care. *New England Journal of Medicine, 351*(1), 13–22.

Hollifield, M., Warner, T. D., Lian, N., Krakow, B., Jenkins, J. H., Kesler, J.,…Westermeyer, J. (2009). Measuring trauma and health status in refugees: A critical review. *Journal of the American Medical Association, 288*(5), 611–621.

Holt, S., Buckley, H., & Whelan, S. (2008). The impact of exposure to domestic violence on children and young people: A review of the literature. *Child Abuse and Neglect, 32*(8), 797–810.

Horowitz, M. J., Siegel, B., Holen, A., Bonanno, G. A., Milbrath, C., & Stinson, C. H. (1997). Diagnostic criteria for complicated grief disorder. *American Journal of Psychiatry, 154*(7), 904–910.

Jenkins, E. J., & Bell, C. C. (1997). Exposure and response to community violence among children and adolescents. In J. Osofsky (Ed.), *Children in a violent society* (pp. 9–31). New York, NY: Guilford.

Johnson, H., & Thompson, A. (2008). The development and maintenance of post-traumatic stress disorder (PTSD) in civilian adult survivors of war trauma and torture: A review. *Clinical Psychology Review, 28*(1), 36–47.

Johnson, S. D., North, C. S., & Smith, E. M. (2002). Psychiatric disorders among victims of a courthouse shooting spree: A three-year follow-up study. *Community Mental Health Journal, 38*(3), 181–194.

Kang, H. K., Bullman, T. A., & Taylor, J. W. (2006). Risk of selected cardiovascular diseases and posttraumatic stress disorder among former World War II prisoners of war. *Annals of Epidemiology, 16*(5), 381–386.

Kang, H. K., Natelson, B. H., Mahan, C. M., Lee, K. Y., & Murphy, F. M. (2003). Post-traumatic stress disorder and chronic fatigue syndrome-like illness among Gulf War veterans: A population-based survey of 30,000 veterans. *American Journal of Epidemiology, 157*(2), 141–148.

Kangas, M., Henry, J. L., & Bryant, R. A. (2007). Correlates of acute stress disorder in cancer patients. *Journal of Traumatic Stress, 20*(3), 325–334.

Karam, E. G., Mneimneh, Z. N., Karam, A. N., Fayyad, J. A., Nasser, S. C., Chatterji, S., & Kessler, R. C. (2006). Prevalence and treatment of mental disorders in Lebanon: A national epidemiological survey. *Lancet, 367*(9515), 1000–1006.

Kazantzis, N., Flett, R. A., Long, N. R., MacDonald, C., Miller, M. & Clark, B. (2009). Traumatic events and mental health in the community: A New Zealand study. *International Journal of Social Psychiatry, 56*(1), 35–49.

Kessler, R. C., Chiu, W. T., Demler, O., Merikangas, K. R., & Walters, E. E. (2005). Prevalence, severity and comorbidity of 12-month DSM-IV disorders in the National Comorbidity Survey replication. *Archives of General Psychiatry, 62*(6), 617–627.

Kessler, R. C., DuPont, R. L., Berglund, P., & Wittchen, H.-U. (1999). Impairment in pure and comorbid generalized anxiety disorder and major depression at 12 months in two national surveys. *American Journal of Psychiatry, 156*(12), 1915–1923.

Kessler, R. C., & Frank, R. G. (1997). The impact of psychiatric disorders on work loss days. *Psychological Medicine, 27*(4), 861–873.

Kessler, R. C., Galea, S., Gruber, M. J., Sampson, N. A., Ursano, R. J., & Wessely, S. (2008). Trends in mental illness and suicidality after Hurricane Katrina. *Molecular Psychiatry, 13*(4), 374–384.

Kessler, R. C., Keane, T. M., Ursano, R. J., Mokdad, A., & Zaslavsky, A. M. (2008). Sample and design considerations in post-disaster mental health needs assessment tracking surveys. *International Journal of Methods in Psychiatric Research, 17*(Suppl. 2), s6–s20.

Kessler, R. C., Sonnega, A., Bromet, E., Hughes, M., & Nelson, C. B. (1995). Posttraumatic stress disorder in the National Comorbidity Survey. *Archives of General Psychiatry, 52*(12), 1048–1060.

Kilpatrick, D. G., & Resnick, H. S. (1993). PTSD associated with exposure to criminal victimization in clinical and community populations. In J. R. T. Davidson & E. B. Foa (Eds.), *Posttraumatic* stress disorder: DSM-IV and beyond (pp. 113–143). Washington, DC: American Psychiatric Press.

Kluznick, J. C., Speed, N., VanValkenburg, C., & Magraw, R. (1986). Forty-year follow-up of United States prisoners of war. American Journal of Psychiatry, 143(11), 1443–1446.

Kohrt, B. A., Jordans, M. J., Tol, W. A., Speckman, R. A., Maharjan, S. M., Worthman, C. M., & Komproe, I. H. (2008). Comparison of mental health between former child soldiers and children never conscripted by armed groups in Nepal. Journal of the American Medical Association, 300(6), 691–702.

Kross, E. K., Gries, C. J., & Curtis, J. R. (2008). Posttraumatic stress disorder following critical illness. Critical Care Clinics, 24(4), 875–887.

Krupnick, J. L., Green, B. L., Stockton, P., Miranda, J., Krause, E., & Mete, M. (2008). Group interpersonal psychotherapy for low-income women with posttraumatic stress disorder. Journal of the Society for Psychotherapy Research, 18(5), 497–507.

Kuch, K., & Cox, B. J. (1992). Symptoms of PTSD in 124 survivors of the Holocaust. American Journal of Psychiatry, 149(3), 337–340.

Kulka, R. A., Schlenger, W. E., Fairbank, J. A., Hough, R. L., Jordan, B. K., Marmar, C. R., & Weiss, D. S. (1990). Trauma and the Vietnam War generation: Report of findings from the National Vietnam Veterans Readjustment Study. New York, NY: Brunner/Mazel.

Kuwert, P., Spitzer, C., Rosenthal, J., & Freyberger, H. J. (2008). Trauma and post-traumatic stress symptoms in former German child soldiers of World War II. International Psychogeriatrics, 20(5), 1014–1018.

Lambert, S. F., Copeland-Linder, N., & Ialongo, N. S. (2008). Longitudinal associations between community violence exposure and suicidality. Journal of Adolescent Health, 43(4), 380–386.

Lasko, N. B., Gurvits, T. V., Kuhne, A. A., Orr, S. P., & Pitman, R. K. (1994). Aggression and its correlates in Vietnam veterans with and without chronic posttraumatic stress disorder. Comprehensive Psychiatry, 35(5), 373–381.

Laugharne, J., Janca, A., & Widiger, T. (2007). Posttraumatic stress disorder and terrorism: Five years after 9/11. Current Opinion in Psychiatry, 20(1), 36–41.

Laugharne, J., van de Watt, G., & Janca, A. (2011). After the fire: The mental health consequences of fire disasters. Current Opinion in Psychiatry, 24(1), 72–77.

Layne, C. M., Pynoos, R. S., Saltzman, W. R., Arslanagić, B., Black, M., Savjak, N.,...Houston, R. (2001). Trauma/grief-focused group psychotherapy: School-based postwar intervention with traumatized Bosnian adolescents. Group Dynamics: Theory, Research and Practice, 5, 277–290.

Layne, C. M., Saltzman, W. R., Poppleton, L., Burlingame, G. M., Pasalic, A., Durakovic, E.,...Pynoos, R. S. (2008). Effectiveness of a school-based group psychotherapy program for war-exposed adolescents: A randomized controlled trial. Journal of the American Academy of Child and Adolescent Psychiatry, 47(9), 1048–1062.

Leeise, M., Pagura, J., Sareen, J., & Bolton, J. M. (2010). The use of alcohol and drugs to self-medicate symptoms of posttraumatic stress disorder. Depression and Anxiety, 27(8), 731–736.

Linehan, M. M. (1993). Cognitive–behavioral treatment of borderline personality disorder. New York, NY: Guilford.

Litz, B. T., Orsillo, S. M., Friedman, M., Ehrlich, P., & Batres, A. (1997). Posttraumatic stress disorder associated with peacekeeping duty in Somalia for U.S. military personnel. American Journal of Psychiatry, 154(2), 178–184.

Lopes Cardozo, B., Vergara, A., Agani, F., & Gotway, C. A. (2000). Mental health, social functioning and attitudes of Kosovar Albanians following the war in Kosovo. Journal of the American Medical Association, 284(5), 569–577.

Mak, I. W., Chu, C. M., Pan, P. C., Yiu, M. G., & Chan, V. L. (2009). Long-term psychiatric morbidities among SARS survivors. General Hospital Psychiatry, 31(4), 318–326.

Mann, J. J., Waternaux, C., Haas, G. L., & Malone, K. M. (1999). Toward a clinical model of suicidal behavior in psychiatric patients. American Journal of Psychiatry, 156(2), 181–189.

Marshall, G. N., Schell, T. L., Elliott, M. N., Berthold, S. M., & Chun, C. A. (2005). Mental health of Cambodian refugees 2 decades after resettlement in the United States. Journal of the American Medical Association, 294(5), 571–579.

Marshall, G. N., Schell, T. L., Elliott, M. N., Rayburn, N. R., & Jaycox, L. H. (2007). Psychiatric disorders among adults seeking emergency disaster assistance after a wildland–urban interface fire. Psychiatric Services, 58(4), 509–514.

May, F. S, Chen, Q. C., Gilbertson, M. W., Shenton, M. E., & Pitman, R. K. (2004). Cavum septum pellucidum in monozygotic twins discordant for combat exposure: Relationship to posttraumatic stress disorder. Biological Psychiatry, 55(6), 656–658.

McFarlane, A. C., & Van Hooff, M. (2009). Impact of childhood exposure to a natural disaster on adult mental health: 20-year longitudinal follow-up study. *British Journal of Psychiatry, 195*(2), 142–148.

McLay, R. N., McBrien, C., Wiederhold, M., & Wiederhold, B. (2010). Exposure therapy with and without virtual reality to treat PTSD while in combat theater: A parallel case series. *Cyberpsychology, Behavior and Social Networking, 13*(1), 37–42.

McWilliams, L. A., Cox, B. J., & Enns, M. W. (2003). Mood and anxiety disorders associated with chronic pain: An examination in a nationally representative sample. *Pain, 106*(1–2), 127–133.

Mehlum, L. & Weisaeth, L. (2002). Predictors of posttraumatic stress reactions in Norwegian U.N. peacekeepers 7 years after service. *Journal of Traumatic Stress, 15*(1), 17–26.

Mehnert, A., & Koch, U. (2007). Prevalence of acute and posttraumatic stress disorder and comorbid mental disorders in breast cancer patients during primary cancer care: A prospective study. *Psycho-oncology, 16*(3), 181–188.

Mellman, T. A., David, D., Bustamante, V., Fins, A. I., & Esposito, K. (2001). Predictors of posttraumatic stress disorder following severe injury. *Depression and Anxiety, 14*(4), 226–231.

Miguel-Tobal, J. J., Cano-Vindel, A., Gonzalez-Ordi, H., Iruarrizaga, I., Rudenstine, S., Vlahov, D., & Galea, S. (2006). PTSD and depression after the Madrid March 11 train bombings. *Journal of Traumatic Stress, 19*(1), 69–80.

Monson, C. M., Friedman, M. J., & La Bash, H. A. J. (2007). A psychological history of PTSD. In M. J. Friedman, T. M. Keane, & P. A. Resick (Eds.), *Handbook of PTSD: Science and practice* (pp. 3–18). New York, NY: Guilford.

Morgan, L., Scourfield, J., Williams, D., Jasper, A., & Lewis, G. (2003). The Aberfan disaster: Thirty-three-year follow-up of survivors. *British Journal of Psychology, 182,* 532–536.

Moscardino, U., Scrimin, S., Capello, F., & Altoè, G. (2010). Social support, sense of community, collectivistic values and depressive symptoms in adolescent survivors of the 2004 Beslan terrorist attack. *Social Science and Medicine, 70*(1), 27–34.

Muhsen, K., Lipsitz, J., Garty-Sandalon, N., Gross, R., & Green, M. S. (2008). Correlates of generalized anxiety disorder, independent of comorbidity with depression: Findings from the first Israeli National Health Interview Survey (2003–2004). *Social Psychiatry and Psychiatric Epidemiology, 43*(11), 898–904.

Murthy, R. S. (2007). Mass violence and mental health—recent epidemiological findings. *International Review of Psychiatry, 19*(3), 183–192.

Nemeroff, C. B. (2004). Early-life adversity, CRF dysregulation, and vulnerability to mood and anxiety disorders. *Psychopharmacology Bulletin, 38*(Suppl. 1), 14–20.

Neria, Y., Gross, R., Litz, B., Maguen, S., Insel, B., Seirmarco, G.,…Marshall, R. D. (2007). Prevalence and psychological correlates of complicated grief among bereaved adults 2.5–3.5 years after September 11th attacks. *Journal of Traumatic Stress, 20*(3), 251–262.

Neumeister, A., Henry, S., & Krystal, J. H. (2007). Neurocircuitry and neuroplasticity in PTSD. In M. J. Friedman, T. M. Keane, & P. A. Resick (Eds.), *Handbook of PTSD: Science and practice* (pp. 151–165). New York, NY: Guilford.

Neuner, F., Onyut, P. L., Ertl, V., Odenwald, M., Schauer, E., & Elbert, T. (2008). Treatment of posttraumatic stress disorder by trained lay counselors in an African refugee settlement: A randomized controlled trial. *Journal of Consulting and Clinical Psychology, 76*(4), 686–694.

Njenga, F. G., Nicholls, P. J., Nyamai, C., Kigamwa, P., & Davidson, J. R. (2004). Post-traumatic stress after terrorist attack. Psychological reactions following the U.S. embassy bombing in Nairobi: Naturalistic study. *British Journal of Psychiatry, 185,* 328–333.

Norman, S. B., Means-Christensen, A. J., Craske, M. G., Sherbourne, C. D., Roy-Byrne, P. P., & Stein, M. B. (2006). Associations between psychological trauma and physical illness in primary care. *Journal of Traumatic Stress, 19*(4), 461–470.

Norris, F. H. (1988, November). *Towards establishing a data base for the prospective study of traumatic stress.* Presented at the National Institute of Mental Health workshop Traumatic Stress: Defining Terms and Instruments, Uniformed Services University of the Health Sciences, Rockville, MD.

Norris, F. H. (1992). Epidemiology of trauma: Frequency and impact of different potentially traumatic events on different demographic groups. *Journal of Consulting and Clinical Psychology, 60*(3), 409–418.

Norris, F. H., Murphy, A. D., Baker, C. K., & Perilla, J. L. (2004). Postdisaster PTSD over four waves of a panel study of Mexico's 1999 flood. *Journal of Traumatic Stress, 17*(4), 283–292.

Norris, F. H., Murphy, A. D., Baker, C. K., Perilla, J. L., Rodriguez, F. G., & Rodriguez Jde, J. (2003). Epidemiology of trauma and posttraumatic stress disorder in Mexico. *Journal of Abnormal Psychology, 112*(4), 646–656.

Norris, F. H., & Murrell, S. A. (1988). Prior experience as a moderator of disaster impact on anxiety symptoms in older adults. *American Journal of Community Psychology, 16*(5), 665–683.

North, C. S., McCutcheon, V., Spitznagel, E. L., & Smith, E. M. (2002). Three-year follow-up of survivors of a mass shooting episode. *Journal of Urban Health, 79*(3), 383–391.

North, C. S., Pfefferbaum, B., Tivis, L., Kawasaki, A., Reddy, C., & Spitznagel, E. L. (2004). The course of posttraumatic stress disorder in a follow-up study of survivors of the Oklahoma City bombing. *Annals of Clinical Psychiatry, 16*(4), 209–215.

Noyes, R., Jr., Kathol, R. G., Debelius-Enemark, P., Williams, J., Mutgi, A., Suelzer, M. T., & Clamon, G. H. (1990). Distress associated with cancer as measured by the Illness Distress Scale. *Psychosomatics, 31*(3), 321–330.

O'Donnell, M. L., Creamer, M., Bryant, R. A., Schnyder, U., & Shalev, A. (2003). Posttraumatic disorders following injury: An empirical and methodological review. *Clinical Psychology Review, 23*(4), 587–603.

O'Donnell, M. L., Creamer, M., & Pattison, P. (2004). Posttraumatic stress disorder and depression following trauma: Understanding comorbidity. *American Journal of Psychiatry, 161*(8), 1390–1396.

Office of Applied Studies. (2008). *Impact of hurricanes Katrina and Rita on substance use and mental health.* Rockville, MD: Substance Abuse and Mental Health Services Administration, US Department of Health and Human Services.

Ohry, A., Solomon, Z., Neria, Y., Waysman, M., Bar-On, Z., & Levy, A. (1994). The aftermath of captivity: An 18-year follow-up of Israeli ex-POWs. *Behavioral Medicine, 20*(1), 27–33.

Ohta, Y., Araki, K., Kawasaki, N., Nakane, Y., Honda, S., & Mine, M. (2003). Psychological distress among evacuees of a volcanic eruption in Japan: A follow-up study. *Psychiatry and Clinical Neurosciences, 57*(1), 105–111.

Ohtani, T., Iwanami, A., Kasai, K., Yamasue, H., Kato, T., Sasaki, T., & Kato, N. (2004). Posttraumatic stress disorder symptoms in victims of Tokyo subway attack: A 5-year follow-up study. *Psychiatry and Clinical Neurosciences, 58*(6), 624–629.

Onder, E., Tural, U., Aker, T., Kiliç, C., & Erdoğan, S. (2006). Prevalence of psychiatric disorders 3 years after the 1999 earthquake in Turkey: Marmara earthquake survey (MES). *Social Psychiatry and Psychiatric Epidemiology, 41*(11), 868–874.

Onyut, L. P., Neuner, F., Ertl, V., Schauer, E., Odenwald, M., & Elbert, T. (2009). Trauma, poverty and mental health among Somali and Rwandese refugees living in an African refugee settlement: An epidemiological study. *Conflict and Health, 26*(3), 6.

Orth, U., & Wieland, E. (2006). Anger, hostility, and posttraumatic stress disorder in trauma-exposed adults: A meta-analysis. *Journal of Consulting and Clinical Psychology, 74*(4), 698–706.

O'Toole, B. I., Marshall, R. P., Grayson, D. A., Shureck, R. J., Dobson, M., Fernech, M., … Vennard, J. (1996). The Australian Vietnam Veterans Health Study III: Psychological health of Vietnam veterans and its relationship to combat. *International Journal of Epidemiology, 25*(2), 331–340.

Ozer, E. J., Best, S. R., Lipsey, T. L., & Weiss, D. S. (2003). Predictors of posttraumatic stress disorder and symptoms in adults: A meta-analysis. *Psychological Bulletin, 129*(1), 52–73.

Ozer, E. J., & Weinstein, R. S. (2004). Urban adolescents' exposure to community violence: The role of support, school safety, and social constraints in a school-based sample of boys and girls. *Journal of Clinical Child and Adolescent Psychology, 33*(3), 463–476.

Palinkas, L. A., Petterson, J. S., Russell, J., & Downs, M. A. (1993). Community patterns of psychiatric disorders after the *Exxon Valdez* oil spill. *American Journal of Psychiatry, 150*(10), 1517–1523.

Palinkas, L. A., Russell, J., Downs, M. A., & Petterson, J. S. (1992). Ethnic differences in stress, coping, and depressive symptoms after the *Exxon Valdez* oil spill. *Journal of Nervous and Mental Disease, 180*(5), 287–295.

Paunovic, N., & Ost, L. S. (2001). Cognitive–behavior therapy versus exposure therapy in the treatment of PTSD in refugees. *Behavior and Research Therapy, 39*(10), 1183–1197.

Perkonigg, A., Kessler, R. C., Storz, S., & Wittchen, H. U. (2000). Traumatic events and posttraumatic stress disorder in the community: Prevalence, risk factors and comorbidity. *Acta Psychiatrica Scandinavica, 101*(1), 46–59.

Pham, P. N., Weinstein, H. M., & Longman, T. (2004). Trauma and PTSD symptoms in Rwanda: Implications for attitudes toward justice and reconciliation. *Journal of the American Medical Association, 292*(5), 602–612.

Raja, M., Onofri, A., Azzoni, A., Borzellino, B., & Melchiorre, N. (2008). Posttraumatic stress disorder among people exposed to the Ventotene street disaster in Rome. *Clinical Practice and Epidemiology in Mental Health, 5*(4), 5.

Raphael, B., Taylor, M., & McAndrew, V. (2008). Women, catastrophe and mental health. *Australian and New Zealand Journal of Psychiatry, 42*(1), 13–23.

Rauch, S. A., Grunfeld, T. E., Yadin, E., Cahill, S. P., Hembree, E., & Foa, E. B. (2008). Changes in reported physical health symptoms and social function with prolonged exposure therapy for chronic posttraumatic stress disorder. *Depression and Anxiety, 26*(8), 732–738.

Ray, R. D. & Webster, R. (2010). Group interpersonal psychotherapy for veterans with posttraumatic stress disorder: A pilot study. *International Journal of Group Psychotherapy, 60*(1), 131–140.

Reagan, L. P., Grillo, C. A., & Piroli, G. G. (2008). The As and Ds of stress: Metabolic, morphological and behavioral consequences. *European Journal of Pharmacology, 585*(1), 64–75.

Rechtman, R. (2004). The rebirth of PTSD: The rise of a new paradigm in psychiatry. *Social Psychiatry and Psychiatric Epidemiology, 39*(11), 913–915.

Renouf, A. G., Kovacs, M., & Mukerji, P. (1997). Relationship of depressive, conduct and comorbid disorders and social functioning in childhood. *Journal of the American Academy of Child and Adolescent Psychiatry, 36*(7), 998–1004.

Richardson, L. K., Frueh, B. C., & Acierno, R. (2010). Prevalence estimates of combat-related posttraumatic stress disorder: Critical review. *Australian and New Zealand Journal of Psychiatry, 44*(1), 4–19.

Rivière, S., Schwoebel, V., Lapierre-Duval, K., Guinard, A., Gardette, V., & Lang, T. (2008). Predictors of symptoms of post-traumatic stress disorder after the AZF chemical factory explosion on 21 September 2001, in Toulouse, France. *Journal of Epidemiology and Community Health, 62*(5), 455–460.Roberts, A. R. (2000). An overview of crisis theory and intervention model. In A. R. Roberts (Ed.), *Crisis intervention handbook* (pp. 3–30). New York, NY: Oxford University Press.

Roberts, B., Damundu, E. Y., Lomoro, O., & Sondorp, E. (2009). Post-conflict mental health needs: A cross-sectional survey of trauma, depression and associated factors in Juba, Southern Sudan. *BMC Psychiatry, 9*, 7.

Robertson, M., Rushton, P., Batrim, D., Moore, E., & Morris, P. (2007). Open trial of interpersonal psychotherapy for chronic post traumatic stress disorder. *Australasian Psychiatry: Bulletin of the Royal Australian and New Zealand College of Psychiatrists, 15*(5), 375–379.

Rosenman, S. (2002). Trauma and posttraumatic stress disorder in Australia: Findings in the population sample of the Australian National Survey of Mental Health and Wellbeing. *Australian and New Zealand Journal of Psychiatry, 36*(4), 515–520.

Rothbaum, B. O., Hodges, L. F., Ready, D., Graap, K., & Alarcon, R. D. (2001). Virtual reality exposure therapy for Vietnam veterans with post-traumatic stress disorder. *Journal of Clinical Psychiatry, 62*(8), 617–622.

Roy, A., Hu, X. Z., Janal, M. N., & Goldman, D. (2007). Interaction between childhood trauma and serotonin transporter gene variation in suicide. *Neuropsychopharmacology, 32*(9), 2046–2052.

Rubonis, A. V., & Bickman, L. (1991). Psychological impairment in the wake of disaster: The disaster–psychopathology relationship. *Psychological Bulletin, 109*(3), 384–399.

Rutherford, A., Zwi, A. B., Grove, N. J., & Butchart, A. (2007). Violence: A priority for public health? (Part 2). *Journal of Epidemiology and Community Health, 61*(9), 764–770.

Sabin, M., Lopes Cardozo, B., Nackerud, L., Kaiser, R., & Varese, L. (2003). Factors associated with poor mental health among Guatemalan refugees living in Mexico 20 years after civil conflict. *Journal of the American Medical Association, 290*(5), 635–642.

Samson, A. Y., Bensen, S., Beck, A., Price, D., & Nimmer, C. (1999). Posttraumatic stress disorder in primary care. *Journal of Family Practice, 48*(3), 222–227.

Sareen, J., Cox, B. J., Afifi, T. O., Stein, M. B., Belik, S. L., Meadows, G., & Asmundson, G. J. (2007). Combat and peacekeeping operations in relation to prevalence of mental disorders and perceived need for mental health care: Findings from a large representative sample of military personnel. *Archives of General Psychiatry, 64*(7), 843–852.

Schlenger, W. E., Caddell, J. M., Ebert, L., Jordan, B. K., Rourke, K. M., Wilson, D.,...Kulka, R. A. (2002). Psychological reactions to terrorist attacks: Findings from the National Study of Americans' Reactions to September 11. *Journal of the American Medical Association, 288*(5), 581–588.

Schlenger, W. E., Kulka, R. A., Fairbank, J. A., Hough, R. L., Jordan, B. K., Marmar, C. R., & Weiss, D. S. (1992). The prevalence of post-traumatic stress disorder in the Vietnam generation: A multimethod, multisource assessment of psychiatric disorder. *Journal of Traumatic Stress, 5*(3), 333–363.

Schnurr, P. P., & Jankowski, M. K. (1999). Physical health and post-traumatic stress disorder: A review and synthesis. *Seminars in Clinical Neuropsychiatry, 4*(4), 295–304.

Scholte, W. F., Olff, M., Ventevogel, P., de Vries, G. J., Jansveld, E., & Cardozo, B. L. (2004). Mental health symptoms following war and repression in eastern Afghanistan. *Journal of the American Medical Association, 292*(5), 585–593.

Segman, R., Shalev, A. Y., & Gelernter, J. (2007). Gene–environment interactions: Twin studies and gene research in the context of PTSD. In M. J. Friedman, T. M. Keane, & P. A. Resick (Eds.), *Handbook of PTSD: Science and practice* (pp. 190–206). New York, NY: Guilford.

Shaffer, D. (1974). Suicide in childhood and early adolescence. *Journal of Child Psychology and Psychiatry, 15*(4), 275–291.

Shafii, M., Steltz-Lenarsky, J., Derrick, A. M., Beckner, C., & Whittinghill, J. R. (1988). Comorbidity of mental disorders in the post-mortem diagnosis of completed suicide in children and adolescents. *Journal of Affective Disorders, 15*(3), 227–233.

Shalev, A. Y., Freedman, S., Peri, T., Brandes, D., Sahar, T., Orr, S. P., & Pitman, R. K. (1998). Prospective study of posttraumatic stress disorder and depression following trauma. *American Journal of Psychiatry, 155*(5), 630–637.

Shariat, S., Mallonee, S., Kruger, E., Farmer, K., & North, C. (1999). A prospective study of long-term health outcomes among Oklahoma City bombing survivors. *Journal of the Oklahoma State Medical Association, 92*(4), 178–186.

Smid, G. E., Mooren, T. T., van der Mast, R. C., Gersons, B. P., & Kleber, R. J. (2009). Delayed posttraumatic stress disorder: Systematic review, meta-analysis, and meta-regression analysis of prospective studies. *Journal of Clinical Psychiatry, 70*(11), 1572–1582.

Smith, P., Yule, W., Perrin, S., Tranah, T., Dalgleish, T., & Clark, D. M. (2007). Cognitive–behavioral therapy for PTSD in children and adolescents: A preliminary randomized controlled trial. *Journal of the American Academy of Child and Adolescent Psychiatry, 46*(8), 1051–1061.

Soeteman, R. J., Yzermans, C. J., Kerssens, J. J., Dirkzwager, A. J., Donker, G. A., ten Veen, P. M.,...van der Zee, J. (2007). Health problems presented to family practices in the Netherlands 1 year before and 1 year after a disaster. *Journal of the American Board of Family Medicine, 20*(6), 548–556.

Solomon, S., & Smith, E. (1994). Social support and perceived controls as moderators of responses to dioxin and flood exposure. In R. J. Ursano, B. G. McCaughey, & C. S. Fullerton (Eds.), *Individual and community responses to trauma and disaster: The structure of human chaos* (pp. 179–200). New York, NY: Cambridge University Press.

Solomon, Z., & Mikulincer, M. (2006). Trajectories of PTSD: A 20-year longitudinal study. *American Journal of Psychiatry, 163*(4), 659–666.

Somasundaram, D. (2002). Child soldiers: Understanding the context. *British Medical Journal, 324*(7348), 1268–1271.

Song, M., Hong, Y. C., Cheong, H. K., Ha, M., Kwon, H., Ha, E. H.,...Kim, E. J. (2009). Psychological health in residents participating in clean-up works of Hebei Spirit oil spill. *Journal of Preventive Medicine and Public Health, 42*(2), 82–88.

Southwick, S. M., Davis, L. L., Aikins, A. R., Rasmusson, A., Barron, J., & Morgan, C. A. (2007). Neurobiological alterations associated with PTSD. In M. J. Friedman, T. M. Keane, & P. A. Resick (Eds.), *Handbook of PTSD: Science and practice* (pp. 166–189). New York: NY: Guilford.

Spitzer, C., Barnow, S., Völzke, H., John, U., Freyberger, H. J., & Grabe, H. J. (2009). Trauma, posttraumatic stress disorder and physical illness: Findings from the general population. *Psychosomatic Medicine, 71*(9), 1012–1017.

Steel, Z., Chey, T., Silove, D., Marnane, C., Bryant, R. A., & van Ommeren, M. (2009). Association of torture and other potentially traumatic events with mental health outcomes among populations exposed to mass conflict and displacement: A systematic review and meta-analysis. *Journal of the American Medical Association, 302*(5), 537–549.

Stein, B. D., Jaycox, L. H., Kataoka, S. H., Wong, M., Tu, W., Elliott, M. N., & Fink, A. (2003). A mental health intervention for schoolchildren exposed to violence: A randomized controlled trial. *Journal of the American Medical Association, 290*(5), 603–611.

Strik, J. J., Lousberg, R., Cheriex, E. C., & Honig, A. (2004). One-year cumulative incidence of depression following myocardial infarction and impact on cardiac outcome. *Journal of Psychosomatic Research 56*(1), 59–66.

Talbot, P. S. (2004). The molecular neuroimaging of anxiety disorders. *Current Psychiatry Reports, 6*(4), 274–279.

Taylor, M. R., Agho, K. E., Stevens, G. J., & Raphael, B. (2008). Factors influencing psychological distress during a disease epidemic: Data from Australia's first outbreak of equine influenza. *BMC Public Health, 8*, 347.

Taylor, S., Asmundson, G. J. G., & Carleton, R. N. (2006). Simple versus complex PTSD: A cluster analytic investigation. *Journal of Anxiety Disorders, 20*(4), 459–472.

Tedeschi, R. G., Park, C. L., & Calhoun, L. G. (Eds.). (1998). *Posttraumatic growth: Positive changes in* the aftermath of crisis. Mahwah, NJ: Lawrence Erlbaum.

Terhakopian, A., Sinaii, N., Engel, C. C., Schnurr, P. P., & Hoge, C. W. (2008). Estimating population prevalence of posttraumatic stress disorder: An example using the PTSD checklist. *Journal of Traumatic Stress, 21*(3), 290–300.

Thabet, A. A., Abu Tawahina, A., El Sarraj, E., & Vostanis, P. (2008). Exposure to war trauma and PTSD among parents and children in the Gaza Strip. *European Child and Adolescent Psychiatry, 17*(4), 191–199.

Thoresen, S., & Mehlum, L. (2008). Traumatic stress and suicidal ideation in Norwegian male peace-keepers. *Journal of Nervous and Mental Disease, 196*(11), 814–821.

Tol, W. A., Komproe, I. H., Susanty, D., Jordans, M. J., Macy, R. D., & De Jong, J. T. (2008). School-based mental health interventions for children affected by political violence in Indonesia: A cluster randomized trial. *Journal of the American Medical Association, 300*(6), 655–662.

Trappler, B., Cohen, C. I., & Tulloo, R. (2007). Impact of early lifetime trauma in later life: Depression among Holocaust survivors 60 years after the liberation of Auschwitz. *American Journal of Geriatric Psychiatry, 15*(1), 79–83.

Turell, S. C., & Armsworth, M. W. (2000). Differentiating incest survivors who self-mutilate. *Child Abuse and Neglect, 24*(2), 237–249.

Udomratn, P. (2008). Mental health and the psychosocial consequences of natural disasters in Asia. *International Review of Psychiatry, 20*(5), 441–444.

United Nations International Strategy for Disaster Reduction Secretariat. (2009). *Global assessment report on disaster risk reduction.* Geneva, Switzerland: United Nations.

US Department of Health and Human Services. (2001). *Mental health: Culture, race, ethnicity. A supplement to Mental health: Report of the surgeon general.* Rockville, MD: Substance Abuse and Mental Health Services Administration, US Department of Health and Human Services.

Van Ameringen, M., Mancini, C., Patterson, B., & Boyle, M. H. (2008). Post-traumatic stress disorder in Canada. *CNS Neuroscience and Therapeutics, 14*(3), 171–181.

van der Kolk, B. A. (2007). The history of trauma in psychiatry. In M. J. Friedman, T. M. Keane, & P. A. Resick (Eds.), *Handbook of PTSD: Science and practice* (pp. 19–36). New York, NY: Guilford.

van der Kolk, B. A., Perry, J. C., & Herman, J. L. (1991). Childhood origins of self-destructive behavior. *American Journal of Psychiatry, 148*(12), 1665–1671.

van Griensven, F., Chakkraband, M. L., Thienkrua, W., Pengjuntr, W., Lopes Cardozo, B., Tantipiwatanaskul, P., ... Tappero, J. W. (2006). Mental health problems among adults in tsunami-affected areas in southern Thailand. *Journal of the American Medical Association, 296*(5), 537–548.

Van Loey, N. E., & Van Son, M. J. (2003). Psychopathology and psychological problems in patients with burn scars: Epidemiology and management. *American Journal of Clinical Dermatology, 4*(4), 245–272.

van Zelst, W. H., de Beurs, E., Beekman, A. T., van Dyck, R., & Deeg, D. D. (2006). Well-being, physical functioning and use of health services in the elderly with PTSD and subthreshold PTSD. *International Journal of Geriatric Psychiatry, 21*(2), 180–188.

Vlahov, D., Galea, S., Ahern, J., Resnick, H., Boscarino, J. A., Gold, J., ... Kilpatrick, D. (2004). Consumption of cigarettes, alcohol, and marijuana among New York City residents six months after the September 11 terrorist attacks. *American Journal of Drug and Alcohol Abuse, 30*(2), 385–407.

Walsh, F. (2007). Traumatic loss and major disasters: Strengthening family and community resilience. *Family Process, 46*(2), 207–227.

Wang, P. S., Gruber, M. J., Powers, R. E., Schoenbaum, M., Speier, A. H., Wells, K. B., & Kessler, R. C. (2008). Disruption in existing mental health treatments and failure to initiate new treatment after Hurricane Katrina. *American Journal of Psychiatry 165*(1), 34–41.

Weaver, I. C., Champagne, F., Brown, S. E., Dymov, S., Sharma, S., Meaney, M. J., & Szyf, M. (2005). Reversal of maternal programming of stress responses in adult offspring through methyl supplementation: Altering epigenetic marking later in life. *Journal of Neuroscience, 25*(47), 11045–11054.

Weaver, I. C., Grant, R. J., & Meaney, M. J. (2002). Maternal behavior regulates long-term hippocampal expression of *BAX* and apoptosis in the offspring. *Journal of Neurochemistry, 82*(4), 998–1002.

Weierich, M. R., & Nock, M. K. (2008). Posttraumatic stress symptoms mediate the relation between childhood sexual abuse and nonsuicidal self-injury. *Journal of Consulting and Clinical Psychology, 76*(1), 39–44.

Weine, S., Kulauzovic, Y., Klebic, A., Besic, S., Mujagic, A., Muzurovic, J., ... Rolland, J. (2008).

Evaluating a multiple-family group access intervention for refugees with PTSD. *Journal of Marital and Family Therapy, 34*(2), 149–164.

Weisler, R. H., Barbee, J. G., 4th, & Townsend, M. H. (2006). Mental health and recovery in the Gulf Coast after hurricanes Katrina and Rita. *Journal of the American Medical Association, 296*(5), 585–588.

Weissman, M., Markowitz, J., & Klerman, G. (2000). *Comprehensive guide to interpersonal psychotherapy*. New York, NY: Basic Books.

Whitlock, J. (2010). Self-injurious behavior in adolescents. *PLoS Medicine, 7*(5). Retrieved from http://www.plosmedicine.org/article/info%3Adoi%2F10.1371%2Fjournal.pmed.1000240

Wilcox, H. C., Storr, C. L., & Breslau, N. (2009). Posttraumatic stress disorder and suicide attempts in a community sample of urban American young adults. *Archives of General Psychiatry, 66*(3), 305–311.

Wilfley, D. E., Agras, W. S., Telch, C. F., Rossiter, E. M., Schneider, J. A., Cole, A. G.,... Raeburn, S. D. (1993). Group cognitive–behavioral therapy and group interpersonal psychotherapy for the nonpurging bulimic individual: A controlled comparison. *Journal of Consulting and Clinical Psychology, 61*(2), 296–305.

Wittchen, H. U., Gloster, A., Beesdo, K., Schönfeld, S., & Peronigg, A. (2009). Posttraumatic stress disorder: Diagnostic and epidemiological perspectives. *CNS Spectrums, 14*(1 Suppl. 1), 5–12.

Wolfe, J., Erickson, D. J., Sharkansky, E. J., King, D. W., & King, L. A. (1999). Course and predictors of posttraumatic stress disorder among Gulf War veterans: A prospective analysis. *Journal of Consulting and Clinical Psychology, 67*(4), 520–528.

Wood, D. P., Webb-Murphy, J., Center, K., McLay, R., Koffman, R., Johnston, S.,... Wiederhold, B. K. (2009). Combat-related post-traumatic stress disorder: A case report using virtual reality graded exposure therapy with physiological monitoring with a female Seabee. *Military Medicine, 174*(11), 1215–1222.

Yehuda, R., Kahana, B., Binder-Brynes, K., Southwick, S. M., Mason, J. W., & Giller, E. L. (1995). Low urinary cortisol excretion in Holocaust survivors with posttraumatic stress disorder. *American Journal of Psychiatry, 152*(7), 982–986.

Yehuda, R., & McFarlane, A. C. (1995). Conflict between current knowledge about posttraumatic stress disorder and its original conceptual basis. *American Journal of Psychiatry, 152*(12), 1705–1713.

Yzermans, C. J., Donker, G. A., Kerssens, J. J., Dirkzwager, A. J., Soeteman, R. J., & Ten Veen, P. M. (2005). Health problems of victims before and after disaster: A longitudinal study in general practice. *International Journal of Epidemiology, 34*(4), 820–826.

Zatzick, D., Jurkovich, G. J., Rivara, F. P., Wang, J., Fan, M. Y., Joesch, J., & Mackenzie, E. (2008). A national US study of posttraumatic stress disorder, depression, and work and functional outcomes after hospitalization for traumatic injury. *Annals of Surgery, 248*(3), 429–437.

Zimmerman, M., & Mattia, J. I. (1999). Is posttraumatic stress disorder underdiagnosed in routine clinical settings? *Journal of Nervous and Mental Disease, 187*(7), 420–428.

Zinzow, H. M., Ruggiero, K. J., Resnick, H., Hanson, R., Smith, D., Saunders, B., & Kilpatrick, D. (2009). Prevalence and mental health correlates of witnessed parental and community violence in a national sample of adolescents. *Journal of Child Psychology and Psychiatry, 50*(4), 441–450.

Zlotnick, C., Johnson, J., Kohn, R., Vicente, B., Rioseco, P., & Saldivia, S. (2006). Epidemiology of trauma, post-traumatic stress disorder (PTSD) and co-morbid disorders in Chile. *Psychological Medicine, 36*(11), 1523–1533.

Zvolensky, M. J., Bernstein, A., Marshall, E. C., & Feldner, M. T. (2006). Panic attacks, panic disorder, and agoraphobia: Associations with substance use, abuse, and dependence. *Current Psychiatry Reports, 8*(4), 279–285.

SECTION V

The Behavioral Health Care Service System

12

Mental Health and the Law

DEBORAH AGUS

Key Points

- The law of the land defines the parameters within which mental health professionals operate.

- The United States Constitution establishes individual rights and limits the authority of the government to create programs that unreasonably interfere with individual liberty.

- People with mental illness are entitled to receive the full protection of the law

- Constitutionally established rights can be limited by government actions or laws only if there is an rational reason related to a valid governmental interest for so doing and there is due process to protect individual citizens

- The rights to consent to treatment and to refuse treatment are examples of the protections created by the Constitution

- The area of forensic law describes the convergence of mental illness and criminal behavior. Issues include competency, criminal responsibility for actions by a person with mental illness, and the expanding population of persons with mental illness in jails and prisons

- The interplay of law and mental health is a key factor affecting public health and the development of systems to prevent and treat mental illness

INTRODUCTION

> We are in bondage to the law so that we
> might be free.
> —**Cicero,** Roman philosopher (106–43 BCE)

Understanding the law and the legal system is crucial to the effective practice of public mental health. Law, after all, is the embodiment of public mores and public policy, both of which act create the underpinnings for building a meaningful system of health care. The law is dynamic and, as it evolves, it both reflects and guides policies and practice. In areas of particular concern to public mental health, such as the right to treatment and the right to refuse treatment, seminal legal cases rely on theories of constitutional law to move the clinical system forward; balancing clinical practice requirements with individual rights. Thus the evolution of the modern public mental health system is fundamentally intertwined with legal principles.

On a practical, day-to-day level, laws guide behavior; they provide a regulatory or enforcement mechanism on which a savvy public mental health professional can rely. There are two broad classes of law: Law can be broadly defined as either "public" or "private" as described below:

- Public law—which defines rules within and between governments and public entities and between those entities and individuals—determines payment systems, professional behavior, individual rights and relationships, and the overall functioning of a health care system.
- Private law—the law of contracts and torts, which add the force of the government to agreements between private individuals— also affects a health care system. The issues of liability and malpractice (torts) and agreements between providers and payers (contracts) are determined by the legal conventions of private law.

At the policy level, mental health and the law also intersect in forensic policy, an area with particular relevance to the practice of public mental health. Unlike individuals with other illnesses, people with serious mental illnesses are affected disproportionately by involvement with the criminal justice system. In fact, in today's era of deinstitutionalization, jails and prisons have become de facto mental facilities (Bureau of Justice Statistics, 2006; Butterfield, 1998; Cox, Morschauser, Banks, & Stone, 2001; Justice Center, 2002). For this reason, development of an effective community mental health system demands a thorough understanding of the criminal justice field as well as the mental health field. Indeed, one might argue convincingly that the historical disconnect between the mental health and criminal justice systems underlies the current warehousing of thousands of mentally ill adults and youth in jails and prisons in lieu of receiving community-based services and supports known to be effective.

Thus this chapter provides an overview of the public, private, and forensic law that can be used to develop more effective systems of mental health care that join a commitment to individual rights with the best clinical practices.

The first section explores the origin and sources of law in the United States and examines the key concepts that underlie public mental health law per se. It is followed by a section highlighting key issues and then a section describing the field of forensic policy, where mental health, public health, and criminal justice intersect. Finally, the chapter explores a number of current mental health issues analyzed using the legal concepts described earlier in the chapter, thus enabling the reader to apply those principles in new situations.

A LEGAL PRIMER

The law is a dynamic set of enforceable rules created over time by courts, legislative officials, and executive staff who write, interpret, and implement law. For the purposes of this chapter, the focus will be primarily on decisions of the US Supreme Court and on enacted federal legislation—the highest laws of the land.

Sources of Law

In the United States, both federal and state law are derived primarily from four sources:

- The Constitution provides the overarching framework and principles for governing.
- Legislation or statutes are enacted by the legislative branches as representatives of the electorate.
- Judicial common law is developed by building on case-by-case legal interpretations by courts by following precedent which is described in legal terms as " stare decisis" which literally means "let the decision stand."
- Regulations are developed by the executive branch (administrators) to spell out the details of implementation of the enacted legislation or statute. For example, if the federal legislature mandates by statute that all domestic meat must be produced in a humane manner, the federal Food and Drug Administration will develop regulations that explain the meaning of humane treatment (e.g., requiring that all chickens be raised without cages). Regulations are promulgated after allowing for public comment.

At the municipal and county levels, mayors and city councils are charged with developing ordinances and regulations affecting day-to-day community management and local issues related to matters such as zoning, police, and regulation of local business.

General Principles Affecting Lawmaking and the Court Structure

The law of supremacy in the United States dictates a hierarchy of lawmaking beginning at the national level and reaching down to the municipal level. Federal law is the supreme law of the land; no state or local law can conflict with federal law, although it may add to it. As with all things legal, however, the law of supremacy is counterbalanced, in this case by the concept of federalism, or shared power between the federal and state governments. Federalism is the principle that underlies the 10th Amendment to the US Constitution, which states that all powers not explicitly granted in the Constitution to the federal government are the provenance of the states. The resulting interplay between federal supremacy

and states' rights affects the dynamics of how laws are developed in all areas, including public health and public mental health, as will be explored later in the chapter.

Just as federal law trumps state or local law, the US Constitution is the highest law of the land at both the federal and state levels; the federal Constitution supersedes all other laws. As a result, no federal or state statute (law) or state court ruling will stand if it conflicts with the US Constitution. The US Supreme Court, the arbiter of the US Constitution, has the final word in determining whether a state or federal statute is either in conflict or consistent with the Constitution. Similarly, each state has a judicial branch parallel to that of the federal level, including a state supreme court.

The hierarchy of the judicial branch, whether at the national or state level, includes three levels. The first, the trial level, is the district court, generally the first place where cases are heard and facts are determined. The middle level, the initial appellate level, the court of appeals, is the first appellate level, the court to which decisions at the district court level may be appealed. There are 11 regional appellate courts across the United States, plus both a District of Columbia and a federal circuit court. The final level is the Supreme Court, the highest level to which lower decisions may be appealed. It is the Supreme Court that makes the final determination when issues of constitutionality are at issue. (See Box 12-1.)

Decisions of the US Supreme Court apply to the entire country. Courts generally make law based on a case with a specific set of facts and a related question or issue Because each decision is limited by the facts of the case being heard, court holdings are explicitly binding only on cases with similar sets of facts. Only under very limited circumstances do courts make decisions or create legal holdings based on hypothetical facts or advisory questions.

Law developed by the courts—common law—builds on both prior decisions as new cases come forward and the law develops based on the rationale of preceding cases. Law developed by legislatures—statutory or civil (or code) law— is developed over time by bodies of lawmakers who consider large problems, do research, and hear testimony to develop systemic solutions

Box 12-1. The Hierarchy of Judicial Review

Marbury v. Madison (1803) was the quintessential case for establishing the hierarchy of judicial review by the Supreme Court. In *Marbury*, the court issued a long, convoluted opinion on the validity of a presidential commission (appointment) that was signed by the former president but not delivered to the proposed appointee before the president left office. With a different person in mind for the position, the new president and Congress tried to block the appointment.

The court declared first that "the government of the US...[is] a government of laws, and not of men." The court continued, "Where the law...directs the performance of an act...neither the heads of departments [executive branch] nor the legislature can thwart the law." They then forcefully explained that "the Constitution is the supreme law of the land, supreme over any ordinary law created by the legislature and that the Court has the authority to interpret the law and must enforce it as interpreted regardless of any Acts by Congress to the contrary."

Thus was established, without doubt, the supremacy of the US Constitution and the power of judicial review.

that are codified in legislation that, when signed by the President, becomes law.

UNITED STATES CONSTITUTION 101

While this chapter focuses primarily on legal issues related to mental health, a general knowledge of several basic legal concepts, such as due process, equal protection, and privacy, provides a necessary foundation for understanding the issues specific to that topic. The contours and definitions of these and other central legal concepts are evolutionary; changing and developing as the court system as a whole decides each new case before it. This section provides a brief summary of these legal concepts, their genesis and their relationship to effective public mental health.

Due Process

Simply stated, due process means fairness. It is a concept first found in the ancient legal codes of Hammurabi and then later in the Magna Carta (The Great Charter). It is the preeminent doctrine of the Constitution of the United States and defines the social contract between the governor and the governed.

The due process clause of the US Constitution emphasizes both fairness and balance. Fairness refers both to procedural fairness (how something is done) and also to substantive fairness (what was done and why). Thus the Fifth Amendment to the Constitution states, "No person shall be...deprived of life, liberty, or property, without due process of law." Similarly, the 14th Amendment says:

All persons born or naturalized in the United States, and subject to the jurisdiction thereof, are citizens of the United States and of the State wherein they reside. No State shall make or enforce any law which shall abridge the privileges or immunities of citizens of the United States; nor shall any State deprive any person of life, liberty, or property, without due process of law; nor deny to any person within its jurisdiction the equal protection of the laws.

Moreover, in the case *In re Gault* (1967), the US Supreme Court stated:

Due process of law is the primary and indispensable foundation of individual freedom. It is the basic and essential term in the social compact which defines the rights of the individual and delimits the powers which the state may exercise. As Justice Frankfurter stated: "The history of American freedom is, in no small measure, the history of procedure. (p. 21)

Equal Protection Under the Law

The 14th Amendment to the US Constitution states, "No *state* shall deny to any person within its jurisdiction the equal protection of the laws." This clause is commonly referred to as the equal protection clause. Although this clause is in the 14th Amendment and thus directed to the actions of a state rather than the federal government, it is now accepted that the Fifth Amendment's due process clause includes equal protection, which is therefore fully applicable to the actions of the federal government.

The clause has been interpreted to mean that a state can treat its citizens differently from one another only if a reasonable state purpose exists for doing so and if the purpose can be achieved in no other, more limited manner. For example, a state law may provide that 16-year-old youth may drive an automobile after following appropriate licensing and testing procedures but that 12-year-olds cannot. Similar age restrictions are imposed on the ability to enter into contracts and to consent to sex, medical treatment, and marriage. Each of these disparities—the product of age discrimination[or different treatment based solely on classification by age]—is perfectly constitutional because it is clearly described and is related to a reasonable state purpose. Most cases fall within this "reasonably related to a rational state purpose" rubric.

However, when the discrimination involves so-called suspect classes of people, the state action is held to a higher legal standard. That standard is one of strict scrutiny, under which the state must be able to demonstrate that the discrimination is a product of a compelling state interest that cannot be accommodated in any other way. This more exacting standard is deliberately difficult to satisfy. Thus, for example, if a state law provides different written (de jure) or applied (de facto) standards for African Americans and for Caucasians, the state will have a heavy burden to demonstrate the law to

Box 12-3. Magna Carta

An early passage of Magna Carta states, "TO ALL FREE MEN OF OUR KINGDOM we have also granted, for us and our heirs for ever, all the liberties written out below, to have and to keep for them and their heirs, of us and our heirs."

Winston Churchill (1956) wrote: "[H]ere is a law which is above the King and which even he must not break. This reaffirmation of a supreme law and its expression in a general charter is the great work of Magna Carta; and this alone justifies the respect in which men have held it."

be valid, since race is a suspect class as determined by the Supreme Court (*Loving v. Virginia*, 1967). Similarly, strict scrutiny will be applied if the rights at issue are fundamental ones, such as the right to vote or freedom of speech or religion (*Murdock v. Pennsylvania*, 1943).

A third standard of scrutiny, falling in the middle, demands both that the state show a compelling interest and that the disparities in treatment be narrow. Currently this middle ground includes distinctions related to gender and disability. Thus individuals with mental illnesses are within the definition of a protected class but are not part of a class granted the highest standards of scrutiny. As a result, a state has a lighter burden of proof in creating legal disparities affecting people with mental illnesses or other defined disabilities than is applicable to distinctions that are racially based. This standard, for example, would enable a state to apply legal standards for people with mental illnesses different from those used for people with physical problems. A disparity of that type would pass constitutional muster as long as the state could show both a rational reason for the difference and no less onerous alternative.

In 1990, Congress enacted the Americans with Disabilities Act (ADA), which specifically heightens protections afforded people with disabilities. This statute is consistent with the tenet that as long as a statute does not conflict with the Constitution, it can be stronger protections beyond the constitutional minimum. Under the ADA, the interests of persons with disabilities now require a state to satisfy a more compelling standard if discrimination or a disparate impact is proved. The ADA has been the foundation for successful litigation relevant to people with mental illnesses in such areas as employment, public benefits, fair housing, and conditions in hospitals and criminal justice facilities. It is a useful tool to promote accommodations and heightened sensitivity to individuals with chronic, disabling mental illnesses.

Note, however, that when a conflict arises between a legislatively created right and the Constitution, the latter prevails. Further, should Congress wish to restrict, add to, or otherwise alter rights it has created, it can amend or repeal the enacted legislation (referred to, when signed by the President, as a statute or law). Thus both public opinion and the will of the electorate are of extreme importance in using a tool like the ADA to protect a class such as people with mental illnesses.

Right to Liberty

The US Constitution clearly and unequivocally states, "...nor shall any person...be deprived of life, liberty, or property, without due process of law." This fundamental right, entitled to the highest procedural protection, safeguards individuals from government actions that will result in a deprivation of their right to life or liberty. The definition of liberty is key, involving such issues as: What is liberty? What restrictions are permissible (i.e., substantive due process)? What process is necessary to implement a restriction (i.e., procedural due process)? Critically, this right to liberty is central both to the development of mental health law and to the treatment process itself.

Creation of a Right to Privacy

Griswold v. Connecticut (1965) concerned the rights of professionals at Planned Parenthood to advise marital couples about birth control, notwithstanding a Connecticut statute that made such activity illegal. The US Supreme Court invalidated the state law, holding that it unconstitutionally violated the privacy rights of married couples. Justice Douglas wrote:

> Though the Constitution does not explicitly protect a general right to privacy, the various guarantees within the Bill of Rights create penumbras, or zones, that establish a right to privacy. Together, the First, Third, Fourth, and Ninth Amendments, create a new constitutional right, the right to privacy in marital relations. The Connecticut statute conflicts with the exercise of this right and is therefore null and void. (p. 484)

The privacy right, as defined in *Griswold*, has considerable relevance to cases involving treatment for mental illnesses. The *Griswold* holding underlies legal issues related to bodily integrity and autonomy, including both consent to treatment and the right to refuse treatment, as will become clear later in this chapter. The rights to liberty and to privacy combine to create a right to autonomy over decisions affecting one's body. This concept of constitutionally protected autonomy strengthens the common-law doctrine of consent to treatment, such that issues of autonomy, privacy, and consent significantly affect the delivery of health care.

Reserved Powers: The 10th Amendment

The lawmaking power of the federal government is limited to the specific grants of power described in the Constitution. The concept of reserved powers refers to the authority conferred on the states by the 10th Amendment to the US Constitution. The 10th Amendment states that "all powers not expressly given to the federal government nor expressly prohibited for the states will go to the states." This is called the States' Rights Amendment and enables the states to establish and enforce their own laws and policies in areas that "protect the safety, health, welfare and morals of the community." The 10th Amendment both reserves some powers for the states and establishes areas of state responsibility, collectively referred to as the police powers of the state. (See below for further explanation of the police power concept.)

However, although the 10th Amendment reserves power for the states and provides a broad police power mandate, disagreements often arise over limits to the reserved powers. In any disagreement in which both the United States and the state have jurisdiction, federal law supersedes state law. For example, the interstate commerce clause of the Constitution gives the federal government the right to make laws on any topic affecting interstate commerce. This broad language has provided the federal government with authority in areas such as education and health that otherwise might be the sole province of the states. Since federal legislation takes precedence in any judicial conflict with a state, states have

an interest in arguing that their jurisdiction in a particular matter is protected under the 10th Amendment.

As in all constitutional matters, the jurisdictional issues are complex, subject to considerable interpretation, and ever evolving. For example, while Article I, Section 8, of the Constitution expressly delineates a number of powers relating to issues of national interest, such as defense, mail, money, and international affairs, the same section ends with a very broad phrase granting the federal govenment the authority "[t]o make all Laws which *shall be necessary and proper for carrying into Execution the foregoing Powers* [emphasis added], and all other Powers vested by this Constitution in the Government of the United States, or in any Department or Officer thereof." While a multitude of cases over the years have been based on the meaning of this "necessary and proper" clause, for the most part the phrase has operated to broaden rather than lessen federal jurisdiction.

POLICE POWERS

Police powers, conferred on the states by the 10th Amendment and in turn delegated by states to their political subdivisions, enable local governments to enact measures to preserve and protect the safety, health, welfare, and morals of the community. Put simply, the Amendment describes the basic right of government to establish laws and regulations for the benefit of its citizens. While establishing a police force as a way to promote public safety and to protect morals is part of the police powers, the term is far broader than that. Protecting the public health by requiring a person to be quarantined to stop the spread of tuberculosis is an example of a state's use of its police powers. Only states have such a broad constitutional mandate; in contrast, the Constitution limits the federal government to powers that are expressly granted. Criminal laws, health regulations, regulation of pornography, and laws against prostitution are a few examples of the powers included in the police power mandate. States use police powers to establish a variety of programs; in fact, public health is an area in which states traditionally exercise a tremendous amount of control. This is important in providing the potential for states to promote innovative and distinctive programming and to test and legislate a variety of models that eventually may find their way to other states or to the national level.

PARENS PATRIAE

The doctrine of parens patriae (translated as "parent of the country") is used to justify a government's ability to act in a custodial or protective capacity for individuals or communities. The doctrine recognizes the inherent power and authority of a government to protect individuals legally unable to act on their own behalf. For purposes of this chapter, the most relevant application of this doctrine is found in the laws and regulations governing the treatment of children and of individuals considered legally unable to manage their own affairs. The concept of parens patriae is broadly used to enable the government to act in the place of a parent; it does not refer to competency decisions made about a particular individual but instead to such things as setting a legal drinking age.

LEGAL ISSUES IN MENTAL HEALTH

Confidentiality

As noted earlier, the Supreme Court has developed a common-law theory of privacy rights, including the right to make decisions about one's body and medical treatment and the right to keep medical information private. The theory that certain conversations are "privileged" (safeguarded from legal disclosure) is based on both these privacy rights and a balance among competing interests. Thus, for

---

Box 12-4. Due Process Hypothetical: The Case of Mr. Smith

Procedural Due Process

Mr. Smith undresses in the middle of the street while believing himself to be talking with a little green Martian and threatening passersby with a big plastic sword. There is little question that this is an emergency situation and that the government has a legal right to pick him up and transport him to the nearest hospital to be involuntarily committed for treatment.

However, the process through which this is accomplished must be fair. The exact procedures to follow will vary from jurisdiction to jurisdiction, but the state must show that there are sufficient, rational procedures to protect his liberty rights to the extent possible and that protect him from unfair deprivation to the extent possible. The state has a right to restrain his liberty, but he has a right to be heard and to the process ensuring this right. How much process is "due," or required, will vary depending on the right at issue or the type of deprivation. Deprivations of liberty and of other fundamental rights such as the free exercise of religion or speech are accorded the highest standards of procedure, and a state must show a compelling interest to restrain such rights.

Substantive Due Process

Whether someone can be committed and the rationale for doing so are the essence of substantive due process. The balance of individual rights against the interests of the state is the content of the fairness issue. Certain rights are specifically delineated in the Constitution, but others or groups of others are inferred from the explicit language or from the panoply of rights taken together. In the case of Mr. Smith, the substantive issue is whether liberty can be restrained in the instance of someone who is mentally ill. The state has a rational and compelling reason for having emergency powers to do so.

---

example, in the absence of a compelling reason, the social interest in promoting treatment is sufficient to protect doctors from being compelled to testify about patients' treatment. The federal and state governments have further advanced the strict confidentiality of medical records for certain conditions, such as mental illnesses and substance use, under the public health theory that preserving patients' rights to treatment in confidential settings promotes engagement in treatment. (See, for example, the Confidentiality of Alcohol and Drug Abuse Patient Records Regulation, 1987.) State confidentiality law provides the structure underlying decisions about what must be kept private and what may be shared. Practitioners who violate those laws may be subject to civil or in some cases criminal proceedings.

Information sharing, however, is necessary to create systems of health care that promote continuity across service settings. Indeed, overall quality of care for behavioral or physical health problems depends in large measure on the continuity of care. To achieve integrated, coordinated care, providers across care settings, state lines, and disciplines must have the ability to freely share relevant information. Yet according to some health care providers, confidentiality laws developed in response to both stigma-related concerns and the right to privacy can compromise the capacity to share information. creating barriers that impede treatment. Creative problem solving can promote systems that both respect reasonable confidentiality and permit necessary information sharing. The goal of a public health leader is to understand both legal rules and best clinical practices and to develop a reasonable, effective compromise.

The ability for health care providers to share information is particularly critical in emergency care, as when an individual arrives at the emergency room and clinical staff have no information about medication history, existing health problems, or current treatment. These complexities are magnified in public health emergencies requiring quick triage and treatment, which could be delayed by limitations on information sharing and issues of confidentiality. Identifying solutions for these types of situations requires familiarity with relevant confidentiality laws, an understanding of the reasoning underlying them, and an exploration of both the potential for sharing within the existing framework and ways to amend the law consistent with constitutional and public health concerns. Exceptions for emergencies, when necessary, are possible but must be markedly limited.

Informed Consent: Treatment

Without consent, medical treatment in non-emergency situations is, deemed to be an unwanted assault on an individual's personal integrity. Consent is required to legitimate the treatment. Common-law history of the consent requirement lies first in cases of torts (a wrongful act) or battery (physical assault). Physical touching of any sort without consent is problematic, and woe to the surgeon who operates without proper consent or whose treatment strays beyond the defined parameters for which consent was given (e.g., amputating the wrong body part).

Another cause of action is found in the negligence doctrine, a common civil-law concept through which liability is created such that

---

Box 12-5. *Schloendorff v. The Society of the New York Hospital* (1914)

In ruling on this case, Justice Cardozo stated: "In the case at hand, the wrong complained of is not merely negligence. It is trespass. Every human being of adult years and sound mind has a right to determine what shall be done with his own body; and a surgeon who performs an operation without his patient's consent, commits an assault, for which he is liable in damages.... This is true except in cases of emergency where the patient is unconscious and where it is necessary to operate before consent can be obtained."

a person who hurts another may be liable for monetary damages to the injured party if the injury is proven to result from the actions. For example, if a passerby breaks a leg after falling into a hole that you dug in the sidewalk and failed to mark before going to the store to buy concrete, you are liable for payment for damages resulting from the broken leg. You are responsible for keeping the sidewalk reasonably safe, and it was reasonable to foresee that an unwarned, innocent passerby might fall in the hole and suffer physical damage. The negligence doctrine applies to treatment that is not authorized by the patient.

As courts broadened the scope of both constitutional privacy rights and the right to autonomy over decisions affecting one's body, the concept of consent to treatment acquired constitutional proportions. This constitutional doctrine means that both federal and state government are markedly limited in the actions they may take that infringe on an individual's rights to privacy and autonomy. Thus treatment by an agent of a government that is provided without consent, such as involuntary treatment in a psychiatric hospital, is strictly limited.

As amplified below, involuntary treatment is permissible only under hazardous or emergent situations, such as those involving imminent danger to life. In all other cases, consent is required. Moreover, that consent must be both voluntary (not coerced) and based on knowledge and understanding of the proposed treatment, including its potential risks and benefits. Consent is a nuanced concept. How much does any patient truly understand, especially given that patients are often anxious and confused? Furthermore, the balance of power in a doctor–patient relationship is not conducive to the existence of a fully empowered patient asking questions sufficient to confirm "true consent." However imperfect, informed consent does provide the patient with some leverage and promotes conversation. For consent to qualify as informed, the consenting individual must be competent to make reasoned decisions and understand what he or she is being told about treatment options. Absent competence, an individual can neither give nor withhold consent. Many times, in such cases, a guardian or other surrogate decision maker will be appointed to advise about and provide consent to treatment.

Competency to Consent

Mental illness and competency can coexist. An individual with a mental disorder may not be competent to make decisions about money, for example, but may have sufficient capacity to decide for or against an operation or the use of a particular psychotropic medication or vice versa. Even individuals who have been involuntarily hospitalized retain a presumption of competency. Consent is taken very seriously by the courts; the right to consent is to be protected. In fact, one recent court decision, *Zinermon v. Burch* (1990), specifically affirmed that health care providers who knowingly

---

Box 12-6. Consent/Enrollment Hypothetical

Describe a situation where an assertive community treatment (ACT) approaches an inpatient who is marginally competent to offer that patient the opportunity for discharge and enrollment in the ACT program. The student is either a public mental health officer or practitioner and must make the decision about the validity of consent in this situation.

Questions: How is it possible to best balance the competing interests between the opportunity to enroll the patient in a terrific program in the community and the need to allow the patient to provide meaningful consent in order to be enrolled, even if that means the patient will remain hospitalized? Do the strictures of the law help or hurt or just more strikingly define the issues?

acquired consent from someone they knew did not have the capacity to understand the issue are guilty of violating the patient's right to consent. As a result of *Zinermon*, a flurry of commentary and changes ensued to better balance the need to protect the right to consent with the need to hospitalize people for treatment when they do not meet the standard of dangerousness required for involuntary admission. Indeed, criteria developed by the American Psychiatric Association (APA) to determine a patient's capacity to consent to hospitalization (APA, 1993) were such that even severely psychotic people were eligible.

Most states have laws on the books that are based on the consent doctrines as they have been enunciated by the US Supreme Court The Court as has provided both the policies underlying the need to protect consent and the procedures to assess decision-making competency. The general rules are similar across states, though the processes and specific definitions vary.

The requirement that consent may be given only by persons competent to do so often leads to a conundrum for community-based public mental health care. For example, some of the most progressive, innovative, consumer-oriented programs will enroll clients only if enrollment is voluntary and given with consent. Yet these programs often treat individuals with the most serious illnesses, thus treading the fine line governing competency to consent on a daily basis. In such cases, the consent bar is lowered, often referred to as "consent with a wink," to enable people with serious mental illnesses to receive voluntary community-based treatment despite their marginal functioning level.

Informed Consent: Research

Research protocols are scrutinized heavily by institutional review boards (IRBs) to safeguard the rights and privacy of individuals participating as research subjects. An IRB is a committee that has been formally designated, often by a university, to approve, monitor, and review biomedical and behavioral research involving humans, with the goal of protecting the rights and safety of the research subjects. Informed consent to participate is a stringent

and valued component of the research protocol itself. Unfortunately, this generally laudable requirement sharply limits research on illnesses affecting the most seriously ill, vulnerable clients precisely because many individuals with those disorders are unable to demonstrate the capacity for informed consent. Moreover, all too often, these most marginalized, at-risk individuals are wary of participating in elaborate research projects. According to many researchers, the result has been a dearth of research on new clinical approaches to serve those most in need of evidence-based care (Teifion, 2001). Is this a desirable result from the public health standpoint?

Given the unfortunate history of abuse in research in the United States, many protective legal structures have been set in place to protect people with serious mental illnesses and others from being unwitting research subjects. One of the most infamous examples of such abuse was the Public Health Service's syphilis research at the Tuskegee Institute, carried out on African American males without their knowledge or consent. After those experiments became public, a huge outcry led to significant reform of research laws and guidelines (Jones, 1981). Bearing in mind the absolute need to protect individuals from unethical practices, this issue nonetheless begs for a more nuanced approach that deftly balances competing needs and crafts an effective solution. Unfortunately, the cumbersome nature of IRBs, coupled with the concomitant pressure to speed research progress, means that the research needs of this population continue to be overlooked. One might argue that in lieu of adopting a subtly nuanced consent-to-research approach, policy makers chose the easiest, strictest route that, while following the letter of the law, establishes an unnecessary barrier to new, effective care options under the otherwise laudatory banner of ethical research protocols.

Right to Refuse Treatment

While it may seem counterintuitive to open a discussion of treatment issues with a discourse on an individual's right to refuse treatment, it is appropriate. The evolution of mental health law, in fact, was propelled by litigation on the right to refuse treatment. These cases provided the very foundation on which the principles underlying a right to effective, humane treatment were built. The civil rights of persons with mental illnesses achieved primacy thanks to court decisions in right-to-refuse litigation; the fundamental tenets that have shaped today's mental health care system are grounded in and opinions laid forth in of case law on the right to refuse treatment.

Court cases in the 1960s and 1970s defined the rights of persons with mental illnesses in ways designed specifically to retain their fundamental liberty interest. In these cases, the constitutional right to liberty provided the rationale not only for the principle of treatment in the least restrictive setting but also for community-based care, expectations of recovery, consumer-directed care, and consent to treatment. Those core values foreshadowed the recovery movement that today underlies the most progressive community systems of care.

Involuntary Commitment to a Hospital

The nearly iconic phrase "dangerous to self or others" articulates the basic principle that determines whether an individual can be committed involuntarily to a hospital for treatment of a mental illness. The standard is set forth in the Supreme Court case *O'Connor v. Donaldson* (1975), in which the court held:

> In short, a State cannot constitutionally confine, without more, a non-dangerous individual who is capable of surviving safely in freedom by himself or with the help of willing and responsible family members or friends. Since the jury found, upon ample evidence, that O'Connor, as an agent of the State, knowingly did so confine Donaldson, it properly concluded that O'Connor violated Donaldson's constitutional right to freedom. (p. 576)

On numerous other occasions, the court has held that "[t]here can be no doubt that involuntary commitment to a mental hospital, like involuntary confinement of an individual for any reason, is a deprivation of liberty which the State cannot accomplish without due process

of law" (*O'Connor*, 1975, p. 580; *Addington v. Texas*, 1979, p. 425).

Of course, even the most fundamental rights can be limited if a compelling state interest exists to do so. The issue is one of balancing optimal commitment to individual rights against the protection of the public interest. In 1905, the US Supreme Court upheld compulsory vaccination as a reasonable exercise of the state police power to protect the health, welfare, and safety of its citizens (*Jacobson v. Massachusetts*, 1905). The decision to proceed with an involuntary commitment must be supported with proof of need to do so. Thus in individual cases, due process must be observed before an individual's rights can be abrogated. In *Jackson v. Indiana* (1972), the Supreme Court unanimously wrote that in the case of civil commitment, "[a]t the least, due process requires that the nature and duration of commitment bear some reasonable relation to the purpose for which the individual is committed" (p. 738).

Whether to protect public safety or as a substitute parent under the doctrine of parens patriae, the state's duty to protect its citizens is the foremost rationale for infringement on an individual's liberty. The Supreme Court has agreed that a state must protect its citizens, but it has also held that in balancing state responsibility with fundamental liberty interest, the Constitution requires that curtailment of liberty be as narrowly drawn as possible, invoked only when the danger is both imminent and extreme. In *O'Connor v. Donaldson* (1975), Justice Stewart, writing for a unanimous court, stated:

> A finding of "mental illness" alone cannot justify a State's locking a person up against his will and keeping him indefinitely in simple custodial confinement...there is still no constitutional basis for confining such persons involuntarily if they are dangerous to no one and can live safely in freedom. (p. 575)

He continued, "In short, a State cannot constitutionally confine without more a non-dangerous individual who is capable of surviving safely in freedom by himself or with the help of willing and responsible family members or friends" (p. 575).

Thus proof of both mental illness and dangerousness (known as substantive due process) must be presented. Moreover, because a fundamental right is at stake, the process used to determine whether a person should be confined must be of the highest order. Accordingly, numerous Supreme Court cases have established that procedural due process related to commitment cases requires, at least, an independent hearing and an opportunity for subsequent hearings to determine whether ongoing commitment remains necessary (*Addington v. Texas*, 1979; *Kansas v. Hendricks*, 1997).

Mental illness is virtually the only disease category under which a diagnosis alone, rather than commission of a criminal act, may result in confinement, a massive curtailment of liberty. Except for short-term quarantine, the idea of taking away a person's liberty based solely on an illness is abhorrent to both the constitutional scheme and the concept of individual freedom. Therefore conditions under which an individual may be confined due to illness alone need to be scrutinized closely and defined as narrowly as possible. For this precise reason, the standard of dangerousness remains unchanged despite substantial litigation. and attempts to change to a more lenient standard.

Refusal of Treatment in a Hospital

Today, the common law is firmly established that persons involuntarily committed to an institution retain a right to liberty that precludes them from being compelled to receive any specific form of treatment without a due process hearing (see above). Administering medication despite the patient's refusal, for example, represents an infringement on the liberty interest to be free from bodily restraint.

Thus before the treatment is permitted, procedural safeguards (e.g., an impartial hearing or substantial medical evidence to justify treatment) must be in place to protect that right. In and of itself, evidence of mental illness is insufficient proof that an individual lacks capacity to refuse treatment.

Before a series of Supreme Court decisions in the 1970s (described later in this chapter), it was assumed that all treatment decisions were the sole purview of medical personnel (Melton, Petrila, & Poythress, 1997). In *Mills v. Rogers* (1982), the Supreme Court granted certiorari (granted a hearing of the issue) to determine whether an individual who was involuntarily committed has a constitutional right to refuse treatment with antipsychotic medications. In *Rogers v. Okin* (1980), the First Circuit Court of Appeals ruled that the right to refuse treatment survives commitment and that a person committed for treatment is not necessarily incompetent to make such a decision. However, the Supreme Court remanded the case to be readjudicated consistent with a Massachusetts ruling that a court should first determine competence and then, if the individual is found to be incompetent, provide substituted judgment about treatment. The only exception was in the case of a life-or-death emergency.

In *Rennie v. Klein* (1981), another federal Court of Appeals came to the identical conclusions as in *Rogers* about the right to refuse treatment. A year later, in *Youngberg v. Romeo* (1982), the Supreme Court determined that an individual who is civilly committed retains "liberty interests in safety and freedom from bodily restraint" (p. 320). While the *Youngberg* decision involved bodily restraint, not forced psychotropic medication, the combination of lower court decisions, the court's remand consistent with both those decisions, and its

Youngberg ruling made a compelling argument that the Supreme Court recognizes that the liberty interest includes the right to refuse treatment by persons involuntarily committed to a mental hospital. Further, *Youngberg* affirmed that hospitalization alone does not render a patient incompetent to make medical decisions. However, the court did recognize the need to accommodate professional judgment about treatment. As a result, since *Youngberg*, it has enunciated a standard that accepts the constitutional right to refuse treatment but permits overriding that right when the treatment team's professional judgment deems the treatment necessary and consistent with accepted standards of care as applied to the individual case (*Youngberg v. Romeo*, 1982; *Rennie v. Klein* on remand, 1981/1983).

Right to Treatment in a Safe and Humane Environment

The absence of a constitutionally recognized right to health care in the United States is a major determinant of the public health landscape and one of the foremost barriers to significant health care reform. In the mental health arena, however, a very limited right to treatment has been recognized in law as a correlate to involuntary confinement. Congress first addressed the right to treatment in a 1964 statute about the rights of hospitalized individuals with mental illnesses that stated that such patients have a right to treatment for both mental and physical disorders while in the psychiatric hospital (Civil Rights Act of 1964). Subsequently enacted statutes have strengthened both the right to treatment and the right to treatment in the least restrictive environment (e.g., Americans with Disabilities Act, 1990; Civil Rights of Institutionalized

---

Box 12-9. Summary of Due Process for Persons Involuntarily Committed

Summary: Because of the liberty interest, except in emergency situations, a patient who has been involuntarily committed to a hospital has the right to due process protection if he refuses specific treatments. This might include a competency hearing, substituted judicial judgment, or a process for medical determination and review.

Persons Act, 1980; and regulations relating to receipt by institutions of Medicaid payments).

While the right-to-treatment issue was brought to the Supreme Court in *O'Connor v. Donaldson* (1975), the court did not specifically address it. Because the court held that the commitment in that case was invalid, it had no need to decide the broader issue. However, *O'Connor* did establish the precedent that a correlation exists between commitment and treatment, noting that the curtailment of liberty permitted in involuntary commitment is specifically intended for the purpose of treatment.

Rights of Institutionalized Persons

As a corollary to the rights to treatment and to due process, the courts have established a right to safe and humane conditions for persons in institutions. The appellate court case *Wyatt v. Stickney* (1971, 1972) challenged the conditions of care for persons with mental retardation who experienced long-term institutionalization. Deplorable conditions and patient maltreatment gave rise to a court case and a demand that the State of Alabama (the defendant) promulgate new operating standards for its facilities that were consistent with constitutional mandates for safe and humane treatment.

The state failed to act. After the defendants failed to formulate "minimum medical and Constitutional standards" for the operation of the three institutions involved in the suit, the district court, on April 13, 1972, established what would become known as the Wyatt standards, several specific requirements for the adequate treatment of both people with mental illnesses and those with mental retardation. The court enjoined the defendants to implement the standards. The former Fifth Circuit affirmed the district court's injunctions (*Wyatt v. Stickney*,1972). Then, using a "consent decree" the parties agreed to a series of principles to govern future actions of the State to solve the problems elucidated in the case. A consent decree is an agreement between the parties often after protracted litigation in a complicated case, that describes future actions and is approved by a court order

and thus enforceable through the Court. The district court thus established judicial oversight to review the state's compliance with the decree. The Wyatt standards for adequate and safe treatment consist of the provisions in the consent decree requiring:

• humane psychological and physical environments
• qualified staff in numbers sufficient to administer adequate treatment
• individualized treatment plans
• services in the least restrictive environment.

After 33 years, in December 2003, compliance was achieved; the State of Alabama was released from the consent decree following the longest mental health case in history. In January 2006, in an article reviewing the convoluted history of *Wyatt*, Clarence Sundram, the final individual appointed to evaluate compliance in the case, wrote:

Finally, after a third of a century, Alabama both had replaced its large institutions with smaller, more patient friendly places and had built a more comprehensive, community-based system of care, enabling more patients to be treated where they live (Sundram, 2004).

The same issue in a slightly different form came before the US Supreme Court in the previously mentioned case of *Youngberg v. Romeo* (1982). Youngberg involved a man with severe mental retardation who was confined to a mental hospital for many years and received little more than custodial care. The facts of the case supported the claim that he had received no treatment and in fact was ill treated. The questions before the Court were whether the Due Process clause of the 14th Amendment includes protected liberty interests to (1) safe conditions, (2) freedom from bodily restraints and (3) minimally adequate training or habilitation [Youngerg at p. 307]

After re-affirming that there is a Constitutionally protect liberty interest to safe conditions and to freedom from bodily restraints [at p. 323], The Court went on to consider whether there is an affirmative 'right' to minimally adequate treatment and then affirmed the lower courts ruling by concluding that "respondent's liberty interests require the State to provide minimally adequate or reasonable training to ensure safety and freedom from undue restraint." [p. 323]. The Court then went on to say, however, that in determining the boundaries of the "right to treatment", there must be a deference to professional judgment to determine what is reasonable treatment in view of the circumstances of an individual case thus providing a balancing test of "reasonableness" and giving deference to professional judgment. [at p. 324]

The 1982 Supreme Court under Chief Justice Warren Burger was not one for blazing new constitutional trails. However, given the egregious facts of the case, the court felt compelled to articulate at least a minimal constitutional right to "reasonably safe conditions...and...minimally adequate training." In doing so, however, the court narrowed the scope of the ruling specifically by adding as many qualifiers of the meaning of "reasonableness" as possible. Thus, while establishing a constitutional right to limited treatment in a safe environment, the court, in large measure, continued to defer to state policy, professional judgment, and budget constraints. Nonetheless, even this otherwise limited ruling advanced the growing body of legal rights afforded individuals confined in mental hospitals and other such facilities.

During the 1972–1982 decade, courts at all levels assumed primacy in laying the groundwork for the rights of and protections for people with serious mental illnesses. The courts established the basic principles underlying rights to treatment and rights while in treatment. Since then, however, relatively few Supreme Court cases have focused on issues affecting persons with mental illnesses; instead, the federal legislature has become more involved, using the earlier judicial standards established in *Wyatt* and *Youngberg* as the basis for laws regarding standards for treatment, advocacy, and equal protection. At the federal level, the ADA (1990), the Civil Rights of Institutionalized Persons Act (1982), and regulations relating to receipt by institutions of Medicaid payments all contain content related to the rights of persons to humane treatment. Additionally, over the past few decades, state legislatures increasingly have taken

action to help protect the rights of persons with mental illnesses. Today, all 50 states have statutes establishing patients' bills of rights and other means of promoting, regulating, and standardizing humane conditions in hospitals and residential facilities of all kinds. Yet even today problems persist; when state budgets are reduced, conditions often fall below expectations. Without constant monitoring, a lack of will and budgetary pressures over time may combine to result in overcrowded and unsafe public hospitals and care facilities.

As abuses are uncovered, the action switches back to the legal arena for enforcement to reestablish the rights of individuals in institutions. Statutes are enforced by the Executive branch through the Department of Justice, including through lawsuits brought by the attorney general. The protection and oversight offered by the legal system can act as a check on unsafe practices, but much still needs to be done.

Consider the very recent case of a resident of a psychiatric hospital in Georgia, as described by local newspaper reporters (Judd & Miller, 2007):

Alone in the darkness of a state mental hospital, Sarah Crider, 14, lay slowly dying. Sarah died lying in her own vomit because of a total and abject failure of the medical staff to provide even minimal monitoring of her health conditions. After investigations by the Atlanta Journal-Constitution, it was discovered that the circumstances of the case were not unique but were related to a string of fatalities in this state psychiatric hospital. Indeed, Sarah was one of at least 115 patients from Georgia's state psychiatric hospitals who have died under suspicious circumstances during the past five years, according to the Atlanta Journal-Constitution. This study revealed a pattern of neglect, abuse and poor medical care in the seven state hospitals, as well as a lack of public accountability for patient deaths. An investigation by the U.S. Justice Department unveiled many violations amounting to statutory and Constitutional abuses. In a 30-page letter describing in detail the violations and relevant law dated December 8, 2009, the Justice Department told the State to initiate reforms or face a federal lawsuit.

A second example was described in a February 2009 *New York Times* article summarizing the history of abuse at a psychiatric unit of a New York City–run hospital (Hartocollis, 2009). According to the article, the New York Civil Liberties Union filed an initial lawsuit in 1997, at which time a federal investigation was initiated. While the case progressed, subsequent deaths at the facility in 1998 provided further evidence of continuing and extremely serious problems. In 2009, after the state agreed to improve conditions, a federal report was released and summarized as follows in the *New York Times* article:

> The federal government has documented a pattern of sexual and other violent assaults among patients at the psychiatric unit of a city-run Brooklyn hospital where a woman died in June on the floor of the emergency waiting room while staff members ignored her. The U.S. Department of Justice responded to a lawsuit by the New York Civil Liberties Union. After a year-long investigation, the Department of Justice portrayed the unit at Kings County Hospital Center as a nightmarish place where patients were not treated for suicidal behavior, were routinely subdued with physical restraints and drugs instead of receiving individualized psychiatric treatment, and were frequently abused by other patients. The investigators found that the psychiatric service operated like a prison. A surveillance video showed Ms. Green, 49, lying on the floor for nearly an hour; during that time, a guard came in to check on her by wheeling his chair along, and another staff member prodded her with a foot. The Justice Department's report said conditions at the psychiatric unit were "highly dangerous and require immediate attention." It added: "Substantial harm occurs regularly due to K.C.H.C.'s failure to properly assess,

diagnose, supervise, monitor and treat its mental health patients.

These are but two of a recent spate of stories about conditions of treatment in mental hospitals and similar facilities. The key question remains, what can be done through available legal tools to protect patient rights in a proactive way over time?

Right to Community Treatment

Is there a constitutional right to mental health treatment in the community? Arguments in the affirmative derive from the concept of least restrictive alternative, established by the Supreme Court as described below. Extrapolating from the right to "least restrictive alternative" supports an argument for a corollary of " right to community-based care". Creating this community care "right" based on the right to least restrictive alternative treatment is best be articulated as follows: If no community treatment is available as an alternative to institutionalization, effectively, no least restrictive alternative exists, thus requiring that services be established to treat the individual in the community. Then by extension, the existence of one right creates the subsequent right to community treatment.

Unfortunately, to date, this argument has failed. No formal, recognized constitutional right to community treatment yet exists in the United States. However, the ADA comes as close as any legal construct today can to creating a right to community-based care. In the landmark case of *Olmstead v. LC* (1999), the Supreme Court considered whether the equal treatment demanded under the ADA requires a state to make sufficient community-based services available to enable anyone in need of treatment for a mental illness to receive it in the community rather than in an institution. The court ruled that the ADA applies to persons with mental illnesses and that the ADA, in fact, does *suggest* that states should offer services that enable individuals to be treated in the least restrictive, most appropriate venue. However, the court also held that as long as a state is making a reasonable effort to accommodate such individuals with community services, the court cannot require wholesale restructuring of a community system or force the state to spend sums to establish a comprehensive community-based system of care. (See box 12-10 below for an overview of the *Olmstead* decision.)

Thus Justice Ginsburg explained that if, for example, a state has a service waiting list that moves reasonably rapidly, that is sufficient to demonstrate that the state is acting in good faith to offer the least restrictive services, consistent with ADA language requiring a state to reasonably accommodate those with disability. Some observers have described the decision as simultaneously creating a right and it by deferring to pragmatism and politics. Notwithstanding its limitations, *Olmstead* did establish a first-time statutory right to community care based on an equal protection claim. Unfortunately, *Olmstead*'s boundaries with respect to the scope of a constitutional right to community-based care have yet to be defined.

Children and Adolescents: Right to Refuse or Consent to Treatment

The concept that an individual attains legal maturity at a particular age stems from ancient times. Historically, in the common law, the age of majority was set at the 21st birthday; today, with a few specific exceptions, it is generally accepted to occur at age 18.

The US Supreme Court has held that under the federal Constitution, children are entitled to protection, but not the full panoply of constitutional protections afforded to adults (*Board v. Barnette*, 1943; *Tinker v. Des Moines*, 1969). Substantial case law has focused on the rights of children and adolescents in the school and juvenile justice systems (*In re Gault*, 1967). For the purposes of this chapter, it is sufficient to note that while children are considered within the penumbra of constitutional protections, the right of the state to limit individuals' rights is given greater weight in the balancing test than when the rights of adults are at issue.

The limits on the rights of children are grounded in the dual concepts of parental rights and the right of the state to assume the parental burden when necessary specifically to increase access to treatment. Thus, for example, adolescents 16 years and older may consent to mental health care but do not have the **right to refuse** treatment. A 16-year-old can walk into a clinic, request a psychiatric assessment, and receive needed subsequent treatment. However, as defined by most states, "voluntary treatment" is related only to whether the parent volunteers. Thus when a parent believes his or her 16-year-old needs treatment for a mental disorder, that parent can commit the youth to an inpatient setting even over the teen's objections. This commitment, because of the parent's decision, is treated as a "voluntary" admission.

Box 12-10. *Olmstead* Decision Overview

- If an individual is involuntarily committed to a hospital because of mental illness, that individual has the right to treatment of that illness in a safe and humane environment.

- Because of their liberty interest, individuals have a right to treatment in the "least restrictive setting."

- The Americans with Disabilities Act requires states to make reasonable efforts to create community-based services so that those individuals who are able and willing to receive services in the community in lieu of a hospital can do so.

- To date, no cases have been adjudicated on whether an individual not committed to an institution has a right to treatment; no case to date establishes an absolute right to treatment in the community.

Under such a circumstance, it is the parent who makes a voluntary decision on behalf of the child based on the legal theory that the parent has a duty and ability to recognize symptoms of illness and to seek and follow medical advice. The parent's right to do so is grounded in the legal definition of family, which acknowledges that parents possess what a child lacks in maturity, experience, and the capacity to make difficult life decisions. More important, historically the law has assumed that natural bonds of affection lead parents to act in the best interests of their children (Blackstone, as cited in *Parham v. J. R.*, 1979; Kent, as cited in *Parham v. J. R.*, 1979).

Some children under age 18 are legally defined as "emancipated minors," and as such are treated as if they were adults for the purposes of decision making. Most states provide that youth age 16 and over who have a child of their own are emancipated minors. Other situations also may give rise to this status. However, since determinations vary from state to state, the law must be reviewed carefully in any given situation.

Rights of Children to Treatment

Under what circumstances, if any, are children guaranteed a constitutional right to mental health care? As a class, children are virtually guaranteed public funding for needed medical treatment. Today, the number of children covered under federal health insurance (Medicaid) is expanding as health reform initiatives continue to move forward. Thus funding for some health care generally is available to children, based on a presumption that minors are entitled to health care provided or supported by the government even though neither the Constitution nor judicial interpretations have enunciated a specific right to treatment. Nonetheless, there is a growing recognition that any children placed under the state's jurisdiction (i.e., wards of the state) are entitled to needed mental health care. This trend is reflected in a series of foster care cases in California.

Many children in foster care have significant unmet mental health needs. In 2002, the Bazelon Center for Mental Health Law filed a lawsuit against the State of California challenging the state's failure to provide home- and community-based mental health services to children either already in the foster care system or at risk for removal from their families. The state agreed to close the worst of its housing institutions and to establish community-based services. However, three years later, in 2005, services were still lacking; the suit continued. Ultimately, the presiding federal judge ordered the parties to meet and report back on how comprehensive services could be covered and billed under Medi-Cal (California's Medicaid program). Only in this way could providers be assured that they would be reimbursed for delivering these critical behavioral health services to children in foster care. The parties finally agreed on how best to provide these services in 2009. Justice had prevailed: Children in foster care now had the right to treatment. And it only took seven years! Over the next few years, it will be interesting to see the national impact of this federal case, if any, on the rights of children under state care to receive appropriate community-based treatment for mental problems under state health programs such as Medicaid.

Responsibility for children in foster care falls under the auspices of state social services or human resource agencies. Children in foster care have done nothing wrong; most are victims of circumstances such as abuse or abandonment. In contrast, children who have run afoul of the law—juvenile offenders—find themselves under the jurisdiction of state juvenile justice agencies. In many cases, children are both wards of the state and under the jurisdiction of juvenile justice agencies. Moreover, many of these young people also experience serious emotional disturbances or substance abuse problems that require public sector treatment.

Juvenile Justice and the Rights of Children

Too often the first contact for a child living at home in poverty or in foster care who exhibits an emotional or substance use problem is a police officer, not a mental health clinician. Sadly, the juvenile justice field is paradigmatic of the adage that "the road to hell is paved with good intentions." Established as a benign alternative to the adult criminal justice system, its purpose was to act as a substitute parent to help youth onto the right path. Because of the concept that the juvenile justice process was a caretaking process rather than an adversarial process, many protections developed as protection in adult trials, were dropped. Thus, because the state was acting like a parent, the courts allowed for scuttling of many constitutional safeguards such as the requirement that the child have a law and rules of evidence. New legal terminology developed to reflect the new reality. Youth would be "placed in" rather than "sentenced to" corrective environments. They would not be found "guilty"; rather, they would be adjudged "delinquent." Their records would be held private.

For a very good summary of the historical development of juvenile law, see *In re Gault* (1967). That case provided a forum for the Supreme Court to establish unequivocally that children arrested for a crime are entitled to due process protection in juvenile proceedings. In the *Gault* case, a 15-year-old boy, Gerald Gault, was arrested for allegedly having made lewd telephone calls. When he was taken from his home by police, his parents were not home; no attempt was made to contact them or to allow Gerald to call them. After hearings before a juvenile court judge, Gerald was ordered committed to the state industrial school as a juvenile delinquent until he reached the age of majority. Based on the facts presented in the case, Gerald had clearly received none of the legal protections afforded to adult defendants, such as the right to have a lawyer present while being questioned.

On taking the case, the Supreme Court first opined that unquestionably a juvenile was entitled to due process before being committed. The question became, how much process is sufficient to meet constitutional standards in a juvenile proceeding? The court explained that wide differences had always existed between the procedural rights accorded adults and those of juveniles. In virtually all jurisdictions, certain rights granted to adults are withheld from juveniles. It also summarized the rationale underlying the juvenile system: A juvenile would benefit from informal court

proceedings as if the court were a wise caretaker ready to steer the juvenile to the right path. The fatherly judge would provide guidance to protect the youth from continuing on a downward path.

However, in *In re Gault*, the court also decried a juvenile system that used a screen of paternalism to deprive juveniles of rights and protections. The court cited studies that made clear that the reality of the juvenile system was sharply at odds with the theory. The court then explained how the system operated in *Gault* to deprive the boy of any protection whatsoever. It stated:

> Ultimately, however, we confront the reality of that portion of the Juvenile Court process with which we deal in this case. A boy is charged with misconduct. The boy is committed to an institution where he may be restrained of liberty for years. It is of no Constitutional consequence and of limited practical meaning that the institution to which he is committed is called an Industrial School. The fact of the matter is that, however euphemistic the title, a "receiving home" or an "industrial school" for juveniles is an institution of confinement in which the child is incarcerated for a greater or lesser time. His world becomes "a building with whitewashed walls, regimented routine and institutional hours...." Instead of mother and father and sisters and brothers and friends and classmates, his world is peopled by guards, custodians, state employees, and "delinquents" confined with him for anything from waywardness to rape and homicide. In view of this, it would be extraordinary if our Constitution did not require the procedural regularity and the exercise of care implied in the phrase "due process." Under our Constitution, the condition of being a boy does not justify a kangaroo court. (*In re Gault*, pp. 26–28)

After clarifying its abhorrence of a juvenile system that used a screen of benevolence to strip children of their rights, the Supreme Court stated that during a delinquency proceeding, juveniles are absolutely entitled at least to the most basic due process protections of the Fifth and 14th Amendments. After the *Gault* decision, it became clear that when fundamental liberties are threatened, a government's good intentions alone are no substitute for constitutional due process.

FORENSICS: THE NEXUS OF MENTAL HEALTH AND CRIMINAL LAW

As described earlier in this chapter, if the standard of dangerousness is reached, persons with mental illnesses can be committed involuntarily to an institution and, in fact, be deprived of their liberty. This is virtually the only situation in which a noncriminal can be institutionalized against his or her will. Thus, while the purpose of confinement is medical treatment, not punishment, the language of civil commitment resonates with the language of constitutional protections in many of the same terms as found in criminal law.

When a person with a mental illness commits a criminal act, the issues become even more complicated. The two worlds of forced treatment and forced punishment collide, raising questions of both good health policy and good justice. For example, is it good public mental health policy to incarcerate individuals whose behaviors result from illnesses? Will such a policy further heighten the stigma associated with mental illnesses and result in still greater reluctance to seek treatment? Should treatment for mental disorders be compulsory as a penalty for committing minor crimes such as trespassing or loitering? Further, what circumstances justify imprisonment of large numbers of persons with mental or substance use disorders for the commission of nonviolent offenses? These questions, and many others, arise from the legal framework erected by the forensic common law and attendant statutes discussed in the balance of this section.

Criminal Law 101

When a person acts in a way defined as illegal under state or federal statute, that individual can be prosecuted and, if found guilty, be punished. Criminal behavior is not a private matter between individuals; it is a matter for the government. Thus if an individual is robbed and reports the robbery to the government, the government, not the individual, takes the robber to court. The victim is a witness. Criminal actions result in punishment by the state, ranging from a fine to a mandate to perform certain actions under court order (such as restitution or community service) to imprisonment.

A person accused of a crime—a defendant—is entitled to a plethora of procedural protections specifically delineated in the Fifth and 14th Amendments of the US Constitution. These include the right to a lawyer, the right to refuse to testify, and the principle that one is considered innocent until proven guilty. The state assumes the burden of proving beyond a reasonable doubt that the crime occurred and that the defendant committed the crime. The defendant need only demonstrate that the burden of proof is not met or, alternatively, provide a defense that absolves the defendant or mitigates his or her guilt. The trial, during which the facts of the case are proved and the defenses are heard, is step one. Step two is a decision about guilt and responsibility, rendered by either judge or jury. The third step, in the case of a finding of guilt, is the assignment of a penalty. Even this step need not end the process; the legal issues argued may be appealed through two further levels of the judicial system. Both state court systems and the federal government provide for appellate court review under certain conditions until the highest court of the state or federal system (the Supreme Court) is reached.

The Insanity Defense

A defendant has the right either to admit or to deny the crime with which he or she is charged. A defendant who admits to the action has a right to provide a defense asserting no guilt based on exonerating factors, such as self-defense. Similarly, after an individual is found to be guilty, the defense can plead special circumstances that could alter the type, duration, or scope of the penalty imposed.

In common law, a doctrine took shape over time enabling a defendant to plead not guilty by reason of insanity. It is based on the premise that to be held liable for one's actions, one must possess intent, the knowledge of what one is doing and that the action is wrong (also referred to as mens rea, translated as "guilty mind"). The earliest accepted enunciation of a standard for such a defense was in M'Naghten (1843).

In 1843, woodworker Daniel M'Naghten, believing he was the target of a conspiracy involving the pope and British Prime Minister Robert Peel, traveled to 10 Downing Street to ambush Peel and mistakenly shot and killed the prime minister's secretary. During the ensuing trial, several psychiatrists testified that M'Naghten was delusional. A jury agreed and declared him not guilty by reason of insanity. In response to the public outrage about the decision, a year later a judicial panel set forth a legal standard that has been the foundation of an insanity defense ever since. Under what has come to be known as the M'Naghten rule, defendants may be acquitted only if they labored "under such defect of reason from disease of the mind" as to not realize what they were doing or why it was a crime. It is sometimes called the right/wrong test.

This relatively strict right/wrong rule became the common-law standard adopted in the United States for both federal and state crimes. Over time, some states added a further behavioral component, enabling a defendant to prove that mental illness had created an "irresistible impulse" to carry out the action. Since then, the stringency of the insanity defense in the United States has waxed and waned.

In 1962, the American Law Institute promulgated an alternative, two-pronged standard, amending the M'Naghten rule and making it easier for a defendant to prevail. Under this standard, a defendant cannot be held criminally responsible if at the time of the act in question and "as a result of a mental disease or defect, he lacks substantial capacity either to appreciate the criminality of his conduct or to conform his conduct to the requirements of the law" (American Law Institute, 1962). Thus a defendant would prevail if he proved lack of understanding or the inability to control his behavior. Many states subsequently

adopted this standard; today, however, only 18 states follow it. While a diagnosis based on the *Diagnostic and Statistical Manual of Mental Disorders* (APA, 1994) may provide evidence to meet insanity defense standards, it is not necessary to substantiate a plea of insanity or mental illness. The clinical and legal standards are related but separate. One is a medical diagnosis to determine treatment and clinical practice; the other is a legal standard regarding the state of mind at the time a criminal act was committed and the rsulting behavior behavior at issue in the crime.

In a 1981 event that eerily paralleled the M'Naghten case, John Hinckley attempted to assassinate then-President Reagan. At trial for the attempted assassination, Hinckley pled not guilty by reason of insanity; the jury agreed. Once again, the public was outraged and called for elimination of the insanity defense. Cooler heads prevailed, and a legislative compromise was crafted and signed into law. The Insanity Defense Reform Act of 1984 restored a stricter standard, once again making it more difficult for a defendant to prevail. The act requires that the mental disease be severe and eliminated the ability to invoke the defense based on the behavioral component alone. Many states followed suit and adopted similarly strict standards.

The most recent twist in the tortured tale of *M'Naghten* and the insanity defense has been the emergence of a wholly new plea: guilty but mentally ill (GBMI). Under this standard, a defendant admits guilt and receives treatment for his or her mental illness (see, for example, Maryland General Code, 1986). In contrast to the insanity defense, under which the prosecutor must prove sanity as an element of the crime, under GBMI the burden falls on the defendant to prove that mental illness was the cause of the criminal action. Moreover, a GBMI verdict means that guilt is a given, without regard to the defendant's status as mentally ill. Thus if treatment is successful, the defendant may still be required to complete a prison sentence.

Subsequently, both the concept of mens rea and the relationship between mental health and criminality have experienced a new wrinkle, due to the Supreme Court's decision in *Roper v. Simmons* (2005). In determining whether the death penalty is an appropriate punishment for juveniles, the Supreme Court added a new dimension to its analysis, ruling that the penalty cannot be assigned to juveniles because their brains are still immature in the areas related to judgment and moral decision making. The court also referred to normative values in other Western countries on this issue. It will be interesting to see the impact this decision has on guilt and sentencing in future cases involving offenders with mental illnesses.

While many are intrigued by this doctrinal evolution that, in many ways, both informs and defines the way people perceive of criminal intent and the alleged dangers posed by mental illnesses, the actual number of major cases involving an insanity defense is relatively small. In fact, a study of cases in Baltimore City (Maryland) circuit courts (Janofsky, Dunn, Roskes, Briskin, & Rudolph, 1996) revealed that of 60,432 indictments filed in the courts, only 190 defendants entered a plea of not criminally responsible. All but 8 dropped the plea before trial. In each of those remaining cases, because both the state and the defense agreed the defendant should be found not criminally responsible, the plea was uncontested at trial. Janofsky and colleagues concluded:

> There were no trials that contested the plea of not criminally responsible. The state and defense agreed with each other for all of the defendants who actually retained the plea at trial. The perception that the insanity defense is overused and misused is not borne out by data. (p. 1464)

These findings are borne out in other studies.

A number of other issues at the intersection of mental illness and criminal justice are perhaps thus more important than the foregoing topics, among them:

- the consequences of pleading, if at all, guilty to minor charges when mentally ill
- the determination of competency to stand trial
- confidentiality, the duty to protect, and the Tarasoff doctrine

- The growing transinstitutionalization of people with mental illnesses from hospitals to jails and prisons.

Each of these is described briefly below.

Pleading Guilty to Minor Charges

Persons who commit minor crimes or misdemeanors for which the sentence is one year or less are sometimes advised to plead guilty but mentally ill. Some of those crimes might be as minor as loitering, urinating in a public place, or talking back to a police officer. In such cases, individuals who otherwise might have been jailed for a relatively short time, if at all, could be institutionalized for years if they are not "cured," despite the fact that under the normal civil commitment standard of dangerousness, they would have been released. The public defenders who often represent such individuals usually have little time and few resources to spend on individual cases. The plea of guilty but mentally ill offers an easy way out. Unfortunately, for the plaintiff it can become a permanent way in, instead.

In *Jones v. U.S.* (1983) the Supreme Court held:

> When a criminal defendant establishes by a preponderance of the evidence that he is not guilty of a crime by reason of insanity, the Constitution permits the Government, on the basis of the insanity judgment, to confine to a mental institution until such time as he has regained his sanity *or* [emphasis added] is no longer a danger to himself or society. (p. 370)

That is, even if an individual does not meet the dangerousness standard required for involuntary civil commitment, he or she can be held in a hospital until found to be "sane." In the case of *Jones*, the plaintiff remained in the hospital far longer than the maximum one-year sentence he could have received for the misdemeanor of petty larceny with which he had been charged. In most cases, virtually no jail time would accompany a first offense of this type. In most states petty larceny means theft of a small amount of money or an object valued at less than $500 without assault or violence. In other words, this misdemeanor would encompass stealing a loaf of bread or shoplifting. Yet Jones was institutionalized for well over a year. Conversely, in *Foucha v. Louisiana* (1984), the Supreme Court held that the defendant, although dangerous, could not be held in a psychiatric hospital because, despite having an antisocial personality, he was not mentally ill.

Competency to Stand Trial

The US Constitution guarantees every defendant the right to be present at trial and to confront witnesses. Further, the right to trial guaranteed by the Sixth Amendment implies that the defendant has a right to meaningfully participate in the defense against the charges. To do so, however, the defendant must be competent to understand the charges and the court proceedings. Unfortunately, that concept is a relatively slippery one. At times, legal reviewers have been heard to say that the standard for competency to stand trial is so low as to be meaningless.

Cynicism aside, it is often the case that a defendant's inability to understand the trial because of incompetence is recognized In such cases, the defendant is committed pretrial to a psychiatric hospital for treatment of the conditions underlying the incompetency. But if treatment is unsuccessful, what happens next?

In *Jackson v. Indiana* (1972) the Supreme Court held:

> Indiana's indefinite commitment of a criminal defendant solely on account of his lack of capacity to stand trial violates due process. Such a defendant cannot be held more than the reasonable period of time necessary to determine whether there is a substantial probability that he will attain competency in the foreseeable future. If it is determined that he will not, the State must either institute civil proceedings applicable to indefinite commitment of those not charged with crime or release the defendant. (p. 738)

The catch is that as soon as the defendant is restored to competency, he or she must be returned to court and tried.

A conundrum presented by the *Jackson* decision is whether a defendant can be medicated forcibly to restore competency sufficient for a trial. As in any case involving forced treatment, due process applies, with the government's interest on one side and the defendant's liberty interest on the other. The government must demonstrate that its interest is of the highest order (i.e., that it represents a compelling interest), that the defendant's liberty interest is protected by a hearing, and that medications will be used only if no less intrusive alternatives are possible. In *Sell v. U.S.* (2003), the Supreme Court determined that the government's interest in both restoring a criminal defendant to competence to stand trial and maintaining the defendant in a competent state so that he or she may be tried is a recognized "compelling interest." Then, based on earlier cases of forced medication in prison, the court declared that medication is permitted if a hearing determines it is clinically appropriate for the individual, no less intrusive treatments or medications will achieve the goal, and medication will not significantly impair the defendant's trial performance. This decision represents an effort to achieve a balance among dangerousness, the seriousness of the crime at issue, the likelihood that the medication will work, and the lack of alternatives.

Duty to Protect: Liability of Clinicians for Potential Criminal Activity of a Patient

Although the privacy rights of individuals and the concomitant right to confidentiality are sacrosanct both in legal doctrine and in medical ethics, at times public health or policy interests override a clinician's professional duty to the patient. In 1976, the Supreme Court of California developed the Tarasoff doctrine on just that topic. In *Tarasoff v. Regents of the University of California* (1976), a university student under psychiatric care declared his intention to buy a gun and shoot a fellow student with whom he previously had a relationship. The treating psychologist warned the appropriate campus security services, who in turn warned the student, named Tarasoff, to stay away from the potential victim. However, after reviewing the file, a psychiatrist working for the security services said no more should be done and destroyed the warning letter from Tarasoff's treating psychiatrist. Shortly thereafter, the potential victim became a real victim, killed by Tarasoff.

The state supreme court ruling held:

> When a therapist determines, or pursuant to the standards of his profession should determine, that his patient presents a serious danger of violence to another, he incurs an obligation to use reasonable care to protect the intended victim against such danger. The discharge of this duty may require the therapist to take one or more of various steps. Thus, it may call for him to warn the intended victim, to notify the police, or to take whatever steps are reasonably necessary under the circumstances. (*Tarasoff v. the Regents of the University of California*, 1976, p. 340)

What is most interesting for the purposes of this chapter is the reasoning behind the decision rather than the liability issues related to practice. The court quoted as precedent that doctors have been held liable for negligent failure to diagnose a contagious disease or failing to warn family members of it. The judge in *Tarasoff* wrote,"The protective privilege ends where the public peril begins" (p. 347). Since that time, 17 states have adopted a Tarasoff-like doctrine.

Many legal scholars and treatment professionals worried that Tarasoff decision would create great upheaval in treatment, but that has not happened. Rather, it has become a basic part of treatment itself that the professional duty to warn and protect the public at times may supersede patient rights when there are clear signs of specific dangerousness.

Transinstitutionalization

More people with mental illnesses are in jails and prisons than are in psychiatric hospitals. Opinions abound about why this is so. To understand the issues and potential solutions, see chapters 13, 14, and 15.

Diverting from Incarceration: Mental Health Courts and Drug Courts

Relatively recently, states and localities across the United States have sought to respond to the problem of increased jail or prison incarceration of people with mental or substance use disorders by creating alternatives that divert such individuals from penal institutions. One popular model establishes specialty courts that enable defendants to voluntarily enter their jurisdiction, plead guilty, and be given a mandatory treatment plan rather than a jail sentence.

Although the substitution of treatment for jail is undeniably laudable, there are potential areas of concern.. For example, if a defendant must plead guilty to qualify for adjudication in these specialized courts and to receive the resulting treatment plan, the defendant is giving up in a relatively coercive setting the right to any kind of a trial or fact determination. Also, the treatment plan might last longer than the duration of any prison or jail sentence. A third concern is that if the treatment plan is violated, the court has the option of sending the defendant back to court for sentencing, and since the defendant already plead guilty as a condition of entering the specialized diversion program, there is no need for trial.

Further, controversy already is beginning to brew over overzealous judges who mandate long treatment plans and then place a person who fails to comply even with a minor part of the treatment protocol in jail for long periods. This is especially worrisome in the case of juvenile drug courts. (For a review and analysis of mental health courts, see Bernstein & Seltzer, 2003.)

All of the foregoing discussion is to demonstrate that in the area of legal custody and abrogation of liberty, care must be taken to create solutions that respect individual rights even while creating new, beneficial systems, as the cautionary lessons of the juvenile justice debacle clearly suggest.

SPECIAL TOPICS

The previous sections described specific areas of law with particular relevance to the practice of behavioral health care. In application, the principles provide the underpinnings for a variety of practical topics facing public mental health professionals. This section provides a sampling of those topics.

Advance Directives

Advance directives have been one of the more promising recent innovations to give patients a greater voice in their treatment for mental illnesses. Completed when patients are competent, advance directives allow patients to make choices about particular treatments and to appoint proxy decision makers, all to be set into motion should patients become incompetent to make decisions for themselves (Appelbaum, 2004). Thus one can make a living will or directive about life support choices before becoming ill and unable to speak or before becoming incompetent. Key for the public mental health system is the right for persons with mental illnesses to sign advance directives to set out their desires regarding treatment during psychiatric crises that result in a loss of competence.

Some lawyers and scholars argue, for example, that it should be possible to use an advance directive proactively to refuse treatment with medication during a later psychotic episode. In *Hargrave v. Vermont* (2003), a woman did just that; however, the hospital and the state sought to override her directive. With a history of paranoid schizophrenia and multiple hospital admissions, Nancy Hargrave had completed an advance directive refusing "any and all antipsychotic...medications." When she was later committed involuntarily, the state sought to override the directive. On her behalf, her lawyers argued that the Vermont statute permitting an override in fact violated the ADA by allowing much broader override authority for directives related to treatment of mental illnesses than for other medical treatment.

The Second Circuit Court of Appeals agreed with Hargrave, leaving a relatively open question about these issues on the national level. Ultimately, a case will reach the Supreme Court and will harken not only to the ADA but also to the constitutional cases about the right to refuse treatment. On the other side will be the issue of whether a state can commit an individual on the grounds of dangerousness but then not render treatment because of a valid advance directive. What does legal precedent suggest by way of resolution? Are the use of advance directives valid as a public health tool? Can an answer be given that serves both needs and is ethical as well? The questions continue to beg for answers.

College Students with Mental Health Care Needs

NOTICE: College Students. Feeling depressed or anxious? Seek help at Counseling Services **BUT** do so at your own risk. Be advised that students seeking help might be subject to disciplinary action or suspended.

That is okay, make sure to come see us—we are here to help.

Strange? Unfortunately, this hypothetical notice reflects the state of affairs on many college campuses today. In the past 10 years, several cases relating to campus mental health care have achieved prominence. The two foremost themes are those of confidentiality when working with seriously ill students and administrative actions taken against students who ask for help.

Cases in this area are best exemplified by that of an MIT student who visited the health service for treatment and ultimately committed suicide. Her parents never knew of her troubles, since confidentiality laws forbid health professionals from sharing. They filed suit in a Massachusetts Superior Court. There the Judge ruled that the parents of Elizabeth H. Shin, an MIT student who committed suicide on the campus in 2000, could proceed with their claims against MIT administrators and staff members for failing to prevent her death, although the plaintiffs cannot seek damages from MIT itself.

> Mr. DeLuca [attorney for the plaintiffs] has argued that MIT officials were negligent in Ms. Shin's death because they knew of her suicide threats but did not immediately attempt to help her on the day she died. Had the defendants in the case hospitalized Ms. Shin, called her parents, or gone to her dormitory room,

the lawyer believes, the student might not have taken her life.

After returning to MIT, Ms. Shin received treatment from numerous campus psychiatrists through the spring of her sophomore year. On April 10, 2000, Ms. Shin told two students in her dormitory that she planned to kill herself that day—a threat she reiterated to her dorm supervisor. At a meeting later that morning, MIT deans and psychiatrists discussed Ms. Shin's condition, including her statements about committing suicide.

Although it is contested what, if any, treatment options were discussed at the meeting, one MIT psychiatrist scheduled an appointment for Ms. Shin at a nearby psychiatric facility for the following day, according to the judge's ruling. The psychiatrist also left Ms. Shin a voice-mail message in which he informed her of the appointment and told her that he was available for the rest of the day. That night Ms. Shin set herself on fire inside her room. She died three days later. [Sontag, NY Times, April 28, 2002; Bombardieri, Boston Globe, July 30, 2005]

This case, like all legal rulings, was decided on its individual facts. Given the specific facts regarding the treating clinicians' behavior, the judge's ruling allowing the claims to move forward because it was reasonably foreseeable that she would harm herself, makes sense. More critical, however, is how this same line of reasoning might be applied in other cases. In the years since the Shin case, judicial rulings have varied. Nonetheless, schools remain particularly concerned about legal liability arising from insufficient action, too much action, or breach of confidentiality when confronting a student's emotional problem.

Some schools or universities have used concerns about liability for harm—whether to the student/patient or to others—as a rationale for removing students who seek mental health care from the campus environment altogether.

Jordan Nott, a 21-year-old former straight A student at George Washington University, sued the institution and several individuals at the university in the Superior Court of the District of Columbia [*Nott v George Washington University*, Civil Case 05–8503court, alleging they "disciplined him, threatened him with criminal prosecution and ultimately ended his college career at the school of his choice" after he sought help for depression at the university's counseling center.

In April 2004, Jordan's very close friend committed suicide by jumping from a window. Jordan and another friend were standing outside the locked door trying to get in. In September he began to experience depression and kept thinking about his friend. He went to University Counseling Services [CSS] for help and eventually was prescribed Ambien and Zoloft. After these sessions, Jordan thought about whether he wanted to commit suicide. He also became anxious that he was having adverse reactions to Zoloft and because he knew that sometimes, patients on Zoloft had heightened symptoms before recovery and were at a greater risk for suicide.

Jordan was nervous that he might become suicidal if left alone and he knew his roommate would be away for the coming weekend increased his fears. As a precaution, he asked his roommate to take him to the George Washington University emergency room for evaluation and they admitted him for evaluation. The UCC then notified Jordan's parents who made plans to travel to D.C. Late that day, October 26, the Dean of Students sent a letter to the hospital explaining the school's policy about "psychological distress in the residence halls" to Jordan. In short, anyone who had suicidal thoughts or emergency psychiatric intervention needed to be "cleared" by the Director of the UCC and Dean of Students before they could return to the dorm. Clearance was dependent on taking many steps and jumping through many hoops before a student could be successful.

In the meantime, the school advised Jordan's mother that they would be sending a Letter of Suspension and that Jordan had to understand the seriousness of the situation. Meanwhile, Jordan received a hand-delivered letter in the hospital notifying him that he had violated the Code of Student Conduct by engaging in endangering behavior. According to the Code, endangering behavior is that which imperils the life or safety of any student including oneself. In other words, by checking himself in to the hospital for evaluation Jordan endangered his life or others and was therefore "indefinitely suspended." He was immediately barred from re-entering his dorm room or any University property and was told that if he did he would be arrested. Not only could he not return to collect his belongings or attend or register for any classes but he was also barred from any public events on campus. This all took place less than 48 hours after he had gone to the emergency room and before his mother even arrived to see him. Jordan was then advised there would be a formal disciplinary hearing on November 3. Jordan was then given a Hobson's choice of withdrawing from school or facing the hearing which would then go on his record if he lost and carry a penalty of expulsion. He withdrew.

In October 2006, GWU entered into a settlement with the Nott family although they never officially acknowledged any wrongdoing. As to the impact on those who might seek help for depression, Jordan's own words that he wrote in a letter to the school's administrators are eloquent:

"If I had known how I would be treated, I never would have checked myself into that hospital....Rather, your actions pushed me into a huge feeling of failure which pushed me further into depression....You did me no favor by removing me from my closest friends and sending me home to an empty town and I can guarantee you that you will do no future student a favor by doing the same to him or her."

In a statement announcing the settlement, "all parties stressed that students should seek professional help in times of need." Joint Statement from the George Washington University and the Bazelon Center for Mental Health Law Regarding the Lawsui by Jordan Nott, October 31, 2006 www.gwnewscenter.org.

According to recent reports, that need is great. Studies suggest that 15% of college students suffer from depression but fewer than 50% receive treatment (Capriccioso, 2006). Could that be related to the stigma reinforced by punitive college policies? Certainly this is a public health challenge; the legal system must help reinforce good public health practice.

Community Housing

A major issue in treating individuals with mental illnesses in the community is housing. Much housing, when available in the first place—whether supervised, supportive, or independent—is unaffordable. When people with serious mental illnesses were institutionalized, as most were until the early 1960s, treatment and housing were one and the same. With the deinstitutionalization movement, many individuals were released to the community, where housing issues began to proliferate.

Here we are concerned with the right of individuals with mental illnesses to safe, habitable, humane housing in the community. Advocates argue that the constitutional right established in *O'Connor v. Donaldson* (1975) to treatment in the least restrictive environment includes housing. The ADA further supports the rights of individuals with mental illnesses to access to housing unfettered by discrimination against people with mental disabilities.

All that aside, adequate housing remains an elusive goal. Many individuals with serious mental illnesses live in substandard, unregulated group homes or in board-and-care homes. In 2009, the *New York Times* reported on a troubling case involving substandard housing conditions in group homes for the mentally ill funded by New York State (Bosman, 2009). The initial legal papers were filed in 2003 and described poorly run adult homes essentially warehousing the inhabitants. The article explained that six years later, the case was still wending its way through federal courts. Abuses and problems continue to be reported in national newspapers. See, for example the New York Times article on fraud and housing (Levy, 2003).

Mental Health During Emergencies: Natural or Man-made Disasters

Today, many jurisdictions are grappling with creating emergency plans in the event of a catastrophic disaster akin to Hurricane Katrina or the September 11 attacks. Such emergency situations give rise to a host of special issues related to the treatment of people with mental illnesses. While this complex topic is beyond the scope of this chapter, public health officials should be aware that the laws attendant to treatment for persons with mental illnesses will significantly affect the scope and content of outreach and care for those special populations in emergencies. For example, when is it permissible to forcibly detain a person suffering a panic attack and unable to move or who is having a delusion that the first responders are aliens intent on harm? Does such a circumstance provide sufficient justification to use force based on imminent danger to the public? Is temporary, severe panic tantamount to a state of incompetence for decision making? The federal Centers for Disease Control and Prevention currently is preparing guidelines on these issues. Questions that might arise in such a circumstance therefore should be referred to a lawyer for help in crafting responses and actions based on those guidelines.

CONCLUDING THOUGHTS

The public health perspective supports a system of care that promotes prevention, continuity of care, integrated care, and a focus on recovery. Many of the landmark legal decision focused on mental health or civil rights of persons with mental illnesses over the last decades directly affect the ability to promote the public's health while strengthening and respecting individual liberty. Because community and individual interests often are in conflict, it is in the purview of the legal system to examine the conflict and explicate the choices. The development of legal protections over the years reveals a tension between the professional medical community and the patient/consumer and highlights issues endemic to public health. A study of the evolution of the law discloses years of efforts to weigh the balance underlying questions fundamental to the development of an effective, humane public health system of care for persons with mental illnesses.

This chapter has explored many of the concepts, cases, and laws that have shaped today's public mental health landscape and that have provided impetus for many of the reforms described in other chapters. As other issues arise and specifically as society continues to address the relationship between behavior and disease in the public health context, the law and the service delivery system will evolve.

However, *plus ça change, plus c'est la même chose* (the more things change, the more they remain the same). The age-old principles of common law will remain as the foundation for decisions impacting public health as we move into the future. Thus a basic understanding of these principles and the importance of balancing individual rights with the public's need will provide a strengthened ability to shape the future of public mental health.

REFERENCES

Addington v. Texas, 441 U.S. 418 (1979).
American Law Institute Model Penal Code § 101 *et seq.* (1962).
American Psychiatric Association. (1994). *Diagnostic and statistical manual of mental disorders* (4th ed.). Washington, DC: Author.
American Psychiatric Association. (1993). *Consent to voluntary hospitalization* (Task Force Report 34). Washington, DC: Author.
American Psychiatric Association. (1998). Guidelines for assessing the decisionmaking capacities of potential research subjects with cognitive impairments. *American Journal of Psychiatry, 155*(11), 1649–1650.
Americans with Disabilities Act, 42 U.S.C. § 12132 (1990).
Appelbaum, P. S. (2004). Psychiatric advance directives and the treatment of committed patients. *Psychiatric Services, 55*(7), 751–763.

Appelbaum, P. S., & Grisso, P. (1998). Assessing patients' capacities to consent to treatment. *New England Journal of Medicine, 319*(25), 1635–1638.

Bernstein, B., & Seltzer, T. (2003, Spring). Criminalization of people with mental illnesses: The role of mental health courts in system reform. *University of the District of Columbia Law Review*, pp. 143–160.

Blackstone, W., Commentaries *447, as cited in Parham v. J. R., 442 U.S. 584 (1979).

Board v. Barnette, 319 U.S. 624 (1943).

Bosman, J., (2009, February 20). Suit progresses on housing for mentally ill. *The New York Times*. Retrieved from http://www.nytimes.com/2009/02/20/nyregion/20adult.html?partner+rss&emc=rss

Bureau of Justice Statistics. (2006). *Special report: Mental health problems of prison and jail inmates*. Washington, DC: US Department of Justice.

Butterfield, F. (1998, March 5). Prisons replace hospitals for the nation's mentally ill. *The New York Times*, A1.

Capriccioso, R. (2006, March 13). Counseling crisis. *Inside Higher Education*. Retrieved from http://www.insidehighered.com/news/2006/03/13/counseling

Civil Rights Act, 42 U.S.C. § 2000 *et seq.* (1964).

Civil Rights of Institutionalized Persons Act, 42 U.S.C. § 1997 (1980).

Confidentiality of Alcohol and Drug Abuse Patient Records Regulation, 42 C.F.R. Pt. 2 (1987).

Cox, J. F., Morschauser, P. C., Banks, S., & Stone, J. L. (2001). A five-year population study of persons involved in the mental health and local correctional systems. *Journal of Behavioral Health Services and Research, 28*(2), 177–187.

Foucha v. Louisiana, 504 U.S. 71 (1984).

Griswold v. Connecticut, 381 U.S. 429 (1965).

Hargrave v. Vermont, 340 F.3d 27 (2d Cir. 2003).

Hartocollis, A. (2009, February 5). Abuse is found at psychiatric unit run by the City. *The New York Times*. Retrieved from http://www.nytimes.com/2009/02/06/nyregion/06kings.html

In re Gault, 387 U.S. 1 (1967).

Insanity Defense Reform Act, 18 U.S.C. § 17 (1984).

Jackson v. Indiana, 406 U.S. 715 (1972).

Jacobson v. Massachusetts, 197 U.S. 11 (1905).

Janofsky, J. S., Dunn, M. H., Roskes, E. J., Briskin, J. K., & Rudolph, M. S. (1996). Insanity defense pleas in Baltimore City: An analysis of outcome. *American Journal of Psychiatry, 153*(11), 1464–1468.

Jones, J. (1981). *Bad blood: The Tuskegee syphilis experiment. A tragedy of race and medicine*. New York, NY: Free Press.

Jones v. U.S., 463 U.S. 354 (1983).

Judd, A., & Miller, A. (2007, January 7). A hidden shame: Death in Georgia's mental hospitals. *The Atlanta Journal-Constitution*, A1. Retrieved from http://psychrights.org/Stories/GeorgiaHiddenShame.htm

Justice Center. (2002). *Fact sheet: The criminal justice and mental health consensus project*. Washington, DC: Council of State Governments.

Kansas v. Hendricks, 521 U.S. 346 (1997).

Kent, J., Commentaries on American Law *190, as cited in Parham v. J. R., 442 U.S. 584 (1979).

Levy, C. (2003, July 3). U.S. indicts doctor in fraud at state homes for mentally ill. *The New York Times*. Retrieved from http://www.nytimes.com/2003/01/07/nyregion/us-indicts-doctor-in-fraud-at-state-homes-for-mentally-ill.html

Loving v. Virginia, 388 U.S. 1 (1967).

Marbury v. Madison, 5 U.S. 137 (1803).

Maryland General Code Ann. §§ 12–108(a) (Supp. 1986).

Melton, G., Petrila, J., & Poythress, N. G. (1997). *Psychological evaluations for the courts: A handbook for mental health professionals and lawyers* (2nd ed.). New York, NY: Guilford.

Mills v. Rogers, 457 U.S. 291 (1982).

M'Naghten's Case, 10 C&F 200 (1843).

Murdock v. Pennsylvania, 319 U.S. 105 (1943).

O'Connor v. Donaldson, 422 U.S. 563 (1975).

Olmstead v. LC, 527 U.S. 581 (1999).

Rennie v. Klein, 653 F.2d 836 (1981), on remand, 722 F.2d 266 (1983).

Rogers v. Okin, 478 F. Supp. 1342 (D. Mass. 1979), 634 F.2d 650 (1st Cir. 1980).

Roper v. Simmons, 543 U.S. 551 (2005).

Mary E. Schloendorff, Appellant, v. The Society of the New York Hospital, Respondent, 211 N.Y. 125; 105 N.E. 92 (1914).

Sell v. U.S., 539 U.S. 166 (2003).

Tarasoff v. Regents of the University of California, 551 P.2d 334 (1976).

Teifion, D. (2001). Informed consent in psychiatric research: A conversation with Donald Steinwachs. *British Journal of Psychiatry, 178*, 297–298.

Tinker v. Des Moines, 393 U.S. 503 (1969).

Wyatt v. Aderholt, 503 F.2d 1305 (5th Cir.1974).

Wyatt v. Stickney, 325 F. Supp. 781 (M.D. Ala. 1971).

Wyatt v. Stickney, 344 F. Supp. 373–386 (M.D. Ala. 1972) (Bryce and Searcy Hospitals); 344 F. Supp. 387–407 (M.D. Ala. 1972) (Partlow State School and Hospital).

Youngberg v. Romeo, 457 U.S. 307 (1982).

Zinermon v. Burch, 494 U.S. 113 (1990).

13

American Mental Health Services: Perspective Through Care Patterns for 100 Adults, with Aggregate Facility, Service, and Cost Estimates

RONALD W. MANDERSCHEID

PIERRE ALEXANDRE

ANITA EVERETT

PHILIP LEAF

BENJAMIN ZABLOTSKY

Key Points

- Mental health services in the United States are provided through four sectors: the specialty sector, the general health care sector, the human service sector, and the self-help sector

- There are more than 4,000 specialty mental health facilities in the United States

- Over the course of 2004 there were more than 2,000,000 admissions to inpatient beds, more than 350,000 to residential beds, and more than 4,000,000 admissions to outpatient programs

- About 10% of persons served in more than 1,000 community health centers receive treatment for mental or behavioral disorders

- Of a random sample of 100 adults in the United States, 32 will experience a mental or substance use disorder during a given year

- Of the 32 persons with a disorder during the year, more than one third will have no health insurance coverage

- Of the original 100 adults, only 20 will participate in some form of behavioral health care over the course of a year

- There is considerable variation in care costs and other social costs across disorders, from an estimated $11 billion per year for simple phobia to over $200 billion per year for alcohol or drug use disorders

INTRODUCTION

Because American mental health services are provided through a number of different care systems, they are both complex and difficult to describe. (See earlier overviews in Schulberg & Manderscheid, 1989; Manderscheid, Henderson, Witkin, & Atay, 2000.) Moreover, mental health service capacity is insufficient to meet the need for care, as noted in a host of epidemiologic studies (Kessler, Demler, et al., 2005). Thus, to simplify the exploration of mental health care patterns in the United States, this chapter describes the mental health epidemiology and service delivery picture for 100 adults drawn at random from the American population.[1] As a corollary, the chapter also presents a description of the characteristics of mental health facilities, their services, available human resources, and aggregate revenues and costs.

Key public health concepts such as prevalence (total number of cases) and incidence (number of new cases) can be applied to service populations as well as to community populations. When examining services, one can speak of the daily and annual prevalences of those receiving treatment, the daily and annual prevalences of persons with specific types of disorders seen in treatment, the daily and annual incidences of cases entering treatment, the daily and annual incidences of cases with specific types of disorders seen in treatment . The balance of this chapter applies these public health concepts to both the population of 100 adults and the mental health service systems themselves.

A SHORT INTRODUCTION TO AMERICAN MENTAL HEALTH SERVICES

Mental health services today are provided primarily through four sectors (Regier et al., 1993).

- The *specialty sector* refers to any setting designed specifically to provide mental health care in which care typically is provided by someone with advanced clinical mental health training (e.g., a community mental health center in which care is provided by a psychiatrist or PhD-level clinical psychologist).
- The *general health care sector* refers to any setting designed to provide primary care in which mental health care usually is provided by a primary care physician or nurse-practitioner (e.g., a community health clinic staffed by family practitioners and nurse-practitioners).
- The *human service sector* refers to any setting that provides social services in which mental health care typically is provided by a social service specialist, most often a social worker with a master's degree in social work (e.g., a multipurpose senior center with a caseworker or a child welfare agency with an outreach worker).
- The *self-help sector* refers to any setting in which a mental health service consumer engages in self-care, typically without assistance other than that provided by a peer support specialist, most often another consumer (e.g., a "clubhouse" or a consumer-run support group).

The specialty mental health sector has evolved dramatically since Colonial times in the United States. Originally, the only sources of mental health care were local: community almshouses and one's family. Gradually the almshouses evolved into state mental hospitals, which have continued in existence to the present day (Stroup and Manderscheid, 1988). Figure 13-1 shows trends in admissions and resident patients[2] for state mental hospitals across the country over the past nearly two centuries, from 1831 to 2005. Between 1831 and 1955, the census of resident patients grew dramatically. After 1955, through a process called deinstitutionalization, the number of resident patients decreased dramatically until 2003. Between 2003 and 2005, however, the inpatient census increased slightly. Admissions to state hospitals followed a similar pattern, rising from 1831 to 1971, then decreasing until 2003.

---

1. When the population analyzed is 100 persons, counts and rates are the same, since the simplest form of a rate is a percent (count per 100 population).

2. "Admissions" refers to the number of entrants to the hospitals over a one-year period; "resident patients" (or census), to the number on the rolls on the last day of a year.

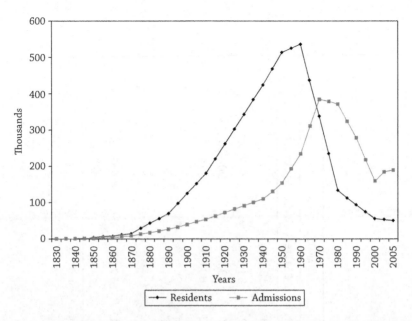

Figure 13-1   **Number of Admissions and Resident Patients in State and County Mental Hospitals, United States.**

Data shown for selected years from 1831 to 2005.
NOTE: The missing years are interpolated.
SOURCE: (1) 1830–1970: Stroup, Atlee L., and Manderscheid, Ronald W., The Development of the State Mental Hospital System in the United States: 1840–1980. *Journal of the Washington Academy of Sciences*, 76(1): 59–68, 1988. (2) 1975: National Institute of Mental Health (NIMH), Statistical Note 132, Table 1. (3) 1980–2003: NIMH and Substance Abuse and Mental Health Services Administration (SAMHSA), *Additions and Resident Patients at End of Year, State and County Mental Hospitals, by Age and Diagnosis, by State, United States*. (4) 2004: SAMHSA, *Background Report, Admissions and Resident Patients, State and County Mental Hospitals, United States, 2004*.

Between 2003 and 2005, admissions increased about 20%, from 150,000 to 190,000.

Between the 1930s and the 1950s, several new types of hospital-based mental health facilities were added: Veterans Administration (now Department of Veterans Affairs) hospitals in the 1930s, general hospitals in the 1940s, and private psychiatric hospitals in the 1950s. As noted above, the deinstitutionalization of people with mental illnesses from state mental hospitals began in earnest in 1955, with the introduction in rapid order of the psychotropic drugs Thorazine and Haldol. Enactment of the Community Mental Health Centers and Mental Retardation Act of 1963 led to a wholesale nationwide expansion of community mental health, with the express purpose of caring for individuals who had been deinstitutionalized. Unfortunately, the law's vision was never fully realized, in part because the mental health centers were required to rely on severely limited insurance reimbursement to support their services. Thus a decade later, in the 1970s, the Community Support Program was developed to fill this and other known gaps in community mental health care for individuals requiring public sector services. The 1980s marked a period of growing emphasis on serving the needs of children with serious emotional disturbances, an emphasis that continues to the present. In the 1990s, a growing number of residential treatment services were established to act as bridges for individuals to make a successful transition from hospital to community-based care. Concurrent with these century-long developments in mental health care has been the rise of both employer-based health coverage and the private practice of mental health care, a care system that continues to operate separately from but parallel to these organized public sector systems (Grob, 1994; Schulberg & Manderscheid, 1989).

Table 13-1 presents a picture of specialty mental health facilities in 2004, the most

Table 13-1. Mental Health Organizations in 2004

TYPE	NUMBER	BEDS		ADMISSIONS		
		INPATIENT	RESIDENTIAL	INPATIENT	RESIDENTIAL	AMBULATORY
State hospital	237	53,539	4,495	252,349	13,223	129,958
Private hospital	264	20,550	7,872	563,639	34,970	447,194
General hospital	1,230	39,820	1,583	1,523,977	9,209	900,404
Residential treatment center	458		33,835		60,620	194,294
Outpatient clinic	1,208					1,234,173
Multiservice organization	702		51,536		254,714	1,761,315
Total	4,099	112,909	99,321	2,339,964	372,736	4,667,338
Overall Total						7,380,038

Source: Unpublished data, Center for Mental Health Services, Substance Abuse and Mental Health Services Administration.

recent year for which data are available. In that year, 4,099 facilities were in operation. The majority of those facilities were general hospital psychiatric services, outpatient clinics, or multiservice mental health organizations.[3] Facilities offering 24-hour care provided 112,909 inpatient hospital beds and 99,321 residential treatment beds. Over that year, 2,339,964 admissions were made to inpatient beds, 372,736 to residential beds, and 4,667,338 to ambulatory (outpatient) programs. In practical terms, the data show that almost one third of over 7.3 million annual admissions were to 24-hour hospital inpatient beds. This last number is notably high, particularly given the long-term effort to develop community-based outpatient services over the last half century.

Bed turnover[4] varied considerably across hospitals providing inpatient services.[5] On average, inpatient beds at state hospitals turned over every 77 days. In contrast, private psychiatric hospitals experienced an average turnover rate of every 13 days; general hospital psychiatric services, every 10 days. Residential treatment beds also showed wide variation in turnover rates: For state mental hospitals, turnover occurred every 124 days; private psychiatric hospitals, every 82 days; general hospitals, every 62 days; and residential treatment centers, every 203 days. In general, these patterns can be attributed to variability in the severity of illness, the dearth of care alternatives, and the wide range of differences across public and private health insurance coverage for mental disorders.

Not surprisingly, then, ambulatory admission rates per facility per year were broadly disparate.[6] For multiservice organizations, the average was 2,508 admissions; for private psychiatric hospitals, 1,693; for outpatient clinics, 1,021; for general hospitals, 732; for state mental hospitals, 548; and for residential treatment centers, 424. As with inpatient services, the differences generally reflect variation in the severity of problems experienced by persons admitted to care and in the size of the programs.

Patterns of care in facilities in the general health sector were markedly different. In 2007, a total of 1,067 community health centers receiving federal grants provided ambulatory care to 13,962,680 persons, 1,357,188 (around 10%) of whom were receiving treatment for mental disorders (Bureau of Primary Health Care, n.d.).

This brief statistical picture would not be complete without an overview of the professional human resources available for specialty care. Table 13-2 shows the numbers of mental health specialty providers by discipline for the indicated year. Based on the latest available data, 515,439 professionals are available to provide specialty mental health care. The majority of these providers are social workers or counselors. Advanced-practice psychiatric nurses (such as nurse-practitioners) and psychiatrists represent the smallest number of specialty providers. Most medications in specialty facilities are prescribed by professionals from these last two disciplines.

Table 13-2. Mental Health Human Resources

DISCIPLINE	NUMBER	YEAR
Psychiatry	43,120	2006
Psychology	92,227	2007
Social work	192,776	2008
Advanced-practice psychiatric nursing	9,764	2006
Counseling	128,886	2008
Marriage/family therapy	48,666	2006
Total	515,439	

Source: Unpublished data provided by each of the mental health disciplines to the Center for Mental Health Services, Substance Abuse and Mental Health Services Administration.

---

3. Multiservice mental health organizations are facilities offering a combination of services, including residential, partial and outpatient care.

4. Bed turnover is defined as number of beds × 365 divided by annual admissions.

5. Results are not shown; turnover rates can be derived from table 13-1.

6. Results are not shown; average admissions can be derived from table 13-1.

SOURCE OF DATA ON PREVALENCE OF DISORDERS AND TREATMENT

The data on which the description of the 100 adults from the community population is based come from the National Comorbidity Survey—Replication (NCS-R) (Kessler, Berglund, et al., 2005; Kessler, Demler, et al., 2005). The initial NCS, supported by the National Institute of Mental Health (NIMH), was undertaken between 1990 and 1992 with a national probability sample from the general household population of the United States of more than 8,000 persons ages 15–54. That effort, administered by lay interviewers, was the first to assess mental illness in a national probability sample and the first to use the World Health Organization Composite International Diagnostic Instrument (CIDI), which is based on the revised third edition of the *Diagnostic and Statistical Manual of Mental Disorders* (American Psychiatric Association [APA], 1987). Annual prevalence was assessed for 14 distinct mental disorders and their treatments. Unfortunately, the NCS did not include a scale for schizophrenia, nor did it collect incidence data for any disorders. Nonetheless, since the original study was conducted, the publicly available NCS data have provided a rich source for researchers to explore a host of mental health issues and as a result have yielded numerous published scientific articles.

Original NCS respondents were reinterviewed in 2001 and 2002, in a study called the NCS-2. Both the NIMH and the Substance Abuse and Mental Health Services Administration (SAMHSA) underwrote the study, which examined the course of mental disorders as well as the relationship between primary mental disorders and secondary substance use disorders. These reinterviews resulted in the collection of incidence data spanning a full decade. Findings from this follow-up study led to development of the concept of a window of opportunity: Between the onset of a primary mental disorder and the onset of a secondary substance use disorder, opportunities exist to prevent the latter from occurring and to reduce the severity of the former.

At about the same time, a new, annual prevalence survey of disorders and treatment, the NCS-R, was conducted in a different national probability sample of 10,000 respondents age 18 and older, using a revised CIDI based on the fourth edition of the *Diagnostic and Statistical Manual of Mental Disorders* (APA, 1994). Results from a parallel annual prevalence study of 10,000 adolescents ages 12–17, the NCS-A (for "adolescents"), are not yet available. Once reported, however, this latest study will be the first to provide detailed annual disorder and treatment prevalence information on a national probability sample of adolescents.

The following sections are based on the mental and substance disorder–related disorder and treatment prevalence findings from the NCS-R for a population sample of 100.

COMMUNITY PREVALENCE OF MENTAL AND SUBSTANCE USE CONDITIONS

Based on the NCS-R findings, 32 individuals in a 100-adult sample will experience a mental or substance use disorder during one year (see figure 13-2). Of them, 19 will have an anxiety disorder; 10, a mood disorder (e.g., depression); 10, an impulse control disorder; and 13, a substance use disorder. While schizophrenia was not measured or reported by the NCS-R, other data sources show that 1 of these 100 persons will experience that disorder (Regier et al., 1993). Other NCS-R–related results show that 7 of the 32 persons with a mental or substance use disorder will experience a second disorder over the course of the year, and another 7 will experience three or more disorders (Kessler, Demler, et al., 2005). Hence, multimorbidity among disorders is more an expectation than an exception.

In contrast to 1-year prevalence, when looking across the lifetime, 57 of the original 100 persons—more than half—will experience one or more mental or substance disorders (results not shown). The original NCS found that over 29 of those individuals will have a history of three or more simultaneous behavioral disorders (Kessler et al., 1994).

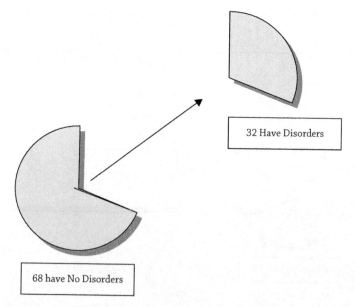

32 Have Disorders

68 have No Disorders

Figure 13-2   **Annual Prevalence of Mental And Substance Use Disorders Among 100 Adults.**

Taken together, these findings are both startling and disturbing. During the course of a single year, each adult in the United States has about a one-in-three chance of experiencing a mental or substance use disorder. Even more disconcerting, over the course of a lifetime, this jumps dramatically to a two-in-three likelihood. In sum, mental and substance use disorders are clearly at epidemic levels in the United States, comparable to those of other chronic disorders such as cancer or heart disease!

Insurance and Treatment Prevalence for Mental and Substance Use Conditions

Of the 32 persons the NCS found to have a mental or substance use disorder during a 12-month period, 11 (more than a third) have no health insurance coverage (see figure 13-3). In contrast, only 12 of the 68 persons without a behavioral disorder lack health insurance. Thus the rate at which individuals lack insurance is almost twice as high for persons with mental or substance use disorders as for persons in the general population.

Of the original 100 adults, 20 will engage in some form of behavioral health care over the course of a year, even though only 13 of the 20 actually will have a diagnosable mental or substance use disorder during that year (see figure 13-4). The remaining 7 will seek care for subclinical symptoms, that is, symptoms that do not rise to the level of a diagnosable illness. (See Wang et al., 2005.) More critically, since 32 of the 100 will have some form of mental or substance use disorder, it is clear that some individuals who actually have mental or substance use disorders of clinical significance do not seek care.

What can be said about patterns of care for the 32 individuals known to experience a mental or substance use disorder during the year? Of the 13 who will seek some form of care, 7 will be treated in a specialty mental health care setting (see figure 13-5). Seven others will get care in a general medical setting, 3 will get care in a human service setting, and 2 will engage in some form of self-care. Clearly, some of the 13 individuals are likely to seek care in more than one care setting.

As noted earlier, 68 persons from the community will not have a mental health or substance use condition over the year. Of the 7 from this group who nonetheless seek some form of care, 3 will receive care in a specialty mental health care setting, 3 will receive care

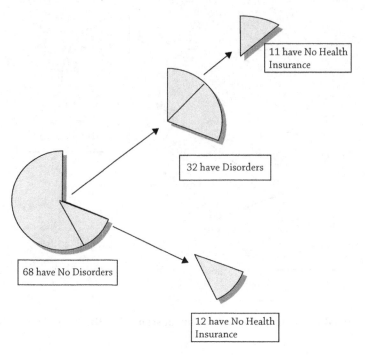

11 have No Health
Insurance

32 have Disorders

68 have No Disorders

12 have No Health
Insurance

Figure 13-3   **Annual Prevalence of Health Insurance Coverage Among 100 Adults.**

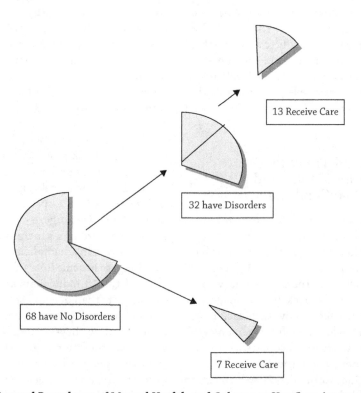

13 Receive Care

32 have Disorders

68 have No Disorders

7 Receive Care

Figure 13-4   **Annual Prevalence of Mental Health and Substance Use Care Among 100 Adults.**

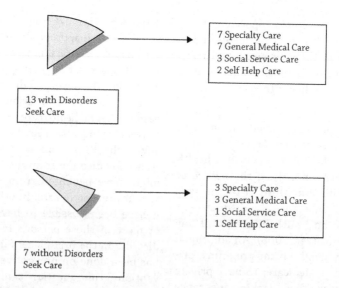

Figure 13-5   Sectors of Mental Health and Substance Use Care Among 100 Adults.

in a general medical setting, 1 will receive care in a human service setting, and 1 will engage in self-care. Only one person will receive care in more than a single setting.

Looking in greater depth at the 10 individuals who receive specialty care (7 with diagnoses and 3 with subclinical symptoms), 6 are likely to receive care from a specialty mental health service facility. In fact, 2 of those 6 are likely will receive inpatient treatment at some point during the year. The remaining 4 are likely to receive outpatient care either from a private practitioner or a group practice. The public, or not-for-profit, system will support the care of at least 5 of the individuals treated in specialty mental health service facilities; 1 will receive care from a for-profit organization. At least 1 of the 6 in care from a specialty mental health facility will be 50 years of age or older and at risk for premature death due to untreated chronic physical health problems (Colton & Manderscheid, 2006). Further, according to Ronald Kessler (personal communication, September 20, 2009), as many as 6 of the 10 individuals in treatment can be expected to drop out of care prematurely, most often for financial reasons.

These findings about patterns of care are as disturbing as those regarding the prevalence of the disorders themselves. The data suggest that in the course of a year, an individual

with a mental or substance use disorder will have only around a one-in-five chance of getting mental health care from a trained clinical specialist and around a two-in-five chance of receiving care at all. Thus the majority of persons experiencing a mental or substance use disorder during one year will get no professional mental health care whatsoever.

Interpreting the Patterns for the 100 Adults

Most striking about the findings that emerge from the 100-adult sample are how many have disorders and how few receive care. The genesis of these results is telling and begins with a closer examination of the pattern of disorders. Of the 32 persons experiencing a mental or substance use disorder over the course of a year, only 6 are likely to have symptoms of sufficient severity to be characterized as experiencing a serious mental illness (Kessler et al., 2004). The SAMHSA (Center for Mental Health Services, n.d.) has defined this population as follows:

Such individuals not only have a diagnosable disorder, but also experience significant functional limitations that affect their ability to function in family, community, or work settings. The public mental health systems operated by state mental health agencies devote the vast majority of their resources to this population and, as a result, a majority of these persons are likely to receive care during the year.

A second important consideration with respect to patterns of care among the 100-adult sample is whether a person has health insurance coverage and, if so, the nature of that coverage. Fully one third of the persons with a mental or substance use disorder—11 of the 32—have no health insurance of any kind (Gilberti & Seltzer, 2008). An additional 8 are covered by public sector programs, primarily Medicaid or Medicare; 13 have private insurance coverage. Those lacking insurance altogether most likely either receive no care or receive crisis care from hospital emergency departments. Individuals with Medicaid or Medicare are most likely to receive care from public or not-for-profit providers; those with private insurance, from private practitioners in either solo or group settings.

Increasingly, a fifth type of mental health service system appears to be emerging, for better or for worse: the adult and juvenile criminal justice systems. The prevalence of mental illnesses among adult and youth populations confined in jails and prisons is an important indicator of the degree to which traditional American mental health service systems are not reaching sizable proportions of the population in need of treatment. A systematic review of the prevalence literature for adults (Fazel & Danesh, 2002; Fazel & Lubbe, 2005) found that in Western nations such as the United States, about one in seven adult prisoners has a diagnosable psychotic illness or major depression; about one in two male and one in five female prison or jail inmates has an antisocial personality disorder. In the United States, these rates translate to a finding that more than 200,000 adult prisoners have psychotic illnesses, major depression, or both. More recent anecdotal evidence from the field suggests this number has increased markedly in the decade since the review was conducted. High prevalence rates of mental illnesses have similarly been observed for children and adolescents involved with the juvenile justice system (Fazel, Doll, & Langstrom,

2008). Alarm is now being raised in several quarters about the inappropriateness of incarcerating persons with mental illnesses for minor offenses as well as about the growing need to establish mental health courts and diversion and reentry programs for these individuals at significant need for mental health care.

Another important consideration is whether any of the 32 persons with a mental or substance use disorder from the 100-adult sample might have benefited from earlier intervention or preventive care. In other words, might it have been possible to have prevented one or more of those persons from developing a disorder in the first place? Since so little work has been done on preventive and early interventions, this question cannot be answered at present. However, it seems clear that much could be done and needs to be done to prevent or mitigate common mental disorders such as depressive illness and anxiety.

COSTS OF MENTAL ILLNESSES

All of these factors—services provided, services needed—affect the overall costs of mental illnesses in direct and indirect ways. The cost estimates presented here should be considered provisional at best, since they are derived from diverse sources with a wide range of methodologies involving an equally wide range of assumptions.

In a targeted review exploring the limited number of relevant US studies conducted in the past 15 years, we sought to obtain data on the total cost of specific mental disorders or the cost per case per year. Credible US estimates were found for major depressive disorder, alcohol abuse or dependence, drug abuse or dependence, schizophrenia, and bipolar disorder. When domestic data were not available, we used total costs from studies conducted outside the United States to estimate per capita costs for the population of US adults. For all disorders considered, the number of adults in the United States in 2005 (222 million) was multiplied by the median annual prevalence; that product then was multiplied by per capita costs to generate total costs in the United

States. Cost estimates were adjusted to 2005 US dollars using an inflation factor, purchasing power parity indices, or both. Costs of childhood disorders were calculated in a similar manner unless otherwise specified.

The cost estimates for specific mental disorders that follow often are based on individual studies, often the single available study of costs associated with a disorder. Perhaps not surprisingly, cost data are not available for all disorders. For example, the single cost study of personality disorders (Soeteman, van Hakkaart, Verheul, & Busschbach, 2008) provided estimated costs solely for persons in treatment. However, the study results have not been included here because the study contained no estimate of the percentage of persons with this diagnosis who need or could benefit from treatment. For similar reasons, there is no estimate available for eating disorders, as studies dedicated to the cost of these disorders in the United States were limited to inpatient and outpatient treatment costs (Striegel-Moore, Leslie, Petrill, Garvin, & Rosenheck, 2000). These deficits in available data caution against making generalizations about the cost data and speak to the potential cost savings that could be realized were more people with these disorders treated.

Despite these caveats, the data yield interesting findings. For example, the estimates reveal considerable cost variation across mental disorders, from $11 billion per year for simple phobia to over $200 billion per year apiece for alcohol and drug use disorders. (See table 13-3 for references.) These cost estimates are composed of direct and indirect costs. The direct costs associated with treating mental and substance use disorders are predominantly treatment costs. The indirect costs include other costs to society, such as the costs of incarceration and lost productivity, and encompass all persons with the disorders, whether in treatment or not. The net effect of these considerations is that the figures in table 13-3 may underestimate the direct costs that would occur if all persons with the disorder were to receive treatment and at the same time overestimate the indirect costs, some portion of which would be saved if all persons were treated.

The cost estimates presented are complex functions of the prevalence and disability associated with each disorder, the costs of its treatment, and its indirect costs. The lowest estimated annual cost ($10.6 billion) is for obsessive–compulsive disorder, an uncommon disorder with a generally lower level of related disability than is experienced by individuals with other mental disorders. While the phobias also have low levels of disability, they are slightly more common disorders, yielding somewhat higher annual cost estimates ($15.7 billion for social phobia and $11.0 billion for simple phobia). Panic disorder, while less common, has higher levels of severity and disability and therefore also higher costs (estimated at $30.4 billion per year). For rare disorders such as schizophrenia and bipolar disorder, single-year costs in the United States total more than $70 billion each, presumably due to the high level of disability associated with those illnesses. Major depressive disorder also gives rise to high costs, resulting primarily from its relatively high prevalence and moderate to severe levels of disability. According to a single study funded by the federal government (Harwood, Fountain, & Fountain, 1999), the costs of substance use disorders (including the use or abuse of drugs, alcohol, or both) are very high. Drug, alcohol, and personality disorders—all externalizing disorders—also incur costs to other people and to society (e.g., for damage to persons and property or involvement with the criminal justice system), costs most often not associated with other mental disorders. Societal costs must similarly account for a substantial proportion of the cost of conduct disorder, which makes estimating that cost difficult. Only one study to date (Foster & Jones, 2005) had explored indirect and direct costs of conduct disorder in the United States and provided a yearly annual estimate per individual. Using the prevalence of the disorder from Costello, Mustillo, Erkanli, Keeler, and Angold (2003) and population estimates from the US census, a figure of $20.3 billion was calculated as the annual cost of conduct disorder.

The childhood autism spectrum disorders and attention deficit hyperactivity disorders

Table 13-3. Total Costs Associated with Specific Mental Disorders

DISORDER	ANNUAL COST (BILLIONS OF DOLLARS)	SOURCE OF COST DATA
DISORDERS IN CHILDREN		
Autism spectrum disorders	35.0	Ganz, 2006[a]
Attention deficit hyperactivity disorder	42.5	Pelham, Foster, & Robb, 2007[a]
Conduct disorder	20.3	Foster & Jones, 2005[a]
Eating disorders	NA	
DISORDERS IN ADULTS		
Panic	30.4	Batelaan et al., 2007[b]
Social phobia	15.7	Andlin-Sobocki & Wittchen, 2005[b]
Simple phobia	11.0	Andlin-Sobocki & Wittchen, 2005[b]
Obsessive–compulsive disorder	10.6	DuPont, Rice, Shiraki, & Rowland, 1995[b]
Major depression	97.3	Donahue & Pincus, 2005[a]
Drug abuse/dependence	201.6	Harwood et al., 1999[a]
Alcohol abuse/dependence	226.0	Harwood et al., 1999[a]
Personality disorders	NA	Soeteman et al., 2008[b]
Schizophrenia	70.0	Wyatt, Henter, Leary, & Taylor, 1996[a]
Bipolar disorder	78.6	Wyatt & Henter, 1995[a]
DISORDERS IN THE ELDERLY		
Dementia (over 65)	76.0	Wimo, Jonsson, & Winblad, 2005[b]

NA, not available. Disability weights used in these analyses taken from Murray and Lopez (1996), annex table 13-3, untreated form, age group 15–44, and from Matthews, Lopez, and Murray (2005); depression is considered at the "moderate" level.

[a]US source. [b]Non-US source; cost estimate extrapolated to United States.

share similar yearly costs at $35.0 billion and $42.5 billion, respectively. The costs of those disorders include not only treatment costs to the family but also lost job productivity for parents who need to attend to their children.

REVENUES TO SUPPORT SERVICES

In 2003, approximately $100 billion was spent on the treatment of mental disorders in the United States, compared with about $55 billion in 1993. Total US spending for all health care in 2003 was $1.6 trillion.

In 2003, a majority (59%) of spending on mental health care came from public sources (see figure 13-6). In contrast, public sources paid for only 45% of all health care spending for all conditions. Medicaid accounted for 27% of all mental health funding in the United States, making it the largest source of such funding among all payers. Slightly more than half of all money expended on mental health

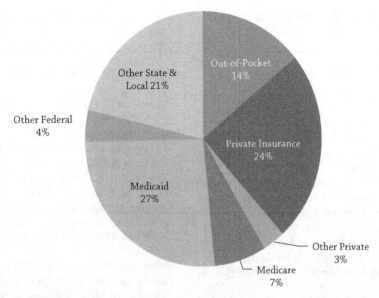

Figure 13-6 Distribution of Mental Health Expenditures by Payer Source, 2003.
Total expenditures were approximately $100 billion.
Source: Mark et al., 2007.

care is at the state level, including the 27% of spending paid for by Medicaid, the 21% from other state and local funding sources, and the 4% from other federal sources. As the admission counts in table 13-1 show, these fundsare used in the main to support care in multiservice mental health organizations, other community mental health services, and psychiatric inpatient care.

In 2003, approximately 41% of all spending for the treatment of mental disorders was by private sector sources (see figure 13-6). Private health insurance accounted for 24% of that spending, individual out-of-pocket payments totaled another 14%, and the remaining 3% was borne by other nonpatient private sources, including philanthropy.

CONCLUSION

By this time it should be clear that unlike many other nations around the globe, America has no single mental health "system." Rather, after years of starts and stops, US mental health care still consists of parallel activities operated by public and private entities across four care sectors. As a result, many individuals who need care do not receive it,

and many who do receive care do not achieve the outcomes they are seeking (see Institute of Medicine, 2006). This chapter's description of the mental health and treatment status of 100 American adults chosen at random from the population clearly demonstrates that many who need care fall through the cracks of the care system or drop out of care after starting it. Costs—including those associated with the dearth of care—are very high. Unquestionably, with the public health of the nation at stake, much more needs to be done much better in the future.

Enactment of the Patient Protection and Affordable Care Act of 2010 holds great promise for achieving the vision of improved care in the future. This national health reform effort will expand insurance and coverage; will promote improved quality and performance assessment through integrated service delivery systems that encompass mental health, substance use, and primary care; and will foster better use of information technology. This landmark legislation has instilled a strong sense of hope in the national mental health advocacy community about a better future. It has the potential to provide care to many persons with mental illness who currently lack health insurance coverage and to improve the quality of care for those who already receive care.

REFERENCES

American Psychiatric Association. (1987). *Diagnostic and statistical manual of mental disorders* (3rd ed., rev.). Washington, DC: Author.

American Psychiatric Association. (1994). *Diagnostic and statistical manual of mental disorders* (4th ed.). Washington, DC: Author.

Andlin-Sobocki, P., & Wittchen, H. U. (2005). Cost of anxiety disorders in Europe. *European Journal of Neurology, 12*(Suppl. 1), 39–44.

Batelaan, N., Smit, F., De, G. R., Van, B. A., Vollebergh, W., & Beekman, A. (2007). Economic costs of full-blown and subthreshold panic disorder. *Journal of Affective Disorders, 104*(1–3), 127–136.

Bureau of Primary Health Care (n.d.). Unpublished data. Rockville, MD: Health Resources and Services Administration.

Center for Mental Health Services (n.d.). Unpublished data report. Rockville, MD: Substance Abuse and Mental Health Services Administration, US Department of Health and Human Services.

Colton, C. W., & Manderscheid, R. W. (2006). Congruencies in increased mortality rates, years of potential life lost, and causes of death among public mental health clients in eight states. *Prevention of Chronic Disease, 3*(2), A42. Retrieved from http://www.cdc.gov/pcd/issues/2006/apr/05_0180.htm

Community Mental Health Centers and Mental Retardation Act, Pub. L. No. 88–164 (1963).

Costello, E. J., Mustillo, S., Erkanli, A., Keeler, G., & Angold, A. (2003). Prevalence and development of psychiatric disorders in childhood and adolescence. *Archives of General Psychiatry, 60*(8), 837–844.

Donahue, J. M., & Pincus, H. A. (2005). Reducing the societal burden of depression: A review of economic costs, quality of care and effects of treatment. *Pharmacoeconomics, 25*(1), 7–24.

DuPont, R. L., Rice, D. P., Shiraki, S., & Rowland, C. R. (1995). Economic costs of obsessive–compulsive disorder. *Medical Interface, 8*(4), 102–109.

Fazel, S., & Danesh, J. (2002). Serious mental disorder in 23,000 prisoners: A systematic review of 62 surveys. *Lancet, 359*(9306), 545–550.

Fazel, S., Doll, H., & Langstrom, N. (2008). Mental disorders among adolescents in juvenile detention and correctional facilities: A systematic review and meta-regression analysis of 25 surveys. *Journal of the American Academy of Child and Adolescent Psychiatry, 47*(9), 1010–1019.

Fazel, S., & Lubbe, S. (2005). Prevalence and characteristics of mental disorders in jails and prisons. *Current Opinion in Psychiatry, 18*(5), 550–554.

Foster, E. M., & Jones, D. E. (2005). The high costs of aggression: Public expenditures resulting from conduct disorder. *American Journal of Public Health, 95*(10), 1767–1772.

Ganz, M. L. (2006). The costs of autism. In S. O. Moldin & Rubenstein, J. L. R. (Eds.). *Understanding autism: From basic neuroscience to treatment* (pp. 475–502). Boca Raton, FL: Taylor and Francis.

Gilberti, M., & Seltzer, T. (2008). *Coverage for all: Inclusion of mental illness and substance use disorders in state healthcare reform initiatives.* Arlington, VA, and Rockville, MD: National Alliance on Mental Illness and National Council on Community Behavioral Healthcare.

Grob, G. N. (1994). *The mad among us: A history of the care of America's mentally ill.* New York, NY: Free Press.

Harwood, H. J., Fountain, D., & Fountain, G. (1999). Economic cost of alcohol and drug abuse in the United States, 1992: A report. *Addiction, 94*(5), 631–635.

Institute of Medicine. (2006). *Improving the quality of health care for mental and substance use conditions.* Washington, DC: National Academies Press.

Kessler, R. C., Berglund, P. A., Demler, O., Jin, R., Merikangas, K. R., & Walters, E. E. (2005). Lifetime prevalence and age-of-onset distributions of DSM-IV disorders in the National Comorbidity Survey Replication (NCS-R). *Archives of General Psychiatry, 62*(6), 593–602.

Kessler, R. C., Chiu, W. T., Colpe, L., Demler, O., Merikangas, K. R., Walters, E. E., & Wang, P. S. (2004). The prevalence and correlates of serious mental illness (SMI) in the National Comorbidity Survey Replication (NCS-R). In R. W. Manderscheid & J. T. Berry (Eds.), *Mental health, United States, 2004* (pp. 34–148). Rockville, MD: Substance Abuse and Mental Health Services Administration, US Department of Health and Human Services.

Kessler, R. C., Demler, O., Frank, R. G., Olfson, M., Pincus, H. A., Walters, E. E., ... Zaslavsky, A. M. (2005). Prevalence and treatment of mental disorders, 1990 to 2003. *New England Journal of Medicine, 352*(24), 2515–2523.

Kessler, R. C., McGonagle, K. A., Zhao, S., Nelson, C. B., Hughes, M., Eshleman, S.,...Kendler, K. S. (1994). Lifetime and 12-month prevalence of DSM-III-R psychiatric disorders in the United States: Results from the National Comorbidity Survey. *Archives of General Psychiatry, 51*(1), 8–19.

Manderscheid, R. W., Henderson, M. J., Witkin, M. J., & Atay, J. E. (2000). Contemporary mental health systems and managed care. In E. A. Dragomirecka & H. Papezova (Eds.), *Social psychiatry in changing times*. Prague, Czech Republic: Psychiatric Center.

Mark, T.L., Levit, K. R., Coffey, R. M., McKusick, D. R., Harwood, H. J., King, E. C.,...Ryan, K. (2007). *National expenditures for mental health services and substance abuse treatment, 1993–2003* (SAMHSA Publication No. SMA 07–4227). Rockville, MD: Substance Abuse and Mental Health Services Administration.

Matthews, C., Lopez, A. D., & Murray, C. (2005). The burden of disease and mortality by condition: Data, methods, and results for 2001. In A. D. Lopez, C. D. Mathers, M. Ezzati, D. T Jamison, & C. J. L. Murray (Eds.), *Global burden of disease and risk factors* (pp. 45–240). New York, NY, and Washington, DC: Oxford University Press and the World Bank.

Murray, C. J. L., & Lopez, A. D. (1996). *The global burden of disease*. Boston, MA: Harvard University Press.

Patient Protection and Affordable Care Act, Pub. L. No. 111–148 (2010).

Pelham, W. E., Foster, E. M., & Robb, J. A. (2007). The economic impact of attention-deficit/hyperactivity disorder in children and adolescents. *Journal of Pediatric Psychology, 32*(6), 711–727.

Regier, D. A., Narrow, W. E., Rae, D. S., Manderscheid, R. W., Locke, B. Z., & Goodwin, F. K. (1993). The de facto U.S. mental and addictive disorders service system: ECA prospective

one-year prevalence rates of disorders and services. *Archives of General Psychiatry, 50*(2), 85–94.

Schulberg, H. C., & Manderscheid, R. W. (1989). The changing network of mental health service delivery. In C. A. Taube, D. Mechanic, & A. A. Hohmann (Eds.), *The future of mental health services research*. Rockville, MD: US Department of Health and Human Services.

Soeteman, D. I., van Hakkaart, R. L., Verheul, R., & Busschbach, J. J. (2008). The economic burden of personality disorders in mental health care. *Journal of Clinical Psychiatry, 69*(2), 259–265.

Striegel-Moore, R. H., Leslie, D., Petrill, S. A., Garvin, V., & Rosenheck, R. A. (2000). One-year use and cost of inpatient and outpatient services among female and male patients with an eating disorder: Evidence from a national database of health insurance claims. *International Journal of Eating Disorders, 27*(4), 381–389.

Stroup, A. L., & Manderscheid, R. W. (1988). The development of the state mental hospital system in the United States: 1840–1980. *Journal of the Washington Academy of Sciences, 76*(1), 59–68.

Wang, P. S., Lane, M., Kessler, R. C., Olfson, M., Pincus, H. A., & Wells, K. B. (2005). Twelve-month use of mental health services in the U.S.: Results from the National Comorbidity Survey replication (NCS-R). *Archives of General Psychiatry, 62*(6), 629–640.

Wimo, A., Jonsson, L., & Winblad, B. (2005). An estimate of the worldwide prevalence and direct costs of dementia in 2003. *Dementia and Geriatric Cognitive Disorders, 21*(3), 175–181.

Wyatt, R. J., & Henter, I. (1995). An economic evaluation of manic–depressive illness: 1991. *Social Psychiatry and Psychiatric Epidemiology, 30*(5), 213–219.

Wyatt, R. J., Henter, I., Leary, M. C., & Taylor, E. (1996). An economic evaluation of schizophrenia: 1991. *Social Psychiatry and Psychiatric Epidemiology, 30*(5), 196–205.

14

Community and Public Mental Health Services in the United States: History and Programs

ANITA EVERETT

SU YEON LEE

Key Points

- By 1890, every state in the United States had funded, constructed, and staffed one or more publicly supported mental hospitals, the total census of which grew concomitantly with the nation's overall population

- The documented abysmal conditions of the state-operated mental hospitals in the 1950s, coupled with the discovery of chlorpromazine, ushered in an era of hope that individuals who were chronically institutionalized might be able to live more successfully in community settings

- In the last 50 years, there has been intensive development of psychoactive medications, psychotherapies, and community support tools

- The President's New Freedom Commission on Mental Health in 2002 embraced the concept of recovery, in which the goal is to enable persons with mental and behavioral disorders to live, work, and participate in the community of their choice

- Community behavioral health organizations (CBHOs) now play a vital role in providing therapeutic and rehabilitative services to persons in the United States with mental and behavioral disorders

- CBHOs provide services across the age spectrum and along the entire continuum of care, from preventive interventions to diagnosis and treatment to long-term rehabilitation and recovery support

- Staff at a CBHO generally include a mix of professionals, paraprofessionals, and administrative personnel

- Important services of CBHOs include case management, assertive community treatment, supported employment, and the clubhouse model

INTRODUCTION

Community behavioral health organizations (CBHOs) are the foundation of mental health service delivery in the United States for the more than 45 million adults age 18 or older with a mental disorder in the past year, among whom 11 million experience serious mental disorders (Substance Abuse and Mental Health Services Administration [SAMHSA], 2010). As discussed in chapter 13, the vast majority of individuals receiving behavioral health care today are served by outpatient community settings; only a small proportion receive care in inpatient facilities. This chapter provides an understanding of the vital role CBHOs play in providing both therapeutic and rehabilitative services to some of the nation's most vulnerable citizens. It outlines the origins of CBHOs within the publicly funded health care system in the United States, provides examples of available programs and services, and delineates the range of challenges faced by contemporary CBHOs as they strive to meet the needs of people with serious mental illnesses.

Today's CBHOs provide a broad array of behavioral health services—from prevention and screening to treatment and rehabilitation—to a wide variety of individuals of all ages who experience mental and behavioral disorders. In chapter 13, Manderscheid and colleagues describe four general sectors through which individuals may receive care for a mental disorder: (1) the general health care sector; (2) the specialty mental health care sector; (3) the human service sector; and (4) the self-help (peer support) sector.

While CBHOs are predominantly specialty mental health care providers, their services often overlap with the activities of providers and organizations in other sectors, such as those in primary care, social and other supportive services, local charities, self-help groups, correctional facilities, and schools. Moreover, CBHOs often serve both individuals with substance use disorders and individuals with mental disorders, in part because mental health systems were set in place long before specialized substance abuse programs and funding became available. In the main, substance abuse programs developed outside and entirely separately from traditional mental health care and services. However, with the growing recognition that mental and behavioral disorders co-occur more often than not, as discussed in chapter 6, the trend is to treat the disorders concurrently rather than separately or sequentially (SAMHSA, 2002). As a result, the term behavioral health care has increasingly been adopted to refer to programs that include treatment for both mental and substance use disorders. This chapter uses the term community behavioral health organization (CBHO) rather than the more traditional term, community mental health center (CMHC), coined by the Kennedy administration in its Mental Retardation Facilities and Community Mental Health Centers Construction Act of 1963 (Surgeon General of the United States, 1999).

Most CBHOs are not single, office-based clinics. Rather, the majority provide a unified management structure for an organized array of affiliated—or collaborating—programs spread across multiple sites throughout a community. Thus today's CBHOs vary widely in number of patients served, size and types of services available, and professional personnel providing care. Many CBHOs, like the CMHCs that preceded them, serve specific geographic catchment areas, usually defined by county or city boundaries; most operate within a single state.

Community behavioral health organizations provide individualized prevention, diagnostic, treatment, and recovery services to individuals of all ages who either have or are at risk for mental illnesses, substance abuse, or both. Traditionally, CBHOs primarily provide services to individuals with long-term (chronic), serious mental illnesses such as schizophrenia, bipolar disorder, and psychotic depression. A second group of persons who have been served includes both individuals of limited income and individuals lacking employer-based health insurance coverage. Thus, much like CMHCs before them, CBHOs have become a central resource among community-based health and social safety net service providers.

Historically, mental health and substance abuse services have not been widely covered by private sector health insurers (SAMHSA, 2011). Thus funding for mental health and substance abuse services—particularly for people with the most serious and disabling chronic behavioral disorders—has come primarily from public sector sources. Among the foremost funders are the federal Substance Abuse Prevention and Treatment Block Grant program of the SAMHSA and, even more critically, the federal–state Medicaid program. CBHOs also have benefited from the allocation of state and municipal public sector dollars. In particular, funding through the Medicaid program has influenced the development and expansion of CBHOs in many ways, as discussed later in this chapter.

In recent years, CBHOs have developed extensive early intervention and treatment services for both children and teens, often linking to schools and child-serving programs to promote community-wide systems of care. Moreover, given the nation's changing demographics—the so-called graying of America—many CBHOs also provide services specifically designed for older adults. Further, CBHOs may provide treatment to those dually diagnosed with mental illnesses and developmental disabilities, acute or chronic physical disorders, or, as already noted, substance use disorders. As key providers to people with the most serious, chronic behavioral disorders, CBHOs reach out with services for individuals who are homeless (many of whom experience mental or substance use disorders), individuals

in correctional settings or court-ordered into community treatment, and people who have experienced trauma (such as a natural or man-made disaster, interpersonal violence, or war).

Community behavioral health organizations provide services across the age spectrum and along the entire continuum of care, from preventive interventions to diagnosis and treatment to long-term rehabilitation and recovery support. Services may include psychiatric diagnosis and assessment, medication management, crisis programs, individual and group therapy, intensive case management, employment coaching, day treatment, and both social and housing supports. The array of settings in which services are provided is equally broad, ranging from health care–related clinics and medical offices to community settings such as schools, homeless shelters, jails, community centers, and private residences. Generally, each CBHO maintains a core of structured clinical services, the majority of which are covered by a state's Medicaid program. Other, more specialized, community-specific services may be funded by what often are time-limited grants from local or state governments or from foundations.

Staff at a CBHO generally include a mix of professionals, paraprofessionals, and administrative personnel. While professionally trained social workers represent the largest proportion of the CBHO workforce, other professionals include psychiatrists, psychologists, and psychiatric nurses; marriage and family counselors; and pastoral counselors. Paraprofessionals, generally with educational backgrounds in social services, may fill roles as case managers, rehabilitation specialists, and outreach staff. In some states, paraprofessional staff must have a college degree; in others, a high school diploma is a sufficient minimum credential. An important recent development in CBHO staffing has been the incorporation of peer support specialists or peer counselors—individuals with a "lived experience" of mental illness who are at a stable point in their lives (in recovery)—employed to engage in community outreach and to support current patients in specific aspects of treatment and recovery. Administrative staff—those who manage staffing, financing, scheduling, and a program's general infrastructure—often have professional clinical backgrounds in service provision or advanced degrees in health services administration. Finally, CBHOs increasingly have been employing health evaluation science professionals with skills in developing, analyzing, and managing quality and performance improvement statistics. Such individuals are critical to providing effectiveness and efficacy data to demonstrate to funders, administrators, and policy makers that the care and services provided by the CBHO are having a beneficial effect on the its patients/clients. Evaluation also can help assure that dollars are supporting evidence-based practices that reflect the service needs of both individuals and the larger community.

HISTORICAL PERSPECTIVE

To understand the role and function of today's CBHOs, a grounding in their genesis as an integral part of the continually evolving system of mental health care in the United States is instructive. Such an understanding not only can provide insight into the current shape of CBHOs but also can point out how their future may be influenced by both changes and advances in science and health policy. The history of public mental health services can be divided into four general eras that this chapter will refer to chronologically as (1) the dark ages, (2) the institutional era, (3) the era of community tools development, and (4) the recovery era. We discuss each within its historical–political context, with an exploration of the services, system structure, workforce, state of clinical care, and available funding sources and mechanisms during the particular period.

The Dark Ages

The Dark Ages, in traditional Western historical accounts, refers to the chronological period from about 500 to 1000 CE, between the fall of the Roman Empire and the Enlightenment. The moniker was applied because the period was marked by stagnation and intellectual "darkness" rather than insightful or creative thought. Sadly, the same term is an apt

descriptor of the state of mental health care and services—and indeed both individual health care and public health services generally—before the start of the 19th century, both in the United States and around the world.

During these dark ages, average life expectancy was relatively short—perhaps around half of what it is in the United States today. In the absence not only of adequate numbers of trained physicians and other health professionals but also of antibiotics, sanitation, and vaccines, common infectious diseases often were fatal. Communicable diseases—such as smallpox, influenza, tuberculosis, diphtheria, and whooping cough—were endemic; they swept virtually unstoppably through communities. Individuals with mental illnesses with generally internalized symptoms (so-called negative symptoms) or social deficits such as those associated with depression, developmental disabilities, anxiety, and some forms of schizophrenia might be allowed simply to live a passive, virtually invisible life in the community. Because such individuals posed no evident danger to others, they likely would be tolerated in the community and would be cared for at home by family members who bore any disease-associated burden and stigma.

In contrast, individuals with mental disorders characterized by loud, intrusive, externalizing presentations likely would be far less tolerated in community settings. Behaviors such as those associated with severe psychotic disorders like many forms of schizophrenia (e.g., grandiose delusions, command hallucinations, psychotic agitation, irritability, paranoia, and emotional instability) might well be perceived as a threat to family and others in the community alike. Most often, such individuals were consigned to facilities designed for involuntary confinement, such as government-operated jailhouses. In some more financially well-off communities in the United States and Europe, community-run poorhouses or almshouses also were employed to house people identified as social dependents, among them individuals with schizophrenia or other serious mental illnesses.

The concept of an asylum specifically for people with the most serious mental illnesses appears to have been created during the 11th-century Islamic Abbasid Dynasty. The concept is believed to have traveled gradually through North Africa and into Europe in the 15th century, at the beginning of the Renaissance (Mora, 1985). Perhaps not surprisingly, the establishment of such a publicly funded asylum for persons with mental illness in the United States predates the secession of the 13 colonies from England and the subsequent signing of the Declaration of Independence in 1776. Indeed, the Virginia colonial legislature allocated public funds on June 4, 1770, specifically to support creation of a dedicated institution for individuals with mental illnesses. Three years later, in 1773, the nation's first public mental hospital, the Williamsburg, VA, Public Hospital for Persons of Insane and Disordered Minds, was ready to accept patients (Eastern State Hospital Archives, n.d.).

In the last quarter of the 18th century—and through the entire 19th and early 20th centuries—virtually no clinical or pharmacologic tools were available to treat the underlying psychiatric conditions of patients. Thus when agitated (or otherwise "difficult" in the eyes of staff), individuals in such facilities were restrained using methods that might include cages, chains, restraint boxes, and seclusion rooms. Similar methods were employed in jails, poorhouses, and hospitals with specialized units for people with serious mental illnesses. These facilities were sometimes in remote areas such as basements and outbuildings. It was not uncommon for a facility to charge a small admission fee to outsiders for the opportunity to observe institutionalized individuals, much as they visited sideshows at the circus. This practice amplified the degrading and punitive situation experienced by the facilities' residents and, at the same time, served to intensify adverse public attitudes toward people with mental illnesses, heightening both stigma and fear of violent behavior.

The overwhelming inhumanity of the conditions in mental hospitals, jails, and almshouses that characterized the dark ages of mental health was brought to light in the early 1800s in a series of reports by Dorothea Dix. Her concern about people housed in such facilities in the United States was influenced by reports about the York Retreat in England, a socially progressive asylum founded by a Quaker community in 1796 and described as a "place in which the unhappy might obtain refuge" (Gollaher, 1995, p. 110). Dix visited,locally operated jails or almshouses for individuals with mental illnesses, penning eyewitness reports (termed "memorials") about the conditions she discovered in those facilities.

As Gollaher (1995) chronicles in his biography of Dix, in testimony before the Massachusetts legislature following the release of her report *Memorial to the Massachusetts Legislature*, she described the state of facilities in the Commonwealth State: "I proceed, Gentleman, briefly to call your attention to the present state of insane persons confined within this commonwealth, in cages, closets, stalls, pens! Chained, naked, beaten with rods and lashed into obedience!" (p. 2). According to Gollaher, "She went on to provide unvarnished sketches of gibbering madmen and madwomen brutalized, smeared with their own excrement, and penned up like animals" (p. 3).

Unquestionably, Dix played a central role as an advocate for persons with mental illnesses, arguing their right to be cared for in clean, orderly, humane settings. She did so at the very time that young federal, state, and local governments in the United States were struggling to define policy and practice on issues relating to the role of government in the lives of individuals—including their health and social welfare. Dix often rose to argue that the true test of an enlightened government is how it meets the service and treatment needs of citizens unable to participate fully in society because of mental disorders.

Repeatedly describing in detail the conditions to which individuals with mental illnesses were subjected, she successfully argued in state legislatures across the United States that the humane treatment of disabled and mentally ill citizens was the moral responsibility of a civilized government. She consistently asserted that an orderly, well-run asylum could restore individuals and urged that state governments assume responsibility for the treatment and welfare of its citizens with mental illnesses.

Her considered opinion was that local governments often were too small and financially unstable to construct and consistently support the type of facility best suited to the treatment of persons with mental illnesses. She posited that state government was the most appropriate level of government to assume the responsibility for the treatment of its residents with mental disorders. Through her work and that of other crusading advocates, there was a subsequent policy shift from local containment of people with mental illnesses in jails and poorhouses to care and treatment in specialty regional- and state-operated asylums. This development marks the end of the behavioral health dark ages, heralding the institutional era in public mental health.

Institutional Era (Circa 1825–1960)

The institutional era in the United States was born of the belief that individuals with mental illnesses—and persons with physical and developmental disabilities, as well—were best treated in clean, well-managed institutions removed from the demands of daily life. The aim was to establish a therapeutic environment within which individuals unable to care for themselves would be housed and cared for with compassion. The intense interest in creating a physical environment that would be therapeutic resulted in considerable, detailed attention to the external architecture and interior organization of space of mental hospitals.

Throughout the early and middle 19th century, the federal and state governments in the United States were embroiled in intense debate about their relative roles in managing public health, social welfare, and education. The War of 1812 affirmed that the young federal government needed to organize and support the national defense, seen as far more important than federal support for Health and social needs. During the same period, Dix and other advocates proposed that state governments should be responsible for the humane treatment of people with mental illnesses or developmental disabilities by sheltering and caring for them in state asylums. To some extent, ironically, the intense debates at the federal and state levels regarding human rights violations associated with slavery helped advance advocacy for mental health reform at the state level. Building a substantial asylum for persons with mental illnesses served as a civilized symbol of compassion and humanitarianism. Asylum construction provided ballast against the far more charged inhumanity and human rights issues associated with the abolition or continuation of slavery.

The number and size of mental asylums around the United States grew markedly from 1825 to 1900. In 1844, asylums had an average census of about 200 patients, for a total of roughly 4,800 nationwide. By 1900, that figure had risen to nearly 70,000 (as shown in figure 13–1 in chapter 13). In 1844, 13 of the nation's 24 asylum superintendents met to create a forum for exchange of ideas regarding treatment and asylum management. This organization, which later became the American Psychiatric Association, is one of the oldest national physician professional organizations in the United States (American Psychiatric Association, n.d.; Deutsch, 1937), and was instrumental in defining living and treatment standards for asylum residents, including optimal censuses and architectural design. By 1890, every state had funded, constructed, and staffed one or more publicly supported mental hospitals, the census of which grew concomitantly with the nation's overall population. Although a few prominent private asylums were built, primarily for the most affluent citizens with mental disorders, people with serious mental disorders generally were consigned to and cared for in facilities established by and maintained with state-appropriated funds. The historical growth in custodial, institution-based care is clearly seen in chapter 13's figure 13–1.

In his history of mental health care in America, Grob (1983) suggests that in the main, treatment provided in these publicly funded facilities sought to maintain order, structure, stability, and cleanliness. To that end, asylum residents were expected to engage in forms of work that not only helped maintain order and cleanliness but also yielded putative therapeutic value. Facility personnel and policy makers alike believed that this type of structured environment could be curative;

those treated ultimately would be able to be restored to sanity and to return to their communities. Being a good asylum resident meant following the rules of the institution. Good patients were compliant with ward programs and schedules; the environment was one in which they experienced little if any control over most aspects of their lives (Grob, 1983). The conditions of persons with serious mental illnesses continued in much the same manner in the United States through the middle of the 20th century.

The early 1950s marked the height of psychiatric institutionalization across the United States. By that time, nearly 500,000 individuals lived as permanent residents of psychiatric institutions. Although some individuals returned to the community, either cured or in remission, the vast majority remained in the facilities for years or decades, often housed in chronic care wards for difficult-to-discharge, seemingly incurable patients.

In the late 1940s and early 1950s, two important events began to reshape public policy and public thinking about institutional care, much as Dix's reports had heightened concern a century earlier. The first was a seminal publication by Albert Deutsch; the second was the introduction in 1952 of a medication, the first of its kind, to treat the symptoms of schizophrenia. Deutsch's *Shame of the States* (1948) described in unvarnished language the conditions and the status of individuals living in state-operated mental hospitals. His accounts stimulated an outpouring of support for the more humane treatment of individuals with mental illnesses. Deutsch's candid descriptions were in the style of Dix's memorials written about 100 years earlier. In the following decades several landmark studies were conducted on the psychological and social effects of institutions which had such complete control over the lives of the individuals living within them. These included concepts such as "institutional neurosis" by Barton (1959), the "total institution" by Goffman (1961), and the "social breakdown syndrome" by Gruenberg, Brandon, and Kasius (1966). These works reinforced the impetus for change.

Shaming and blaming alone, however, were not sufficient to alter the situation. What was demanded was a greater understanding of the mechanisms of mental illnesses and the identification of viable treatment tools for specific serious mental disorders. Thus even more than the exposés of the state hospital systems, impetus and hope for change came in the form of a medication found to alleviate some of the most disturbing symptoms of schizophrenia. That medication, chlorpromazine, was first used in Europe to facilitate anesthesia; subsequently it was found to abate hallucinations and delusions in persons with schizophrenia. It was introduced specifically for use in individuals with that diagnosis in 1952. As a result, the small pharmaceutical budgets for state mental hospitals began to grow as state legislatures allocated resources to pay for the wide-scale use of chlorpromazine and other, later introduced antipsychotic medications for patients in those facilities (Swazey, 1974). The perceived failure of psychiatric institutions, coupled with the new availability of medications and a growing armamentarium of non-somatic interventions to treat persons with schizophrenia and, increasingly, other serious mental disorders, helped usher in a new era of hope that individuals who were chronically institutionalized might be able to live more successfully in community settings and not in mental hospitals.

Community Tools Development (Circa 1960–2000)

In his last State of the Union address, President John Kennedy (1963) told the American people, "I believe that the abandonment of the mentally ill and the mentally retarded to the grim mercy of custodial institutions too often inflicts on them and on their families a needless cruelty which this Nation should not endure." Within nine months of that statement, he signed into law the Mental Retardation Facilities and Community Mental Health Centers Construction Act of 1963 (CMHC Act). Title II of that law both provided funds to build CMHCs across the country and established a clear federal role in the treatment of individuals with mental illnesses. Thus with this law, the 1960s—an era of social change and attention to human rights—also marked the birth of the community behavioral health movement in the United States (Goode, 1992).

Under the CMHC Act, the United States was divided into catchment areas of approximately 75,000 to 200,000 persons, each of which ideally would contain a CMHC to serve those in need. Federal funding to build and organize the CMHCs was made available through competitive grants to local governments. It was not unusual for CMHCs to be created as branches of local or county health departments. Populations to be served by these programs included not only low-income individuals in need of assessment, diagnosis, and treatment for mental disorders but also persons who were returning to the community from state mental hospitals. To be eligible for federal grant funding, CMHCs were required to provide five essential services: (1) inpatient services, (2) outpatient services, (3) day treatment, (4) emergency services, and (5) consultation and education (prevention) services. Many CMHCs, as part of local government, had the capacity to provide a broad array of services—what today would be described as spanning prevention through rehabilitation and recovery. Further, CMHCs often undertook local community behavioral health promotion and illness prevention (Caplan, 1961,1964).

During these early years of CMHC development, considerable attention was paid to creating the clinical and social support tools best able to help provide individuals with serious mental illnesses with the tools, treatment, and skills needed live in community settings. These tools are grouped into three types:

• biologics and pharmacologics
• psychological and psychotherapeutic interventions
• rehabilitation and community supports.

PSYCHOACTIVE MEDICATIONS

Several broad categories of medications are commonly used to treat a range of mental illnesses; among the most common are antipsychotics, antidepressants, mood stabilizers, and anxiolytic (antianxiety) agents. Following the introduction of chlorpromazine in the 1950s, the number and range of medications continued to grow exponentially during the community tools era.

By 1975, the year in which the antipsychotic loxapine was introduced in the United States, about 15 different antipsychotic agents were in regular use, among them thioridazine, chlorpromazine, thiothixene, and haloperidol. These medications were defined and ranked in potency by their affinity to dopamine receptors in the brain.

A significant change in the range of medications available to treat the signs and symptoms of schizophrenia began to take shape in 1990 with the availability of a new medication, clozapine. While known to have superior efficacy to its predecessor medications, clozapine has been of limited use because of its significant untoward side effects (Crilly, 2007). However, beginning in 1992, a second generation of antipsychotic medications—among them risperidone, olanzapine, and quetiapine—began to come onto the market. Unlike predecessor agents, these new antipsychotic medications interact with a wide variety of neuroreceptors in the brain, not just those for dopamine. While increasingly effective, the improved efficacy of these multifactorial agents dashed the hope that schizophrenia could be explained by a defect in a single neurochemical circuit.

Rapid development of drugs to treat depressive disorders was also under way during this period. At the outset of the community tools era, the predominant type of antidepressants available were the tricyclic agents, known to be highly sedating and fraught with multiple, difficult-to-tolerate adverse side effects. Fluoxetine (released under the trade name of Prozac in 1985) was the first of many in a new class of antidepressants: selective serotonin reuptake inhibitors (SSRIs). Since that time, a number of well-tolerated SSRIs and similar medications have become available.

Medications to stabilize mood available at the outset of the community tools era were limited primarily to lithium. Since then, a number of mood stabilizer agents have become available, many of which also act as antiseizure agents, among them valproic acid, carbamazepine, and lamotrigine. The benzodiazepines—diazepam and alprazolam—are the mainstays of pharmacologic treatment for anxiety disorders. While very effective in the treatment of anxiety, the benzodiazepines also have significant abuse potential. For that reason, more often than not a combination of modern antidepressants, even antipsychotic agents, may be used in lieu of the benzodiazepines to treat individuals with anxiety disorders.

Whether antipsychotics, anxiolytics, or antidepressants, these new pharmacologic treatments, while generally more effective than their predecessors, are also considerably more expensive. CBHOs and their funders, including local, state, and federal sources, were thus confronted with a dilemma. Historically, medication costs for patients being discharged into the community often were borne by state governments as part of state hospital budgets. As newer, much more expensive medications were released, continued state funding of medication costs became an increasing challenge.

PSYCHOTHERAPIES

Psychotherapies—initially referred to as "talking therapies"—are the second key set of services to help treat persons with serious mental illnesses that underwent significant refinement during the community tools development era. Psychotherapy as first conceptualized by Sigmund Freud has broadened markedly in its nature, scope, and practice.. Indeed, a variety of schools of thought grew and diverged from Freud's work that turned out to benefit, with some range of efficacy, people with serious mental disorders. The psychotherapies were sometimes used alone and sometimes in combination with somatic therapies.

Among the therapies that have proven effective in the treatment of persons with serious mental disorders are cognitive behavioral therapy (CBT), interpersonal psychotherapy (IPT), dialectical behavioral therapy (DBT), and behavioral activation therapy(BAT) (Dewan, Steenbarger, & Greenberg, 2004). Many of these psychotherapeutic interventions have been carefully described in detailed instructional manuals to help standardize their use in individual or group settings. At the same time, they can be individualized to serve the specialized needs of each person in care.

During the tools development era, substantial advances also were made in specialized substance abuse treatments. By the early 1980s, most communities had at least one inpatient addiction treatment center providing intensive treatment based on a 28-day model. Thereafter, substance abuse treatment services were broadened to include an array of options, among them individual outpatient counseling and intensive, multisession, group programs that provide both treatment and education. Many of these services remain in place today, along with increased use of medications—from methadone to buprenorphine—to counteract addictive cravings.

COMMUNITY SUPPORT TOOLS

A third set of tools was developed in this era: community support tools, often referred to as rehabilitation or habilitation services. Such tools are designed to give individuals with serious mental illnesses what they need to sustain meaningful, productive, and engaged lives in a community setting. An array of community support programs were implemented during the tools development era, among them the clubhouse (a place for people "to be" in the community) and case management (providing both outreach and services support). Both are described in greater detail later in this chapter.

As CBHOs expanded and became more specialized, so, too, did the types of programs and interventions available to individuals they served. Increasingly, CBHOs began to make available services that extended beyond the somatic and nonsomatic therapies, among them crisis programs, supported housing, sheltered workshops and employment, community integration groups, and individualized, community-based interventions (e.g., assertive community treatment and intensive outpatient services). Specialty community behavioral health services for children, developed along similar lines, often included after-school programs, in-home care, and other wraparound supports that together addressed an individual child's specific needs within the context of the family, school, and community.

Rehabilitative services also underwent extensive development and refinement during this era. In the 1950s, few community mental health services were available to meet the needs of discharged state hospital patients. By the turn of the millennium, however, an extensive array of specialized community behavioral health services and programs had become available across the nation. During the interim, and continuing to this day, the capacity of systems of community care in place during the era of deinstitutionalization (shown in figure 13–1 of chapter 13) was not equal to the pace of discharge of individuals from custodial era mental hospitals into community settings, leading to problems such as a high proportion of homelessness among the mentally ill (Fischer & Breakey, 1986; Koegel, Burnam, &Farr, 1988. The problems of the predictable custodial environment of the institutional era were exchanged for the possibility of a much less predictable environment, sometimes entailing homelessness, in the era of deinstitutionalization.

CHANGE AGENTS

Three federal programs enacted during the tools development era had tremendous impact on the delivery of behavioral health services and the rise of CBHOs: Social Security, Medicare, and Medicaid (the last, a federal–state partnership). The original Social Security Act, signed into law in 1935 by President Franklin D. Roosevelt, made retirement benefits available to individuals who had paid into the program during their working years; benefits also were available to individuals' spouses and offspring. In addition, two distinct programs within the original Social Security framework provide payments to individuals with disabilities that prohibit them from performing "substantial gainful employment." The Supplemental Security Disability Income (SSDI) program provides support to disabled individuals who have worked; payments are proportional to previous employment income. The Supplemental Security Income (SSI)program provides minimal cash assistance to low-income (often no-income) individuals who are so disabled that they are unable to work at all.

Mental conditions are allowed as an eligible condition for disability determination. Frank and Glied (2006) suggest that these federal programs are a lifeline providing basic financial support that brings individuals with mental illnesses up to the federal poverty level, removing them from the extreme poverty under which such persons lived before disability benefits under Social Security became available.

With President Lyndon B. Johnson's signature in 1965, Medicare became public law, providing health insurance to individuals over age 65 and to adults of any age who are eligible for SSDI. Persons who have been found to be disabled under the SSDI program are eligible for Medicare benefits two years after receiving SSDI benefits. Medicare benefits include inpatient, outpatient, and medication coverage for the treatment of mental illnesses, though initially not at the same level as available for other illnesses.

The federal health program with the greatest impact on the form, content, and growth of community mental health services in this period is the federal–state collaboration known as Medicaid. Signed into law on July 30, 1965, the program provides health insurance coverage for low-income children and adults meeting specific income requirements. Certain basic services must be provided as a condition of Medicaid participation, but because the program is operated as a partnership between individual states and the federal government, states may opt to provide (or exclude) a much broader range of health and support services, among them mental health services. Consistent with efforts to encourage community-based care, one of Medicaid's particular emphases is on community alternatives to long-term care in nursing homes.

The financing of Medicaid, too, is a federal–state partnership. The percentage of federal funds available for state matching is based on a state's overall personal income level. Thus states with greater poverty receive a higher federal match; states with low poverty have a dollar-to-dollar, or 50%, federal match. For example, in 2010, Mississippi had the highest federal match at 84.6 federal dollars and 16.4 state dollars for every 100 dollars spent on Medicaid health benefits (Kaiser Family Foundation, 2012). By the end of the 20th century, each of the 50 states provided some type of mental health coverage for its Medicaid-eligible populations of all ages.

The community tools development era was a significant and active period in the development and refinement of community mental health services. Many tools, policies, and programs were developed that helped support the ability of persons with mental illnesses to live safe and satisfying lives in community settings. These advances are the foundation on which today's community mental and behavioral health services and programs have been built.

Recovery Era

At the close of the 20th century, in an interim report to President George W. Bush (Hogan, 2002), the chair of the President's New Freedom Commission on Mental Health characterized the mental health system in the United States as a "patchwork relic—the result of disjointed reforms and policies." In the letter transmitting the final report to the president the following year (New Freedom Commission on Mental Health, 2003), the chair observed that "instead of ready access to quality care, the system presents barriers that all too often add to the burden of mental illnesses for individuals, their families and our communities." The commission called for increased national attention to the services and health care of Americans with or at risk for mental disorders. Foremost, however, the report firmly embraced recovery as an essential goal for all behavioral health services and programs.

The concept of recovery is consistent with the aim of contemporary disability policy in the United States to establish a level playing field for individuals with disabilities. The goal is to enable persons with disabilities to live, work, and participate in the community of their choice. For people with mental disorders, much as for people with other chronic, remitting illnesses, recovery includes not only management of specific symptoms but also community support mechanisms that promote integration of individuals with mental illness into the social, behavioral, and economic fabric of their environments. To support recovery, communities and workplaces are expected to make adaptations and accommodations as necessary for the management of features of a mental illness, just as they would accommodate specialized needs of an individual in a wheelchair or with a visual or auditory impairment. (For a discussion about the health needs of persons with disabilities of all kinds, see US Department of Health and Human Services, 2012.)

The recovery era for behavioral health services was bolstered by enactment of the federal Mental Health Parity and Addiction Equity Act of 2008, which sought to eliminate existing disparities between coverage for behavioral and physical health care. This movement toward parity was reinforced further during the Obama administration in the form of health care reform legislation enacted in 2010 as the Patient Protection and Affordable Care Act.

The clinical tools of this current era place emphasis on services and techniques that both are supported by evidence of efficacy and encourage active patient participation in their own care. Newer medications such as second-generation antipsychotics are in common use, and growing attention is being paid to novel delivery systems and mechanisms, such as long-acting injections that foster consistent adherence to effective medication dosages.

The recovery concept holds great promise both for promoting the engagement of the consumer as a partner in treatment and for reducing the stigma that continues to be associated with mental illnesses. Indeed, a growing number of CBHOs include consumers of mental health services themselves among their professional and paraprofessional staff. These individuals work in volunteer or paid capacities to provide peer support and other services, including the provision of both outreach services and community integration promotion. Only time will tell whether the concepts that underlie recovery will ultimately be found to improve access, quality, and coordination of CBHO service delivery.

EXEMPLAR SERVICES DELIVERED THROUGH CBHOS

This section explores types of services that frequently are provided to persons with serious mental illnesses by contemporary CBHOs in the United States. This information is intended to be useful for students of mental health who are not clinical practitioners and may not have seen these services firsthand. It may be useful to clinicians as well by providing a full orientation and background on these services.

Case Management

The foremost goal of case management is to enable individuals in need of mental health care to navigate complex, often fragmented service systems to ensure they have access to health, mental health, and other needed supportive and social services (Kersbergen, 1996). The concept and practice of case management actually dates to 1863, when nurses and social service providers sought to respond to a growing public health crisis among the increasing poor and immigrant populations in urban areas of the United States. The introduction of case management was designed to improve collaboration and coordination across traditionally parallel, unintegrated health care and human services sectors (Kersbergen, 1996). In its earliest incarnation, case management focused on advocating for services to meet the full range of an individual family's needs as well as on larger environmental and neighborhood concerns (Kersbergen, 1996).

Over time, both the value of and the need for case management grew, particularly with the commensurate growth in human services programs to serve returning World War II veterans in the 1940s, to respond to the war on poverty, and to meet the challenges of advancing the civil rights and the deinstitutionalization movements alike in the 1960s and beyond. Case management also changed the treatment of individuals in need of or seeking care, helping to move them from social dependence to active participation in their own care. This active, consumer-based mentality has helped to change the relationship between consumers and service providers (Kersbergen, 1996).

Case management demanded specialized staff able to provide outreach to persons in need of behavioral health and supportive

---

Box 14-1. A CBHO Case Example

Maryanne is a 35-year-old woman with a 15-year history of schizophrenia. Her condition began in college with paranoid delusions that centered on a belief that she was receiving encoded messages through calculus equations about a secret mission she was to undertake on behalf of her math professor. The first several years of her illness were marked by multiple psychiatric hospitalizations and rounds of homelessness, during which she was the victim of two rapes and a mugging. Over the years, she became progressively alienated from family and friends. Then, at age 27, she was referred to a CBHO, where she was assessed, diagnosed, and received intensive services for the next five years. Those services included assertive community treatment and psychiatric care that centered on community support services and supported housing. As a part of her recovery, she took several classes at a local community college; she eventually entered a training program to become a peer support specialist. Most recently, she was certified by her state as a peer support specialist, enabling her to help provide community support services to other people at the very CBHO from which she first received care. Her current ambition is to facilitate the recovery of others so that they do not experience the same difficulties she did early in her illness. She also is working actively to redevelop relationships with family and past friends.

services, to identify the range of any one individual's service needs, and to piece providers, programs, and service systems together to meet those individual needs. As long-term inpatients from state mental hospitals were moved into community settings beginning in the 1960s, they often were confronted by complex social services and health care systems that were neither readily accessed nor well coordinated to meet an individual's varied needs. Recognizing the problem, in the early 1970s the US Department of Health, Education, and Welfare (now known as the Department of Health and Human Services) sought to improve coordination across health and supportive service programs through evaluation of a variety of service coordination models at the local and state levels (Vincent, 2005). From these early explorations of coordinated care, the National Institute of Mental Health, part of the US Department of Health and Human Services, developed the concept of the community support system, designed to facilitate improved service integration for people with mental disorders. Subsequently, service integration was mandated under the Developmentally Disabled Assistance and Bill of Rights Acts of 1975 and 1978. The former statute required that each client be assigned to a program coordinator; the latter further stipulated that case management services were to play the central role in coordinating services.

Today, CBHO case managers often serve as focal points for organizing and facilitating access to a wide variety of services, including behavioral health, rehabilitation, physical health, social services, and even housing, employment, and education. CBHOs generally provide case management services based on one of three models, each of which emphasizes the individualization of care:

- Brokered case management model: The case manager links the patient to services (Intagliata, 1982; Rohland, Rohrer, & Tzou, 2004).
- Clinical case management model: The case manager serves in a blended role to provide limited clinical, therapeutic support and to link the patient to needed services (Kanter,1989).

- Strengths model: The case manager functions as an advocate to support the strengths and preferences of the patient (Brun & Rapp, 2001).

Case managers represent hands-on staff with clearly delineated roles who are critical to assuring the availability and functioning of the full complement of specific services needed to support an individual's successful integration into community living.

Assertive Community Treatment

In the early 1970s, a group of innovative investigators at the Mendota State Hospital in Madison, Wisconsin, sought to establish a program to meet the needs of patients in community settings, particularly since rates of patient dropout and loss to follow-up in community day hospitals and psychosocial rehabilitation centers were found to be very high. These researchers first created a program called "Total In-Community Treatment" to teach coping skills in the community, to instruct in ways to reduce the likelihood of rehospitalization, and to establish close working relationships with multiple agencies to help secure housing and supportive services for clients (Stein, Test, & Marx, 1975). This evolved into the Assertive Community Treatment (ACT) program (Stein & Santos, 1998; Stein &Test, 1980). The investigators determined that the most significant problems confronting hard-to-discharge patients, regardless of diagnosis, included poor problem-solving skills, vulnerability to stress, and dependence on caregivers (Stein & Santos, 1998). By the mid-1970s, the Mendota State Hospital began operating the first formally described and organized Program for Assertive Community Treatment (PACT). That program both acknowledged the chronic nature of mental illness and emphasized the development of interpersonal relationships, negotiation of practical everyday problems, employment-sustaining housing, and the need for regular adherence to prescription of psychiatric medication. By 1980, the program had evolved so that the first formal ACT program began as a mobile community treatment (MCT) program of the Dane

County, Wisconsin, Mental Health Center. Today, ACT has become one of the most prominent community-based treatment models for individuals with severe mental disorders. Assertive community treatment is a well-defined intervention for people with severe mental disorders and also has been adapted for populations with added special needs, such as persons with co-occurring substance abuse disorders (Stein & Santos, 1998).

At its core, ACT is structured to resemble an inpatient treatment team; it simply functions in the outpatient, community-based setting. Not surprisingly, ACT often is referred to as a "hospital without walls." The treatment team meets daily to review the status and needs of individual patients and make plans for that day's activities and interventions. A typical team includes a psychiatrist, a therapist, several psychiatric nurses, case managers, and care coordinators who together treat a fixed number of individuals. Increasingly ACT team staffing includes consumers who serve as peer support specialists. Treatment teams support a range of individual recovery goals and often work directly with issues surrounding medication (McGrew & Bond, 1995). Interactions generally take place in a community location, at patients' homes, and only occasionally in an office setting. On a given day, a single patient may be seen once or multiple times; ACT teams see particularly fragile clients more often than more stable patients.

Several randomized controlled trials have used clinical, social, and economic measures to determine the effectiveness of ACT compared with standard community care for people with serious mental illnesses (Marshall & Lockwood, 1998). Research consistently has demonstrated that patients engaged with ACT have fewer hospital admissions and, when hospitalized, have shorter stays. They are more likely than those receiving standard care to remain engaged with mental health services. Moreover, ACT provides increased housing stability, as measured by greater likelihood and duration of independent housing (Latimer, 1999). Clinical and social measures such as employment and patient satisfaction were significantly better among those participating in ACT than among those in standard

community care. The ACT approach has been found to be cost-effective as an intervention both for individuals who are homeless and for others with high service utilization compared with those in standard care or receiving solely case management. Among individuals with mental illnesses who also are homeless, Wolff and colleagues (1997) reported that ACT was more cost-effective than brokered case management for making service contacts, managing symptoms, and providing satisfactory services. Further, successful use of ACT was found to lead patients, over time, to less costly forms of care (Clark & Samnaliev, 2005).

The clinical effectiveness of ACT has been demonstrated, particularly among individuals with high numbers of long-stay hospital admissions, in many (Burns & Santos, 1995; Lehman, Dixon, Kernan, DeForge, & Postrado, 1997) but not all (Killaspy et al., 2009) evaluations. Unfortunately, its regular use in community-based settings has been limited by its higher start-up costs compared with case management. Its cost-effectiveness arises over time, from reduced use of other mental health, social, and hospital care services (Salkever et al., 1999). Nonetheless, ACT is increasingly an important foundation of services provided by CBHOs.

Clubhouse Model

A clubhouse is a community center for people with mental illnesses to socialize and work together. The clubhouse functions as an intentional therapeutic community with the goal of helping clients regain self-confidence, promoting rights for people with mental illness, and overcoming stigma.

The model has its roots in a program called We Are Not Alone, which began as a support group for former patients of the Rockland State Hospital in New York. Although individuals wanted to remain in the community, many former patients found it difficult because of social isolation, a dearth of independent housing, and limited employment opportunities. In 1948, with the help of volunteers and a donation from the National Council of Jewish Women, the program purchased a house in midtown Manhattan which had a small garden that included a fountain—and Fountain House was born (Fountain House, 1999).

From its inception, Fountain House and subsequent clubhouses have been founded and operated by members as a club. Potentially stigmatizing terms are avoided, participants are referred to as members, and specific diagnoses are unimportant. The clubhouse model emphasizes relationships between and among members and staff. The model does not provide behavioral or physical health care services, though some clubhouses are affiliated with clinical facilities. Members have lifetime membership, are involved in tasks essential to clubhouse operation, have the right to choose the type of work they participate in, and help in selecting staff.

The clubhouse model creates an environment in which members feel wanted and appreciated for who they are. This sense of belonging, along with the potential for work, empowers each member to become a respected coworker, neighbor, and friend. Members are accepted without regard to psychiatric symptoms, and they are not required to show improvement in their symptoms to maintain membership. The length of stay, which differentiates the clubhouse model from many other psychosocial programs, allows members to participate indefinitely, regardless of their clinical state. Once a member of a clubhouse, one is a member for life.

Fountain House has become a model for psychiatric rehabilitation not only in the United States but also around the world. Today, the International Center for Clubhouse Development (ICCD) both maintains standards for the clubhouse model and provides training for staff to ensure consistent application of the program approach and philosophy. The ICCD works with people with mental illness, professionals in mental health, family members, volunteers, and local government to disseminate information about the clubhouse model broadly.

Based on ICCD international surveys in 1999 (see Macias, Jackson, Schroeder, & Wang, 1999), a typical clubhouse in the United States is between 4 and 123 years old and has from 65 to 150 active members. About 40% of members attend the clubhouse daily. The average staff-to-member ratio is 1:12.8. Half of the staff are bachelor-level social workers, and 10% are consumers, people with serious mental illness themselves. Staff receive a three-week-long model-specific training conducted by the ICCD. The staff turnover rate in clubhouses was found to be very low, an indication of job satisfaction. The majority (77%) of clubhouses also provide case management services, which play an integral role in assuring members' access to resources in the community that are not available in the clubhouse (Fountain House, 1999).

The heart of a clubhouse program is the "work-ordered day," which encourages members to work side by side with staff in the clubhouse building. Tasks generally fall into one of three work units. The maintenance work unit supports the building and undertakes activities such as grounds maintenance and repairs. The clerical work unit answers the phone and manages other communications, often including production of a newsletter for the community. The kitchen work unit generally plans and prepares a noontime meal every day. The work-ordered day is not intended as job training for specific skills; rather, its purpose is to help participants regain self-worth and confidence through making a contribution.

Since its inception at Fountain House, the clubhouse program has been a grassroots phenomenon. In 1999, Fountain House and the ICCD started more formal evaluation and research of the approach, though much of the work remains qualitative and descriptive. Nonetheless, a few studies have compared vocational and social outcomes of the ACT and clubhouse models. Stein, Barry, Van Dien, Hollingsworth, and Sweeney (1999) found strong similarities between ACT and clubhouse participants in vocational activities, social rehabilitation, social networks, and community integration. A long-term experimental comparison of participants' employment status between an ACT program and an ICCD-certified clubhouse in the northeastern United States reported that both were successful in generating employment opportunities (Macias et al., 2006). The ACT program was slightly better at engaging and retaining clients. This result likely reflects the assertive nature and aggressive outreach of ACT teams, whereas clubhouses rely on members' daily personal motivation to participate. But even though the proportion of employment achievement initially was higher for the ACT program, this difference diminished over the study period. Clubhouse members were found to work more total days and to receive higher hourly wages. Moreover, clubhouse members were not as likely to engage in basic labor; they generally attained longer-lasting, career-oriented employment.

The clubhouse model has played an invaluable role in the development of a humanistic model for psychiatric rehabilitation of individuals with enduring mental illnesses who otherwise might be relegated to long-term hospitalization or social isolation in communities. However, the role of the clubhouse in the spectrum of psychosocial rehabilitation services has been drawn into question for a variety of reasons. A significant issue, for example, is the priority the model places on voluntary attendance and participation. After all, isolation, difficulty engaging in social relationships, lack of motivation, easily being discouraged, and vulnerability to illicit drug use in the community are symptoms of an array of mental illnesses that may thwart motivation to participate in programming of any kind and render regular participation a particular challenge. In the clubhouse model, it is easy for individuals to be absent, drop out, and disengage. In contrast, ACT staff typically visit clients in their homes and engage in intense, hands-on follow-up and outreach.

Another factor that has impeded clubhouse programs may be the high priority today's consumers place on obtaining employment. The core of the clubhouse model provides a work-ordered day but does not necessarily provide entry into competitive employment. While the clubhouse model has a place in a community that is unable to offer a full range of rehabilitative services, in other communities its role may be supplanted by programs such as supported employment programs that offer direct links to regular competitive employment (discussed below) and by ACT, which is better able

to reach out to individuals who have difficulty maintaining participation.

Supported Employment

In another effort to promote community-based living in the mid-1970s, vocational rehabilitation services were developed to better integrate people with severe disabilities of all kinds into specialized types of community employment. The emphasis of vocational services at the time was primarily on individuals with physical and developmental disabilities (Wehman & Kregel, 1985); little if any attention was paid to people with serious mental illnesses. This imbalance in both public awareness and support for people with mental illnesses further marginalized their job opportunities, opportunities already compromised by the fear and stigma associated with these disorders. Although, thanks to these initiatives, the overall employment rate increased among people with disabilities, the rate during the same period actually decreased by 3% among persons with mental illnesses (Skelley, 1980).

In response to the dearth of vocational programming for persons with serious mental disorders, a few psychosocial rehabilitative programs began to develop transitional employment programs. Distinct from traditional vocational rehabilitation programs, these programs focused entirely on people with mental disorders and provided on-site coaching in actual job settings (Becker, Whitley, Bailey, & Drake, 2007).

Over the last 30 years, tremendous advances have been made in the development of successful strategies to help individuals with even the most severe mental conditions achieve some degree of competitive employment. Debate continues, however, regarding the best method to facilitate job attainment; an answer may lie in the capacity to differentiate the level of service based on individual factors such as education, prior work history, mental condition, and age of onset of mental condition.

The intense focus and scrutiny that employment services have been given over the decades is a fundamental element in the transition from the tools development era to the current, recovery era. Rather than being satisfied with just being quiet and symptom free in a noninstitutional setting, today consumers with serious mental conditions are actively engaged in the workforce and are participating in increasingly meaningful ways in the community of their choice.

CONCLUSION

Mental health services in the United States have evolved markedly through four distinct periods over the nation's history. The evolution began in the dark ages, during which scant specific treatment was available and containment of persons perceived to be unstable in a community setting was a central priority. The second, institutional era was associated with great humanitarian ideas manifested in part by the construction of specialized regional institutions intended to provide treatment and restorative asylum to individuals with serious mental illnesses, who also were considered to be incapable of social independence. The third, community tools era was associated with the development of a growing array of clinical and rehabilitative services designed to enable individuals with serious mental illnesses to adapt successfully to community living. The current, fourth era—the recovery era—builds on the significant strides made during the community tools era, placing emphasis on long-term, supported recovery for persons with serious mental disorders and the achievement of lives that are full, meaningful, and productive. Specific services that promote recovery include case management, ACT, and psychosocial rehabilitative programs such as clubhouse and supported employment programs.

Today, more is known than ever before about the causes of and effective treatments and services for mental illnesses. More is known about the need for individualized care and the importance of integrated, concurrent treatment for individuals with co-occurring mental and substance use disorders or mental and physical illnesses. Until mental illnesses can be prevented altogether, services will continue to grow in sophistication and capacity to reduce the adverse impact of these long-term disorders on individuals, their families, their communities, and their nation. Community behavioral health organizations represent the bedrock of essential community support and recovery services for persons with serious mental illnesses.

REFERENCES

American Psychiatric Association. (n.d.). *APA history*. Retrieved from http://psych.org/MainMenu/EducationCareerDevelopment/Library/APAHistory.aspx

Barton, R. (1959). *Institutional neurosis*. Bristol, UK: John Wright and Sons.

Becker, D., Whitley, R., Bailey, E. L., & Drake, R. E. (2007). Long-term employment trajectories among participants with severe mental illness in supported employment. *Psychiatric Services, 58*(7), 922–928.

Brun, C., & Rapp, R. C. (2001). Strengths-based case management: Individuals' perspectives on strengths and the case manager relationship. *Social Work, 46*(3), 278–288.

Burns, B. J., & Santos, A. B. (1995). Assertive community treatment: An update of randomized trials. *Psychiatric Services, 46*(7), 669–675.

Caplan, G. (1961). *An approach to community mental health*. New York, NY: Grune and Stratton.

Caplan, G. (1964). *Principles of preventive psychiatry*. New York, NY: Basic Books.

Clark, R. E., & Samnaliev, M. (2005). Psychosocial treatment in the 21st century. *International Journal of Law and Psychiatry, 28*(5), 532–544.

Crilly, J. (2007). The history of clozapine in the U.S. and its emergence in the U.S. market: A review and analysis. *History of Psychiatry, 18*(1), 39–60.

Deutsch, A. (1937). *The mentally ill in America: A history of their care and treatment from colonial times*. New York, NY: Columbia University Press.

Deutsch, A. (1948). *Shame of the states. Mental illness and social policy: The American experience*. North Stratford, NH: Ayer.

Developmentally Disabled Assistance and Bill of Rights Act, Pub. L. No. 94–103 (1975).

Developmentally Disabled Assistance and Bill Of Rights Act, Pub. L. No. 95–602 (1978).

Dewan, M. J., Steenbarger, B. N., & Greenberg, R. P. (Eds.). (2004). *The art and science of brief psychotherapies: A practitioner's guide*. Arlington, VA: American Psychiatric Publishing.

Eastern State Hospital Archives. (n.d.). *The history of Eastern State*. Retrieved from http://www.esh.dmhmrsas.virginia.gov/

Fischer, P. J., & Breakey, W. R. (1986). Homelessness and mental health: An overview. *International Journal of Mental Health, 14,* 6–41.

Frank, R. G., & Glied, S. A. (2006). *Better but not well: Mental health policy in the United States since 1950.* Baltimore, MD: Johns Hopkins University Press.

Fountain House. (1999). Gold award: The wellspring of the clubhouse model for social and vocational adjustment of persons with serious mental illness. *Psychiatric Services, 50*(11), 1473–1476.

Goffman, E. (1961). *Asylums: Essays on the social situation of mental patients and other inmates.* New York, NY: Anchor.

Gollaher, D. (1995). *Voice for the mad: The life of Dorothea Dix.* New York, NY: Free Press.

Goode, E. (1992). *Collective behavior.* Fort Worth, TX: Harcourt-Brace-Jovanovich.

Grob, G. N. (1983). *Mental illness in American society, 1875 to 1940.* Princeton, NJ: Princeton University Press.

Gruenberg, E. M., Brandon, S., & Kasius, R. V. (1966). Identifying cases of the social breakdown syndrome. *Milbank Memorial Fund Quarterly, 44*(1), 150–155.

Hogan, M. (2002) *Interim report of the President's New Freedom Commission on Mental Health.* Rockville, MD: Substance Abuse and Mental Health Services Administration, US Department of Health and Human Services.

Intagliata, J. (1982). Improving the quality of community care for the chronically mentally disabled: The role of case management. *Schizophrenia Bulletin, 8*(4), 655–674.

Kaiser Family Foundation. (n.d.). *State health facts.* Retrieved March 21, 2012 from http://www.statehealthfacts.org

Kanter, J. (1989). Clinical case management: Definition, principles, components. *Hospital and Community Psychiatry, 40*(1), 361–368.

Kennedy, J. F. (1963, January 14). *State of the Union address.* Boston, MA: John F. Kennedy Presidential Library and Museum. Retrieved from http://www.jfklibrary.org/Historical+Resources/Archives/Reference+Desk/Speeches

Kersbergen, A. (1996). Case management: A rich history of coordinating care to control costs. *Nursing Outlook, 44*(4), 169–172.

Killaspy, H., Kingett, S., Bebbington, P., Blizard, R., Johnson, S., Nolan, F.,...King, M. (2009). Randomised evaluation of assertive community treatment: Three-year outcomes. *British Journal of Psychiatry, 195,* 81–82.

Koegel, P., Burnam, M. A., & Farr, R. K. (1988). The prevalence of specific psychiatric disorders among homeless individuals in the inner-city of Los Angeles. *Archives of General Psychiatry, 45*(12), 1085–1092.

Latimer, E. (1999). Economic impacts of assertive community treatment: A review of the literature. *Canadian Journal of Psychiatry, 44*(5), 443–454.

Lehman, A. F., Dixon, L. B., Kernan, E., DeForge, B. R., & Postrado, L. T. (1997). A randomized trial of assertive community treatment for homeless persons with severe mental illness. *Archives of General Psychiatry, 54*(11), 1038–1043.

Macias, C., Jackson, R., Schroeder, C., & Wang, Q. (1999). What is a clubhouse? Report on the ICCD 1996 survey of USA clubhouses. *Community Mental Health Journal, 35*(2), 181–190.

Macias, C., Rodican, C. F., Hargreaves, W. A., Jones, D. R., Barreira, P. J., & Wang, Q. (2006). Supported employment outcomes of a randomized controlled trial of ACT and clubhouse models. *Psychiatric Services, 57*(10), 1406–1415.

Marshall, M., & Lockwood, A. (1998). Assertive community treatment for people with severe mental disorders. In C. Adams, C. Anderson, & J. De Jesus Mari (Eds.), *Schizophrenia Module, Cochrane Database of Systematic Reviews.* London, UK: BMJ Publishing.

McGrew, J. H., & Bond, G. R. (1995). Critical ingredients of assertive community treatment: Judgments of the experts. *Journal of Mental Health Administration, 22*(2), 113–125.

Mental Health Parity and Addiction Equity Act of 2008, Public Law No. 110–343, 122 Stat. 3765 (2008).

Mental Retardation Facilities and Community Mental Health Centers Construction Act of 1963, Public Law No. 88–184, 42 U.S.C. § 2689–2689e (1963).

Mora, G. (1985). History of psychiatry. In H. I. Kaplan & B. J. Sadock (Eds.), *Comprehensive textbook of psychiatry* (4th ed., pp. 2034–2054). Baltimore, MD: Williams & Wilkins.

New Freedom Commission on Mental Health. (2003). *Achieving the promise: Transforming mental health care in America. Final report.* Rockville, MD: Substance Abuse and Mental Health Services Administration, US Department of Health and Human Services.

Patient Protection and Affordable Care Act, Public Law No. 111–148, 124 Stat. 119–124 (2010).

Rohland, B. M., Rohrer, J. E., & Tzou, H. (2004). Broker model of case management for persons with serious mental illness in rural areas. *Administration and Policy in Mental Health and Mental Health Services Research, 25*(5), 549–553.

Salkever, D., Domino, M. E., Burns, B. J., Santos, A. B., Deci, P. A., Dias, J., ... Paolone, J. (1999). Assertive community treatment for people with severe mental illness: The effect on hospital use and costs. *Health Services Research, 34*(2), 577–601.

Sharfstein, S. S. (2000). Whatever happened to community mental health? *Psychiatric Services, 51*(5), 616–620.

Shen, W. W. (1999). A history of antipsychotic drug development. *Comprehensive Psychiatry, 40*(6), 407–414.

Skelley, T. J. (1980). National developments in rehabilitation: A rehabilitation services perspective. *Rehabilitation Counseling Bulletin, 24,* 22–23.

Stein, L. I., Barry, K. K., Van Dien, G., Hollingsworth, E. J., & Sweeney, J. K. (1999). Work and social support: A comparison of consumers who have stability in ACT and clubhouse programs. *Community Mental Health Journal, 35*(2), 193–204.

Stein, L., & Santos, A. (1998). *Assertive community treatment of persons with severe mental illness.* New York, NY: W. W. Norton.

Stein, L. I., & Test, M. A. (1980). Alternative to mental hospital treatment: I. Conceptual model, treatment program, and clinical evaluation. *Archives of General Psychiatry, 37*(4), 392–397.

Stein, L. I., Test, M. A., & Marx, A. J. (1975). Alternative to the hospital: A controlled study. *American Journal of Psychiatry, 132*(5), 517–522.

Substance Abuse and Mental Health Services Administration. (2002). *Report to Congress on the prevention and treatment of co-occurring substance abuse disorders and mental disorders.* Rockville, MD: Substance Abuse and Mental Health Services Administration, US Department of Health and Human Services.

Substance Abuse and Mental Health Services Administration. (2010). *Results of the 2009 National Survey on Drug Use and Health: Mental health findings.* Rockville, MD: Substance Abuse and Mental Health Services Administration, US Department of Health and Human Services.

Substance Abuse and Mental Health Services Administration. (2011). *National expenditures for mental health services and substance abuse treatment, 1986–2005.* Rockville, MD: Substance Abuse and Mental Health Services Administration, US Department of Health and Human Services.

Surgeon General of the United States. (1999). *Mental health: A report of the surgeon general.* Rockville, MD: Substance Abuse and Mental Health Services Administration, US Department of Health and Human Services.

Swazey, J. P. (1974). *Chlorpromazine in psychiatry: A study of therapeutic innovation.* Cambridge, MA: MIT Press.

U.S. Department of Health & Human Services, Office on Disability: Health, Wellness, and Disability (retrieved March 21, 2012, from http://www.hhs.gov/od/about/fact_sheets/healthwellnessdisability.html.

Vincent, C. (2005). *The "superwaiver" proposal and service integration: A history of federal initiatives.* Washington, DC: Congressional Research Service, US Library of Congress.

Wehman, P., & Kregel, J. (1985). A supported work approach to competitive employment of individuals with moderate and severe handicaps, *Journal of the Association for Persons with Severe Handicaps,10*(1), 3–11.

Wolff, N., Helminiak, T., Morse, G., Calsyn, R., Klinkenberg, W., & Trusty, M. (1997). Cost-effectiveness evaluation of three approaches to case management for homeless mentally ill clients. *American Journal of Psychiatry, 154*(3), 341–348.

15

Pathways to Care: Need, Attitudes, Barriers

RAMIN MOJTABAI

WILLIAM W. EATON

PALLAB K. MAULIK

Key Points

- The *treatment gap* is commonly defined as the discrepancy between the large number of people with mental disorders and the much smaller number who seek treatment for them

- The treatment gap has narrowed in industrialized countries in recent years, but it persists as a public health challenge

- Addressing the unmet need for mental health care requires a better understanding of the process of seeking mental health treatment

- Seeking mental health treatment can be understood as a decisional balance between perceived need for mental health care and perceived barriers

- Stigma and financial difficulties are prominent examples of barriers to care

- These barriers have been reduced somewhat by public antistigma campaigns and legislative initiatives in health care financing

WHY STUDY TREATMENT-SEEKING BEHAVIOR?

Public concern about the high prevalence of untreated mental disorders in the United States was raised to significant levels, perhaps for the first time, in the 1950s with the publication of the Midtown Manhattan study (Srole & Fischer, 1975). The study found that as many as 25% of the population experienced marked or severe impairment due to mental illness and that over 50% suffered from moderate to mild psychological problems. These unanticipated findings suggested a great level of unmet need for mental health care. An even more alarming study finding was the low rates of treatment among individuals with the most significant impairments. Just over one fourth (26.7%) of those experiencing marked or severe mental health impairments had been treated at any point in their lives (Srole & Fischer, 1975).

Since the Midtown Manhattan study over five decades ago, much has transpired in the mental health field, in science, in programs development, and in policy. The capacity of the mental health care system in the United States has dramatically expanded, especially with regard to the size, training, and scope of the workforce. The number of psychiatrists in the United States has increased markedly, from around 5,500 in 1950 (Joint Commission on Mental Illness and Health, 1961) to just over 41,000 by 2002 (Duffy et al., 2006), a number that has remained relatively constant since that time (Smart, 2010). In addition, hundreds of thousands of psychologists, social workers, and counselors have joined the mental health clinical workforce since the 1950s. Even more dramatic than the growth in the number of mental health professionals have been the rising numbers of individuals who seek mental health care not from specialists but from clinicians in the general medical sector. The 2001–2003 National Comorbidity Survey Replication (NCS-R) study reported that individuals with common mental disorders sought treatment from general medical providers (including primary care doctors and other nonpsychiatrist physicians) at a slightly greater rate than from mental health care providers (23% vs. 22%) (Wang, Lane, et al., 2005).

This reliance on care from the general medical sector not only adds to the ranks of professionals who provide mental health care but also suggests an ongoing shift in the nature of mental health care itself. General medical providers are more likely than specialty sector mental health providers to rely predominantly on medications rather than on psychodynamic or behavioral treatments, a trend buttressed by the explosion of knowledge about the impact of brain chemistry on behavior and mental illnesses.

The growth of knowledge in the decades since the Midtown Manhattan study has led to important innovations in the technology (including new medications) for treatment of mental disorders. While the introduction of new short-term psychotherapies has provided increasingly efficient tools to meet individual treatment needs of patients in outpatient settings, the role of medications has became increasingly critical, particularly for people with the most serious mental disorders. The introduction of chlorpromazine, the first antipsychotic medication, not only dramatically changed care for individuals with schizophrenia but also is widely credited for the deinstitutionalization of people with the most severe mental illnesses (Joint Commission on Mental Illness and Health, 1961). Tricyclic antidepressant medications, introduced in the late 1960s, had a similarly dramatic impact on outpatient psychiatric treatment for depression and anxiety disorders. Finally, the introduction of selective serotonin reuptake inhibitors in the late 1980s and early 1990s greatly helped to expand the involvement of the primary health care sector in the treatment of depression and other common mental disorders. By the early 2000s, over 70% of antidepressant prescriptions in the United States were by general medical providers (Mojtabai & Olfson, 2008).

These significant advances in both pharmacologic and psychosocial interventions to treat mental disorders make the ongoing disparity between need for care and receipt of treatment for mental disorders all the more noteworthy. Apparently the field has had greater success in creating more effective treatments for mental disorders than it has in breaking through the various barriers, including fear and misunderstanding that keep people in need of treatment for mental disorders from seeking it. Based on data from the 1992–1993 National Comorbidity Survey (NCS), only 20% of individuals who met criteria for a mental disorder in the year prior to being interviewed sought care of any kind (Kessler et al., 2005). That figure rose to 32% a decade later in the 2001–2003 NCS replication (NCS-R, Kessler et al., 2005). Even among people with the most severe mental illnesses (5–6% of respondents), only 24% (in NCS) and 41% (in NCS-R) had sought treatment. These findings suggest that a large number of people who potentially could benefit from treatment neither seek nor receive care. As a result, the advances in the technologies of mental health treatment are mostly lost to the majority of individuals in greatest need of treatment whose illnesses give rise to significant social, economic, and health burden at the individual, community, and national levels.

This so-called treatment gap is not unique to the United States. An international study of mental disorders and their treatment in the early 2000s, the World Health Organization's World Mental Health Surveys, found that many individuals with serious mental conditions, whether living in the Americas, Europe, the Middle East, Africa, or Asia, did not receive any mental health treatment in the preceding year (Demyttenaere et al., 2004). (See table 15-1.) Even among those who ultimately do receive care, the time lag between illness onset and first treatment may be surprisingly long: from 6 to 10 years for many common, disabling mood and anxiety disorders, such as major depression and panic disorder (Wang, Berglund, Olfson, & Kessler, 2004; Wang, Berglund, et al., 2005).

While the mental health field has actively sought to discern the causes of mental disorders and to develop treatments for them, it has been slow both to recognize and to address the gap between prevalence of these disorders and treatment. In most cases this gap represents a valid, unmet need for care. Moreover, individuals who self-identify with mental disorders in general population surveys *do* experience negative social, financial, and health outcomes when they do not receive treatment. As both the public health and social implications of

this unmet need have been elucidated, numerous attempts have been made to address the problem and increase treatment seeking for common mental disorders.

Efforts have focused on two types of barriers: stigma and financial barriers. The stigma associated with mental illness is pervasive and commonly thought to be a significant barrier to the social integration of people with mental illness into the fabric of the society. Self-stigma, the internalized negative feelings individuals with mental illness have about their own value and abilities, adds a further impediment to treatment seeking (Vogel, Wade, & Hackler, 2007). Many individuals with common mental disorders may feel embarrassed disclosing their feelings and experiences to family, friends, or clinicians. In recognition of this issue, public education information and media campaigns have sought to reduce the stigma associated with mental illnesses and their treatments and to improve public recognition and understanding that mental health treatments can be effective. Later in the chapter we discuss some of these programs. At the same time, legislative initiatives have been undertaken to remove financial impediments to care for those who do seek treatment. In the United States, a recent prominent example of such an initiative is the Mental Health Parity and Addiction Equity Act of 2008, which aimed to expand insurance coverage of mental health care for employees.

Addressing the unmet need for mental health care requires a better understanding of both treatment seeking and barriers to service use. This chapter first presents an overview of the process of seeking mental health treatment in community-based settings and briefly discusses stigma and financial barriers to mental health care. Attempts to overcome these barriers have been at the forefront of the public mental health agenda for many years, with varying degrees of success. The chapter then explores some of the most significant public health campaigns targeting the stigma associated with mental illness and treatment seeking. Finally, it examines a range of policy initiatives that have sought to eliminate or reduce financial barriers that stand between treatment need and treatment receipt.

Table15-1. Percentage of Participants with Serious, Moderate or Mild Conditions Who Received Treatment in the Prior Year in the WHO World Mental Health Surveys

COUNTRY	SERIOUS % (95% CONFIDENCE INTERRVAL)	MODERATE % (95% CONFIDENCE INTERVAL)	MILD % (95% CONFIDENCE INTERVAL)
AMERICAS			
Colombia	23.7 (15.2–32.3)	11.5 (6.6–16.5)	8.4 (4.5–12.4)
Mexico	20.2 (12.7–27.8)	18.6 (12.5–24.8)	10.2 (5.5–14.9)
United States	52.3 (48.5–56.1)	34.1 (30.9–37.4)	22.5 (19.0–26.1)
EUROPE			
Belgium	53.9 (25.2–82.5)	50.0 (35.8–64.2)	28.2 (14.9–41.4)
France	63.3 (38.6–88.1)	35.7 (21.4–49.9)	22.3 (15.8–28.9)
Germany	49.7 (26.6–72.8)	30.5 (18.5–42.5)	27.9 (14.5–41.3)
Italy	...	30.5 (19.3–41.7)	18.9 (11.3–26.6)
Netherlands	50.2 (29.5–70.8)	35.0 (15.7–54.2)	26.5 (15.6–37.4)
Spain	64.5 (49.2–79.7)	37.9 (26.8–49.0)	35.2 (23.8–46.6)
Ukraine	19.7 (13.9–25.6)	17.1 (9.7–24.4)	7.1 (1.2–13.0)
MIDDLE EAST AND AFRICA			
Lebanon	14.6 (5.8–23.4)	9.7 (2.6–16.7)	4.5 (0.6–8.5)
Nigeria	...	...	10.3 (3.7–17.0)
ASIA			
Japan	...	16.7 (4.5–28.9)	11.2 (0.1–22.3)
PEOPLE'S REPUBLIC OF CHINA			
Beijing	...	11.9 (0.0–26.2)	2.0 (0.0–4.8)
Shanghai	...	...	0.5 (0.0–1.7)

For a description of how severity levels were defined see Demyttenaere et al., 2004. Ellipses indicate that the results were not reported because of sparse data (<30 at the severity level).

Source: Adapted from Demyttenaere et al., 2004, table 5.

MODELS OF TREATMENT-SEEKING BEHAVIOR

Treatment seeking is a complex phenomenon involving motivational, cognitive, social, and cultural factors. Furthermore, formal treatment seeking involves interactions between the individual and the treatment system. Over the years, a number of theoretical models have been proposed to explain treatment seeking and determine the factors that affect it. This section reviews some of the better-known theoretical models of mental health treatment–seeking behavior and discusses strengths and limitations of those models.

"Sick Role" and "Illness Behavior"

Attention to treatment-seeking behavior is not unique to the mental health field. Practitioners in other health care fields have been interested in treatment-seeking behavior as an important factor in community-based care for common physical disorders (Dankner, Geulayov, Olmer, & Kaplan, 2009; Petrella &

Campbell, 2005). Sociological studies of health and illness were among the earliest to assess the concept of treatment-seeking behavior. The sociologist Talcott Parsons, a pioneer in this tradition, posited that sick individuals adopt a social role associated with a set of expected behaviors from both the individual inhabiting the "sick role" and his or her social circle. Thus Parsons saw illness not solely as a medical condition but also as a social role conveying rights and responsibilities both for the person in the sick role and for the larger society (Parsons, 1951). Sick persons are exempted from normal social obligations and responsibilities and are not held responsible for their health status. The sick person, however, is expected to be motivated toward achieving improved health and therefore is held responsible for seeking treatment.

In Parsons's view, the sick role represents a form of motivated social deviance; the treating professional is viewed as an agent of social control (Parsons, 1951). Yet it is unclear how this social constructionist view of the sick role explains the behavior of many individuals with mood and anxiety disorders, who consider themselves neither sick nor in need of treatment. Nonetheless, Parsons's conceptualization of the sick role both influenced the work of subsequent theorists and drew attention to social factors that may influence treatment-seeking behavior.

In the early 1960s, the sociologist David Mechanic (1962) described a set of behaviors, termed "illness behavior,", which could explain variations in treatment-seeking behavior. He defined illness behavior as

the ways in which given symptoms may be differentially perceived, evaluated, and acted (or not acted) upon by different kinds of persons. Whether by reason of earlier experiences with illness, differential training in respect to symptoms, or whatever, some persons will make light of symptoms, shrug them off, and avoid seeking medical care; others will respond to the slightest twinges of pain or discomfort by quickly seeking such medical care as is available....Variables affecting illness behavior come into play prior to medical scrutiny and treatment,

but after etiological processes have been initiated. In this sense, illness behavior even determines whether diagnosis and treatment will begin at all. (p. 189)

Mechanic identified a number of factors that characterize a problem as an illness in need of treatment, among them:

• visibility, frequency, and chronicity of symptoms
• perceived seriousness of the problem
• disruption in role functioning
• knowledge, cultural assumptions, and alternative explanations for the problem
• competing needs
• treatment availability.

Illness behavior becomes a useful framework to help explain individual variations in responses to the distress of common psychiatric disorders. This framework also illuminates the roles that social factors, attitudes, and various personal evaluations play in the treatment-seeking process.

Social Network Perspective

While family and other social networks are featured in Mechanic's illness behavior model (Mechanic, 1962), they are even more prominent in the work of proponents of the social network perspective, such as Charles Kadushin. An early proponent, Kadushin (1969) discovered the impact of a person's social circle—what he called the "friends and supporters of psychotherapy"—on treatment seeking among patients in psychoanalytic clinics in New York City.

The impact of social networks also features prominently in the work of sociologist Bernice Pescosolido, who proposed a dynamic, network-episode model of treatment seeking. According to this model, which draws on elements of many other treatment-seeking models, "dealing with health problems is a social process that is managed through the contacts (or social networks) that individuals have in the community, the treatment system and the social service agencies" (Pescosolido & Boyer, 1999, p. 406.) This model, unlike others, recognizes the use of mental health services as a dynamic process incorporating sociodemographic and economic factors; illness characteristics; social networks and social support; coping skills; attitudes toward mental illness and assessment of need; and treatment system–related factors such as quality, accessibility, equity, and previous experience with service use. By working to capture the various factors that influence each other continuously and evolve with time, this model represents an advance over previous single-episode, unidirectional models of mental health treatment–seeking.

Andersen's Sociobehavioral Model

Perhaps no model of treatment seeking matches the popularity achieved by the sociobehavioral model introduced in the 1960s by Ronald Andersen (Andersen, 1968; Andersen & Newman, 1973) (Figure 15-1). The model details three sets of factors involved in treatment seeking:

- need factors that are experienced as uncomfortable, necessitating professional help (e.g., distress or pain)
- predisposing factors, which include the social and cultural factors that influence the decision to seek professional help (e.g., gender, race, education, and health beliefs)
- enabling factors that facilitate or hinder access to services (e.g., geographical distance and insurance coverage) (Andersen, 1995).

Despite criticisms and further elaborations (Andersen, 1995), the original Andersen model

is commonly used as a template for organizing the factors that affect the treatment-seeking process. That the terms need, predisposing, and enabling factors have permeated the study of treatment seeking is a testimony to the model's popularity.

Theory of Reasoned Action

The foregoing theoretical models originated primarily from sociology. However, psychologists and other mental health specialists also have articulated or contributed to the development of models of treatment-seeking behavior. For example, Fishbein's well-known theory of reasoned action has been applied to a wide range of health behaviors (Ajzen, 1980; Albarracin, Johnson, Fishbein, & Muellerleile, 2001; Bayer & Peay, 1997; Fishbein, Ajzen, & Hornik, 2007; Lierman, Young, Kasprzyk, & Benoleil, 1990). As the term reasoned action implies, the theory assumes that human behavior follows reasonably (though not necessarily rationally) from beliefs about performing that behavior, attitudes associated with those beliefs, and anticipated outcomes. (See figure 15-2.) Under the model, behavioral beliefs influence attitudes about the behavior, including costs, benefits and outcome expectancies. Normative beliefs influence perceived norms (such as social expectations and social pressure), and control beliefs influence perceived self-efficacy. Together, these attitudes influence intention to act (Fishbein, 2008; Fishbein & Ajzen, 1975; Fishbein et al., 2007).

Unlike some sociological theories of treatment seeking, the theory of reasoned action

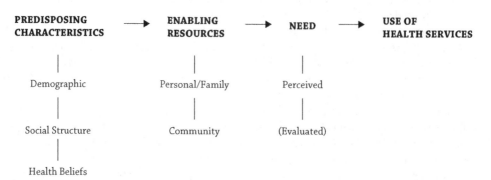

Figure 15-1   Andersen's Original Sociobehavioral Model of Health Service Use.
Source: Reprinted with permission from Andersen, 1995, figure 1.

Theory of Reasoned Action

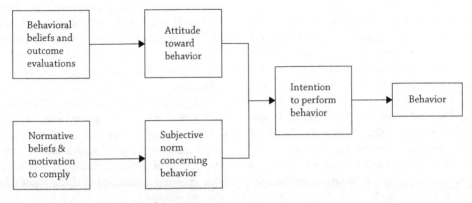

Figure 15-2   **Theory of Reasoned Action.**
Source: Adapted with permission from Fishbein & Ajzen, 1975.

focuses on individuals' beliefs, attitudes, and expectations as decisive factors in treatment-seeking decisions. (Some of these evaluative factors are included in Mechanic's model of illness behavior as well.) The theory of reasoned action does not deny the influence of access to care and social factors in treatment-seeking; rather, it encompasses those factors as elements within an individual's attitudes, evaluations, and belief system.

In all, the theory of reasoned action provides a powerful context for understanding and predicting personal health behaviors (such as the use of condoms or the use of preventive health services such as colonoscopy and mammography) (Fishbein, 2008). Yet despite its broad use, the model's explanatory power with respect to seeking help for an illness is limited, primarily because it omits factors, such as pain, distress, and disability, that affect a perceived need for care. Unlike individuals who opt to use a preventive service or to adopt a particular health-preserving behavior, those who seek help for a mental or physical illness often are both distressed and impaired, two of the most consistent, powerful predictors of mental health treatment seeking. Indeed, these two factors often drive perceived need for care and may profoundly affect or alter attitudes toward mental health treatment–seeking behavior (Mojtabai, Olfson, & Mechanic, 2002). They simply cannot be relegated to the role of background influences. Nevertheless,

despite its deficiencies, the theory of reasoned action provides a detailed representation of the more proximal processes involved in treatment-seeking decisions.

Mental Health Care Seeking as a Decisional Balance

The multiplicity of models that attempt to explicate treatment seeking is perhaps testament to the elusive nature of the treatment-seeking process itself. As a behavior, mental health treatment seeking is influenced by a host of factors, including an individual's psychopathology, self-evaluation of his or her mental state, attitudes toward and previous experiences with the mental health care system, reactions and attitudes of the immediate and the larger social circle, and assessments of the economic and personal costs and benefits of treatment seeking. Many models have striven to accommodate these factors. Some have incorporated change over time as an element in treatment-seeking stages, episodes, or careers (Pescosolido & Boyer, 1999). Further complicating efforts to explicate treatment seeking for mental disorders is that pathways to treatment vary by the severity and nature of mental disorders and by stage in the life span. Models that attempt to incorporate all of these factors generally lack parsimony—an important virtue for any explanatory model. In contrast, significantly parsimonious models, by necessity, are reductive and do not reflect the full complexity of the process.

Over the last three decades, findings from large, general population surveys on the prevalence of treatment seeking, perceived need for care, attitudes toward treatment, and perception of barriers to care have provided new insights into the treatment-seeking process (Leaf, Livingston-Bruce, Tischler, & Holzer, 1987; Mojtabai, 2005, 2009b; Regier et al., 1993). A common finding from many surveys in the United States and abroad is that perception of need for mental health services plays a central role in seeking such care (Edlund, Unutzer, & Curran, 2006; Mojtabai et al., 2002; Van Voorhees et al., 2006). Perceived need for treatment is influenced by the severity of distress, knowledge of treatment resources, and attitudes toward mental health treatments (Edlund et al., 2006; Mojtabai et al., 2002; Van Voorhees et al., 2006). Similarly, perceptions about barriers to mental health care are based on assessing the factors that can compromise access to care (e.g., geographic distance, cost of or limits to care, insufficient or absent insurance coverage, or limited financial resources) as well as perceptions of norms, social attitudes and stigma. Whether or not

an individual decides to seek treatment is the product of balancing the perceived need for treatment against the perceived barriers that impede treatment seeking (see figure 15-3). Thus the decision to seek mental health care most often is the result of these countervailing influences.

This approach to understanding mental health treatment seeking combines psychological factors (attitudes and expectations) and social and structural factors (social stigma, availability of services, financial accessibility) with the important added dimension of perception of need.

PATHWAYS TO MENTAL HEALTH CARE

Models of mental health treatment seeking generally do not distinguish among different sources of care. In some countries, such as the United Kingdom, primary care physicians serve as gatekeepers for all specialty care, including mental health care (Goldberg & Huxley, 1992; Issakidis & Andrews, 2006). Some managed care organizations in the United States have adopted a similar model, requiring prior authorization and referral before specialty care may be provided. In such settings, patients have little choice regarding the source of care. In settings in which patients have greater choice among sources of care, the choice of provider is influenced by a range of factors, including gender, age, and severity of illness (Ettner & Hermann, 1997; Frank & Kamlet, 1989; Leaf et al., 1988; Mainous & Reed, 1993; Sturm, Meredith, & Wells, 1996). Much of the past research has focused on the choice between seeking care in the specialty mental health sector or in the primary care sector, where a growing share of treatment for mental health problems is delivered. Some research has found that women, older adults, and individuals with physical illnesses are more likely to seek mental health treatment from general medical providers than from mental health specialists (Leaf et al., 1988; Wang et al., 2006), perhaps because they are more likely than other population groups to have contact with general medical providers. The multiplicity of potential service providers adds a new dimension to the

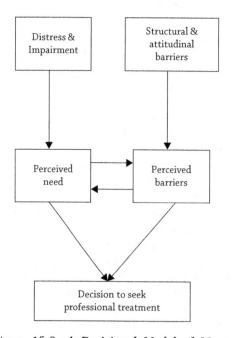

Figure 15-3 A Decisional Model of Mental Health Treatment Seeking.

treatment-seeking models discussed earlier. With the growing diversification of both providers and treatment settings (Frank & Glied, 2007; Wang et al., 2006), future models of mental health treatment-seeking must take account of choice of provider and setting as well as the factors that influence those choices.

Barriers to Care

Over the years, many barriers to mental health care have been recognized. Such barriers often have been characterized as either attitudinal barriers (such as stigma and negative beliefs about the effectiveness of mental health treatments) or structural barriers (such as geographical distance, physical inaccessibility of services and providers, and disparate or insufficient insurance coverage for treatment of mental disorders). From a global perspective, the availability of services and providers is perhaps a more significant deterrent to use of mental health services than are attitudinal and financial barriers. Data from the World Health Organization's Project Atlas (World Health Organization [WHO], 2011) have shown remarkable variation in the availability of services and providers around the world. The median distribution of psychiatrists, for example, was found to vary from 0.05 per 100,000 population in the African region to 8.6 per 100,000 in the European region. The numbers of other mental health professionals, such as psychologists, psychiatric nurses, and social workers similarly varied across the low- and the high-income countries.

However, in high-income countries, where services are more readily available than in the low-income countries, factors such as stigma, low rates of perceived treatment need, and inadequate or disparate insurance coverage likely play a more prominent role. The balance of this chapter explores stigma and financial barriers, both of which have been subjects of growing attention in recent years, including a number of public health policy initiatives in the United States.

Stigma of Mental Illness and Treatment-Seeking Behaviors

An ample body of evidence affirms that many individuals suffering from mental illnesses are subject to stigma and discrimination in many aspects of their lives (Chong et al., 2007; Corrigan, Watson, & Miller, 2006; Crisp, Gelder, Rix, Meltzer, & Rowlands, 2000; Gaebel, Baumann, Witte, & Zaeske, 2002; Kleinman & Hall-Clifford, 2009; Link & Phelan 1999; Link, Yang, Phelan, & Collins, 2004; Phelan & Link, 1998; Saravanan et al., 2008; Thara & Srinivasan, 2000). In part as a result of both social and internalized stigma, many choose not to seek mental health care despite an acknowledged need for such care (Corrigan, 2004). In a 27-nation study, people with schizophrenia said they experienced adverse discrimination in a variety of ways and milieus (Thornicroft et al., 2009). Almost half reported experiencing stigma in their relationships with friends and family, and almost 30% in intimate relationships, in the workplace, or in job searches. Other studies have found that stigma plays an adverse role in adherence to treatments among individuals receiving care (Sirey et al., 2001).

These individuals are not misperceiving the attitudes of those around them; most surveys of public attitudes toward people with mental illnesses corroborate these reports. Results of the 2006 Eurobarometer survey of a general population sample in European Union countries, for example, found that large proportions of the community regarded the mentally ill as unpredictable or dangerous (Directorate-General of Health and Consumer Protection (SANCO)–European Commission, 2006). (See figure 15-4.) In another survey of adults in the United Kingdom, Crisp and colleagues (2000) found that the lay public believed people with schizophrenia, alcoholism, or drug addiction to be dangerous. A similar result was found in a population sample of Germans who were asked to characterize individuals with schizophrenia (Angermeyer & Matschinger, 2003).

The stigma that surrounds mental illness is not limited to the mental disorders that are perceived to be severe and disabling, such as schizophrenia. The public also evidences negative attitudes toward what are perceived to be less severe disorders, such as depression and anxiety (Alonso, Buron, Bruffaerts, et al., 2009; Alonso, Buron, Rojas-Farreras, et al., 2009).

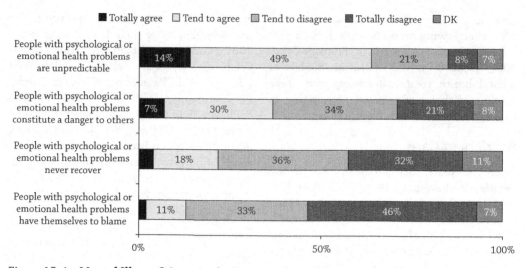

People with psychological or emotional health problems are unpredictable: 14% | 49% | 21% | 8% | 7%

People with psychological or emotional health problems constitute a danger to others: 7% | 30% | 34% | 21% | 8%

People with psychological or emotional health problems never recover: 18% | 36% | 32% | 11%

People with psychological or emotional health problems have themselves to blame: 11% | 33% | 46% | 7%

0%   50%   100%

Figure 15-4   Mental Illness Stigma in the European Union Countries.
Source: Reprinted with permission from Directorate-General of Health and Consumer Protection (SANCO)–European Union, 2006.

The issue of stigma appears more pronounced in non-Western societies in which traditional beliefs persist and information about mental illnesses is not disseminated as widely as in Western nations. Studies from India (Thara & Srinivasan, 2000), Ethiopia (Shibre et al., 2001), and China (Phillips, Pearson, Li, Xu, & Yang, 2002) have found that the stigma of mental illness extends beyond the individual. Members of the individual's family may have difficulty gaining employment, finding mates for their children, and being accepted by their communities. Stigmatizing attitudes also have an effect on treatment-seeking behaviors. In fact, such negative attitudes toward both mental illnesses and their treatments are among the most significant attitudinal barriers to help-seeking behavior (Mechanic, 2002). In a qualitative study of African Americans, stigma was the reason most commonly cited for choosing not to seek care for a known mental health problem (Cruz, Pincus, Harman, Reynolds, & Post, 2008). Among young adults, negative attitudes toward mental disorders were found to be associated with reduced acceptance of a diagnosis of depression and agreement to treatment (Van Voorhees et al., 2005). Perceived social stigma may give rise to self-stigma as well, which further contributes to reluctance to seek mental health treatment (Vogel et al., 2007).

When it comes to the stigma toward care-seeking behavior, the choice of provider or setting matters. Typically, more stigma is associated with seeking help from specialty mental health care providers than from general medical providers. A national study on the stigma of childhood mental disorders found that even among individuals who correctly identified serious childhood mental disorders like attention deficit hyperactivity disorder and depression, most preferred to access care from general practitioners, teachers, family, friends, and nonmedical counselors than from a psychiatrist or psychologist or in a specialty setting (Pescosolido et al., 2008). In a large study in Chile, only 6% of those with a mental disorder were found to have received specialty mental health care; 44% had seen another type of treatment provider (Vicente, Kohn, Saldivia, Rioseco, & Torres, 2005). The study found that stigma was one of the key barriers to seeking care from mental health specialists.

Public Mental Health Campaigns to Fight Stigma

The first recommendation of the widely publicized 2003 United States President's New Freedom Commission on Mental Health was to "[a]dvance and implement a national campaign to reduce the stigma of seeking care"

(p. 17). This was not the first call to action or the first recognition that stigma needs to be combatted. In fact, over the years, recognition of the large gaps between the significant need for mental health care and markedly lower levels of service use gave rise to a number of public information campaigns (Aseltine, Schilling, James, Murray, & Jacobs, 2008; Buist et al., 2007; Hickie, 2004; Jacobs, 1995; Jorm, Christensen, & Griffiths, 2005, 2006a; Morgan & Jorm, 2007; Olfson et al., 2002; Paykel, Hart, & Priest, 1998; Paykel et al., 1997; Rix et al., 1999). The aims of many of these initiatives were to increase public recognition and understanding of mental illnesses, provide information about available community-based treatment resources, and dispel common myths and stigma associated with those disorders and their treatment.

One of these programs in the United States is the National Anxiety Disorders Screening Day (Olfson et al., 2002). Initiated in 1993 and sponsored by a number of organizations including the American Psychiatric Association, the American Psychological Association, and the National Institute of Mental Health (NIMH), the program is designed to screen people for symptoms of common anxiety disorders. The program is conducted annually during the first week of May in sites across the 50 states and the District of Columbia. In advance of the designated screening day, each screening site receives an information packet describing recommended screening procedures and providing advice on how to publicize the event (Olfson et al., 2002). On the screening day, participants are invited to view an educational video about common anxiety disorders and major depression; they are then asked to complete a screening questionnaire. A mental health professional reviews the responses with each participant, gathering further information about symptoms and determining whether referral for treatment is indicated. Large proportions of participants receive referrals after being found to meet diagnostic criteria for the common mood and anxiety disorders. However, neither follow-up rates nor broader effects of the program on public knowledge, attitudes, and treatment seeking have been investigated.

The Defeat Depression campaign, sponsored by the Royal College of Psychiatrists and the Royal College of General Practitioners in the United Kingdom, is another prominent public mental health campaign (Paykel et al., 1997, 1998). The five-year (1992–1996) campaign, part of a broader initiative to improve prevention, detection, and treatment of depression in the United Kingdom, was designed to enhance public awareness of the nature, course, and treatment of depression and to improve the skills of general practitioners in detecting and treating depression (Paykel et al., 1997, 1998; Rix et al., 1999). The campaign's public elements included distribution of books, audiotapes, leaflets, and fact sheets in English and other languages; publication of magazine and newspaper articles; and participation of mental health professionals in educational television and radio interviews and in press conferences. General practitioners received practice guidelines, other publications, and videotapes to amplify their ability to recognize and manage depression in patients. General population surveys in 1991, 1995, and 1997 found a rise in the proportion of individuals reporting experience with depression themselves or in a close friend, from 22% and 13%, respectively, in 1991, before initiation of the program, to 25% and 18% in 1997 (Paykel et al., 1997, 1998; Rix et al., 1999). The surveys also disclosed an increase in the proportion of people who thought that:

- "Depression is a medical condition like other illnesses" (rising from 73% in 1991 to 81% in 1997).
- People suffering from depression should be offered antidepressants (up from 16% to 24%).
- Antidepressants are an effective treatment (rising from 46% to 60%) (Paykel et al., 1998).

An earlier, somewhat similar US public health campaign focused on depression was the Depression Awareness, Recognition, and Treatment Program (or D/ART for short), sponsored in the 1980s by the NIMH (Regier et al., 1988). D/ART included a multiphase information and education campaign to help improve the knowledge of both health professionals and the general public about depressive disorders and the availability of community-based treatment options. This effort was followed in the coming years by other public and private initiatives. A more recent example is the "Real Men. Real Depression" campaign that ran from 2003 through 2005 and included a series of television and radio public service announcements as well as print media featuring men telling how depression affected their lives. During the campaign's lifetime, the NIMH distributed nearly one million copies of various printed material in English and Spanish to individuals and organizations. In addition, there were 14 million hits on the web site, and over 150,000 copies of the material were downloaded from the web. There were also nearly 5,000 e-mails and phone calls to the information hotline (NIMH, 2009).

Among the ongoing national mental health awareness campaigns, Australia's Beyondblue is perhaps the most extensive (Jorm et al., 2005). (See figure 15-5.) Since its inception in 2000 under the aegis of the Australian national government and its state and territorial governments, Beyondblue has enjoyed wide support, including significant unsolicited donations from Australian businesses and individuals (Beyondblue, 2008). The central campaign aim is to increase awareness of and to destigmatize mental illnesses and their treatments. Reaching out through traditional and nontraditional print and electronic media outlets, the campaign makes a special effort to reach both students and individuals in rural areas, groups known to have less access to mental health services. In 2008, the Beyondblue web site (http://www.beyondblue.org) was reported to be the most visited lay or professional health-related web site in Australia (Beyondblue, 2008). A number of surveys have documented an Australia-wide increase in public awareness both of mental disorders and of the Beyondblue initiative itself (Beyondblue, 2008; Jorm et al., 2005, 2006a; Morgan & Jorm, 2007). For example, 56% of respondents to a 2007–2008 survey spontaneously mentioned depression as a major mental health problem, up from 49% in a survey five years earlier (Beyondblue,

2008). Similarly, 10% of those surveyed in 2007–2008 mentioned bipolar disorder as a major mental health problem, up from a zero rate of recognition in 2002. Awareness of the Beyondblue campaign also has increased across the years. Fewer than one third of respondents (31%) were aware of the campaign in 2002; by 2007–2008, over three fourths (76%) were (Beyondblue, 2008). Notwithstanding these positive findings, recognition of mental disorders as major health problems in Australia remains low. As late as the 2007–2008 survey, only 8% identified mental health as a major health issue. In contrast, 59% identified obesity as a major health issue, 46% identified cancer, 35% identified heart disease, and 24% identified diabetes (Beyondblue, 2008).

Beyond these and other nationwide public campaigns designed to improve recognition and treatment of common mental disorders, a number of international initiatives have targeted efforts on reducing the stigma associated with mental disorders. In 1996, the WHO launched a program in over 20 countries designed to combat the stigma associated with schizophrenia (Sartorius, Schulze, & Global Programme of the World Psychiatric Association, 2005). While specific program content varied from country to country, most sites undertook a survey of public knowledge and attitudes; public education through newspaper and magazine articles and school-based programs; and training and continuing education for health care providers (Sartorius & Schulze, 2005).

The expansion of the Internet and the growing use of this electronic medium as a source of health information has provided information campaigns with a new means of reaching an even larger audience. A panoply of web-based public education programs about mental health issues , sponsored by a broad array of public and private agencies, are ongoing in the United States, such as Depression Is Real (www.depressionisreal.org) and CBS Cares (www.cbs.com/cbs_cares/topics/?sec=5) http://wwwapps.nimh.nih.gov/health/publications/real-men-real-depression.shtml). The number of such resources is likely to increase exponentially in coming years.

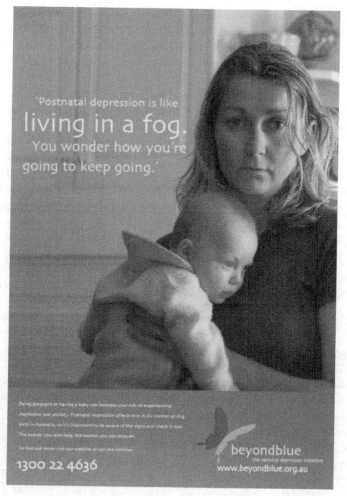

Figure 15-5 Antistigma Poster from the Beyondblue Initiative.
Source: From http://www.beyondblue.org.au/index.aspx?link_id=105.903

Changes in Public Attitudes Toward Mental Health Treatment Seeking

A 2007 US study based on data from the NCS and the NCS-R found a modest but significant positive change in public attitudes toward treatment seeking for mental disorders (Mojtabai, 2007). For example, 41.4% of NCS-R participants reported that they would definitely go for professional help, compared with 35.6% in 1990–1992. NCS-R respondents also reported greater comfort talking with a professional about personal problems (32.4% compared with 27.1% in 1990–92); they also felt less embarrassed if others found out about their doing so (40.3% compared with 33.7% in

1990–1992) (Mojtabai, 2007). These changes in attitude were particularly prominent among younger age groups.

Similar attitude changes have been noted in other parts of the world (Angermeyer & Matschinger, 2005; Jorm, Christensen & Griffiths, 2006b). For example, using data from two surveys, Angermeyer and Matschinger (2005) found that between 1990 and 2001, the German public became more inclined to recommend that in the case of schizophrenia or major depression, help be sought from psychiatrists or psychotherapists. It is tempting to attribute these attitude changes to public mental health campaigns such as those described earlier. The more significant change in the opinions of the younger generation found in the US study suggests that the educational system or the popular media (to which the young are heavily exposed) may play a part in public attitude changes. However, untangling the causes underlying changes in attitude toward mental health service use in recent years is not a simple proposition. Individual attitudes likely are influenced by far more than public education campaigns, formal education system or media. The attitudes of others in one's social network, the changing beliefs regarding the etiology of mental disorders and socioeconomic factors all may play a role.

Growing Medicalization of Public Attitudes About Mental Illness

Thanks to decades of basic and clinical research, the public increasingly believes that mental illnesses are biologically based (Blumner & Marcus, 2009). Data from the 2006 US General Social Survey, for example, demonstrate that 88% of participants in 2006 believed depression to be attributable to biological causes, up from 77% a decade earlier (Blumner & Marcus, 2009). Similarly, attitudes about the treatment of depression have become more positive. In 2006, 60% of participants in that study thought going to a general practitioner or psychiatrist or using prescription medications was an appropriate first treatment for the disorder, up from 48% in 1996; 41% thought talking with a therapist, counselor, clergy member, or other religious leader or joining a self-help group was an appropriate first treatment, down from 52% in 1996 (Blumner & Marcus, 2009).

This and other studies of public attitudes about mental illnesses conducted in the United States (Mojtabai, 2009a), Germany (Angermeyer & Matschinger, 2005), and Australia (Jorm et al., 2006b) have detected a similar uptick from the 1990s to the 2000s in positive evaluation of the benefits of medications in treating a broad array of mental disorders. According to the 2006 US General Social Survey, 76% of participants agreed or strongly agreed that taking psychiatric medications makes relations easier with family and friends, up from 68% eight years prior. The study also

found people more willing to use psychiatric medications in 2006 (49.1%) than in 1998 (41.2%) (Mojtabai, 2009a). Similarly, a 2001 German survey found that 40% of the general public recommended psychiatric medications for treatment of depression, up from 29% a decade earlier (Angermeyer & Matschinger, 2005).

Reasons underlying these changed views and attitudes about the use of medications remain poorly understood. Many of the previously discussed public information and education campaigns emphasize that most mental disorders have a biological base. With the explosion of research in the 1990s, declared the Decade of the Brain by then-President George H. W. Bush (1990), significant advances in knowledge of the genetic and physiological underpinnings of mental disorders were publicized broadly in the mass media. At the same time, a growing literature has focused on the organic bases of psychological and social stressors (Grassi-Oliveira, Ashy, & Stein, 2008; Shea, Walsh, MacMillan, & Steiner, 2005) and on the organic correlates of psychosocial treatments for mental disorders (de Lange et al., 2008; McClure et al., 2007; Siegle, Carter, & Thase, 2006; Straube, Glauer, Dilger, Mentzel, & Miltner, 2006). This growing medicalization of mental disorders has likely contributed to the growing popularity of medication treatments for mental disorders.

Trends in Psychiatric Medications and Direct-to-Consumer Pharmaceutical Advertising

Changes in public attitudes toward mental illnesses appear to correspond to the increased use of psychiatric medications. For example, in the United States, the use of antidepressants quadrupled from 1990–1992 to 2001–2003, primarily because of increased use of selective serotonin reuptake inhibitors (Mojtabai, 2008). In the period from 2001 to 2003, more than 1 in 10 American adults reported having taken an antidepressant medication in the past year. More recent US medication marketing data show that in 2007, antidepressants were the most commonly prescribed class of medications (Jorm & Wright, 2007). Over

70% of antidepressants are prescribed by primary care and other general medical providers, not by psychiatrists (Mojtabai & Olfson, 2008).

Aggressive pharmaceutical marketing and highly visible direct-to-consumer (DTC) advertising of psychiatric medications in the United States[1] in recent years may well have contributed to more positive public attitudes toward those medications and to their increased use. In 2005, spending on DTC advertising of all prescription drugs in the United States was estimated at over $4 billion, up from less than $1 billion in 1996 (Donohue, Cevasco, & Rosenthal, 2007). Direct-to-consumer ads frequently are framed as public service announcements that emphasize that mental illnesses are medical disorders, that viewers should discuss their symptoms with their physicians, and that the particular medication should be considered a treatment of choice. (See figure 15-6.)

Exposure to DTC advertisements for medications is remarkably widespread in the United States. Many more individuals are likely exposed to DTC ads than to any of the public campaigns for mental health discussed earlier in this chapter. For example, a 2001–2002 survey of a nationally representative sample of 3,000 American adults found that 86% of respondents had heard or seen a drug advertisement in the previous year, and about 35% were prompted by an advertisement to discuss the advertised medication or other health concerns with their physicians. In 43% of these visits, the physician prescribed the advertised drug (Weissman et al., 2003).

Psychiatric medications, particularly antidepressants, are among the most commonly advertised—and prescribed—medications in the United States. In a general population telephone phone survey in the early 2000s, 79% of the 300 people interviewed recalled seeing or hearing an advertisement for an antidepressant in the prior six months; 25% remembered at least one brand name (An, 2008). Individuals exposed to DTC antidepressant advertising also estimated the prevalence of clinical depression in the population at significantly higher rates than did those who were not exposed to such advertisements (An, 2008).

The effects of DTC marketing are dramatically demonstrated in a study by Kravitz and colleagues (2005), who sent actors with rehearsed complaints (standardized patients) to see family physicians and internists. Each physician saw a single standardized patient, who presented either with symptoms of major depression and wrist pain or with adjustment disorder and back pain. In one third of the visits, the patient–actors requested a specific, brand-name medication, saying: "I saw this ad on TV the other night. It was about Paxil. Some things about the ad really struck me. I was wondering if you thought Paxil might help." In another third of the visits, the patient–actors made a more generic request for medication, saying: "I was watching this TV program about depression the other night. It really got me thinking. I was wondering if you thought a medicine might help me." In the final third of the visits, patient–actors made no request for medication.

In 101 visits with depression symptoms in which a brand-specific or general request for medication was made, 65% of patient–actors received a prescription for an antidepressant. In contrast, fewer than one third (31%) of the 48 patient–actors who did not request medication for the same complaints received such a prescription. The results were comparable for patient–actor visits presenting with adjustment disorder symptoms (Kravitz et al., 2005). Overall, the study found that a request for a medication was a stronger predictor for getting a prescription than were the presenting symptoms.

From the perspectives of both treatment and health economics, the increased use of antidepressants resulting from DTC advertising has been a double-edged sword. While these prescribing practices may have helped reduce the unmet need for treatment among individuals with serious mental disorders, they also may have exposed a much larger group of individuals with mild to moderate psychopathology to the adverse effects of medications. At the same

---

1. Direct-to-consumer advertising is legal only in the United States and New Zealand at this time.

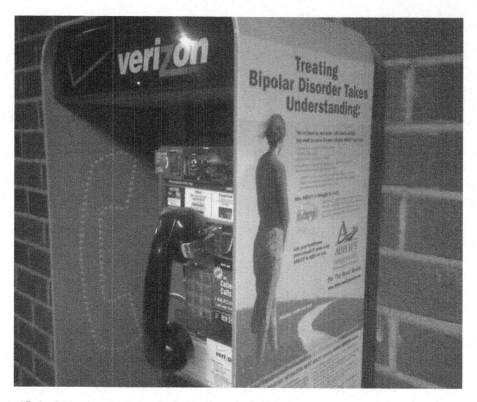

Figure 15-6   **Direct-to-Consumer Advertising of Pharmaceuticals.**
Source: From Google Picasaweb at http://picasaweb.google.com/ShrinkRapRoy/BlogPics#5066145849910761794

time, over the past decade, the contribution of psychiatric medications to overall mental health care costs has increased markedly. As noted by a group of mental health economists and researchers, "[p]rescription drug spending is the key driver of spending growth in mental health care" (Frank, Goldman, & McGuire, 2009, p. 655). Whether or not the benefits of treating a larger number of historically undertreated people with mental illnesses outweigh the human and economic costs of increased use of psychiatric medications has not yet been determined (Block, 2007; Jureidini, Mintzes, & Raven, 2008).

Financial Barriers to Mental Health Treatment Seeking

The effect of financial barriers on the use of mental health care was well illustrated by the multisite Rand health insurance study (Wells et al., 1984)—the sole large-scale randomized trial of the effect of patient-borne coinsurance on service use in the United States. Observational studies exploring the effect of insurance coverage on service use are difficult to interpret, particularly given adverse selection (i.e., selective enrollment in programs with more generous coverage by individuals with a greater need for health services).

Compared with free patient coverage, the Rand study found that imposition of a 95% patient-borne copayment was associated with a 47% reduction in the use of outpatient mental health services and a 33% reduction in the use of outpatient general medical services (Wells et al., 1984). Thus while reduced service use was not unique to mental health, the reduction was more pronounced in this area than in other areas of health care. At its heart, the study found that reducing financial disincentives to care—deductibles, copayments, and caps on benefits—was associated with increased use of both medical and mental health services, with a somewhat larger effect on mental health services.

Trends in Financial Barriers

Improvements in state and federal parity laws and in insurers' voluntary parity initiatives over the past two decades have led to somewhat lower out-of-pocket payments for mental health care in the United States. Between 1996 and 2003, out-of-pocket expenditures for outpatient mental health care dropped from 39% to 35% (Zuvekas & Meyerhoefer, 2006). However, the reduction in out-of-pocket costs was even greater for physical health care visits, dropping from 31% to 26%. Thus despite some progress, the ratio of out-of-pockets costs remained significantly higher for mental health care than for physical health care.

Moreover, the modest decline in out-of-pocket costs for outpatient mental health care has been overtaken by increases in overall patient-borne mental health costs (Frank et al., 2009). Rising costs for psychiatric medications have been particularly pronounced, tripling in the decade from 1996 to 2006, with no appreciable reduction in out-of-pocket expenditures for medications over the same period (Zuvekas & Meyerhoefer, 2006). (See figure 15-7.)

These escalating costs have translated into serious financial barriers to care for a growing number of individuals with mental disorders who need such care (Mojtabai, 2005). According to one study of mental health treatment seeking and unmet need for care, while contact with mental health professionals increased from 29.1% to 35.5% from 1997 through 2002, the cost-related unmet need for care also rose during the same period (Mojtabai, 2005).

In recent years, the impact of cost-related barriers to care has taken on increased importance commensurate with the growth in both costs of care and out-of-pocket expenditures. In 2005–2006, individuals reporting both major depression and a need for treatment most frequently cited cost barriers as the reason for not seeking needed care (Mojtabai, 2009b). (See figure 15-8.) The growing role of cost as a barrier to care is not unique to the United States. A study across Spain, Israel, Australia, Brazil, Russia, and the United States found that out-of-pocket costs were the most commonly reported barrier to receiving care for depression (Simon, Fleck, Lucas, & Bushnell, 2004). Although, the prevalence varied considerably from 24% in Spain to 75% in Russia.

The cost-related barriers to care faced by people in the United States with health coverage, while significant, are eclipsed by another, perhaps even more pressing issue: the financial barriers facing uninsured people with mental illnesses. One third of Americans under age 65 went without health insurance for at least

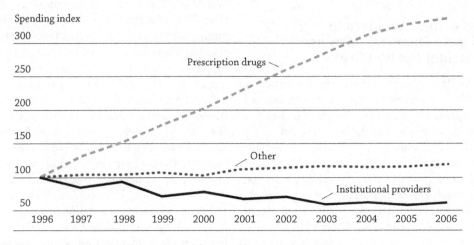

Figure 15-7   **Growth In US Mental Health Spending, 1996–2006.**
Data are indexed to 1996.
Source: Adapted with permission from Frank, Goldman, & McGuire, 2009.

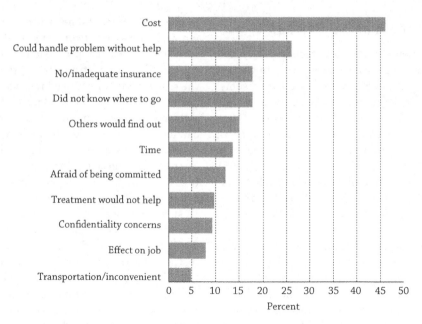

Figure 15-8   **Barriers to Seeking Mental Health Treatment Among Adults with Major Depression.**
Source: Reprin ted with permission from Mojtabai, 2009b.

part of the two-year period from 2007 through 2008 (Baily, 2009). In most studies of mental health care use, people who are uninsured lag behind those with even the most limited public or private insurance coverage (Kataoka, Zhang, & Wells, 2002; Landerman, Burns, Swarz, Wagner, & George, 1994; McAlpine & Mechanic, 2000).

Legislative Initiatives to Address Financial Barriers to Mental Health Care

In the United States and elsewhere around the world, the past few decades have been marked by significant advances in mental health–related laws and regulations. Project Atlas (WHO, 2011) found that 71% of countries have enacted laws related to mental health in general, or in areas of welfare, disability benefits, and employment opportunities for persons with mental disorders. Still, significant global variation in access to such benefits persists. A dedicated mental health legislation is found in more than 75% of high income countries but only in less than 40% of low income countries. Further, the presence of mental health–related

laws does not necessarily mitigate the personal financial burden associated with seeking and receiving care for a mental disorder. Worldwide out-of-pocket expenditures for mental health services remain significant, accounting for between 30% and 40% of total payments in some of the poorest parts of the world, including some African and Southeast Asian nations (WHO, 2005). While some populous countries, like India and Pakistan, make subsidized public sector care available, treatments in these settings are often rudimentary; private sector care is possible only with significant out-of-pocket supplemental payments. The integration of mental health care into publicly funded general medical health care by Canada, the United Kingdom, and other European nations has often been lauded as a way to surmount both cost barriers to mental health care and disparities between mental and physical health care coverage. Yet even in those nations, access to care remains a challenge, in part as a result of rationing and long waiting lists, leading to gradual introduction of private health care options in some countries

In the United States, a history of unsuccessful attempts to mandate parity in third-party reimbursement for the treatment of mental disorders and physical disorders at the federal level (Daly, 2008b) led a number of states to enact their own parity laws. The result was a pastiche of disparate statutes, many of which fell short of full parity in coverage (Daly, 2006). All that changed with enactment of the landmark Mental Health Parity and Addiction Equity Act of 2008 (Daly 2008a; Edwards, 2008; Sipkoff, 2008).

The absence of parity between mental and physical health has its genesis in the long history of health care policy, the structure of treatment programs, and research that artificially separated body and mind. When insurance for inpatient medical care first became available in the 1930s, people with serious mental illnesses most often were housed in state-run facilities where effective treatments were limited, at best. With new developments in somatic and psychological treatments in the 1940s and 1950s, the locus of mental health care gradually began to shift to outpatient settings and to incorporate patients with less severe disorders. The trend toward outpatient care picked up momentum in the late 1950s and early 1960s with the introduction of antipsychotic medications and the growth of the deinstitutionalization movement. Yet insurance coverage of mental health care lagged behind (Sharfstein, Muszynski, & Myers, 1984).

Various factors played a role in this ongoing disparity. In the era before publication of the third edition of the *Diagnostic and Statistical Manual of Mental Disorders* (American Psychiatric Association, 1980), the lack of clear clinical distinctions between diagnosable mental illnesses and transient, subclinical emotional problems made determinations of the need for treatment uncertain. The greater cost elasticity of the demand for mental health services compared with that for the treatment of physical problems raised the specter of uncontainable costs of care (Wells et al., 1984). The social and institutional stigma associated with mental illness coupled with pessimism about the efficacy of treatment further contributed to the disparity.

Over time, however, advocacy efforts, increased recognition that mental disorders are real, treatable illnesses, and the growing demand for mental health care led to increased, albeit not equal, insurance coverage for mental disorders. The trend toward increased mental health coverage continued though the 1970s and 1980s in state legislation (Barry, Huskamp, & Goldman, 2010). In 1977, about 87% of individuals with private health insurance coverage had some mental health coverage.

One of the earliest attempts at parity was President Kennedy's 1961 call for mental health insurance parity for federal employees (Hustead, Sharfstein, Muyszynski, Brady, & Cahill, 1985). Nevertheless, even in public insurance programs, the gap between coverage of mental and physical health care persisted. When enacted in 1965, Medicare's Part B limited outpatient coverage for the treatment of mental disorders to a maximum of $500 a year, which, coupled with a 50% copayment, created a functional annual ceiling on outpatient treatment for mental illnesses. The potential impact of the 2008 law that finally brought mental and physical health care to coverage parity will become evident in the coming years.

Enactment of the Patient Protection and Affordable Care Act (ACA) in the United States in 2010 was another major legislative achievement in the first decade of the 21st century. While the full impact of the ACA on access to care by individuals with mental disorders will not be known for a few years, the law's expansion of health insurance coverage is likely to reduce or eliminate existing inadequate access to care among the uninsured or underinsured, including many people with mental illnesses. Further, other ACA provisions, such as expanding Medicaid to the near poor and maintaining the current Child Health Insurance Plan, will also likely have a positive impact on care for individuals with severe and persistent mental illnesses and for children with significant mental health needs. As of this writing, the fate of ACA remains uncertain due to a number of legal challenges.

THE WAY AHEAD

Mental health care seeking is a complex process that is not entirely the result of an individual's experience of distress and impairment associated with a mental illness. Rather, a decision to seek treatment is most often the product of a combination of attitudinal, social, and structural factors. Among these, stigma and financial barriers play significant roles. Antistigma campaigns and policy initiatives to reduce financial barriers to mental health care have been at the forefront of public health initiatives to improve mental health treatment seeking at the population level and likely will continue to be so in the coming years. Other factors, such as geographical distance, perceived benefits and risks of treatment, fear of adverse effects of psychiatric medications, and prior experience with the mental health care system all influence an individual's decision to seek help. A person's social network is another complicating factor in treatment-seeking behavior (Maulik, Eaton, & Bradshaw, 2010).

Undoubtedly, treatment seeking cannot be understood fully without an exploration of service delivery itself. Simply put, efforts to reduce stigma and improve financial accessibility to care are useless in settings where services and providers don't exist in the first place. In fact, in many resource-poor nations, the dearth of both providers and services is probably the most salient barrier to adequate treatment of mental disorders. Moreover, with poverty and poor physical health affecting large segments of the population, mental health remains a low priority in many of those countries. The ability to improve treatment seeking in these parts of the world demands not only increased funding but also the availability of behavioral health services at the primary care level.

Integrating mental and physical health care makes good practical and policy sense. Linking mental health care with the care of prevalent physical conditions such as HIV, malaria, tuberculosis, and hepatitis in resource-poor nations might provide an efficient solution to the problem of poor access to mental health care services (Prince et al., 2007). Integrated care of this type is equally relevant for high income nations, where the comorbidity of chronic medical conditions with mental disorders is increasingly recognized (Felker, Yazel, & Short, 1996). The linkage of mental and physical health care— the reunification of the mind and body—also can help ameliorate the stigma too often associated with the use of mental health services.

Addressing the need–treatment gap in mental health care calls for a concerted effort to eradicate the attitudinal, knowledge, and financial barriers to seeking such care and to create responsive, accessible, affordable, and effective services in communities in the United States and around the world.

REFERENCES

Ajzen, I. (1980). *Understanding attitudes and predicting social behavior.* Englewood Cliffs, NJ: Prentice-Hall.

Albarracin, D., Johnson, B. T., Fishbein, M., & Muellerleile, P. A. (2001). Theories of reasoned action and planned behavior as models of condom use: A meta-analysis. *Psychological Bulletin, 127*(1), 142–161.

Al-Krenawi, A. (2005). Mental health practice in Arab countries. *Current Opinions in Psychiatry, 18*(5), 560–564.

Alonso, J., Buron, A., Bruffaerts, R., He, Y., Posada-Villa, J., Lepine, J. P.,...Von Korff, M. (2009). Association of perceived stigma and mood and anxiety disorders: Results from the World Mental Health Surveys. *Acta Psychiatrica Scandinavica, 118*(4), 305–314.

Alonso, J., Buron, A., Rojas-Farreras, S., de Graaf, R., Haro, J. M., de Girolamo, G.,...the ESEMeD/ MHEDEA 2000 Investigators. (2009). Perceived stigma among individuals with common mental disorders. *Journal of Affective Disorders, 118*(1–3), 180–186.

American Psychiatric Association. (1980). *Diagnostic and statistical manual of mental disorders* (3rd ed.). Washington, DC: Author.

American Psychiatric Association. (1994). *Diagnostic and statistical manual of mental disorders* (4th ed.). Washington, DC: Author.

An, S. (2008). Antidepressant direct-to-consumer advertising and social perception of the prevalence of depression: Application of the availability heuristic. *Health Communications, 23*(6), 499–505.

Andersen, R. (1968). *A behavioral model of families' use of health services (Center for Health Administration Studies Research Series).* Chicago, IL: University of Chicago Press.

Andersen, R. M. (1995). Revisiting the behavioral model and access to medical care: Does it matter? *Journal of Health and Social Behavior, 36*(1), 1–10.

Andersen, R., & Newman, J. F. (1973). Societal and individual determinants of medical care utilization in the United States. *Milbank Quarterly, 51*(1), 95–124.

Angermeyer, M. C., & Matschinger, H. (2003). The stigma of mental illness: Effects of labelling on public attitudes towards people with mental disorder. *Acta Psychiatrica Scandinavica, 108*(4), 304–309.

Angermeyer, M. C., & Matschinger, H. (2005). Have there been any changes in the public's attitudes towards psychiatric treatment? Results from representative population surveys in Germany in the years 1990 and 2001. *Acta Psychiatrica Scandinavica, 111*(1), 68–73.

Aseltine, R. H., Jr., Schilling, E. A., James, A., Murray, M., & Jacobs, D. G. (2008). An evaluation of National Alcohol Screening Day. *Alcohol and Alcoholism, 43*(1), 97–103.

Baily, K. (2009). Americans at risk: One in three uninsured. Washington, DC: Families USA. Retrieved from http://www.familiesusa.org/assets/pdfs/americans-at-risk.pdf

Barry, C. L., Huskamp, H. A., & Goldman, H. H. (2010). A political history of federal mental health and addiction insurance parity. *Milbank Quarterly, 88*(3), 404–433.

Bayer, J. K., & Peay, M. Y. (1997). Predicting intentions to seek help from professional mental health services. *Australian and New Zealand Journal of Psychiatry, 31*(4), 504–513.

Beyondblue (2008). *2007/2008 annual report. Beyondblue: The national depression initiative.* Retrieved from http://www.beyondblue.org.au/index.aspx?link_id=2.24

Block, A. E. (2007). Costs and benefits of direct-to-consumer advertising: The case of depression. *Pharmacoeconomics, 25*(6), 511–521.

Blumner, K. H., & Marcus, S. C. (2009). Changing perceptions of depression: Ten-year trends from the General Social Survey. *Psychiatric Services, 60*(3), 306–312.

Buist, A., Ellwood, D., Brooks, J., Milgram, J., Hayes, B. A., Sved-Williams, A.,...Bilszta, J. (2007). National program for depression associated with childbirth: The Australian experience. *Best Practices and Research in Clinical Obstetrics and Gynaecology, 21*(2), 193–206.

Bush, G. H. W. (1990, July 17). *Presidential proclamation 6158.* Retrieved March 23, 2011, from http:/www.loc.gov/loc/brain/proclaim.html

Chong, S. A., Verma, S., Vaingankar, J. A., Chan, Y. H., Wong, L. Y., & Heng, B. H. (2007). Perception of the public towards the mentally ill in developed Asian country. *Social Psychiatry and Psychiatric Epidemiology, 42*(9), 734–739.

Corrigan, P. (2004). How stigma interferes with mental health care. *American Psychologist, 59*(7), 614–625.

Corrigan, P. W., Watson, A. C., & Miller, F. E. (2006). Blame, shame, and contamination: The impact of mental illness and drug dependence stigma on family members. *Journal of Family Psychology, 20*(2), 239–246.

Crisp, A. H., Gelder, M. G., Rix, S., Meltzer, H. I., & Rowlands, O. J. (2000). Stigmatisation of people with mental illnesses. *British Journal of Psychiatry, 177*, 4–7.

Cruz, M., Pincus, H. A., Harman, J. S., Reynolds, C. F., & Post, E. P. (2008). Barriers to care-seeking for depressed African Americans. *International Journal of Psychiatry and Medicine, 38*(1), 71–80.

Daly, R. (2006). Several states take action on insurance parity. *Psychiatric News, 41*, 4.

Daly, R. (2008a). Parity advocates gather to celebrate victory. *Psychiatric News, 43*, 7.

Daly, R. (2008b). Parity victory was long, winding road. *Psychiatric News, 43*, 7.

Dankner, R., Geulayov, G., Olmer, L., & Kaplan, G. (2009). Undetected type 2 diabetes in older adults. *Age and Ageing, 30*(1), 56–62.

de Lange, F. P., Koers, A., Kalkman, J. S., Bleijenberg, G., Hagoort, P., van der Meer, J. W. M., & Toni, I. (2008). Increase in prefrontal cortical volume following cognitive behavioural therapy in patients with chronic fatigue syndrome. *Brain, 131*(8), 2172–2180.

Demyttenaere, K., Bruffaerts, R., Posada-Villa, J., Gasquet, I., Kovess, V., Lepine, J. P.,...Chatterji, S. (2004). Prevalence, severity, and unmet need for treatment of mental disorders in the World Health Organzation World Mental Health Surveys. *Journal of the American Medical Association, 291*(21), 2581–2590.

Directorate-General of Health and Consumer Protection (SANCO)–European Union. (2006). *Special Eurobarometer 248, Wave 64.4. Eurobarometer survey on mental well-being.* Brussels, Belgium: European Union. Retrieved from http://ec.europa.eu/health/ph_information/documents/ebs_248_en.pdf

Donohue, J. M., Cevasco, M., & Rosenthal, M. B. (2007). A decade of direct-to-consumer advertising of prescription drugs. *New England Journal of Medicine, 357*(7), 673–681.

Duffy, F. F., Wilk, J., West, J. C., Narrow, W. E., Rae, D. S., Hall, R.,...Manderscheid, R. W. (2006). Mental health practitioners and trainees (pp. 256–309). In R. W. Manderscheid & J. T. Berry (Eds.). *Mental health, United States, 2004.* Rockville, MD: Substance Abuse and Mental Health Services Administration, US Department of Health and Human Services.

Edlund, M. J., Unutzer, J., & Curran, G. M. (2006). Perceived need for alcohol, drug, and mental health treatment. *Social Psychiatry and Psychiatric Epidemiology, 41*(6), 480–487.

Edwards, D. J. (2008). Parity at last. Business and insurance groups' support was key to its passage. *Behavioral Healthcare, 28*(11), 12–17.

Ettner, S. L., & Hermann, R. C. (1997). Provider specialty choice among Medicare beneficiaries treated for psychiatric disorders. *Health Care Financing Review, 18*(3), 43–59.

Felker, B., Yazel, J. J., & Short, D. (1996). Mortality and medical comorbidity among psychiatric patients: A review. *Psychiatric Services, 47*(12), 1356–1363.

Fishbein, M. (2008) A reasoned action approach to health promotion. *Medical Decision Making, 28*(6), 834–844.

Fishbein, M., & Ajzen, I. (1975). *Belief, attitude, intention, and behavior: An introduction to theory and research.* Reading, MA: Addison-Wesley.

Fishbein, M., Ajzen, I., & Hornik, R. C. (2007). *Prediction and change of health behavior: Applying the reasoned action approach.* Mahwah, NJ: Lawrence Erlbaum.

Frank, R. G., & Glied, S. (2007). *Better, but not well.* Baltimore, MD: Johns Hopkins University Press.

Frank, R. G., Goldman, H. H., & McGuire, T. G. (2009). Trends in mental health cost growth: An expanded role for management? *Health Affairs, 28*(3), 649–659.

Frank, R. G., & Kamlet, M. S. (1989). Determining provider choice for the treatment of mental disorder: The role of health and mental health status. *Health Services Research, 24*(1), 83–103.

Gaebel, W., Baumann, A., Witte, A. M., & Zaeske, H. (2002). Public attitudes towards people with mental illness in six German cities: Results of a public survey under special consideration of schizophrenia. *European Archives of Psychiatry and Clinical Neuroscience, 252*(6), 278–287.

Goldberg, D. P., & Huxley, P. (1992). *Common mental disorders: A bio-social model.* London, UK: Tavistock/Routledge.

Grassi-Oliveira, R., Ashy, R. M., & Stein, L. M. (2008). Psychobiology of childhood maltreatment: Effects of allostatic load? *Revista Brasileira de Psiquiatria, 30*(1), 60–68.

Hickie, I. (2004). Can we reduce the burden of depression? The Australian experience with Beyondblue: the national depression initiative. *Australasian Psychiatry, 12*(Suppl.), s38–s46.

Hustead, E., Sharfstein, S. S., Muszynski, S., Brady, J., & Cahill, J. (1985). Reductions in coverage for mental and nervous illness in the Federal Employees Health Benefits Program, 1980–1984. *American Journal of Psychiatry, 142*(2),181–186.

Issakidis, C., & Andrews, G. (2006). Who treats whom? An application of the Pathways to Care model in Australia. *Australian and New Zealand Journal of Psychiatry, 40*(1), 74–86.

Jacobs, D. G. (1995). National Depression Screening Day: Educating the public, reaching those in need of treatment, and broadening professional understanding. *Harvard Review of Psychiatry, 3*(3), 156–159.

Joint Commission on Mental Illness and Health. (1961). *Action for mental health: Final report.* New York, NY: Basic Books.

Jorm, A. F., Christensen, H., & Griffiths, K. M. (2005). The impact of Beyondblue: the national depression initiative on the Australian public's recognition of depression and beliefs about treatments. *Australian and New Zealand Journal of Psychiatry, 39*(4), 248–254.

Jorm, A. F., Christensen, H., & Griffiths, K. M. (2006a). Changes in depression awareness and attitudes in Australia: The impact of Beyondblue, the national depression initiative. *Australian and New Zealand Journal of Psychiatry, 40*(1), 42–46.

Jorm, A. F., Christensen, H., & Griffiths K. M. (2006b). The public's ability to recognize mental disorders and their beliefs about treatment: Changes in Australia over 8 years. *Australian and New Zealand Journal of Psychiatry, 40*(1), 36–41.

Jorm, A. F., & Wright, A. (2007). Beliefs of young people and their parents about the effectiveness of interventions for mental disorders. *Australian and New Zealand Journal of Psychiatry, 41*(8), 656–666.

Jureidini, J., Mintzes, B., & Raven, M. (2008). Does direct-to-consumer advertising of antidepressants lead to a net social benefit? *Pharmacoeconomics, 26*(7), 557–568.

Kadushin, C. (1969). *Why People Go to Psychiatrists.* New York, NY: Atherton Press.

Kataoka, S. H., Zhang, L., & Wells, K. B. (2002). Unmet need for mental health care among U.S. children: Variation by ethnicity and insurance status. *American Journal of Psychiatry, 159*(9), 1548–1555.

Kessler, R. C., Demler, O., Frank, R. G., Olfson, M., Pincus, H. A., Walters, E. E., ...Zaslavsky, A. M. (2005). Prevalence and treatment of mental disorders, 1990 to 2003. *New England Journal of Medicine, 352*(24), 2515–2523.

Kleinman, A., & Hall-Clifford, R. (2009). Stigma: A social, cultural and moral process. *Journal* of Epidemiology and Community Health, 63(6), 418–419.

Kravitz, R. L., Epstein, R. M., Feldman, M. D., Franz, C. E., Azari, R., Wilkes, M. S., . . . Franks, P. (2005). Influence of patients' requests for direct-to-consumer advertised antidepressants: A randomized controlled trial. Journal of the American Medical Association, 293(16), 1995–2002.

Landerman, L. R., Burns, B. J., Swarz, M. S., Wagner, H. R., & George, L. K. (1994). The relationship between insurance coverage and psychiatric disorder in predicting use of mental health services. American Journal of Psychiatry, 151(12), 1785–1790.

Leaf, P. J., Bruce, M. L., Tischler, G. L., Freeman, D. H., Weissman, M. M., & Myers, J. K. (1988). Factors affecting the utilization of specialty and general medical mental health services. Medical Care, 26(1), 9–26.

Leaf, P. J., Livingston-Bruce, M., Tischler, G. L., & Holzer, C. E. (1987). The relationship between demographic factors and attitudes toward mental health services. Journal of Community Psychology, 15(2), 275–284.

Lierman, L. M., Young, H. M., Kasprzyk, D., & Benoleil, J. Q. (1990). Predicting breast self-examination using the theory of reasoned action. Nursing Research, 39(2), 97–101.

Link, B. G., & Phelan, J. C. (1999) The labeling theory of mental disorder (II): The consequences of labeling. In A. V. Horwitz & T. L. Scheid (Eds.), A handbook for the study of mental health (pp. 361–376). New York, NY: Cambridge University Press.

Link, B. G., Yang, L. H., Phelan, J. C., & Collins, P. Y. (2004). Measuring mental illness stigma. Schizophrenia Bulletin, 30(3), 511–541.

Mainous, A. G., & Reed, E. L. (1993). Choice of provider. Hospital and Community Psychiatry, 44(3), 289.

Maulik, P. K., Eaton, W. W., & Bradshaw, C. P. (2010). The effect of social networks and social support on mental health services use, following a life event, among the Baltimore Epidemiologic Catchment Area cohort. Journal of Behavioral Health Services, 38(1), 29–50.

McAlpine, D. D., & Mechanic, D. (2000). Utilization of specialty mental health care among persons with severe mental illness: The roles of demographics, need, insurance, and risk. Health Services Research, 35(1, Pt. 2), 277–292.

McClure, E. B., Adler, A., Monk, C., Cameron, J., Smith, J., Nelson, S., . . . Pine, D. (2007). fMRI predictors of treatment outcome in pediatric anxiety disorders. Psychopharmacology, 191(1), 97–105.

Mechanic, D. (1962). The concept of illness behavior. Journal of Chronic Disease, 15, 189–194.

Mechanic, D. (2002). Removing barriers to care among persons with psychiatric symptoms. Health Affairs, 21(3), 137–147.

Mental Health Parity and Addiction Equity Act, Pub. L. No. 110–343 (2008).

Mojtabai, R. (2005). Trends in contacts with mental health professionals and cost barriers to mental health care among adults with significant psychological distress in the United States: 1997–2002. American Journal of Public Health, 95(11), 2009–2014.

Mojtabai, R. (2007). Americans' attitudes toward mental health treatment seeking: 1990–2003. Psychiatric Services, 58(5), 642–651.

Mojtabai, R. (2008). Increase in antidepressant medication in the U.S. adult population between 1990 and 2003. Psychotherapy and Psychosomatics, 77(2), 83–92.

Mojtabai, R. (2009a). Americans' attitudes towards psychiatric medications: 1998–2006. Psychiatric Services, 60(8), 1015–1023.

Mojtabai, R. (2009b). Unmet need for treatment of major depression in the United States. Psychiatric Services, 60(3), 297–305.

Mojtabai, R., & Olfson, M. (2008). National patterns in antidepressant treatment by psychiatrists and general medical providers: Results from the National Comorbidity Survey replication. Journal of Clinical Psychiatry, 69(7), 1064–1074.

Mojtabai, R., Olfson, M., & Mechanic, D. (2002). Perceived need and help-seeking in adults with mood, anxiety, or substance use disorders. Archives of General Psychiatry, 59(1), 77–84.

Morgan, A., & Jorm, A. (2007). Awareness of Beyondblue: the national depression initiative in Australian young people. Australasian Psychiatry, 15(4), 329–333.

National Institute of Mental Health (2009). Background on education materials. Bethesda, MD: Author. Retrieved on March 31, 2009, from http://www.nimh.nih.gov/health/topics/depression/men-and-depression/background-on-education-materials.shtml

Olfson, M., Marcus, S. C., Druss, B., Elinson, L., Tanielian, T., & Pincus, H. A. (2002). National trends in the outpatient treatment of depression. Journal of the American Medical Association, 287(2), 203–209.

Parsons, T. (1951). Illness and the role of the physician: A sociological perspective. American Journal of Orthopsychiatry, 21(3), 452–460.

Patient Protection and Affordable Care Act, Publ. L. No. 111–148 (2010).

Patel, V., Musara, T., Butau, T., Maramba, P., & Fuyane, S. (1995). Concepts of mental illness and medical pluralism in Harare. *Psychological Medicine, 25*(3), 485–493.

Paykel, E. S., Hart, D., & Priest, R. G. (1998). Changes in public attitudes to depression during the Defeat Depression campaign. *British Journal of Psychiatry, 173*, 519–522.

Paykel, E. S., Tylee, A., Wright, A., Priest, R. G., Rix, S, & Hart D. (1997). The Defeat Depression campaign: Psychiatry in the public arena. *American Journal of Psychiatry, 154*(6, Suppl.), 59–65.

Pescosolido, B., & Boyer, C. A. (1999). How do people come to use mental health services? Current knowledge and changing perspectives. In A. V. Horwitz & T. L. Scheid (Eds.), *A handbook for the study of mental health* (pp. 392–411). New York, NY: Cambridge University Press.

Pescosolido, B. A., Jensen, P. S., Martink, J. K., Perry, B. L., Olafsdottir, S., & Fettes, D. (2008). Public knowledge and assessment of child mental health problems: Findings from the National Stigma Study–Children. *Journal of the American Academy of Child and Adolescent Psychiatry, 47*(3), 339–349.

Petrella, R. J., & Campbell, N. R. (2005). Awareness and misconception of hypertension in Canada: Results of a national survey. *Canadian Journal of Cardiology, 21*(7), 589–593.

Phelan, J. C., & Link, B. G. (1998). The growing belief that people with mental illnesses are violent: The role of the dangerousness criterion for civil commitment. *Social Psychiatry and Psychiatric Epidemiology, 33*(Suppl. 1), s7–s12.

Phillips, M. R., Pearson, V., Li, F., Xu, M., & Yang, L. (2002). Stigma and expressed emotion: A study of people with schizophrenia and their family members in China. *British Journal of Psychiatry, 181*, 488–493.

President's New Freedom Commission on Mental Health. (2003). *Achieving the promise: Transforming mental health care in America. Final report.* Rockville, MD: Substance Abuse and Mental Health Services Administration, US Department of Health and Human Services.

Prince, M., Patel, V., Saxena, S., Maj, M., Maselko, J., Phillips, M. R., & Rahman, A. (2007). No health without mental health. *Lancet, 370*(9590), 859–877.

Regier, D. A., Hirschfeld, R. M., Goodwin, F. K., Burke, J. D., Lazar, J. B., & Judd, L. L. (1988). The NIMH Depression Awareness, Recognition, and Treatment Program: Structure, aims, and scientific basis. *American Journal of Psychiatry, 145*(11), 1351–1357.

Regier, D. A., Narrow, W. E., Rae, D. S., Manderscheid, R. M., Locke, B. Z., & Goodwin, F. K. (1993). The de facto US mental and addictive disorders service system: Epidemiologic catchment area prospective 1-year prevalence rates of disorders and services. *Archives of General Psychiatry, 50*(2), 85–94.

Rix, S., Paykel, E. S., Lelliott, P., Tylee, A., Freeling, P., Gask, L., & Hart, D. (1999). Impact of a national campaign on GP education: An evaluation of the Defeat Depression campaign. *British Journal of General Practice, 49*(439), 99–102.

Saravanan, B., Jacob, K. S., Deepak, M. G., Prince, M., David, A., & Bhugra, D. (2008). Perceptions about psychosis and psychiatric services: A qualitative study from Vellore, India. *Social Psychiatry and Psychiatric Epidemiology, 43*(3), 231–238.

Sartorius, N., Schulze, H., & Global Programme of the World Psychiatric Association. (2005). *Reducing the stigma of mental illness: A report from a global programme of the World Psychiatric Association.* New York, NY: Cambridge University Press.

Sharfstein, S. S., Muszynski, S., & Myers, E. (1984). *Health insurance and psychiatric care: Update and appraisal.* Washington, DC: American Psychiatric Press.

Shea, A., Walsh, C., MacMillan, H., & Steiner, M. (2005). Child maltreatment and HPA axis dysregulation: Relationship to major depressive disorder and post traumatic stress disorder in females. *Psychoneuroendocrinology, 30*(2), 162–178.

Shibre, T., Negash, A., Kullgren, G., Kedebe, D., Alem, A., Fekadu, A., ... Jacobsson, L. (2001). Perception of stigma among family members of individuals with schizophrenia and major affective disorders in rural Ethiopia. *Social Psychiatry and Psychiatric Epidemiology, 36*(6), 299–303.

Siegle, G. J., Carter, C. S., & Thase, M. E. (2006). Use of fMRI to predict recovery from unipolar depression with cognitive behavior therapy. *American Journal of Psychiatry, 163*(4), 735–738.

Simon, G. E., Fleck, M., Lucas, R., & Bushnell, D. M. (2004). Prevalence and predictors of depression treatment in an international primary care study. *American Journal of Psychiatry, 161*(9), 1626–1634.

Sipkoff, M. (2008). Mental health parity at long last? *Managed Care, 17*(4), 14–16, 25–27.

Sirey, J. A., Bruce, M. L., Alexopoulos, G. S., Perlick, D. A., Friedman, S. J., & Meyers, B. S. (2001). Stigma as a barrier to recovery: Perceived stigma and patient-rated severity of illness as predictors of antidepressant drug adherence. *Psychiatric Services, 52*(12), 1615–1620.

Smart, D. R. (2010). *Physician characteristics and distribution in the U.S.* Chicago, IL: American Medical Association Press.

Srole, L., & Fischer, A. K. (1975). *Mental health in the metropolis: The Midtown Manhattan study* (rev., enlarged ed.). New York, NY: Harper & Row.

Straube, T., Glauer, M., Dilger, S., Mentzel, H.-J., & Miltner, W. H. R. (2006). Effects of cognitive-behavioral therapy on brain activation in specific phobia. *NeuroImage, 29*(1), 125–135.

Sturm, R., Meredith, L. S., & Wells, K. B. (1996). Provider choice and continuity for the treatment of depression. *Medical Care, 34*(7), 723–734.

Thara, R., & Srinivasan, T. N. (2000). How stigmatising is schizophrenia in India? *International Journal of Social Psychiatry, 46*(2), 135–141.

Thornicroft, G., Brohan, E., Rose, D., Sartorius, N., Leese, M., & INDIGO Study Group. (2009). Global pattern of experienced and anticipated discrimination against people with schizophrenia: A cross-sectional survey. *Lancet, 373*(9661), 408–415.

Van Voorhees, B. W., Fogel, J., Houston, T. K., Cooper, L. A., Wang, N.-Y., & Ford, D. E. (2005). Beliefs and attitudes associated with the intention to not accept the diagnosis of depression among young adults. *Annals of Family Medicine, 3*(1), 38–46.

Van Voorhees, B. W., Fogel, J., Houston, T. K., Cooper, L. A., Wang, N.-Y., & Ford, D. E. (2006). Attitudes and illness factors associated with low perceived need for depression treatment among young adults. *Social Psychiatry and Psychiatric Epidemiology, 41*(9), 746–754.

Vicente, B., Kohn, R., Saldivia, S., Rioseco, P., & Torres, S. (2005). Service use patterns among adults with mental health problems in Chile. *Revista Panamerica Salud Publica, 18*(4–5), 263–270.

Vogel, D. L., Wade, N. G., & Hackler, A. H. (2007). Perceived public stigma and the willingness to seek counseling: The mediating roles of self-stigma and attitudes toward counseling. *Journal of Counseling Psychology, 54*(1), 40–50.

Wang, P. S., Berglund, P. A., Olfson, M., & Kessler, R. C. (2004). Delays in initial treatment contact after first onset of a mental disorder. *Health Services Research, 39*(2), 393–415.

Wang, P. S., Berglund, P., Olfson, M., Pincus, H. A., Wells, K. B., & Kessler, R. C. (2005). Failure and delay in initial treatment contact after first onset of mental disorders in the National Comorbidity Survey replication. *Archives of General Psychiatry, 62*(6), 603–613.

Wang, P. S., Demler, O., Olfson, M., Pincus, H. A., Wells, K. B., & Kessler, R. C. (2006). Changing profiles of service sectors used for mental health care in the United States. *American Journal of Psychiatry, 163*(7), 1187–1198.

Wang, P. S., Lane, M., Olfson, M., Pincus, H. A., Wells, K. B., & Kessler, R. C. (2005). Twelve-month use of mental health services in the United States: Results from the National Comorbidity Survey replication. *Archives of General Psychiatry, 62*(6), 629–640.

Weissman, J. S., Blumenthal, D., Silk, A. J., Zapert, K., Newman, M., & Leitman, R. (2003). Consumers' reports on the health effects of direct-to-consumer drug advertising. *Health Affairs*, Suppl. Web Exclusives, W3–82–95. Retrieved from http://content.healthaffairs.org/cgi/content/abstract/hlthaff.w3.82v1

Wells, K. B., Manning, W. G., Jr., Duan, N., Newhouse, J. P., Ware, J. E., & Benjamin, B. (1984). The sensitivity of mental health care use and cost estimates to methods effects. *Medical Care, 22*(9), 783–788.

World Health Organziation. (2001). *The world health report 2001—Mental health: New understanding, new hope.* Geneva, Switzerland: Author.

World Health Organization. (2005). *Mental health Atlas 2005.* Geneva, Switzerland: Author.

World Health Organization. (2011). *Mental health Atlas 2011.* Geneva, Switzerland.

Yang, L. H., Kleinman, A., Link, B. G., Phelan, J. C., Lee, S., & Good, B. (2007). Culture and stigma: Adding moral experience to stigma theory. *Social Science and Medicine, 64*(7), 1524–1535.

Zola, I. K. (1973). Pathways to the doctor—from person to patient. *Social Science and Medicine, 7*(9), 677–689.

Zuvekas, S. H., & Meyerhoefer, C. D. (2006). Coverage for mental health treatment: Do the gaps still persist? *Journal of Mental Health Policy and Economics, 9*(3), 155–163.

16

Mental Health Systems
Around the World

SHEKHAR SAXENA

JUDITH K. BASS

ANITA EVERETT

WILLIAM W. EATON

ATIEH NOVIN

Key Points

- Systematic and comparable information on mental health systems around the world is not available

- Mental health systems in most low- and middle-income countries are underdeveloped and underresourced

- Mental health systems in low- and middle-income countries tend to be vertical, not well integrated within the overall health systems, and oriented toward hospital care

- In recent years, the World Health Organization projects like the Mental Health Atlas and the Assessment Instrument for Mental Health Systems have published data on key variables of mental health systems in the world

- Integration of mental health care within the primary health care system has been identified as the most immediate need for strengthening mental health systems in low- and middle-income countries

INTRODUCTION

Mental disorders affect a large number of people worldwide; based on the disability-adjusted life methodology, these illnesses cause approximately 12% of the global burden of disease (Prince et al., 2007). However, the majority of persons with mental disorders do not receive mental health care (Demyttenaere et al., 2004; Kohn, Saxena, Levav, & Saraceno, 2004). Moreover, resources devoted to the diagnosis and treatment of these conditions are scarce, inequitably distributed, and inefficiently utilized (Saxena, Thornicroft, Knapp, & Whiteford, 2007). Together, the global prevalence of these disorders, the significant gaps in care, and the marked impact on individuals and communities underscore the need for exploration of global mental health systems from a public mental health perspective.

The first section of this chapter discusses the concepts, definitions, measurement instruments, and sources of data bearing on global mental health and mental illness. That information provides background for the balance of the discussion by exposing the dearth of system-level instruments and readily comparable global data to help guide international public mental health policy. This is followed by an exploration of selected data on mental health systems around the world. Finally, the chapter presents a brief summary of mental health–related activities by leading international agencies.

MENTAL HEALTH SYSTEMS: CONCEPT AND DEFINITIONS

The concept of a mental health system is analogous to that of the overall health system, which the World Health Organization (WHO) defines as the body of organizations, people, and actions whose primary intent is to promote, restore, or maintain health (WHO, 2000). The goals of a health system are to improve health and health equity in ways that are responsive, are financially fair, and make the best (or most efficient) use of available resources. Based on this same framework, a mental health system can be defined as those organizations, people, and actions whose primary intent is to promote, restore, or maintain mental health. The next sections outline six building blocks of a successful health system (WHO, 2010) that are equally applicable to mental health systems.

Service Delivery

Service delivery is the provision of effective, efficient, appropriate, and high-quality health interventions to anyone in need, whenever and wherever needed. From a public health perspective, service delivery by mental health systems includes individual and public health interventions focused on both the promotion of mental health and the prevention and treatment of mental disorders. Thus, the range of interventions encompasses policy as well as psychosocial and pharmacologic interventions.

Health Workforce

Given available resources and circumstances, the mental health workforce should be responsive, fair, efficient, and of sufficient numbers to meet the service need. To that end, the workforce should include specialty and non-specialty personnel engaged in the delivery of mental health interventions. Thus, for example, in low-income nations or settings, the majority of mental health care is provided by general health personnel; other nations may amplify specialty care through the use of peer services, paraprofessionals, and trained family members. These are integral and essential parts of the mental health system. Moreover, while many key mental illness prevention and mental health promotion activities are conducted by individuals outside the health care sector, too often such service providers are not recognized appropriately as contributing parts of the mental health system.

Health Information

A well-functioning health or mental health care system attends to the production, analysis, dissemination, and use of reliable and timely information about health determinants, health system performance, and health status. To help ensure that the mental health service system is functioning appropriately and in the best interests of the people it serves, data need to be collected in a systematic, reliable way. They need to capture information not only on the mental health of communities but also on the incidence, prevalence, patterns, and determinants of mental health problems and disorders. These data should also encompass information about availability, use, and effectiveness of mental health resources (including treatment and other services). Moreover, to ensure both reliability and comparability within and across systems and services, all indicators should be based on clear, uniform definitions and examined using solid, evidence-based measures.

Medical Technologies

Medical technologies include products and procedures of assured quality, safety, and efficacy that are known to be both scientifically sound and cost-effective to use. While mental health care is not highly dependent on technology, the availability of medicines and equipment for diagnosis and management is critical to an effective mental health system. Recent developments in telemedicine are opening new opportunities to provide mental health care to populations distant from existing facilities and to enhance the effective use of precious specialized mental health expertise.

Health Financing

Issues of funding often affect access to and quality of care available to people in need. Health financing practices markedly affect whether people can use needed services and are protected from financial catastrophe or impoverishment associated with the cost of care. Historically, funding for mental health care has been a challenge for communities worldwide, without regard to their economic status. Mental illness remains on the periphery of health resource allocation because of a lack of full appreciation of the burden it causes and also because of stigma around mental health issues. From a public health perspective, mental health financing should include not only the costs of direct services but also the costs of supportive care for affected individuals and their families. Moreover, since many mental disorders are chronic, the need for care often is long term, necessitating ongoing, dependable financing.

Leadership and Governance

Both leadership and governance are needed to establish a strategic health policy framework as well as effective oversight, coalition building, accountability, regulations, incentives, and attention to system design. Similarly, systems of mental health care demand clear policy and legislative infrastructures that acknowledge mental illnesses as treatable disorders from which people can recover. Moreover, mental health care leadership must respond to issues of legal and human rights, complying with international and national human rights standards for persons with mental disorders and their families.

While each of the foregoing building blocks is essential for a mental health system, none is sufficient on its own to ensure a smoothly functioning system that meets care needs. The synergy and multiple relationships among these building blocks determine the functioning and effectiveness of the system and its capacity to deliver successful outcomes. Only through that synergy can the key attributes of a successful system—access, quality, coverage, and safety—be achieved, leading to the public health outcome of improved mental health.

MENTAL HEALTH SYSTEMS: INDICATORS AND INFORMATION SYSTEMS

The multiple attributes and dimensions of mental health systems make it difficult to assess a system's structure or functions. However, such assessments are essential if comparison across systems or detection of change in a single system over time is to be undertaken. To that end, proxy measures—indicators—have been developed to garner information on health-related variables that can be used to assess change resulting from particular actions or the passage of time. Since diverse disciplines address mental health issues, the indicators vary widely. However, from a public health perspective, a specific list of indicators is of particular value. Saxena, van Ommeren, Lora, and Saraceno (2006) define a public mental health indicator scheme as a systematic collection of brief proxy measures that represent summary information on variables that are potentially influenced by or relevant to mental health systems, programs, and services.

Critically, such a mental health indicator scheme is not a mental health information system, described by WHO (2005c) as "a system for collecting, processing, analyzing and using information about a mental health service and the mental health needs of the population" (p. 1). Nonetheless, such information systems may be of considerable value to public mental health indicator schemes. As repositories of detailed data on such topics as who is being treated by whom, at what location, at what estimated cost, and with what estimated outcome, mental health information systems may provide the very types of information needed by public mental health indicator schemes.

For example, a mental health information system may provide detailed information on each discharged and readmitted patient for each hospital in a particular geographic region. That information can be aggregated as summary information—an indicator—of overall readmission rates for patients discharged in the region. In turn, the indicator can track and provide key information on the impact of a policy designed to decrease readmissions. Similarly, a mental health information system may provide data on the sums spent on inpatient and outpatient mental health services in a particular region or health catchment area. From this information, one can craft an indicator to monitor the relative amount of mental health services money spent on inpatient care in the region over a set period of time. Thus while public mental health indicator schemes ideally should be designed in advance of mental health information systems, it is possible to derive data on individual mental health indicators from preexisting mental health information systems.

Many public mental health information systems are not linked to specific public mental health indicators and thus not structured to monitor key policy, plan, and program indicators. Nonetheless, such unlinked mental health information systems have value. In fact, on occasion they may provide data to help track the impact of policy change. For example, retrospective analyses of data from the US National Reporting Program for Mental Health Statistics, the oldest continuous data

collection program in mental health in the world (enumerating data on persons with mental disorders in the United States since 1840), have rich value in work to monitor policy changes over time (Manderscheid, Witkin, Rosenstein, & Bass, 1986).

Other important public mental health indicator systems include:

- Performance Indicators for Mental Health Trusts in England (Commission for Health Improvement, 2003)
- Mental Health Report Card in the United States (Mental Health Statistics Improvement Program (MHSIP) Task Force on a Consumer-Oriented Mental Health Report Card, 1996)
- Healthy People 2010 to assess national mental health in the United States (US Department of Health and Human Services, 2000)
- European Community Health Indicators (European Community Health Indicator Project, 2001).

Characteristics and limitations of these schemes have been described and compared by Saxena, van Ommeren, and colleagues (2006).

INTERNATIONAL DATA SOURCES ON MENTAL HEALTH SYSTEMS

Comparable data on mental health systems across the world are scarce. Thus WHO has taken a lead in this area, developing both the Mental Health Atlas (WHO, 2001a, 2005b) and the Assessment Instrument for Mental Health Systems (WHO-AIMS) (WHO, 2005d) projects to help buttress worldwide mental health data aggregation and availability. These and a number of other initiatives are briefly described below.

Mental Health Atlas

The WHO began the Mental Health Atlas project in 2000 to collect essential information on mental health resources, particularly from low- or middle-income nations. The first atlas was published in 2001 (WHO, 2001a), followed by a revision in 2005 (WHO, 2005b). The next revision is slated for 2011. The project's objective is to collect and make available comparable mental health data across countries and over a period of time by using both explicit definitions and protocols. Several areas are covered, including general national information; epidemiology (specifically for low- and middle-income countries); mental health policy, programs, and legislation; financing; facilities and beds; mental health professionals and other providers; and mental health–engaged nongovernmental organizations. Other areas of interest include mechanisms for data gathering and the availability and types of programs for special populations. Data collection occurs through mail questionnaires and accompanying instructions sent to ministries of health around the world. The information received then is triangulated with that available from other data sources.

The most recent Mental Health Atlas, with data from 193 WHO member countries, is available both in print (WHO, 2005b) and on an interactive website containing a variety of tables, charts, maps, and country profiles (http://www.who.int/mental_health/evidence/atlas/en/).

WHO Assessment Instrument for Mental Health Systems

Given the importance of assessing and monitoring mental health systems in low- or middle-income countries and the dearth of suitable indicator schemes, WHO once again stepped in to fill the breach, developing WHO-AIMS in 2004 (WHO, 2005d). The development of WHO-AIMS was the result of an iterative process to identify appropriate, feasible indicators for mental health systems in low-income settings. The 10 recommendations of the World Health Report 2001 (WHO, 2001b) served as the foundation for WHO-AIMS.

Today, an updated version (WHO-AIMS 2.2) is being used to collect and report essential mental health data from around the world across six domains:

1. Policy and legislative framework
2. Mental health services

3. Mental health in primary care
4. Human resources
5. Public information and links with other sectors
6. Monitoring and research.

Spanning 28 facets and 155 items, all six of the domains must be assessed to yield a basic yet broad picture of a nation's mental health system, with a focus on health sector activities. The current instrument includes supporting documentation (such as answers to frequently asked questions, guidance on data collection, and definitions of frequently used terms), a data entry program, and a template for writing country reports. In addition, WHO-AIMS 2.2 includes a briefer instrument (WHO-AIMS-Brief) that can be used when a rapid assessment of one or more mental health system is warranted.

WHO-AIMS was created to help in assessing mental health systems in low- or middle-income countries and may be implemented for an entire nation or for a region, state, or province of a large country such as Brazil, China and India. Moreover, most elements of the instrument are both relevant and applicable to resource-poor areas within otherwise high-income countries. The instrument also may help provide a more comprehensive picture of the mental health system in high-income countries than is captured by an assessment of specialty mental health services alone.

In most cases, country investigators are identified, approved, or both by their ministry of health. Relying on explicit directions and definitions, country teams collect WHO-AIMS data using all available sources and both iterative and triangulation processes to ensure reliability. The country team works closely with the WHO team on data collection and compilation. In many cases, data are subjected to several rounds of review before they are finalized.

Developed to assess key components of a mental health system, WHO-AIMS provides information essential to strengthening individual mental health systems. Because it was designed for the needs of developing mental health systems in low- and middle-income countries, the instrument's scope, objectives, structure, contents, and data collection methods differ significantly from those of other existing indicator schemes. For example, while most monitoring instruments focus narrowly on the psychiatric service sector, WHO-AIMS can provide a comprehensive assessment of the mental health system, including services and support for people with mental disorders that are provided outside the psychiatric services sector (e.g., mental health in primary care).

The objectives of WHO-AIMS also differ from those of other mental health indicator schemes. The instrument was designed to map all of the essential formal mental health resources in a country, while most other instruments measure the quality or performance of mental health services or a particular service facility. In fact, the very structure of WHO-AIMS is distinct from that of other common indicator schemes. Many indicator schemes include a large number of outcome measures. In contrast, since many low- and middle-income countries lack a basic mental health infrastructure (e.g., community-based services) and a functioning information system, it is extremely difficult to collect outcome data, which are essential for assessing effectiveness. Thus, WHO-AIMS includes input *and* process indicators. (The former are resources for developing or modifying systems and services; the latter assess service use and aspects of program quality.)

Other Data Sources

BASELINE SURVEY IN EUROPE

The European Office of the WHO has published a report on mental health policies and practices in Europe (WHO, European Office, 2008) based on data collected in a 42-country project—the Baseline Survey—undertaken by the WHO and cofunded by the European Commission. Information was collected on such topics as mental health policy and legislation, mental health promotion and illness prevention, mental health in primary care, and issues in both mental health services and workforce. Additionally, data were amassed on mental health service funding, social inclusion

and welfare, service users and careers, human rights and mental health, and mental health information and research. The data were collected using a 90-item questionnaire focused on the 12 milestones of the Mental Health Action Plan for Europe (WHO, European Office, 2005). Responses were provided by national mental health coordinators in each of the surveyed countries; in some cases, data were aggregated across provinces based on clearly defined rules. The Baseline Survey report adds to the data already available through the WHO Mental Health Atlas; a particular strength is its inclusion of data on mental health promotion and illness prevention activities.

PUBLISHED LITERATURE

Numerous scientific journals publish analyses of countrywide data on mental health systems. *International Psychiatry* is a particularly rich source of data and information, with a section on country profiles that has featured more than 80 countries in just the first seven years of publication. Unfortunately, data presented in the profiles cannot be compared across countries. An even more recently launched journal, the *International Journal of Mental Health Systems*, is dedicated entirely to mental health systems.

MENTAL HEALTH POLICY, PLANS, AND LEGISLATION

Throughout the world, the essential infrastructure for mental health is built on the tripartite foundation of mental health policy, plans, and legislation.

Mental health policy is the organized set of values, principles, and objectives dedicated to improving mental health and reducing the burden of mental disorders in a population. Generally formulated to span many years of activity and programs, written mental health policy serves a variety of important functions. First, it sets out a specific model for action to guide mental health services toward a delineated vision for the future, providing a general blueprint and describing the objectives to be achieved. A policy perspective also can help place mental disorders alongside both the disease burden that they represent and the effective interventions available to treat them. Policy also can improve procedures for developing and prioritizing mental health services and activities within the context of other health and social policies. Policy identifies the principal mental health stakeholders, articulates their roles and responsibilities, and promotes collaboration and action among disparate stakeholders. A number of key action areas in national mental health policy have been recognized, ranging from coordinating unit and service organization to human resources and training and from adequate funding, advocacy, and quality improvement to research, collaboration, and the arc of services themselves.

A mental health plan is a detailed, preformulated design for implementing strategic actions favoring the promotion of mental health and the prevention of, treatment for, and rehabilitation from mental disorders. Such a plan fosters implementation of the vision, values, principles, and objectives articulated in mental health policy. A plan usually contains pragmatic, stepwise strategies and time frames, resource needs, targets to be met, indicators, and activities.

Most often, a mental health plan corresponds to the analogous milestones and organizational structure found in the mental health policy. The plan usually builds on the knowledge base underlying the policy, such as population needs, current services, evidence, exchanges with other countries, consultation, and negotiation. Each action area in the plan is grounded in setting priorities based on strengths, weaknesses, opportunities, and threats associated with existing services. The steps to achieve each strategy are delineated together with details of how, when, and by whom the process will be managed. Targets and indicators not only give clear direction to the plan but also allow each strategy to be monitored and evaluated. Both costs and resources needed to undertake each strategy are calculated and plans developed accordingly.

Mental health laws and regulations provide the legal basis under which policy goals are achieved and the health and safety of people with mental disorders are protected. People with mental disorders are subject to a number of unique vulnerabilities. These disorders can affect how people think and behave,

their capacity to protect their own interests and, on rare occasions, their capacity for decision making. Moreover, persons with mental disorders face stigma, discrimination, and marginalization in most societies. The stigma associated with mental illnesses increases the probability that need for care will not translate into care received. Moreover, marginalization and discrimination increase the risk for violation of an individual's civil, political, economic, social, and cultural rights.

On rare occasion, people with mental disorders may pose a risk to themselves or others due to impairments in their decision-making capacities, with potential consequences for family members, neighbors, work colleagues, and society at large. However, the risk of violence or harm associated with mental disorders is relatively small. Common misconceptions about the dangerousness of persons with these disorders should not influence the focus of mental health policy, statutes, or regulations.

Data from the WHO Mental Health Atlas (WHO, 2005b) demonstrate that many countries have yet to establish even the most rudimentary mental health policy (see figure 16-1). In fact, globally, more than one third of all countries have no identified mental health policy. In the African region, the proportion is nearly 50%. While 78% of countries (representing 69% of the world's population) have mental health laws in place (see figure 16-2), worldwide nearly one in three individuals remains without specific legal protection if experiencing a mental disorder.

Moreover, about half of existing mental health laws are more than 15 years old; 16% were enacted before 1960, a period before the deinstitutionalization movement began and during which the human rights of people with severe mental disorders received little attention. Even today, discrimination against people with mental disorders is widespread, sometimes even formalized or codified in law. The issue of disability benefits provides just one example. While most countries provide some sort of disability benefits to their populations, people with mental illnesses often are excluded from such entitlements. Indeed, 20% of all nations provide no disability coverage for people with these disorders; in low-income

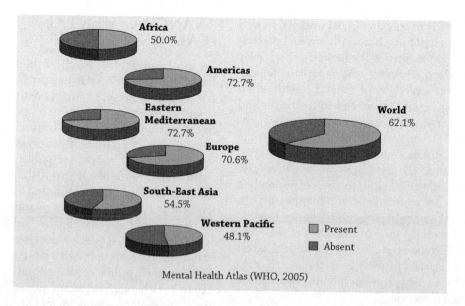

Mental Health Atlas (WHO, 2005)

Figure 16-1   **Presence of Mental Health Policy in Each WHO Region and the World, 2005 (N = 201).**
Source: Reprinted with permission from World Health Organization, 2005b.

nations, the proportion can be as high as 55%. Another example of the type of systematic discrimination faced by people with mental disorders is their exclusion from or limited coverage by some social and private insurance in the United States, some European countries, and China, among other countries.

HUMAN RESOURCES FOR MENTAL HEALTH

In the vast majority of cases, mental health care requires neither advanced technology nor equipment. Mental health professionals form the backbone of mental health care systems, among them psychiatrists, psychologists,

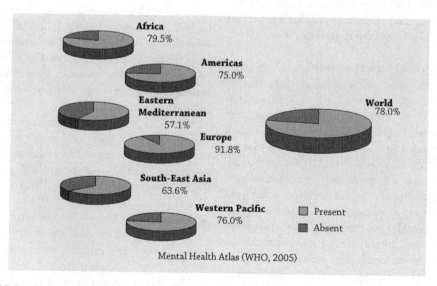

Mental Health Atlas (WHO, 2005)

Figure 16-2   **Presence of Law in the Field of Mental Health in Each WHO Region and the World, 2005 (N = 181).**
Source: Reprinted with permission from World Health Organization, 2005b.

psychiatric nurses, and social workers, as well as a variety of psychosocially trained personnel (e.g., occupational therapists and peer counselors). However, the dearth of human resources expertise in mental health is an ongoing, significant barrier to treatment and care in most low- and middle-income countries. The median number of psychiatrists in low-income countries is 0.05 per 100,000 population; for psychiatric nurses, it is 0.16. In high-income nations, the corresponding figures are approximately 200 times higher. Fewer than one psychiatric nurse per 100,000 population is found in over 75% of all countries (Saxena et al., 2007). These data attest to the marked disparities in the distribution of human resources for mental health care around the world.

Studies in several African countries affirm that inadequate numbers of professionals are the major limiting factor in psychiatric care (Jacob et al., 2007; Saxena et al., 2007). For example, Chad, Eritrea, and Liberia, with populations of 9, 4.2, and 3.5 million, respectively, each have only one in-country psychiatrist. Rwanda and Togo (with populations of 8.5 and 5 million, respectively) are little better off, with two psychiatrists in active service in each nation. Recent WHO data further confirm the serious shortfall of mental health professionals; the median rate of mental health professionals in 11 low-income countries totaled only 1.4 per 100,000 population (Saxena et al., 2007).

Migration of mental health professionals from low- and middle-income countries to more affluent areas is also a serious concern (Saxena et al., 2007). This phenomenon, part of a larger migratory pattern among health professionals in general, is especially disruptive to care in low- and middle-income countries, given their already underdeveloped mental health systems. A review of education and training of current mental health professionals reveals that the availability and extent of training facilities within those economically challenged countries are grossly inadequate to meet the existing shortfall of professionals, even if there were no migratory depletion (WHO, 2005a).

FINANCING MENTAL HEALTH

The availability of a specified budget for mental health within a nation's public health care system represents an opportunity to achieve needed mental health objectives for the nation's population. Unfortunately, today almost one third of countries (31%) lack a designated budget for public mental health (WHO, 2005b). Of the 101 countries with such a budget, 21% (spanning a population of more than one billion people) spent less than 1% of their total health budgets on mental health. WHO data analysis revealed that in the main, nations with low per capita gross domestic products also allocated little of their health budgets toward mental health care. These data amply demonstrate the double disadvantage facing mental health in low-income countries: Economically challenged countries spend a lower proportion of their scarce resources on mental health compared with economically advantaged countries (Saxena et al., 2007).

Comparing the relative burden of mental disorders with the relative budget assigned to mental health is instructive. Because infectious disease poses a significant burden in low- and middle income countries, the proportionate burden of mental disorders is less than in high-income nations. However, the budget for mental health in middle-income countries is even smaller in comparison with high-income countries. Given the availability of effective and affordable interventions, a strong case can be made for narrowing the gap between burden and budget.

Globally, the most common means of financing health care as a whole are regular government sources (60%), followed by social insurance (19%), out-of-pocket payments (16%), external grants (3%), and voluntary insurance (2%) (WHO, 2005b). However, while only 3% of high-income countries rely on out-of-pocket care as a primary payment source, over one third of low-income nations do so.

Moreover, even the small public funds available for mental health are not used efficiently in most countries. In 34 countries for which data were available, 80% of the total mental health budget supported mental hospitals, leaving only 20% for community-based or other mental health care, including care provided in general hospital settings (WHO, 2009).

Though enhanced investments are sorely needed in low- and middle-income countries, much can be achieved with relatively small economic allocations. Only two US dollars per person per year could provide persons in low-income countries with basic mental health care. For middle-income nations, that figure is around three to four US dollars per person per year. Both are modest expenditures, particularly compared with the costs of scaling up services to treat other major contributors to the global burden of disease (Lancet Global Mental Health Group, 2007). The incremental expenditures per person needed in selected low- and moderate-income countries are presented in figure 16-3.

MENTAL HEALTH CARE IN PRIMARY HEALTH CARE

Given the scarcity of specialized mental health professionals in most low- and middle-income countries, the only feasible solution to provide care to people who need it is to integrate mental health care with primary care. However, a substantial proportion of disadvantaged nations have not yet done so (see figure 16-4). Integration of mental health with primary health care also highlights the human and economic benefits of community-based care over hospitalization for people with mental disorders.

Integrated Care Improves Access

When mental health and primary care are consolidated, people can access mental health services closer to home, helping to keep families together and maintain daily activities. Integrated care also facilitates both community outreach and mental health promotion; it improves the capacity for long-term monitoring and management of individuals with chronic mental and physical disorders.

Integrated Care Promotes Respect for Human Rights

Providing mental health services within primary care settings can reduce the stigma and discrimination associated with mental illnesses, encouraging more people in need of care to seek it. Integrated care also can

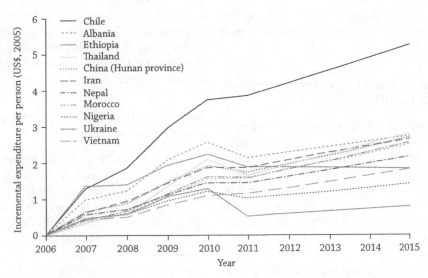

Figure 16-3 **Incremental Expenditures for a Core Package of Mental Health Interventions, 2006–2015.**

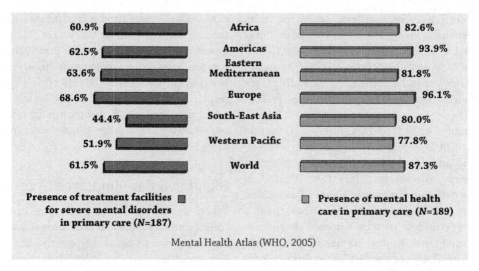

60.9%	Africa	82.6%
62.5%	Americas	93.9%
63.6%	Eastern Mediterranean	81.8%
68.6%	Europe	96.1%
44.4%	South-East Asia	80.0%
51.9%	Western Pacific	77.8%
61.5%	World	87.3%

Presence of treatment facilities ■
for severe mental disorders
in primary care (N=187)

■ Presence of mental health
care in primary care (N=189)

Mental Health Atlas (WHO, 2005)

Figure 16-4 Presence of Mental Health Care Facilities and Treatment Facilities for Severe Mental Disorders in Primary Care in Each WHO Region and the World, 2005.
Source: Reprinted with permission from World Health Organization, 2005b.

help curb inappropriate practices and human rights violations that may be associated with psychiatric hospitalizations in some countries.

Integrated Care is Both Affordable and Cost-effective

Integrated primary and mental health care provided in community-based settings is far less expensive and most often far more effective than care in psychiatric hospitals, not only for patients but also for communities and governments.

Integrated Care Generates Improved Overall Health Outcomes

The majority of people with mental disorders who receive care for those disorders within primary care settings have positive outcomes with regard to both their behavioral and physical health issues. When linked to a network of community-based supports, positive outcomes can be sustained over time and co-occurring morbidities reduced.

Unfortunately, the ability to provide high-quality, effective integrated care for people with mental disorders within a primary care setting poses a host of policy and program challenges. Careful attention must be paid to a

number of issues to enhance the likelihood of creating successfully integrated care programs (WHO, 2008).

Policy and Plans Need to Embrace the Concept of Integrated Care

A government's commitment to integrated mental health care should be codified through formal enactment of legislation to help safeguard the system's success. Integration can be facilitated not only through enactment of mental health policy but also by adoption of general health policy that emphasizes the importance of mental health services whether in facilities or in the community.

Advocacy Can Help Shift Attitudes and Behavior

Advocacy is an important component in moving toward integrated primary and mental health care. Information can be used in deliberate and strategic ways to encourage change—from explaining the effectiveness of treatment for mental disorders to the public and general health care providers to demonstrating the cost savings of integrated care. Time and effort are required to sensitize national and local policy makers, health authorities and management, and primary care providers about the importance of mental health integration. Providing estimates of the prevalence of mental disorders and describing the human and economic burdens of untreated disorders, the human rights violations that often occur in psychiatric hospitals, and the existence of effective primary care–based treatments are often important arguments.

Adequate Training of Primary Care Providers Is Required

Clinical education and training of primary care providers on the prevention, diagnosis, and treatment of mental illnesses are prerequisites for mental health integration. However, primary care providers also must practice behavioral health care skills and engage in ongoing training and specialist supervision. Collaborative or shared care models, in which consultations and treatments are undertaken in tandem by primary care providers and mental health specialists, represent a particularly promising means of providing high-quality care along with ongoing training and support.

The Role of Primary Care Providers in Mental Health Must Be Discrete and Circumscribed

Typically, primary care providers will function best when their role in the diagnosis and treatment of mental problems is both limited and doable. Specific areas of responsibility must be identified based on consultation with the community, assessment of human and financial resources, and careful examination of the strengths and weaknesses of the current health system's capacity to address mental health. The functions of primary care providers may be expanded as they gain skills and confidence in the conduct of mental health care.

Mental Health Professionals and Facilities Must Be Available to Support Primary Care

The integration of mental health services into primary care must be accompanied by the availability of specialized care providers to which primary care providers can turn for referrals, support, and supervision. This support can come from community mental health centers, secondary-level hospitals, or specialty mental health practitioners—psychiatrists, psychologists, social workers, and psychiatric nurses—working specifically within the primary care system.

Patients Must Have Access to Needed Psychoactive Medications

While psychoactive medications are not always required to treat individuals with diagnosed mental disorders, the new generations of these agents can be of significant benefit to many such people. That is why the ability to prescribe and monitor those medications— and to ensure against interactions with other medicines—is essential to the successful integration of mental health care into primary care. Laws, regulations, and rules of practices will need to be reviewed and, if necessary, revised to permit primary care providers to prescribe and dispense psychotropic medications, particularly in areas with few mental health specialists.

Integration Is a Process, Not an Event

Even when policies and procedures are in place to foster integrated mental and primary health care, integration takes time and typically involves a series of stages and steps. For example, meetings with a range of concerned parties are essential, particularly given the likelihood that considerable skepticism or resistance will need to be overcome. Health providers need training, and additional staff may need to be hired. Critically, budgets require revision, appropriation, and allocation.

A Mental Health Service Coordinator Is Crucial

Integration of mental health care into primary care can be incremental and opportunistic, reversing or changing directions. Unexpected problems sometimes can threaten the program's outcomes or its very survival. On-site mental health service coordinators can steer programs around these challenges and drive the integration process.

Collaboration with Nonhealth Sectors, Nongovernmental Organizations, Community Health Workers, and Volunteers Is Required

Government agencies of all kinds can work effectively with primary care to help patients with mental disorders gain access to educational, social, and employment opportunities that can promote recovery and community integration.

Integration Demands Both Financial and Human Resources

While establishing and maintaining cost-effective integrated care services requires financial resources, training costs also need to be covered, and additional primary and community health workers may be needed. Mental health specialists who provide support and supervision also must be given dedicated time for such activities.

RESEARCH INFRASTRUCTURE

The benefits of research range from the general advancement of science and knowledge to improving equity in care and ultimately to improved prevention, diagnosis, and treatment of the illnesses that arise in people of all ages around the world. Although not specific to the mental health field, research also is important to policy development, program planning, and the provision of appropriate, effective services.

Notwithstanding the explosion of basic and applied research, the mental health field continues to experience a significant and special kind of research gap. Most available evidence about mental illnesses and mental health is based on European and North American cultural norms (Lancet Global Mental Health Group, 2007). In

fact, several recent studies have found that little of the published literature on mental health originates in middle- or low-income countries (Patel & Sumathipala 2001; Saxena, Paraje, Sharan, Karam, & Sadana, 2006, Sharan et al., 2009). An imbalance exists between the magnitude of mental health problems in some nations and the resources devoted to addressing them. The Global Forum for Health Research (2000) has identified what it calls the 10/90 gap, in which only 10% of global spending on health-related research is directed toward the problems that affect the poorest 90% of the world's population.

Low- and middle-income countries have certain built-in barriers, among the most significant of which is the scarcity of financial resources and qualified staff to meet the behavioral health challenges these nations face. In addition, changing research funding policies and inefficient use of resources when made available combine to make research agendas even more difficult to implement (Saxena et al., 2007). Most low- and middle-income countries spend less than 1% of their gross domestic products on research and development (El Tayeb, 2005). The migration of research scientists to countries where funding and opportunities seem plentiful also has been found to pose a challenge to adequate research planning (Global Forum for Health Research and WHO, 2007; Sharan et al., 2009).

To help address the gaps in the conduct of research and implementation of research findings faced by low- and middle-income countries, members of the Lancet Global Mental Health Group (2007) iterated and set priorities for a series of research investment options across four categories: schizophrenia and other major psychotic disorders, major depressive disorder and other common mental disorders, alcohol abuse and other substance abuse disorders, and child and adolescent mental disorders (Lancet Global Mental Health Group, 2007; Razzouk et al., 2010). A study by Tomlinson and colleagues (2009) found that the greatest priorities for research funding were in health policy and systems, epidemiology, and improved delivery of cost-effective interventions.

INTERNATIONAL AGENCY PROGRAMS TO STRENGTHEN MENTAL HEALTH SYSTEMS

A number of international organizations, including agencies of the United Nations, nongovernmental organizations, and professional associations, are active in the area of mental health. A few representative examples are summarized below.

World Health Organization

Created in 1948, WHO is a specialized agency of the United Nations with primary responsibility for international health matters and public health. Through this organization, health professionals of 194 countries exchange health knowledge and experience with the goal of attaining a level of global health that enables citizens of the world to attain and maintain socially and economically productive lives.

The WHO's Department of Mental Health and Substance Abuse provides leadership and guidance to help achieve two broad objectives: (a) close the gap between needed and available services to reduce the burden of mental disorders worldwide, and (b) promote mental health. The recently launched mental health Global Action Program emphasizes creating and sustaining strategic partnerships to enhance the capacity of individual nations to combat stigma, reduce the burden of mental disorders, and promote mental health. The program works to reinforce commitments by governments, international organizations, and other stakeholders to increase the allocation of financial and human resources for care of mental disorders. A further objective is to broaden the availability of key interventions in countries with low and lower-middle incomes and a large proportion of the global burden of mental disorders. With priorities based on the best available scientific and epidemiologic evidence, the program attempts to deliver an integrated package of interventions, taking into account current and potential barriers to scaling up care.

These objectives are pursued through strong linkages within WHO, through collaboration with regional and country offices and more than 60 centers around the world, and through combined action in education, social welfare, justice, rural development, and women's affairs.

United Nations International Children's Educational Fund

With its historic focus on children, the United Nations International Children's Educational Fund (UNICEF) emphasizes both mental health promotion and health education. Skills-based mental health education can be included as part of a broader effort to create a healthy psychosocial environment at school and thereby help to reduce risk factors for emotional difficulties and mental disorders. A healthy school environment has been shown to enhance students' psychosocial and emotional well-being and learning outcomes when it promotes cooperation rather than competition, facilitates supportive, open communication, views the provision of creative opportunities as important, and prevents physical punishment, bullying, harassment, and violence. For example, Australia's Gatehouse Project (http://www.rch.org.au/gatehouseproject/) has been developing and evaluating a school-based mental health promotion strategy since 1996.

United Nations High Commissioner for Refugees

The Office of the United Nations High Commissioner for Refugees (UNHCR), established in 1950 by the United Nations General Assembly, leads and coordinates international action to protect refugees and resolve refugee problems worldwide. Its primary purpose is to safeguard the rights and well-being of refugees. To that end, it strives to ensure that everyone can exercise the right to seek asylum and find safe refuge, with the option to return home voluntarily, integrate locally, or resettle in a third country. It also has a mandate to help stateless people. To address mental health issues among refugee populations, the UNCHR provides guidelines on the development and implementation of relevant psychosocial and mental health programs.

CBM

An international development organization, CBM is committed to improving the quality of life for persons with physical or behavioral disabilities living in the poorest countries around the world. It works with partner organizations to enable such persons in the developing world to gain access to affordable and comprehensive health care and rehabilitation programs, quality education programs, and livelihood opportunities. CBM's vision is of an inclusive world in which all persons with disabilities enjoy their rights and achieve their full potential.

The organization's history is over a century in the making, dating to its founding in 1908 by the German pastor Ernst Jakob Christoffel. Since then, CBM has become one of the leading professional organizations serving people with disabilities worldwide. Beginning with a focus on people with visual disabilities, the organization's work now spans the education, rehabilitation, and inclusion of people with physical, psychosocial, and intellectual disabilities. CBM implements its programs—including a growing number with a mental health focus— in collaboration with local partners. With over 1,000 projects in more than 100 countries in Africa, Asia, and Latin America, among other regions, CBM's financial resources, know-how, and staff support enable partners in developing countries to gradually become sustainable and independent of foreign aid.

BasicNeeds

BasicNeeds (http://www.basicneeds.org/) is an international nongovernmental organization that works to bring about lasting change in the lives of individuals with mental illnesses in many countries. By working with, not just for, people with mental disorders, BasicNeeds has built an innovative approach that tackles poverty as well as the illnesses experienced by these individuals. The program's goal is to help people with mental illnesses earn as they work toward recovery through a community-based service system. The organization also works with communities to overcome the stigma and misunderstanding that still pervade the issue of mental illness. However, the heart of BasicNeed's work is grounded in the drive to help people with mental disorders to solve their problems, recover, and become productive, engaged members of their communities.

World Psychiatric Association

The World Psychiatric Association (WPA) (http://www.wpanet.org/) is a global confederation of national psychiatric societies that works to increase the medical knowledge and skills required to meet the diagnostic, treatment, and recovery needs of people with mental illnesses worldwide. It includes 135 member societies spanning 117 different countries and representing more than 200,000 psychiatrists. The WPA convenes the World Congress of Psychiatry every three years and also organizes international and regional congresses and meetings as well as thematic conferences. Its 65 scientific sections disseminate information about and promote collaborative work in specific domains of psychiatry. In addition to producing several educational programs and book series, the WPA has developed ethical guidelines for psychiatric practice.

International Union of Psychological Sciences

The International Union of Psychological Sciences (http://www.iupsys.net/) works to promote "the development, representation and advancement of psychology as a basic and applied science nationally, regionally, and internationally" (International Union of Psychological Sciences, 2011, article 5, IUPsyS statutes). Representing psychology as both a science and a profession, the union aims to:

• enhance and promote the development of the science and profession of psychology
• exchange ideas and scientific information between psychologists of different countries
• organize the International Congresses of Psychology and other meetings on subjects of general or special interest in psychology

- contribute to psychological knowledge through publishing activities
- foster the exchange of publications and other communications among different countries
- promote excellence in standards for education, training, research, and the applications of psychology
- enable the development of psychological scientists and national associations through capacity-building activities
- foster international exchange, especially among students and young researchers
- collaborate with other international, regional, and national organizations in matters of mutual interest.

It can be seen from the foregoing brief summary that a number of international organizations, including professional federations and nongovernmental organizations, are active in efforts to strengthen mental health systems worldwide.

CONCLUSIONS

Mental health systems around the world differ widely, primarily as a result of differences in economic and social resources but also as a product of the historical development of health and mental health care patterns and priorities. Most of the low- and middle-income countries have relatively underdeveloped systems characterized by scarcity of resources, their inequitable distribution, and their inefficient utilization. Often the systems are hospital based, and development of community-based care has been slow and uneven.

Relatively little information and evidence have been available to guide practice and policy in mental health systems, though the last 10 years have seen rapid progress. Global mental health has been recognized as a discipline and has acquired credibility. The challenges are to further increase the availability of information and evidence and to ensure their use, especially by countries where the needs are large and immediate.

REFERENCES

Commission for Health Improvement. (2003). *Final performance indicators for mental health trusts, 2002/2003*. London, UK: Author. Retrieved from http://www.chi.nhs.uk/Ratings/Trust/Indicator/indicators.asp?trustType=3

Demyttenaere, K., Bruffaerts, R., Posada-Villa, J., Gasquet, I., Kovess, V., Lepine, J. P., ... Chatterji, S. (2004). Prevalence, severity, and unmet need for treatment of mental disorders in the World Health Organization World Mental Health Surveys. *Journal of the American Medical Association, 291*(21), 2581–2590.

El Tayeb, M. (Ed.). (2005). *UNESCO science report 2005*. Paris, France: United Nations Education, Science and Cultural Organization. Retrieved from http://www.unesco.org/new/fileadmin/MULTIMEDIA/HQ/SC/pdf/sc_usr05_full_en.pdf

European Community Health Indicator Project. (2001). *Minimum data set of European mental health indicators*. Helsinki, Finland: Stakes. Retrieved from http://groups.stakes.fi/NR/rdonlyres/6FB78EA1-C444-4396-90F5-3672754700F5/0/minimum.pdf

Global Forum for Health Research. (2000). *10/90 report*. Geneva, Switzerland: Author.

Global Forum for Health Research and World Health Organization. (2007). *Research capacity for mental health in low- and middle-income countries: Results of a mapping project*. Geneva, Switzerland: Global Forum for Health Research.

International Union of Psychological Science. (2011). *Aims of the IUPsyS*. Toronto: IUPsyS. Retrieved from http://www.iupsys.net/index.php/about/aims

Jacob, K. S., Sharan, P., Mirza, I., Garrido-Cumbrera, M., Seedat, S., Mari, J. J., ... Saxena, S. (2007). Mental health systems in countries: Where are we now? *Lancet, 370*(9592), 1061–1077.

Kohn, R., Saxena, S., Levav, I., & Saraceno, B. (2004). Treatment gap in mental health care. *Bulletin of the World Health Organization, 82*(11), 858–866.

Lancet Global Mental Health Group. (2007). Scale-up services for mental disorders: A call for action. *Lancet, 370*(9594), 1241–1252.

Manderscheid, R. W., Witkin, M. J., Rosenstein, M. J., & Bass, R. D. (1986). The National Reporting Program for Mental Health Statistics: History and findings. *Public Health Reports, 101*(5), 532–539.

Mental Health Statistics Improvement Program (MHSIP) Task Force on a Consumer-Oriented Mental Health Report Card. (1996). *Consumer-oriented report card: Final report of the Mental Health Statistics Improvement Program*. Rockville, MD: Substance Abuse and Mental Health

Services Administration, US Department of Health and Human Services.

Patel, V. & Sumathipala, A. (2001) International representation in psychiatric literature: Survey of six leading journals. *British Journal of Psychiatry, 178,* 406–409.

Prince, M., Patel, V., Saxena, S., Maj, M., Maselko, J., Phillips, M. R., & Rahman, A. (2007). No health without mental health. *Lancet, 370*(9590), 859–877.

Razzouk, D., Sharan, P., Gallo, C., Gureje, O., Lamberte, E., Mari, J., ... Saxena, S. (2010). Scarcity and inequity of mental health research resources in low and middle income countries: A global survey. *Health Policy, 94*(3), 211–220.

Saxena, S., Paraje, G., Sharan, P., Karam, G., & Sadana, R. (2006). The 10/90 divide in mental health research: Trends over a 10-year period. *British Journal of Psychiatry, 188,* 81–82.

Saxena, S., Thornicroft, G., Knapp, M., & Whiteford, H. (2007). Resources for mental health: Scarcity, inequity, and inefficiency. *Lancet, 370*(9590), 878–889.

Saxena, S., van Ommeren, M., Lora, A., & Saraceno, B. (2006). Monitoring of mental health systems and services: Comparison of four existing indicator schemes. *Social Psychiatry and Psychiatric Epidemiology, 41*(6), 488–497.

Sharan, P., Gallo, C., Gureje, O., Lamberte, E., Mari, J., Mazzotti, G., ... Saxena, S. (2009). Mental health research priorities in low and middle income countries of Africa, Asia, Latin America and the Caribbean. *British Journal of Psychiatry, 195*(4), 354–363.

Tomlinson, M., Rudan, I., Saxena, S., Swartz, L., Tsai, A., & Patel, V. (2009). Setting priorities for global mental health research. *Bulletin of the World Health Organization, 87*(6), 438–446.

US Department of Health and Human Services. (2000). *Healthy people 2010: Understanding and improving health* (2nd ed.). Washington, DC: Government Printing Office.

World Health Organization. (2000). *World health report. Health systems: Improving performance.* Geneva, Switzerland: Author.

World Health Organization. (2001a). *Mental health atlas.* Geneva, Switzerland: Author.

World Health Organization. (2001b). *Mental health: New understanding, new hope.* Geneva, Switzerland: Author.

World Health Organization. (2005a). *Atlas: Psychiatric education and training across the world 2005.* Geneva, Switzerland: Author.

World Health Organization. (2005b). *Mental health atlas.* Geneva, Switzerland: Author.

World Health Organization. (2005c). *Mental health information systems: WHO mental health policy and service guidance package—module 12.* Geneva, Switzerland: Author.

World Health Organization. (2005d). *World Health Organization Assessment Instrument for Mental Health Systems (WHO-AIMS).* Geneva, Switzerland: Author.

World Health Organization. (2008). *Integrating mental health into primary care: A global perspective.* Geneva, Switzerland: Author.

World Health Organization. (2009). *Mental health systems in selected low and middle income countries: A WHO-AIMS cross national analysis.* Geneva, Switzerland: Author.

World Health Organization. (2010). *Key components of a well functioning health system.* Geneva, Switzerland: Author.

World Health Organization, European Office. (2005). *Mental health action plan for Europe.* Copenhagen, Denmark: World Health Organization.

World Health Organization, European Office. (2008). *Policies and practices for mental health in Europe.* Copenhagen, Denmark: World Health Organization.

SECTION VI

Prevention and The Future

17

The Logic and Practice of the Prevention of Mental Disorders

TAMAR MENDELSON

ELISE T. PAS

JULIE A. LEIS

CATHERINE P. BRADSHAW

GEORGE W. REBOK

WALLACE MANDELL

Key Points

- There is a strong logic for efforts to prevent the occurrence of mental and behavioral disorders

- There are dramatic historical examples of success in prevention of mental disorders

- In its 1994 monograph *Reducing Risks for Mental Disorders*, the Institute of Medicine proposed a three-tiered prevention framework of *universal, selective*, and *indicated* prevention programs

- Research on epidemiology, life course development, and intervention trials forms the basis for prevention efforts

- Important statistical developments in designing and evaluating prevention trials have occurred in the two last decades

- There are documented successful prevention efforts at the level of the individual, small group, family, school, workplace, community, and society

- There are documented successful prevention efforts for nearly the entire range of mental and behavioral disorders

- The Internet provides a new vehicle for prevention of mental and behavioral disorders

- There is a need to integrate prevention trials with long-term follow-up, cost–benefit analysis, and advances in genetics and biology

- The results of prevention trials have not been sufficiently disseminated

INTRODUCTION

The field of public health has a long, successful history of health promotion and disease prevention, including efforts relevant to mental health problems. Recent years have been marked by a dramatic increase in the development, implementation, and assessment of approaches to prevent the incidence of mental disorders. Scientists in both public health and behavioral health are exploring prevention strategies for a broad array of mental, emotional, and behavioral disorders characterized by multiple risk factors and complex causal pathways. This chapter examines the rationale for prevention, the theories and methods that inform prevention science, the prevention strategies being employed across developmental stages and at multiple ecological levels, and emerging directions for the prevention field.

The Rationale for Prevention

Epidemiologic surveys in the United States report high rates of mental disorders in the general population. In the 1990s, more than one quarter of the population sample reported signs and symptoms consistent with a mental disorder in the National Comorbidity Survey (Kessler et al., 1997); nearly one third of individuals did so in the National Comorbidity Survey Replication approximately 10 years later (Kessler, Chiu, Demler, & Walters, 2005). Most recently, the National Survey on Drug Use and Health (Substance Abuse and Mental Health Services Administration [SAMHSA], 2010) found that 45.1 million American adults in the United States (19.9% of the population) had experienced mental illness in the year prior to being surveyed. Of them, 11 million (4.8% of the population) had a serious mental illness—a diagnosable mental disorder that substantially interfered with or limited one

or more major life activities. Similar rates are reported in many countries around the world.

As described in chapter 1, because mental disorders can result in significant impairment and disability, the disease burden caused by these disorders is substantial (Albee, 1985; Muñoz, Le, Clarke, & Jaycox, 2002). Unfortunately, the dearth of trained mental health professionals to meet service demand has combined with a host of other barriers—economic, social and, cultural—to impede access to care. As a result, treatment reaches only a small proportion of individuals suffering from mental, emotional, and behavioral disorders in the United States and around the world, as discussed in greater detail in chapters 13, 15, and 16. The 2009 National Survey on Drug Use and Health (SAMHSA, 2010) found that fewer than 4 in 10 (37.9%) of adults with mental illness in the United States in the prior year actually got care. Moreover, among those who get treatment, many individuals either do not adhere to it or do not benefit from it. For example, as many as one third of individuals receiving treatment for depression do not improve (Depression Guideline Panel, 1993b). Australian studies have found that neither behavioral nor pharmacologic treatments were able to reduce the burden of depressive disorders by more than 35%, even under optimal circumstances (G. Andrews, Issakidis, Sanderson, Corry, & Lapsley, 2004; G. Andrews & Wilkinson, 2002).

Because many mental disorders follow a chronic course of exacerbation and remission, once an initial episode has occurred, treatment needs are likely to recur. The recurrence rate for major depressive disorder, for example, is approximately 50% after a single episode, 70% after two episodes, and 90% after three episodes (Depression Guideline Panel, 1993a; Judd, 1997). A recent population-based study found that among individuals with an initial major depressive episode, 38% had had a recurrence over the ensuing 10 years; an additional 15% had not ever recovered within the 20 years subsequent to the depressive episode (Eaton et al., 2008). Thus the prevention of an initial depressive episode, or even its delay, may reduce lifetime mental health care needs substantially (Cuijpers, van Straten, Smit, Mihalopoulos, & Beekman, 2008).

The burden of mental disorders is even greater than prevalence rates alone suggest, in part because disorders such as depression can increase the risk for poor nutrition, risky sexual behavior, and involvement with the criminal justice system (Muñoz, 2001). Research has shown that prevention of one mental disorder may delay or prevent the subsequent onset of a second, comorbid disorder. Anxiety problems, for example, tend to emerge early in the life course, preceding and predicting other disorders such as depression (Wittchen, Beesdo, Bittner, & Goodwin, 2003). Preventing anxiety problems may forestall the incidence of subsequent depression, reducing potential morbidity and mortality and improving health across multiple domains of functioning.

From an ethical standpoint, prevention is both intuitive and compelling. As epidemiologist Geoffrey Rose (1992) argued: "It is better to be healthy than ill or dead. That is the beginning and the end of the only real argument for preventive medicine. It is sufficient" (p. 4). Alleviating potential suffering on a population basis is consistent with both the goals of public health and humanitarian values (Institute of Medicine [IOM], 2009; Rose, 1992). Prevention also may offer significant economic benefits (Aos, Lieb, Mayfield, Miller, & Pennucci, 2004). Effective prevention programs could realize considerable cost savings, given the impact of mental disorders not only on afflicted individuals but also on their families and other members of society (Anderson, Chisholm, & Fuhr, 2009; Cuijpers et al., 2008; Zechmeister, Kilian, & McDaid, 2008). Those savings may be seen in expenditures associated with health care, reduced workplace productivity, and missed days at work; in costs of the criminal justice and juvenile justice systems; and in costs associated with lost educational opportunities and the need for special education. Thus far, however, the complexities inherent in cost–benefit analyses of prevention programs—including the difficulty of placing monetary values on quality-of-life indicators—have made it difficult to quantify the economic benefits of prevention with rigor (IOM, 2009).

A Historical Perspective on Prevention of Mental Disorders

Public health has a successful history of preventing diseases and disorders that may affect or influence mental health functioning. A few examples are illustrative.

SCURVY

Scurvy, a disease resulting from vitamin C deficiency, leads to depression as well as to discoloration of the legs, bleeding from mucous membranes, spongy gums, and partial immobilization. In the 18th century, scurvy was rife among sailors away at sea for extended periods of time; the illness became a matter of concern to the British navy (Carpenter, 1988). Based on an earlier hypothesis that scurvy might be related to insufficient intake of fresh fruit and vegetables, Sir James Lind conducted one of the first clinical experiments in the history of medicine. In 1747, he randomly assigned a dozen sailors with scurvy to receive one of six options in addition to their regular diet: cider, sulfuric acid, vinegar, seawater, two oranges and one lemon, and barley water. After six days, only the men assigned to consume cider or fresh fruit showed symptomatic improvement. This study and others subsequent to it demonstrated that scurvy not only could be treated but also could be prevented by adding vitamin C to the diet. As a result, the British navy mandated that sailors' diets include fresh lemons or other sources of ascorbic acid. This policy and adoption of a diet rich in lime juice resulted in British sailors being called limeys, a nickname still heard today (Jukes, 1989).

DELIRIUM TREMENS

Delirium tremens—severe alcohol withdrawal syndrome—can be manifested in a variety of symptoms: tremors, confusion, fever, agitation, hypertension, rapid heart rate, acute and severe loss of mental functions, sleeplessness, emotional instability, excitement, fear, hallucinations, increased activity, restlessness, and seizures (Erwin, Williams, & Speir, 1998). In 1813, Samuel Pearson, a British physician, was one of the first to describe the set of symptoms now known as delirium tremens, a term coined that same year by Thomas Sutton (Osborn, 2006). Delirium tremens was found to coincide with withdrawal from sustained excessive alcohol consumption. Early prevention strategies advocated abstinence from alcohol (Wills, 1930); current strategies include the administration of benzodiazepines to individuals in the early stages of alcohol withdrawal (DeBellis, Smith, Choi, & Malloy, 2005).

PELLAGRA

Pellagra, another disease related to nutritional deficiency, was endemic in Europe for centuries before it arose in epidemic proportions in the early 1900s in the southern United States (Rajakumar, 2000). The illness can give rise to dermatitis, skin lesions, weakness, diarrhea, emotional distress, dementia, and, in a minority of cases, psychosis (Cooper & Morgan, 1973; Hegyi, Schwartz, & Hegyi, 2004). From observations of individuals in mental institutions, orphanages, and prison farms, a US Public Health Service officer, Joseph Goldberger, hypothesized that diet was implicated in pellagra (Goldberger, 1914). He confirmed this theory in a series of well-designed experiments that demonstrated that dietary manipulation could prevent or induce pellagra (Cooper & Morgan, 1973). Goldberger's further experimentation led to the finding that niacin (vitamin B3) deficiency causes the disease. Thanks to a long-term prevention program in which grain products are fortified with niacin, pellagra has been eliminated in the United States for many years.

GENERAL PARESIS

The introduction of antibiotics that could eliminate the syphilis spirochete, preventing the onset of general paresis (a form of psychosis), is an important example of the successful public health–related prevention of psychosis. In the 19th century, thousands of individuals with this type of psychosis were relegated to mental hospitals. By the 1950s, the disorder had been prevented so effectively that the diagnostic category virtually went unused (Albert, 1999).

Other public health prevention models effective in reducing neurologic disorders and their mental health repercussions include programs of immunization, diet enrichment, and parent education, all of which promote physically and psychologically supportive environments for children. Such interventions have effected society-level changes with powerful preventive effects. Table 17-1 offers examples of successful prevention approaches with relevance to mental health in the areas of nutrition, congenital vulnerabilities, and hazardous environmental exposures. Many mental health–related prevention programs are based on models that have prevented or reduced other acute and chronic diseases using public health tools, including environmental modifications to reduce and ultimately eliminate disease risk factors. When cost or other circumstances make it impossible to eliminate environmental risk factors altogether, efforts have sought to reduce them using such methods as public health advisories to inform the public about risk factors, identification and labeling of health hazards; mass media campaigns, and school-based programs to promote healthy behaviors.

Defining Prevention and Setting Goals

Researchers, clinicians, and public health practitioners have long wrestled with how to define prevention in the context of mental health and how to develop a coherent framework and approach to the prevention of mental disorders. G. Caplan (1964) provided an initial conceptual framework for prevention science in public health, distinguishing among primary, secondary, and tertiary prevention:

• Primary prevention reduces or eliminates the incidence of a disorder.

Table 17-1. Examples of Successful Prevention Approaches with Relevance for Mental Health

DISORDER	RISK FACTORS	PREVENTION METHODS
Wernicke-Korsakoff syndrome	Severe deficiency of thiamine (vitamin B1) associated with prolonged alcohol consumption; Gastric disorders including carcinoma, chronic gastritis, and repetitive vomiting	Public health dietary advisories; Mandatory school-based alcohol abuse prevention education; Vitamin supplementation for alcoholic patients
Intellectual disability	Congenital infection including toxoplasmosis, rubella, herpes simplex, and cytomegalovirus	Maternal education; Maternal immunization
Down syndrome/ trisomy 21	Presence of all or part of an extra 21st chromosome	Early screening of pregnant women at increased risk of having a child with Down syndrome; Prenatal screens including amniocentesis, chorionic villus sampling, and percutaneous umbilical cord blood sampling
Phenylketonuria (PKU)	Autosomal recessive genetic disorder characterized by a deficiency in the hepatic enzyme phenylalanine hydroxylase	Mandatory newborn screening; PKU clinics optimize phenylalanine hydroxylase levels through dietary intake management
Iodine deficiency disorder (cretinism)	Iodine Deficiency	Mandated adoption of the use of iodized salt, requiring education and regulation of salt producers and sellers
Mercury poisoning	Mercury exposure	Governmental regulation of occupational exposure to mercury and mercury compounds; Publication of advisories about protective health practices
Cognitive deficits (including dementia, learning disorders, and attention deficit disorders)	Traumatic brain injury caused by falls, vehicular accidents, interpersonal violence, and military combat	Enactment of laws to reduce accidents through speed limitation; Prohibition of driving under the influence of alcohol or drugs; Court-mandated participation in driver safety education programs; Regulations mandating use of technology to protect the brain, including seat belts and window guards; Mandatory school-based education to prevent drinking and driving; Helmets and armored vehicles
Meningitis	Infection with viruses, bacteria, or other microorganisms	Immunization; Quarantine of infected individuals to prevent transmission
Neural tube defects	Folic acid deficiency	Regulations requiring the addition of folic acid to breads, cereals, flour, and other grain products; Folic acid supplementation for women who are pregnant or could become pregnant

- Secondary prevention focuses on early identification and treatment of the disorder.
- Tertiary prevention emphasizes the reduction of disorder-related impairment and disability.

Caplan's framework has been challenged. Cowen (1977, 1980), for example, posited that the primary prevention category is overly inclusive; Gordon (1983) argued that some might consider tertiary prevention to be treatment. Nevertheless, Caplan's categorizations provided a useful way to conceptualize public health prevention efforts at the time.

The early 1990s witnessed dynamic strides in prevention science. The year 1991 marked the establishment of the Society for Prevention Research, a nonprofit professional organization dedicated to creating a "scientific, multidisciplinary forum for prevention science" (http://www.preventionresearch.org/about.php) that continues to promote and disseminate prevention research through meetings and its flagship journal, *Prevention Science*. Around the same time, the National Institute of Mental Health (NIMH) Prevention Research Steering Committee's (1994) report, *The Prevention of Mental Disorders: A National Research Agenda*, laid the groundwork for a prevention science that integrates the perspectives of epidemiology and life span development (Kellam, Koretz, & Mościcki, 1999). At the request of the US Congress, the IOM's Committee on Prevention of Mental Disorders built on the NIMH effort in a two-year review of mental health prevention research, culminating in the 1994 publication *Reducing Risks for Mental Disorders: Frontiers for Preventive Intervention Research* (Mrazek & Haggerty, 1994), which summarized theory and research on the prevention of mental disorders and recommended directions for future work.

The report proposed that the term *prevention* be reserved for interventions administered before onset of a clinically diagnosable disorder. In contrast, *treatment* is the provision of services designed to improve symptoms of or cure an existing disorder. Finally, *maintenance* enhances rehabilitation and reduces the risk for recurrence following resolution of an episode of acute mental disorder (Muñoz, Mrazek,

& Haggerty, 1996). The IOM report recommended adoption of a modification of Gordon's (1983) three-tiered prevention framework for mental disorders:

- Universal preventive interventions target an entire population group (e.g., school-wide coping skills training to prevent depression).
- Selective preventive interventions target high-risk subpopulations as determined by biological, psychological, or social factors empirically associated with the onset of a disorder (e.g., coping skills training for children of depressed parents).
- Indicated preventive interventions target individuals at highest risk for developing the disorder based on subclinical signs that do not yet meet full diagnostic criteria (e.g., mood management for high school students with elevated depression symptoms) (Muñoz et al., 1996).

The IOM report galvanized other prevention-related behavioral health activities, including a 1994 workshop, "A Scientific Structure for the Emerging Field of Prevention Research," jointly sponsored by NIMH and the Johns Hopkins Prevention Research Center. To focus more specifically on prevention, in subsequent years the Centers for Disease Control and Prevention (CDC) of the US Department of Health and Human Services identified key behavioral targets for prevention initiatives, including:

- substance use and abuse
- risky sexual behaviors
- tobacco use
- behaviors that result in purposeful or accidental harm to others
- unhealthy dietary choices
- physical inactivity (CDC, 2003).

These behaviors often arise together and co-occur with mental disorders; they can be targeted through individual, family, or community prevention efforts.

The IOM revisited the science of prevention in behavioral health in a 2009 report summarizing the considerable progress made since publication of the 1994 report. The 2009 report recommended further steps to advance prevention science in behavioral health (IOM, 2009). While retaining the three-level classification system adopted in 1994, the 2009 report also presented an argument for increased emphasis on mental health promotion, defined as "efforts to enhance individuals' ability to achieve developmentally appropriate tasks (competence) and a positive sense of self-esteem, mastery, well-being, and social inclusion and to strengthen their ability to cope with adversity" (p. 67).

Mental health promotion generally targets entire populations (e.g., schools or workplaces); its assessed outcomes relate to adaptive, positive aspects of functioning. The 2009 report argued that conceptually, mental health promotion is well aligned with the prevention of mental disorders, that it is consistent with the goals of a public health perspective, and that emerging evidence supports the feasibility and effectiveness of such promotion approaches (IOM, 2009). As displayed in figure 17-1, the prevention continuum in mental health ranges from the promotion of positive mental health in the general population to the maintenance of

treatment gains among those being treated for mental disorders.

An Integrated Prevention Framework

To link prevention with both epidemiology and life course development, Kellam and colleagues proposed an integrated prevention framework that serves as a useful basis for the development, evaluation, and dissemination of effective preventive interventions (Ialongo, Kellam, & Poduska, 2000; Kellam et al., 1999; Kellam & Rebok, 1992).

EPIDEMIOLOGY

As defined by Last (2001), "[e]pidemiology is the study of the distribution and determinants of health-related states or events in specified populations, and the application of this study to control of health problems" (p. 62). Prevention science is rooted in epidemiologic research on the factors that increase risk and the factors that protect against risk for developing problem behaviors or mental disorders

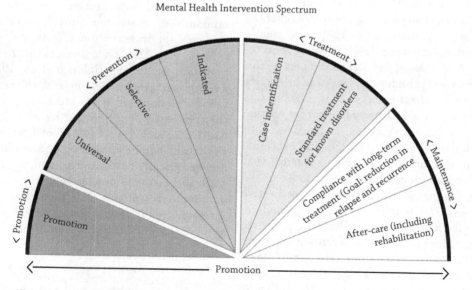

Figure 17-1 **Mental Health Intervention Spectrum**

Source: Reprinted with permission from Institute of Medicine, 2009, p. 67.

(Flay et al., 2005). Knowledge gleaned from epidemiologic studies provides the direction and rationale for developing and undertaking prevention programs in particular areas and evaluating their effectiveness (Lilienfeld & Lilienfeld, 1980).

The public health approach to prevention assumes that the etiology of most mental disorders is multifactorial, with interacting biological, environmental, psychological, and sociocultural components. The approach is further based on the assumption that mental disorders are not randomly distributed in a population. Epidemiologic methods such as studies of the natural history of a disease, cohort studies, case–control studies, and cross-sectional studies can identify risk factors for a disorder that are related to variance in its distribution over time, place (environment), and person (age, race, and ethnicity) (Lilienfeld & Lilienfeld, 1980). Further, identification of differences in a disorder's prevalence or incidence in comparable populations can help provide an estimate of potential results of preventive interventions.

LIFE COURSE DEVELOPMENT

Life course epidemiology (Kuh & Ben-Schlomo, 1997) examines the disparate factors affecting healthy and pathologic outcomes over the life span. As discussed in chapter 6, mental disorders have long developmental trajectories. A life course, developmental perspective offers a way to understand risk and protective factors (moderators) as well as other factors along the causal pathway to disorder (mediators). Such an approach emphasizes both critical developmental periods and exacerbations of commonly occurring behaviors that sometimes progress to or contribute to the risk for mental disorders. This perspective can help clarify the extent to which moderators and mediators are malleable, appropriate targets for preventive interventions. In turn, well-designed prevention trials can inform and advance developmental theory (Ialongo et al., 1999; Kellam et al., 1999; Kellam & Rebok, 1992).

INTERVENTION TRIALS RESEARCH

Well-designed prevention trials play an important role in understanding and assessing the long-term impact of a preventive intervention. As noted by Kellam and colleagues (1999), two key questions often are asked when evaluating preventive intervention trials: "Can the risk or protective factor be changed by the intervention? And, if so, does the change result in a changed developmental trajectory in the predicted direction?" (p. 470). Using randomized controlled designs, researchers can make causal inferences about the effects of a preventive intervention. Longitudinal outcome assessment can provide valuable information about the intervention's impact on individual functioning over time and can also facilitate exploration of the effects of mediators of the intervention.[1]

PREVENTION RESEARCH METHODOLOGIES

While the effects of preventive interventions can be evaluated through a variety of study designs, randomized controlled trials are the gold standard for assessing causal effects on desired outcomes (Flay et al., 2005). When implemented within the context of a rigorous process of risk factor identification and intervention development, randomized trials can provide powerful evidence for intervention effects and also serve to evaluate developmental theories of pathways to disorder (Ialongo et al., 1999). As summarized by Kellam and colleagues (1999), randomized trials are a key part of the *preventive intervention research cycle*, which also includes reliable identification of the disorder to be prevented, a theoretically and empirically based understanding of the malleable risk and protective factors, intervention development and pilot testing of intervention efficacy, large-scale field trials, and subsequent dissemination of outcomes

---

1. For examples, see the 2008 special issue of the *Journal of Drug and Alcohol Dependence* (Vol. 95, Suppl. 1) that focused on a series of rigorous longitudinal studies that applied this integrated prevention framework.

and findings (Kellam et al., 1999; Koretz & Mościcki, 1997).

Interest is also growing in a number of other strategies for assessing prevention effects:

- aggregation of data across multiple studies to assess the impact of preventive interventions on low-prevalence disorders (e.g., suicide and schizophrenia)
- analyses of specific intervention components in a multicomponent prevention program using design or statistical strategies
- staging of multiple cohorts to test effectiveness, sustainability, and scalability in a single trial (IOM, 2009).

Nonrandomized designs also are common in prevention research, particularly given the often formidable logistical and financial challenges to implementing randomized controlled trials in community settings. Alternatives to randomization include both interrupted time series designs and regression discontinuity designs (Shadish, Cook, & Campbell, 2002; Wagner, Soumerai, Zhang, & Ross-Degnan, 2002). As discussed in chapter 5, statistical methods such as matching, weighting, and propensity scores also can be used to select similar treatment and control units when randomization is not possible or is unsuccessful.

Since publication of the 1994 IOM report, advances in statistical methodologies have enhanced the capacity to assess prevention program outcomes as well as potential mediators and moderators of program effects (Fairchild & MacKinnon, 2009). (See chapter 5.) For example, multilevel modeling approaches have improved analysis of data clustered at multiple levels (e.g., interventions delivered within different classrooms or across different schools). Multilevel mixture modeling has facilitated analysis of both longitudinal and clustered data (Asparouhov & Muthén, 2008; Muthén & Asparouhov, 2006; Raudenbush & Bryk, 2002). Growth modeling techniques enable researchers to model changes in the outcome over multiple points in time, thereby elucidating the potential developmental trajectories of symptoms (Muthén, 2004; Muthén et al., 2002; Muthén & Curran, 1997; Nagin, 2005).

Separate growth trajectories can be modeled (e.g., by growth mixture modeling) for groups of individuals with similar patterns of change over time, trajectories that may be associated with different risk characteristics or different levels of responsiveness to the preventive intervention (Muthén, 2004; Muthén et al., 2002; C. Wang, Brown, & Bandeen-Roche, 2005). Advances have also been made in methods for accommodating missing data in longitudinal trials (Dempster, Laird, & Rubin, 1977) and for incorporating intervention dosage and adherence into analyses of outcomes.

The Current Status of Prevention for Specific Mental Disorders

In recent years, a number of preventive interventions for a variety of mental disorders have been introduced, with generally promising results. Some of these interventions have been evaluated in multiple randomized trials, have been shown to be effective in real-world settings, and have been adapted for use across a variety of populations and settings (IOM, 2009). A meta-analysis of 13 randomized mental disorder prevention trials reported that those preventive interventions reduced the risk for new cases of mental disorder (overall relative risk = 0.73, 95% confidence interval = [0.56, 0.95]) (Cuijpers, van Straten, & Smit, 2006). The majority of prevention studies have centered on behavioral problems and substance abuse in youth and on depressive disorders in youth and adults. As a result, those areas of prevention have the most extensive base of empirical support. Prevention of other mental illnesses, such as anxiety disorders and schizophrenia, is acquiring a growing research base (Cuijpers, 2009).

THE PRACTICE OF PREVENTION

Prevention science is informed by ecological theory, which emphasizes the continuous influence of the environment on behavior (Bronfenbrenner & Morris, 1998; Kelly, Ryan, Altman, & Stelzner, 2000). Bronfenbrenner's (1977, 1979) ecological theory focuses on the reciprocal interactions of individuals with their immediate social contexts (e.g., family) and more distal contexts (e.g., neighborhood and society) in a dynamic fashion over the life course. Risk and protective factors on which prevention efforts focus are embedded within those various levels of social context. Thus prevention strategies—whether universal, selective, or indicated—must be designed with consideration for the most appropriate environmental level at which to intervene and must be implemented in carefully selected settings within that ecology, as displayed in figure 17-2.

Behavior is shaped not only by environmental context but also by an individual's unfolding development across the life span. The timing of prodrome and first episodes varies widely across mental disorders. For instance, the onset of anxiety and impulse control disorders tends to occur in childhood (median onset at age 11); substance use disorders are more likely to emerge in late adolescence or young adulthood (median onset at age 20); and mood disorders like depression and bipolar disorder tend to have onsets in adulthood (median onset at age 30) (Kessler et al., 2005). Thus, guided by developmental research on the onsets and courses of mental disorders, preventive interventions must be timed carefully across the life course so they can be of greatest effect in the prevention of the target mental disorder. Indeed, preventive interventions known to be effective at a specific point in the life course may have no effect, or even an iatrogenic effect, when implemented at another developmental stage (Zandi & Rebok, 2007).

The timing of preventive interventions during the life course also is critical because these strategies may yield downstream benefits across multiple domains of functioning. In particular, preventive interventions early in the life course may have a unique capacity to modify risk factors that underlie a host

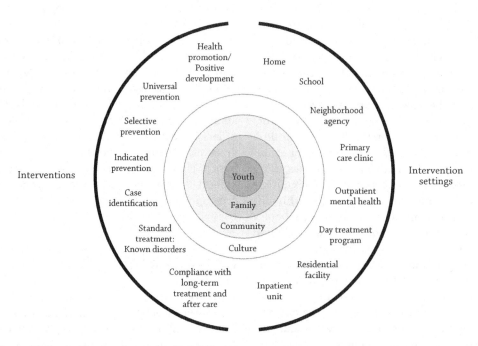

Figure 17-2   **An Ecodevelopmental Model of Prevention.**

Source: Adapted from Weisz, Sandler, Durlak, & Anton, 2005, with permission of the *American Psychologist*.

of adverse mental health outcomes, thereby enhancing development into adulthood (Zandi & Rebok, 2007). Aggressiveness in children as young as age 5, for example, is known to predict later substance abuse (Kellam, Rebok, Ialongo, & Mayer, 1994); similarly, association with deviant peers is strongly predictive of substance use in adolescence and early adulthood (Dishion, 1990). Early preventive interventions have the capacity to alter each of these trajectories by modifying its risk factors.

Evidence from the Nurse–Family Partnership (NFP), which targets mothers during the first two years of the child's life, shows that family-focused prevention programs produce several significant proximal impacts for mothers and children (e.g., reduced rates of domestic violence) as well as distal impacts for children up to 20 years later (e.g., reduced aggressive behavior and criminality) (Eckenrode et al., 2010; Olds, 2006). The life course perspective offers a multitude of opportunities to prevent mental disorders at different life stages, from interventions to promote maternal and fetal well-being at the start of life to the prevention of physical and emotional sequelae of dementia in late life. Thus the ultimate goal of a public health prevention framework should be to embed prevention principles into the structure of everyday life activities and into community structures to enhance development across the life span (Rapp-Paglisi & Dulmas, 2005).

The following sections of this chapter highlight examples of prevention programs implemented across the life course and at various levels of the social ecology, ranging from individual and family to school, workplace, and public health policy. Each of the three types of prevention—universal, selective, and indicated—can be implemented at any ecological level. However, broadly speaking, preventive interventions at the societal level (e.g., federal or state policy) tend to be universal, while interventions targeting individual or family tend to be selective or indicated. Systematic review of all existing prevention programs for mental disorders is beyond this chapter's scope; instead, we provide an overview, highlighting effective models and areas for further inquiry.

Prevention Targeting Individuals or Small Groups

This section offers an overview of interventions to prevent mental disorders that focus strategies on individuals or small groups drawn from a target population. Preventive interventions targeted to other ecological levels—family, school, work, community, and society—are described in subsequent sections. As already noted, prevention programs at the level of the individual commonly use selective or indicated approaches that target individuals with known risk factors for or early symptoms of a particular disorder. Although universal approaches to prevention of mental disorders that are focused on the individual are theoretically possible (e.g., universal screening for depression in primary care), they have not been widely researched or implemented.

This section concentrates on the prevention of depression, schizophrenia, and cognitive decline in Alzheimer's disease, areas of prevention research in which most efforts are focused at the individual level. As will be seen, the prevention programs are implemented at different developmental stages, from childhood through late life. Many of the prevention approaches are adapted from individual- and group-based psychosocial treatment strategies. Although the prevention of other mental disorders, such as anxiety and conduct disorders, includes programs targeting individuals, most work in those areas is directed toward family- and school-based approaches.

PREVENTION OF DEPRESSION

Studies of depression prevention programs have yielded encouraging results. A meta-analysis of research on the reduction of subsyndromal (preclinical) symptoms of depression reported that the 69 studies assessing preventive interventions yielded an 11% improvement in depressive symptoms (Jané-Llopis, Hosman, Jenkins, & Anderson, 2003). Horowitz and Garber's (2006) meta-analysis of 30 studies on the prevention of depressive symptoms in children and adolescents found that selective and indicated programs produced small to moderate effects in symptom reduction. Selective programs performed better than universal programs post intervention; both selective and indicated programs performed better than universal programs at follow-up (Horowitz & Garber, 2006). A more recent meta-analysis of interventions to prevent the onset of mental disorders reported that preventive interventions reduced the incidence of depressive disorders by 22% compared with control conditions (Cuijpers et al., 2008). Similar to earlier findings, selective and indicated interventions were found to be comparable in effectiveness and more effective than universal interventions.[2] On the basis of existing data, a number of researchers have concluded that the prevention of new cases of depression is feasible and can be implemented effectively (Barrera, Torres, & Muñoz, 2007; Cuijpers & Smit, 2008; Cuijpers et al., 2008).

Six randomized controlled studies have assessed whether the onset of major depressive disorder can be prevented using approaches derived from the Coping with Depression (CWD) course (Lewinsohn, Antonuccio, Steinmetz, & Teri, 1984), a group-based behavioral intervention that includes an emphasis on increasing pleasant activities. Two of the studies explored depression prevention among adolescents, one among pregnant women, and three among adult men and women. A recent meta-analysis found that CWD course participants had a 38% lower chance of developing a depressive disorder than controls ($p < 0.05$) (Cuijpers, Muñoz, Clarke, & Lewinsohn, 2009).

A growing number of studies have begun examining the prevention of postpartum depression among pregnant women with subclinical depressive symptoms or histories of depression. While research is still in its early stages, findings from small randomized controlled trials suggest promising outcomes for group-based interventions using interpersonal (Crockett, Zlotnick, Davis, Payne, & Washington, 2008; Zlotnick, Miller, Pearlstein, Howard, & Sweeney, 2006) or cognitive behavioral (Muñoz et al., 2007;

Tandon, Perry, Mendelson, Kemp, & Leis, 2011) approaches that target pregnant at-risk women. Prevention of depression among new mothers has the potential not only to improve functioning for the women but also to promote positive social and emotional development for their offspring.

PREVENTION OF SCHIZOPHRENIA

Schizophrenia is a relatively uncommon disorder, with a lifetime prevalence of approximately 1%, but its course generally is both chronic and deteriorating. The personal and societal burdens of the disorder are considerable (Murray, Lopez, Mathers, & Stein, 2001). Universal and selective prevention approaches to schizophrenia are not viable, given the disorder's low incidence and because current knowledge precludes accurate prediction of onset based specifically on identifiable risk factors (Klosterkötter, Schultze-Lutter, & Ruhrmann, 2008). However, the ability to predict onset on the basis of early signs and symptoms has grown markedly in recent years, prompting the development of indicated approaches to prevent schizophrenia (Klosterkötter et al., 2008; Yung et al., 2007). Sequential screening of multiple risk factors to identify persons at ultrahigh risk for developing psychosis has been employed with encouraging results (Yung et al., 2003, 2007). Age is included in this risk calculation, since peak onset of schizophrenia occurs in late adolescence and early adulthood (Kaplan, Sadock, & Grebb, 1994). Using ultrahigh-risk criteria, approximately 35% of persons identified as at risk were found to have developed a diagnosable psychotic disorder in the following 12 months, a rate 1,000 times that in the general population (Yung et al., 2007). Other symptom-based approaches to the prospective identification of the onset of psychosis also have demonstrated promise (Yung et al., 2007).

Thanks to these and other advances in screening, there is growing interest in the indicated prevention of schizophrenia via implementation of interventions during the prodromal stage, including cognitive behavioral therapy, psychoeducation, and the administration of pharmacologic agents. A meta-analysis of studies

---

2. Conclusions regarding universal interventions must be made with caution, however, since only two studies of universal interventions met inclusion criteria for the meta-analysis.

assessing such interventions reported that the onset of schizophrenia arose in approximately 11% of individuals receiving preventive interventions, compared with 36% in control individuals at risk for schizophrenia (McFarlane, 2007). The 2009 IOM report concludes that while study limitations and the risk of adverse effects preclude broad dissemination of existing preventive interventions for schizophrenia, the promising new findings warrant further funding and development (IOM, 2009).

PREVENTION OF COGNITIVE DECLINE AND ALZHEIMER'S DISEASE

Over 50% of community-residing older adults report cognitive decline (Blazer, Hays, Fillenbaum, & Gold, 1997). Longitudinal studies have found that a decline in cognitive functioning results in loss of functional abilities, such as declines in activities of daily living, and an increased risk for institutionalization (Bharucha, Pandav, Shen, Dodge, & Ganguli, 2004) and, ultimately, mortality (Lavery, Dodge, Snitz, & Ganguli, 2009). Epidemiologic studies have found that increased leisure time with cognitive, social, and physical activities is associated consistently with better cognitive and functional health (see Studenski et al., 2006). Observational studies of this kind, however, limit the ability to draw causal inferences between increased physical and mental activity and the amelioration of age-related cognitive decline, impairment, and disability. Recent programs to help stimulate activity by engaging older adults as volunteers in public schools show considerable promise. For example, in a randomized, pilot trial of Experience Corps, a senior health promotion program, Fried and her colleagues demonstrated that high-intensity volunteering in elementary schools can lead both to cognitive and other health benefits for senior volunteers (Carlson et al., 2008, 2009; Fried et al., 2004) and to educational and behavioral gains for the children (Rebok et al., 2004).

A growing number of reports reveal the value of cognitive training for the maintenance or improvement of cognitive function in healthy older adults. (For recent reviews,

see Hertzog, Kramer, Wilson, & Lindenberger, 2009; Papp, Walsh, & Snyder, 2009; Rebok, 2008.) The majority of these studies aim to modify specific aspects of cognition, such as memory, reasoning, perceptual-spatial ability, or speed of information processing, each of which is affected by age-related mental decline. Findings indicate that training effects can last months or in some cases years; further, training gains may prevent distal adverse outcomes in everyday cognitive functioning (Craik et al., 2007; Willis et al., 2006), everyday behavior (Studenski et al., 2006), and quality of life (Wolinsky et al., 2006).

The Advanced Cognitive Training for Independent and Vital Elderly (ACTIVE) intervention trial (Ball et al., 2002; Willis et al., 2006), the largest documented study to date, is a multisite randomized controlled trial of a large ($N = 2,802$), ethnically diverse sample of community-residing adults ages 65 and older in six US sites. Its primary objective has been to test the effects of three cognitive interventions—targeting memory, reasoning, and speed of information processing—on outcome measures of mentally demanding activities of daily living, such as medication management, telephone use, driving, and financial management. Early findings demonstrated that participants in all three interventions improved in the specific training domain; for example, individuals trained in memory improved only on memory measures, not in speed of processing or reasoning. Training effects simply did not transfer across domains (Ball et al., 2002). Recent evidence, however, suggests that training gains in memory, reasoning, and speed of processing may transfer to more distal cognitive functioning outcomes related to more nuanced, instrumental activities of daily living, such as safer driving, increased mobility, and improved health-related quality of life (Roenker, Cissell, Ball, Wadley, & Edwards, 2003; Willis et al., 2006; Wolinsky et al., 2006). These findings suggest both that the impact of cognitive training may be greater than once believed and that the training has real-world consequences for older adults that eventually may prevent the age-related functional losses that often lead to nursing home admissions and hospitalizations.

Cognitive decline is the clinical hallmark of Alzheimer's disease and related dementing illnesses, all of which disproportionally affect older adults. While late-life cognitive decline is a defining feature of Alzheimer's disease, support is growing for a life course approach that focuses on early- and midlife factors associated with risk for the disorder (Hughes & Ganguli, 2009; Launer, 2005; Whalley, Dick, & McNeill, 2006). The need for more effective prevention and treatment is paramount amid rising concerns about the impact of Alzheimer's disease as a major public health problem affecting increasing numbers of older adults and their families across the United States and around the world. Against this backdrop, the National Institutes of Health (2010) convened a consensus conference, "Preventing Alzheimer's Disease and Cognitive Decline," supported by a review of the evidence-based research literature (Williams, Plassman, Burke, Holsinger, & Benjamin, 2010). Surprisingly, the review yielded little evidence to support prevention: "Considering our results on concordance, the quality of evidence, and gaps in evidence more broadly, currently available evidence does not support recommendations for interventions to delay or prevent cognitive decline or Alzheimer's disease" (Williams et al., 2010, p. 109). More recently, however, some researchers have suggested that that conclusion is both premature and based on a highly selective, cursory review of available evidence. For example, Flicker, Ambrose, and Kramer (2011) argue that the report and its supporting review too readily discounted the empirical evidence supporting the benefits of smoking cessation and physical activity, particularly aerobic activity, for improving cognition and preventing Alzheimer's disease and a multitude of other diseases. They suggest that continued research is warranted to discover safe, effective, affordable ways to prevent this common and devastating condition for older adults. Among the most important future studies will be those focused not only on individuals with preclinical signs and symptoms or mild cognitive impairment but also on individuals in early and mid-adulthood who are at high risk for Alzheimer's and related disorders due to overweight, hypertension, or sedentary lifestyles (Hughes & Ganguli, 2009).

Prevention at the Family Level

The family plays a central role in shaping a child's developmental trajectory, including building his or her capacities for secure attachment, healthy cognitive and emotion regulation, a sense of mastery, and social–emotional competence (see Bowlby, 1982; W. A. Collins, Maccoby, Steinberg, Hetherington, & Bornstein, 2000). Not surprisingly, many significant risk and protective factors for an individual's later mental health originate with both early development and the family, making this ecological unit an important target for prevention efforts. Across cultures, youth spend a great deal of time with their caregivers; families often continue to influence offspring through adolescence and young adulthood (W. A. Collins et al., 2000). Thus family-based interventions can be delivered across an array of developmental periods, from before conception through adolescence.

Family-based interventions offer several advantageous features. They have the potential to modify early risk factors before they give rise to the development of mental, emotional, or behavioral disorders (Eckenrode et al., 2010). Interventions early in the life of a child may be among the most beneficial, because they can disrupt an adverse developmental course before behavioral and emotional problems become entrenched (IOM, 2009). Moreover, interventions that modify parent or caretaker behaviors, a primary and ongoing source of environmental influence, may produce long-lasting benefits for youth. In contrast, the benefits of attending an after-school or school-based preventive intervention may be more short-lived, particularly if the skills and messages are not reinforced over time (IOM, 2009).

However, implementation of family-based interventions poses special challenges. At-risk families must be identified before selective or indicated interventions can be introduced. In extreme cases, families may come to a state's attention based on abuse or neglect reports. In less extreme cases, families may be more difficult to identify, given a lack of standardized family-based screening procedures to identify specific sources of behavioral health risks. Moreover, when a child's early emotional or behavioral symptoms are identified in a school or pediatric setting, the intervention must be sufficiently attractive and accessible that families want to participate (Bradshaw, Zmuda, Kellam, & Ialongo, 2009). Impediments such as stigma, lack of time, and limited financial resources may act as barriers to family engagement in preventive interventions.

A broad array of preventive interventions have been developed and delivered in the family context. These interventions target problems at different periods of the life course, employing strategies from broad-based family education to parenting training to home visits with pregnant women. Most family-oriented prevention efforts are selective (i.e., targeted to families with a member at high risk for a particular emotional or mental disorder) or indicated (i.e., targeted to families in which a member exhibits subclinical signs or symptoms).

Many preventive interventions focus on positive outcomes such as promoting healthy pregnancy and birth; fostering infant attachment; and reducing child maltreatment, child emotional and behavioral problems, and HIV transmission (IOM, 2009). Areas of family-focused prevention vary widely with respect to the number of interventions that have been developed to address the targeted outcome, the number and rigor of studies conducted to evaluate those interventions, and the extent of evidence to support intervention efficacy. Parent training programs, for example, have a particularly long history of development and implementation; their ability to reduce or prevent youth emotional and behavioral problems has been well documented (e.g., Eckenrode et al., 2010; Ireland, Sanders, & Markie-Dadds, 2003; Webster-Stratton & Hammond, 1997; Webster-Stratton & Herman, 2008).

The following discussion highlights programs in three areas of family-based prevention in which interventions have been evaluated through randomized clinical trials with longitudinal follow-up assessments: (1) home visiting, (2) parenting training, and (3) reduction of adverse child outcomes following parental divorce or death. The intention is not to provide an exhaustive summary of family-based programs in these areas but rather to showcase a number of promising programs and to illustrate the methods and approaches employed.

HOME VISITING

Home visiting, a type of home-based intervention, generally involves regular visits to pregnant women or new mothers by health professionals such as nurses and social workers. These programs target a host of public health concerns, such as preterm delivery, low birth weight, infant mortality, child abuse and neglect, childhood injuries, parenting skills, intimate partner violence, and child and parent mental health (Bair-Merritt et al., 2010; Barnet, Liu, DeVoe, Alperovitz-Bichell, & Duggan, 2007; Duggan et al., 1999). While home visiting models and goals vary, all deliver services in families' homes and share the goal of improving family functioning and parent and child outcomes.

The NFP, designed to reduce negative outcomes for mother and child by improving maternal health and behavior, is the most widely researched and disseminated home visiting model in the United States (Olds, 2006). Development of the program was informed by research on and theories of human ecology, self-efficacy, and attachment. Three longitudinal randomized controlled trials of the NFP intervention have been conducted with high-risk families from New York, Tennessee, and Colorado (Eckenrode et al., 2010; Kitzman et al., 2000, 2010; Olds et al., 1998, 1999, 2002, 2007, 2010; Olds, Kitzman, et al., 2004; Olds, Robinson, et al., 2004). In each, women in the intervention groups received home visits from nurses beginning the second trimester of pregnancy though 24 months postpartum. The goal of the visits was to:

• improve maternal behaviors associated with pregnancy and child outcomes

- assist women in building supportive relationships
- link families with other health services and resources.

The trials found the NFP model to be associated with a decrease in child behavior problems at age 6 (Olds, Kitzman, et al., 2004) and internalizing disorders at age 12 (Kitzman et al., 2010) as well as a decrease in maternal substance abuse and child early-onset antisocial behavior at age 15 (Olds et al., 1998, 1999). The most recent outcomes suggest that the greatest effects were among girls, who by age 19 had fewer children and were less likely to have been arrested or to be reliant on Medicaid than their peers who didn't participate in the NFP program (Eckenrode et al., 2010). Few significant effects were found among boys of the same ages. The NFP is being implemented in 28 states in the United States and elsewhere around the world; a large federal initiative is under way to expand use of the NFP model to children across the United States.

Marcenko and Spence (1994) tested a modified version of the NFP with pregnant women whose newborns would be at risk for out-of-home placement. Six months postpartum, after approximately 10 months of home visits, women in the intervention group reported lower levels of psychological distress and higher levels of social support than at baseline, whereas distress and social support levels remained essentially unchanged among women in the control group. Unfortunately, by the children's first birthdays, the sense of increased social support was not maintained, perhaps because the number of home visits was reduced following the six-month assessment (Marcenko, Spence, & Samost, 1996).

Other home visiting preventive interventions have been used to improve mental health outcomes in high-risk families. Koniak-Griffin and colleagues used a public health nursing model to prevent adverse health and social outcomes among adolescent mothers (Koniak-Griffin, Anderson, Verzemnieks, & Brecht 2000, Koniak-Griffin et al., 2002, 2003). At 12 months postpartum, both intervention and control groups reported decreased depressive symptoms and increased self-esteem since

pregnancy. Although both groups displayed increased substance use, rates of use did not return to prepregnancy levels (Koniak-Griffin et al., 2002). The comparable pattern of improvement across the groups may reflect the high level of contact between nurse home visitors and control participants. At two years postpartum, adolescents in the intervention group were less likely to use marijuana than control participants (Koniak-Griffin et al., 2003).

Using a program of parenting education, skills building, and emotional support, Butz and colleagues sought to prevent emotional and behavioral problems among children exposed to drugs in utero (Butz, Lears, O'Neil, & Lukk, 1998; Butz et al., 2001). Women who had used drugs during pregnancy received either standard care or 16 home visits by a nurse from the child's birth through 18 months postpartum. By two to three years after birth, the nurse-visited children had fewer anxiety- and depression-related problems, fewer internalizing and externalizing problems, and fewer total problems than children in the comparison group (Butz et al., 2001). While promising, these findings should be interpreted with caution, given both significant loss to follow-up and the absence of study replication.

In Finland, Aronen and Kurkela (1996) conducted one of the few home visiting studies to deliver an intervention for more than two years and to investigate the long-term effects of home visiting on child mental health. They found that home visits by a psychiatric nurse designed to improve family interaction and child management during the first five years of life can prevent psychiatric symptoms in adolescence (Aronen & Kurkela, 1996) and young adulthood (Aronen & Arajärvi, 2000).

PARENTING TRAINING

Programs to enhance parenting behaviors and practices are common; many have yielded positive effects on children (Barlow & Stewart-Brown, 2000) and short-term improvement in maternal psychosocial functioning (Barlow & Coren, 2004). The majority of these parenting training programs have their theoretical roots in the work of Patterson, DeBaryshe, and

Ramsey (1989) on the negative consequences of harsh and inconsistent parenting. These programs aim to increase positive parent–child activities and interactions and to teach parents to reinforce children's desirable behavior and to impose consistent, but mild, consequences for undesirable behavior (IOM, 2009).

An exploration of all prevention-oriented parent training models is beyond the scope of this chapter. The following discussion focuses on four exemplar programs, each with an extensive empirical basis, two targeting children and two focusing on young adolescents.

The Incredible Years (Webster-Stratton, 1990) has shown efficacy as a selective and indicated prevention program to reduce child aggression and other behavior problems (Gardner, Burton, & Klimes, 2006; J. B. Reid, Eddy, Fetrow, & Stoolmiller, 1999; M. J. Reid, Webster-Stratton, & Hammond, 2003; Webster-Stratton & Herman, 2008). The program uses videotaped vignettes to illustrate positive parenting behaviors to parents and also includes teacher and skills training components.

The Positive Parenting Program (also called Triple P) includes five levels of parenting training, from an initial universal component using mass media to disseminate information about effective parenting strategies, to a selective skills training component for parents of children with behavior problems, to an indicated component ("standard" Triple P) of up to 12 sessions for parents with children manifesting serious behavioral problems. This third level addresses such issues as marital problems and parental depression. Multiple trials have found the overall program to be effective in reducing child behavior problems (Ireland et al., 2003; Prinz, Sanders, Shapiro, Whitaker, & Lutzker, 2009; Sanders, Markie-Dadds, Tully, & Bor, 2000; Sanders et al., 2004).

The Strengthening Families Program is a universal, family-based program designed to prevent adolescent substance use. Randomized controlled trials of an adaptation of the program found that the intervention reduced substance use and had a positive effect on both delinquency and internalizing problems (Spoth, Redmond, & Lepper, 1999; Spoth, Redmond, & Shin, 2000; Spoth, Shin,

Guyll, Redmond, & Azevedo, 2006; Trudeau, Spoth, Randall, & Azevedo, 2007).

The Adolescent Transitions Program is a multilevel program to reduce and prevent adolescent substance use and antisocial behavior, which has universal, selective, and indicated components (Dishion & Kavanagh, 2003; Dishion et al., 2003). Various versions of the program have shown benefits for adolescents, such as reductions in aggressive behaviors, school problems, and substance use (D. W. Andrews & Dishion, 1995; Connell, Dishion, Yasui, & Kavanagh, 2007; Dishion & Stormshak, 2007; Dishion, Kavanagh, Schneiger, Nelson, & Kaufman, 2002; Irvine, Biglan, Smolkowski, Metzler, & Ary, 1999). Both the Strengthening Families Program and the Adolescent Transitions Program also have been found to be cost-effective preventive interventions, producing positive adolescent outcomes for which benefits or savings exceeded program costs (Aos et al., 2004).

REDUCING ADVERSE OUTCOMES OF PARENTAL DIVORCE OR DEATH OF A PARENT

Both parental divorce and the death of a parent can result in serious emotional turmoil for children, increasing the risk for subsequent emotional and behavioral problems (Amato & Keith, 1991; Hetherington & Stanley-Hagan, 1999; Tremblay & Israel, 1998). A number of family-based interventions have sought to reduce the likelihood of these problems (see IOM, 2009). One promising program is Parenting Through Change (Forgatch, 1994), a group-based program that works with divorced mothers. The program's development was informed by coercion theory, which posits that poor child outcomes may be the result of divorce-related disruptions in parenting practices (Patterson, Reid, & Dishion, 1992). Parenting Through Change includes training in positive parenting practices and in other areas, such as affect regulation. A randomized trial of mothers of elementary school–age boys found that the intervention improved effective parenting practices, reduced coercive practices, and was associated with improved child-, mother-, and teacher-rated child outcomes (Forgatch &

DeGarmo, 1999). Follow-up assessment showed that the intervention gave rise to sustained gains in positive parenting and reductions in child noncompliance at 30 months (Martinez & Forgatch, 2001). Improved parenting practices were associated with reduced maternal depression, which predicted maintenance of good outcomes at 30 months (Patterson, DeGarmo, & Forgatch, 2004).

Another program, New Beginnings, evaluated two versions of a preventive intervention for children of divorced parents—one providing individual and group sessions for divorcing mothers, the other providing individual sessions to mothers and group sessions to mothers and their children—against a literature-only control group (Wolchik et al., 2000). The intervention was informed by cognitive behavioral, social-cognitive, and social learning principles. Compared with the control group, middle school–age children (ages 9–12) whose mothers participated in the program showed improvements in their relationships with their mothers and reductions in both internalizing and externalizing problems. Reductions in externalizing problems were sustained at six-month follow-up (Wolchik et al., 2000). Longer term positive program effects for children, including lower prevalence of diagnosed mental disorders and fewer sexual partners, were evident at six-year follow-up (Wolchik et al., 2002).

Few rigorously designed trials have been undertaken to assess prevention programs for children experiencing the death of a parent. One of those few is the Family Bereavement Program (Sandler et al., 2008), a prevention program for bereaved children that has demonstrated encouraging findings in a randomized trial of 156 families. The program includes separate groups for caregivers, adolescents, and children, each of which meets for 12 group sessions. The intervention, which incorporates behavioral change methods, targets modifiable risk factors for poor outcomes. Family and individual functioning were found to improve following the intervention (Sandler et al., 2003). Girls and children with baseline mental health problems maintained reductions in internalizing and externalizing behaviors at 11-month follow-up (Sandler et al., 2003). Longitudinal growth curve models indicated that the rate of recovery was significantly different for girls in the intervention group and girls in the control group (Schmiege, Khoo, Sandler, Ayers, & Wolchik, 2006). Intervention gains, including reductions in clinical levels of grief, were evident at six-year follow-up (Sandler et al., 2010).

Prevention at the School Level

Schools have received considerable attention in the prevention literature (Kellam, Branch, Agrawal, & Ensminger, 1975). Since most children in the United States attend school for approximately six hours a day for 12 years, schools are a desirable setting in which to implement preventive interventions. In addition to the amount of time that children and youth spend in school, educational systems play an important socializing role in multiple aspects of children's academic, social, and emotional development, with both direct and indirect influences on their mental health. Furthermore, the growing recognition that learning problems, school failure, and school dropout often co-occur with mental problems (Bradshaw, Buckley, & Ialongo, 2008)—as either a cause or consequence—highlights the need for preventive mental health interventions in schools (Zins, Weissberg, Wang, & Walberg, 2004).

The past two decades have witnessed great progress in school-based behavioral health promotion and mental disorder prevention (Greenberg, 2004). Recent reviews and meta-analyses have found a growing number of programs that effectively promote positive youth development (Catalano, Berglund, Ryan, Lonczak, & Hawkins, 2002) and that prevent substance abuse (Blitz, Arthur & Hawkins, 2002; D. C. Gottfredson & Wilson, 2003; Lochman & van den Steenhoven, 2002), aggressive and disruptive behavior problems (Hahn et al., 2007; Park-Higgerson, Perumean-Chaney, Bartolucci, Grimley, & Singh, 2008; Ringwalt et al., 2002; S. J. Wilson & Lipsey, 2007; S. J. Wilson, Lipsey & Derzon, 2003), and mental problems (Greenberg, Domitrovich, & Bumbarger, 2001; Hoagwood et al., 2007).

Although effective school-based preventive interventions exist at the universal, selective, and indicated levels, the majority of research has focused on universal prevention programs implemented during the early elementary school years (Greenberg et al., 2001). Drawing on prevention science and public health models, many of these evidence-based programs target risk and protective factors to help reduce disruptive behavior problems in childhood and adolescence (S. J. Wilson & Lipsey, 2007). Fewer interventions focus on reducing internalizing problems. Most current effective interventions neither integrate prevention and treatment nor work across the three IOM levels of prevention (Greenberg, 2004; Weisz, Sandler, Durlak, & Anton, 2005).

Most school-based preventive interventions are manualized programs created to be delivered by teachers or other school-based staff. However, increasing demands on teachers to optimize instruction time and to prepare students for standardized tests as a result of government initiatives such as the No Child Left Behind Act (2002) limit class time available to implement universal social–emotional prevention programs or more intensive selective and indicated programs for targeted children at increased risk for mental problems. As a result, among educators, the most attractive prevention programs tend to be those with positive proximal effects on academic achievement and externalizing behavior problems (see Durlak, Weissberg, Dymnicki, Taylor, & Schellinger, 2011). Thus many prevention-oriented school-based programs are broad in scope, yielding a variety of positive academic, emotional, and behavioral outcomes for students and schools. For this reason, the programs reviewed in this section are organized by level of prevention rather than by targeted outcome. The programs span developmental periods, targeting students from preschool to college.

UNIVERSAL SCHOOL-BASED PREVENTION PROGRAMS

Most effective universal programs draw heavily on developmental theory and research on risk and protective factors for mental problems. Several programs, for example, target early elementary school–age children to help enhance social–emotional functioning and promote effective conflict resolution and adaptive coping skills. Promoting Alternative Thinking Strategies (PATHS) (Greenberg, Kusche, & Mihalic, 1998) is one such universal, school-based, social–emotional learning curriculum that has demonstrated positive effects on elementary school–age children. Using a developmentally appropriate curriculum and activities that teach self-control and emotion regulation skills, the program has been found to reduce both internalizing and externalizing behavior one year after the intervention (Kam, Greenberg, & Kusche, 2004; Riggs, Greenberg, Kusche, & Pentz, 2006). A large, multisite trial of children from high-risk neighborhoods resulted in improved prosocial behavior as well as significantly reduced aggressive behavior, inattention, and poor academic behavior (Conduct Problems Prevention Research Group [CPPRG], 2010).

The Good Behavior Game (Barrish, Saunders, & Wolf, 1969) is another school-based universal preventive intervention that has been subjected to considerable empirical scrutiny. This classroom-based behavior management strategy based on social learning principles is designed to improve academic instruction by reducing student aggressive, disruptive, and off-task behavior. Using a whole-class strategy, the program assigns children to teams; only teams that do not exceed a specified criterion of precisely defined off-task, disruptive, and aggressive behaviors are allowed to "win." The team-based approach enables teachers to use positive peer pressure to help manage both class and individual student behavior.

The long-term effects of the Good Behavior Game, both alone and in combination with academic interventions, have been tested in a series of large-scale randomized controlled trials. When delivered in first grade, the Good Behavior Game was associated with reductions in aggressive and disruptive behavior (Dolan et al., 1993) as well as in diagnoses of conduct disorder in fourth grade (Brown et al., 2008) through middle school (Kellam, Ling, Merisca, Brown & Ialongo, 1998; Kellam et al., 1994). Longer-term benefits, evident at ages

19–21, included reduced rates of antisocial personality disorder, drug and alcohol abuse and dependence, and tobacco use (Kellam et al., 2008); less frequent use of school-based mental health services (Poduska et al., 2008); and decreased violent behavior (Petras et al., 2008). For the most part, the Good Behavior Game has the greatest effect on males who on entering first grade exhibited aggressive or disruptive behavior.[3]

When combined with instructional components and delivered in first grade, the Good Behavior Game had a short-term effect on aggressive or disruptive behavior as well as on achievement (Ialongo et al., 1999). At sixth-grade follow-up, the same children were less likely to have a diagnosis of conduct disorder and were found by teachers to have fewer conduct problems than controls. Moreover, children who participated in the Good Behavior Game were less likely to have been suspended from school or to need or receive behavioral health services (Ialongo, Poduska, Werthamer, & Kellam, 2001). Finally, exposure to the Good Behavior Game and educational enhancements was found to reduce special education service needs, increase both high school graduation and college attendance, and improve performance on standardized tests (Bradshaw, Zmuda, et al., 2009).

The LifeSkills training program (Botvin, Griffin, & Nichols, 2006; Botvin, Mihalic, & Grotpeter, 1998) is an interactive, skills-based universal prevention program designed to lower substance use and promote adaptive skills. Trials of LifeSkills found it had a significant impact on reducing substance use and violence among middle schools students (Botvin et al., 2006; Griffin, Botvin, Nichols, & Doyle, 2003). A recently developed high school version of the program uses developmentally appropriate, collaborative learning strategies to help students achieve competency (see http://www.lifeskillstraining.com/lst_hs.php). While the high school program has yet to be tested in randomized controlled trials, program evaluations have

demonstrated promising outcomes on substance use among high school students.

INDICATED SCHOOL-BASED PREVENTION PROGRAMS

The Coping Power program (Lochman & Wells, 1996), a school-based, indicated preventive intervention, has produced significant effects among preadolescent students with aggressive or disruptive behavior problems. This multicomponent program applies a contextual, social-cognitive framework addressing both parenting processes and children's sequential cognitive processing. Delivered to parents and students over one to one and a half academic years, the intervention provides training in social skills and problem solving and addresses the social-cognitive factors and mechanisms involved in aggressive and disruptive behaviors. Randomized trials of the program have indicated that relative to a comparison group, participants experienced lower rates of substance use and proactive aggression, improved levels of social competence, and significant teacher-rated behavioral improvement (Lochman & Wells, 2002). The Coping Power intervention was found to have positive effects 1 year following program delivery, including improved teacher-rated behaviors and parent-rated substance use (Lochman & Wells, 2004).

The Penn Resiliency Program (PRP; Gillham, Reivich, & Jaycox, 2008) is a depression prevention program for youths 10–14 years old. The program is grounded in cognitive behavioral principals. It is delivered in a group format, is typically implemented in school contexts, and has been widely studied. Evaluated in the context of universal, selective, and indicated studies, PRP demonstrated larger effects on the reduction of depressive symptoms in trials involving children already showing elevated depressive symptoms than in universal trials (Brunwasser, Gillham, & Kim, 2009). This finding is consistent with a more recent systematic review of 42 randomized controlled trials evaluating school-based depression prevention programs (Calear & Christensen, 2010). The review found that indicated programs were more effective than universal and

---

3. See the June 1, 2008, special issue of the journal of *Drug and Alcohol Dependence* (Vol. 95, Suppl. 1) for additional review of the findings of the Good Behavior Game.

selective programs and were more likely to have positive effects at both postintervention and follow-up.

INTEGRATED MODELS OF SCHOOL-BASED PREVENTION

Integrated prevention programs—a strategy increasingly being adopted—fuse separate strategies or programs into a single, enhanced intervention effort (Domitrovich et al., 2009; Walker et al., 1996) designed to target multiple risk and protective factors in a coordinated, synergistic fashion. Such integration may be horizontal (e.g., combining two universal programs) or vertical (e.g., integrating universal, selected, and indicated programs into a single, multitiered approach) (Sugai & Horner, 2006; Walker et al., 1996). Critical to the success of an integrated model is the adoption of a common implementation language and process that makes use of commonalities and connections among the original programs. In contrast to integrated programs, implementing multiple, uncoordinated programs more likely than not will contribute to program fatigue and washout, as noted in several large-scale studies of programs most often implemented in schools (e.g., Fixsen, Naoom, Blase, Friedman, & Wallace, 2005; G. D. Gottfredson & Gottfredson, 2001). Integrating programs also may benefit more students; because no single prevention program benefits all youth equally, combined interventions may positively affect a broader range of students with different needs. In fact, growing evidence suggests that the impact of universal interventions can vary widely based on children's symptom patterns (van Lier, Verhulst, & Crijnen, 2003) or trajectories (Kellam & Rebok, 1992), since some children may require more intensive interventions than are available in a universal program.

Dynamic treatment designs, or adaptive models, are an increasingly popular program delivery system designed to meet the needs of higher-risk individuals (L. M. Collins, Murphy, & Bierman, 2004). Based in substance abuse treatment and prevention (Breslin et al., 1999; Prochaska, Velicer, Fava, Rossi, & Tsioh, 2001; Sobell & Sobell, 2000), these models more

recently have been applied to help prevent disruptive behaviors in children (CPPRG, 2002a, 2002b; Dishion & Kavanagh, 2003; Dishion & Stormshak, 2007). In an adaptive approach, a set of pretreatment, individual- and family-level "tailoring variables" is identified and matched with components of the intervention to meet a child's specific needs. Identification of these tailoring variables is typically based on secondary analysis of intervention trial data and review of both the theorized program targets and the empirical literature on risk and protective factors. By identifying in advance the interventions most likely to benefit specific individuals under particular circumstances, the adaptive or dynamic treatment is thought to boost program effectiveness, resulting in higher-quality, dynamic preventive interventions (L. M. Collins et al., 2004; L. M. Collins, Murphy, Nair, & Strecher, 2005).

The developmental-phased Fast Track program, designed to prevent serious forms of aggressive behavior in children and adolescents, arguably has been the most comprehensive school-based prevention program developed to date (CPPRG, 2002a, 2002b, 2004, 2007). The program delivered a series of developmentally appropriate interventions through multiple classroom, group, and family-focused activities to a cohort of high-risk first-grade children. The aim was to address risk and protective factors such as child competencies, parenting style, the school environment, and school–family communication. Program components, integrated and tailored to meet each child's level of need, were implemented over a period of 10 years. Fast Track, tested in a multisite design, demonstrated several significant effects during the elementary school years on social-cognitive skills, aggressive behavior, academic performance (CPPRG, 2004, 2007), and receipt of mental health, pediatric, and emergency health services (Jones et al., 2010). However, more recent findings suggest that by middle school, several of the foremost intervention effects were no longer significant (Lochman et al., 2010); nonetheless, a few subgroups remained responsive to the program over time. In many ways, the Fast Track trial was a groundbreaking prevention study. It greatly informed prevention research on conduct problems and contributed significantly to the understanding not only of risk and protective factors but also of potential mediators and moderators associated with aggressive behaviors in early childhood through adolescence (CPPRG, 2002a, 2002b).

The Positive Behavioral Interventions and Supports program (PBIS) is a school-based, integrated, tiered prevention initiative that applies social learning and behavioral and organizational principles to the management of the school environment and the implementation of prevention programs and services (Sugai & Horner, 2006). In the PBIS program, a universal intervention is established school-wide to reduce overall levels of behavior problems. The universal effort is theorized to meet the needs of approximately 80% of students in the school. Some 10–15% will require selected interventions; another 5–10% will require indicated interventions (Walker et al., 1996). Students who do not respond adequately to the universal program of positive behavior support (Sugai & Horner, 2006) receive targeted or individually tailored preventive interventions based on systematic assessment of their specific needs (Sugai, Horner, & Gresham, 2002). Improved systems of support for these students are critical, since they account for the majority of children suspended from school and are at greatest risk for both academic failure and future violence (Mayer, 1995; Tobin, Sugai, & Colvin, 1996).

Randomized controlled trials of the universal PBIS intervention have indicated that it improves a school's organizational environment (Bradshaw, Koth, Bevans, Ialongo, & Leaf, 2008; Bradshaw, Koth, Thornton, & Leaf, 2009) and reduces disruptive behavior problems (Bradshaw, Mitchell, & Leaf, 2010; Horner et al., 2009). Some evidence also suggests the universal program has a relatively small but significant positive impact on teacher ratings of students' aggressive behaviors and of their problems with concentration and emotion regulation, as well as on prosocial behavior and numbers of referrals to the principal's office (e.g., Waasdorp, Bradshaw, & Leaf, 2012). These effects likely also translate into increased academic success (Bradshaw et al., 2010; Horner et al., 2009), reduced rates of school dropout, and improved mental health functioning. As many as 13,000 schools, in no fewer than 45 states in the United States, are implementing the universal PBIS program, making it the most commonly used evidence-based prevention program across all service sectors (Fixsen, Blase, Horner, & Sugai, 2009).

School systems and communities are reaching beyond specific prevention programs and models to create comprehensive systems of school-based prevention programs and services that meet the needs of all students (Adelman & Taylor, 2003; Strein, Hoagwood, & Cohn, 2003; Weist, 2001). The three-tiered PBIS provides a framework for connecting multiple programs and initiatives. To achieve this end, however, schools need to develop internal organizational structures that can both manage and facilitate systematic program implementation (Devaney, O'Brien, Resnik, Keister, & Weissberg, 2006; Sugai & Horner, 2006). Parallel structures at the district and state levels should be set in place to provide technical assistance and overall program coordination and assessment (Barrett, Bradshaw, & Lewis-Palmer, 2008). This in turn can help reduce duplication in programs and staffing, competition for scarce resources, and program burnout, turnover, or both (Fixsen et al., 2005).

Workplace Prevention

The negative effects of mental disorders on occupational productivity give rise to substantial financial and social burdens on workers, employers, and society itself. Mental disorders are associated with decreased productivity and reductions in hours worked (Kessler & Frank, 1997). For example, Kessler and Frank (1997) determined that annually, affective disorder is associated with over four million days of work lost in the United States. Comorbidity involving at least two mental disorders is associated with over 15 million days of work lost. Interventions such as depression screening, outreach, and treatment have been shown to yield financial benefits for employers and personal benefits for employees (P. S. Wang et al., 2006, 2007; P. S. Wang, Simon, & Kessler, 2008). Thus the workplace is a logical setting in which to deliver preventive interventions to adult populations. However, the stigma associated with mental disorders poses unique challenges to implementing mental disorder prevention programs in the workplace. As a result, one of the most common strategies employed to manage mental health problems in the workplace has been to embed mental health topics into less stigmatizing efforts and programs such as stress management courses and wellness interventions (Cook & Schlenger, 2002). While workplace-based mental disorder prevention programs are not yet common, several programs have been implemented with promising outcomes.

Heirich and Sieck (2000) implemented a successful workplace prevention program using a cardiovascular disease risk–reduction program to address alcohol use. Employees at a large manufacturing plant, recruited through cardiovascular disease screening, were randomly assigned to either a series of health education classes or a program of individual outreach in which workers were contacted every six months for health risk monitoring and behavior change counseling. Changes in plant organization resulted in a more complex study design (i.e., four comparison groups, three of which received varying levels of exposure to individual counseling). At the end of three years, overall alcohol consumption had decreased in all groups, and 43% of workers identified as high risk at baseline had reduced their alcohol consumption to low-risk levels. Individual health counseling was found more effective than health education classes in reducing the proportion of heavy drinkers during the intervention period. Results are encouraging, but the lack of a separate control site and the possible confounding effects of a voluntary fitness program offered during the study period limit to some extent conclusions regarding program effectiveness.

Because web-based programs can be accessed privately and anonymously, they may be particularly helpful in overcoming the stigma associated with mental and substance abuse problems (Billings, Cook, Hendrickson, & Dove, 2008). Check Your Drinking, a web-based program based on theories of motivational enhancement and social norming, is a personalized, normative feedback program to prevent and reduce high-risk alcohol use targeting working adults ages 18–24 years (Cunningham, Humphreys, & Koski- Jännes, 2000). A randomized controlled trial indicated that the program was effective in both preventing and reducing workplace alcohol use; the program produced significant decreases in weekend drinking, frequency of drinking to intoxication, and peak alcohol consumption among young adult workers, with particularly pronounced gains for high-risk individuals (Doumas & Hannah, 2008). The absence of long-term follow-up or assessment of work-related outcomes, however, limits the conclusions that can be drawn from this research.

Another web-based prevention program, Stress and Mood Management (Billings et al., 2008), was designed to help employed adults manage stress, prevent depression and anxiety, and reduce substance use. The intervention begins with a stress management module, including an assessment instrument that screens for potential problems, and creates an individualized program based on the results. A variety of techniques, including cognitive behavioral strategies, relaxation, problem-solving and time management skills, are coupled with psychoeducation and other resources to achieve program goals. To evaluate the Stress and Mood Management program, a randomized controlled trial assigned participants either to three-month access to the program or to a waiting list. Following the three months, participants in the intervention condition, as compared with participants in the control group, reported increased knowledge about stress, anxiety, and depression; a more positive attitude toward help seeking; decreased stress and binge drinking; and marginally significant improvements in work productivity (Billings et al., 2008). While these results are promising, further follow-up is necessary to ascertain if the intervention is able to prevent depression and anxiety.

Other workplace-based interventions to prevent or reduce alcohol use or mental health problems that have been evaluated include:

• team-oriented social health promotion training (Bennett, Lehman, & Reynolds,

2000; Bennett, Patterson, Reynolds, Wiitala, & Lehman, 2004)
- mindfulness-based stress reduction programs (Cohen-Katz et al., 2005; Cohen-Katz, Wiley, Capuano, Baker, & Shapiro, 2004)
- a program to increase coping skills and social support (Heaney, 1991; Heaney, Price, & Rafferty, 1995).

The JOBS program is a preventive intervention focused on reducing depression related to unemployment. Developed by R. D. Caplan, Vinokur, Price, and van Ryn (1989) and implemented outside the workplace, the JOBS program was designed to reduce the likelihood of unemployment-related depression and to increase the probability of reemployment. The intervention—a series of eight three-hour group sessions delivered over two weeks—is aimed at enhancing job-seeking skills and motivation, building confidence and self-efficacy, and improving mental health. The first evaluation of the program demonstrated that one month after program completion, participants in the intervention group were significantly more likely to be reemployed and to have lower levels of anxious and depressive symptomatology than participants in the control group (R. D. Caplan et al., 1989). Subsequent evaluations found that two and a half years following the intervention, high-risk participants who received the intervention had significantly lower levels of depressive symptomatology than those in the control group (Price, van Ryn, & Vinokur, 1992). A second trial of the program that modified the number and length of sessions and oversampled unemployed persons at higher risk for depressive symptoms yielded similar positive results (Vinokur, Price, & Schul, 1995; Vinokur, Schul, Vuori, & Price, 2000). Findings of a test of JOBS in Finland also point to the program's effectiveness in lowering psychological distress among unemployed persons (Vuori, Silvonen, Vinokur, & Price, 2002).

Both the JOBS program and the body of research exploring its effectiveness have multiple strengths. Vinokur, van Ryn, Gramlich, and Price (1991) built the program on a solid theoretical approach; findings of the first trial have been replicated at home and abroad;

the US trials following participants over an extended period showed longer term positive results; and finally, a cost–benefit analysis indicates the JOBS preventive intervention to be cost-effective (Vinokur et al., 1991). For these reasons and others, the JOBS program has been implemented in sites in Michigan, California, Maryland, China, Ireland, and Israel.

Prevention at the Community Level

In recent years, increasing attention has been paid to the ways in which community-level factors contribute to residents' mental and physical health. Local social stressors, such as environmental disorganization, can combine with insufficient access to resources to yield greater risks for poor mental health and for externalizing and internalizing problems in both children and adults (Caughy, Nettles, & O'Campo, 2008; Dupere & Perkins, 2007; Leventhal & Brooks-Gunn, 2000; Sampson, Morenoff, & Earls, 1999; Sampson, Raudenbush, & Earls, 1997). These community-related factors have an effect on mental health that is distinct from effects of individual risk factors.

Because they are a source of multiple behavioral influences, local communities and neighborhoods are advantageous places to implement prevention. According to Leventhal and Brooks-Gunn (2000), successful neighborhood initiatives can target risk factors for mental disorders (e.g., poverty and lack of safety) by providing needed "resources, stability and safety" (p. 332). One simultaneously can reduce risk factors and promote protective factors through community-based intervention, by employing a variety of approaches to affect a broad array of factors (IOM, 2009). Moreover, neighborhoods generally offer samples of sufficient size to test findings about potential population-wide effects (IOM, 2009).

Some researchers have argued that despite an understanding of the theoretical frameworks for implementing large-scale, partnership-focused, community-based initiatives, too little is known about their effectiveness to warrant their broad-based implementation. Spoth and Greenberg (2005), for example, have identified five ways in which community-based programs may fall short:

- a narrow focus on a single outcome
- lack of a positive, developmental approach
- insufficient use of and coordination among community agencies and resources
- not connecting across communities to share resources
- inadequate research–practitioner collaboration.

Moreover, researchers often struggle to precisely measure community-related prevention variables. Despite evidence of effectiveness for some community-based prevention programs, implementation fidelity and intervention sustainability are often poor, highlighting the need for development of more sustainable approaches (Sandler et al., 2005).

Although community-level programs generally take a universal approach to prevention, on occasion both selective and indicated strategies are implemented, as in programs that mentor at-risk youth or that provide community counseling or mediation. However, larger scale interventions often are required to affect prevalence rates of adverse behaviors (Spoth & Greenberg, 2005). Some community-based programs, such as youth-mentoring initiatives, emphasize outcome improvements for a specific age group. Others, such as housing programs and violence prevention initiatives, are more broadly focused. Of note, community-based prevention programs have the potential for simultaneous effects on the health of community members of diverse developmental stages. Successful violence prevention strategies, for example, can improve mental health outcomes for community members from early childhood to late life by lowering trauma exposure and reducing the risk for victimization. The sections that follow describe different community-based prevention approaches.

BROAD-BASED COMMUNITY APPROACHES

Communities around the country have established coalitions to respond to issues such as youth violence, substance abuse, and crime, particularly when available resources do not seem to effect the change needed (Feinberg, Greenberg, & Osgood, 2004). These collaborations of community leaders and citizens promote change through citizen-based problem solving (Watson-Thompson, Fawcett, & Schultz, 2008). Because this problem-solving effort results in the selection of interventions, its effectiveness is crucial to the success of the larger initiative. Unfortunately, difficulties affecting recruitment, random assignment, and measurement have limited the availability of empirical research on the effectiveness of coalition processes or on the programs subsequently set in place (Feinberg et al., 2004; Watson-Thompson et al., 2008). Coalitions operate in complex ways; many elements contribute to their effectiveness, including community readiness, coalition functioning, knowledge and attitudes of leaders, and level of implementation (Feinberg et al., 2004)

Communities That Care (CTC) (Developmental Research and Programs, 1997; Hawkins & Catalano, 2004) is an evidence-based, comprehensive approach that encourages the collection and systematic use of community-level data to identify areas of strength and need and to guide plans for preventive strategies based on a community's specific profile (Hawkins, Catalano, & Arthur, 2002). Emphasis is placed on areas of greatest need, not those with the largest populations, and because schools typically are included, CTC frequently explicitly targets school-age children and adolescents. The program is built on the tenets underlying both social control and social learning theories, which hold that individuals' behaviors are influenced by the groups to which they belong. Interventions based on these theories aim to create prosocial norms and community bonds both by providing opportunities and teaching the skills to be involved with a group and by creating a system of recognition for positive behaviors (Hawkins et al., 2002). The CTC approach accomplishes those goals by increasing communication among community members, guiding community mobilization, and providing training. In each country in which it has been implemented, including the United tates, the United Kingdom, the Netherlands, and Australia, a central organization has provided the manualized intervention and guides as well as training and technical assistance. The end goal is to ensure healthy outcomes by having the involved community take ownership of the process.

Studies of CTC in four states (Hawkins et al., 2002; Manger, Hawkins, Haggerty, & Catalano, 1992) consistently have documented that even with limited funding, communities can implement the CTC process, including being trained in a five-phase, data-driven, analytic problem-solving approach, forming an action plan, selecting evidence-based interventions, and implementing them. Compared with non-CTC sites, CTC communities were more likely to select evidence-based prevention programs for implementation. Moreover, when adopted and evaluated by the US Department of Justice's Office of Juvenile Justice and Delinquency Prevention, CTC gave rise to better interagency collaboration and less service overlap and redundancy than had existed previously. Behaviors targeted by communities have included substance abuse, violence and crime, parenting skills, and school outcomes. In a five-year randomized controlled trial across seven states and 24 communities, CTC sites implemented at least 75% of the objectives or core components of the programs chosen in the first year, deviated minimally from the programs, and provided the appropriate intervention at the required dosage (frequency and duration) (Fagan, Hanson, Hawkins, & Arthur, 2008). Program attendance and retention was quite high; universal programs reached nearly all targeted middle school students. However, training initiatives reached fewer than 10% of parents. Findings were mixed with respect to parental knowledge, attitudes, and behavior. While parent training showed the most positive effects, selection bias may have confounded the findings; further, only one school-based program had positive effects (Fagan et al., 2008).

Other community-level prevention activities both target specific outcomes and use a particular program or framework. The following section explores examples of this research, grouped by the targeted outcomes.

VIOLENCE PREVENTION

Violence prevention has been one of the foremost targets of community-based preventive initiatives. As noted previously, neighborhood stressors relating to safety and violence affect the prevalence of internalizing and externalizing disorders (Leventhal & Brooks-Gunn, 2000). While violence prevention programs can influence individuals across the life span, youth and young adults most often are targeted explicitly. For example, the CeaseFire program, an Illinois-based community mobilization effort, aims to prevent violence by communicating the social and personal costs of violence, changing community norms, and providing alternatives to violence (Skogan, Hartnett, Bump, & Dubois, 2008). The program uses a number of techniques to achieve its goals, among them dissemination of educational materials designed to raise broad-based community awareness. Further, following any homicide in the community, stakeholders conduct marches, rallies, and prayer vigils to demonstrate community solidarity against the violent act. Both selected and indicated program components engage outreach workers who provide counseling, mentoring, and mediation to gang members, community members affected by gun violence, and those likely to resort to gun violence (i.e., those identified as high risk).

A quasiexperimental, matched-comparison evaluation of CeaseFire in Chicago, Illinois (Skogan et al., 2008), found that mentoring helped "high-risk" clients—individuals reporting problems such as previous arrests, time in jail, gang involvement, and/or failure to continue beyond grade school—to be successful in achieving vocational and educational goals. Violence was reduced over time in six of the seven matched CeaseFire sites. The number of shootings and individuals shot also was lower in the CeaseFire sites. Finally, gang activity, retaliatory shootings, and overall shootings attributed to gangs were reduced. In assessing the validity of these findings, however, consideration should be given to the issue of selection, since program involvement was the result of community and individual self-selection.

A modified version of CeaseFire, called Safe Streets, was implemented in Baltimore, Maryland (Webster, Vernick, & Mendel, 2009). A quasiexperimental, matched-comparison study found that, after one year, two of three neighborhoods successfully implemented the program and broadened the numbers of both outreach workers and clients. The neighborhood with the most thorough implementation showed significantly less tolerance of violence as well as a downturn in homicide trends.

Operation Ceasefire, a problem-solving initiative developed and implemented in Boston, Massachusetts, in the mid-1990s, addressed the growing rate of youth homicide (Braga, Kennedy, Waring, & Piehl, 2001). A large-scale, interagency investigation found that 60% of youth homicides were committed by the city's gang members using semiautomatic weapons. Those youth comprised fewer than 1% of the youth population in the Boston area. Operation Ceasefire pursued a twofold approach that included both a law enforcement crackdown on weapons traffickers and an outreach effort sending a clear message of intolerance for violence to gang members. Unlike the Chicago and Baltimore programs, which emphasized mentoring, this program sent a message about the immediate and intense consequences imposed by law enforcement agents on perpetrators of violence. Study results indicated that in the year following implementation, youth homicide rates were the lowest they had been in 20 years. Using time-series data, a 63% reduction from the preintervention to postintervention time series was identified in the monthly incidence of homicide; significant reductions were also found in gun assaults and "shot fired" calls to the police after controlling for other causal factors. While a recent evaluation of an Operation Ceasefire–like program conducted in Pittsburgh reported mixed results (J. M. Wilson, Chermack, & McGarrell, 2010), the study included significant departures from the Boston model that may well explain its less favorable outcomes (J. M. Wilson et al., 2010). Taken together, the extant research suggests

a substantial need for additional, systematic evaluation of both the process and effects of implementing community-based youth violence prevention models.

A different approach to neighborhood violence prevention seeks to alter environmental factors to reduce opportunities for the commission of crimes (Mair & Mair, 2003). Such changes have included requiring exact bus fares to reduce robberies, using bright exterior sodium vapor lighting, redesigning spaces such as subways and nightclubs to reduce crowding and hiding places, and erecting traffic barriers to prevent easy escape from high-crime areas (Mair & Mair, 2003). This type of prevention has the potential to help reduce event-triggered anxiety, trauma, and other mental illness by reducing the occurrence of adverse events.

ENHANCING RESOURCES FOR THE UNDERSERVED

Housing has important links to physical and mental health, particularly because residence location largely determines the availability of public resources. Low-income neighborhoods often lack resources to support child development owing to the link among income, taxes, and neighborhood-based public institutions. Low-income families who live in mixed-income neighborhoods can benefit from resources they otherwise might not have, such as access to schools and libraries that could better foster their children's development (Keels, 2008)

The first major evaluation of a housing-based prevention initiative was the Gautreaux program, the product of a court decision in 1976 that led the Chicago Housing Authority to provide African American families in public housing or on wait lists for housing with a voucher enabling them to move to lower poverty areas through 1998 (Fisher, 2005). The voucher program was found have positive educational effects on children who were relocated to less impoverished communities (Kaufman & Rosenbaum, 1992). In the long term, mothers felt their children's safety, development, and education improved when they lived in the suburbs compared with public housing in the city (Keels, 2008). While they reported some difficulty adjusting to the move, most felt it was worth that cost.

The landmark Moving to Opportunities project was sponsored by the US Department of Housing and Urban Development (HUD) specifically to provide a larger scale assessment of the effects of moving low-income residents into higher income neighborhoods than was possible in the Gautreaux program (Orr et al., 2003). This evaluation, spanning the years 1994–1998, randomly assigned people in Baltimore, Boston, Chicago, Los Angeles, and New York City into one of three groups: (1) an experimental group, in which families were given a voucher, provided with housing assistance, and required to move to a "low-poverty" neighborhood (an area where 10% or fewer people were in poverty) for at least one year; (2) a comparison group, in which people were given vouchers to move where they chose; and (3) a control group, who continued to receive public housing and assistance (Orr et al., 2003).

Multiple evaluations across sites have provided a mixed picture from the HUD initiative. The 10-year outcome report prepared for HUD (Orr et al., 2003) disclosed that once given vouchers, almost 50% of the experimental group and 60% of the comparison group moved; however, many in the comparison group moved to other impoverished areas. When the two voucher recipient groups were compared with the control group on measures of mental health, experimental-group adults showed decreased psychological stress and depression, experimental-group girls showed decreased stress, comparison-group girls showed decreased depression, and girls in both voucher groups showed very large reductions in the incidence of generalized anxiety disorder. However, parent and self-reports of problem behaviors did not decrease as a result of being in the voucher groups. Indeed, boys in the experimental and comparison groups self-reported increased problem behaviors and smoking. Boys in the voucher groups also had a higher frequency of arrests, due either to increased criminal activity or to improved policing, than those in the control group. Girls in the experimental group had reductions in their self-reported rates of marijuana and tobacco use, and girls in the comparison voucher group had large reductions in the incidence of arrests for violent crime (but not for other crimes). Neither voucher group displayed significant changes in educational achievement, employment, or self-sufficiency (Orr et al., 2003).

Analyses of HUD data collected in Baltimore found that participants in the experimental group, who received housing assistance and counseling, were more successful in and satisfied with their relocation than were those in the comparison group (Bembry & Norris, 2005), suggesting that the provision of housing vouchers alone does not ensure improved housing or subsequent improvements in mental health or education. In a follow-up study in New York City (Leventhal & Brooks-Gunn, 2004), three years after relocation male students in low-poverty schools were more likely to be retained in grade. While no gender gap in reading and math achievement test scores was observed in schools of the experimental group, in the control group female students outperformed male students in school. Analyses indicated that relocation to low-poverty neighborhoods increased the amount of time male students spent on homework and had a positive effect on school safety, which in turn improved achievement. Two years later, unfortunately, the positive effects of relocation on student achievement were no longer discernible (Leventhal, Fauth, & Brooks-Gunn, 2005).

YOUTH PROTECTIVE FACTORS

Youth mentoring has become a popular way to provide youth with positive relationships with adults, which act as a powerful protective factor (Dubois, Holloway, Valentine, & Cooper, 2002). A meta-analysis of 59 studies examining the effects of one-on-one youth mentoring relationships found that mentoring by adults or older peers was associated with small positive effects (Dubois et al., 2002). Mentored youth achieved higher outcome scores than those who did not receive mentoring (average $d = 0.14$) (Dubois et al., 2002). While many variables were examined for their moderating effects on mentoring outcomes, few were significant. Mentoring effects were not moderated by most mentor and youth demographic characteristics (e.g., gender and race) nor by whether the mentor was paid, where the mentoring took place, how mentors were matched to youth, frequency and duration of mentoring, or type of mentoring program (Dubois et al., 2002). An individual, randomized trial of the Big Brothers/Big Sisters program found that youth mentored for one or more years reported the most improvement; those whose mentors terminated their participation after a short time reported reduced functioning (Grossman & Rhodes, 2002). Both youth characteristics (e.g., older age or being a victim of abuse) and mentor characteristics (younger age, being married, and having a lower income) were predictive of early termination.

The most positive effects in the meta-analysis were found among mentors trained in a "helping" profession and in programs that provided ongoing training to mentors, used evidence-based practices, offered structured activities, and were not school based. Effects were largest when mentoring programs targeted at-risk youth and when parents were involved in the programs (Dubois et al., 2002). However, for some variables the analyses included only a small subset of the 59 available studies and thus may have lacked strong predictive power. Nonetheless, the findings of the meta-analysis support the use of community- rather than school-based youth mentoring programs to help reduce or prevent behavioral problems.

PREVENTION OF SUBSTANCE USE AND ABUSE

Substance use and abuse are the focus of prevention efforts at multiple levels of the social ecology, including schools, family, society, and policy. While few community-based initiatives have reported success in preventing substance use and abuse, effects are improved when efforts are embedded in larger community efforts such as Communities That Care. Hallfors, Cho, Livert, and Kadushin (2002) designed a community-based initiative to combat substance abuse, which began by enabling each community to develop and implement its own substance abuse reduction strategy. Not

a single one of the strategies implemented across 12 communities (and 12,000 randomly selected individuals) was found effective in reducing substance abuse. However, another program, Communities Mobilizing for Change on Alcohol (Wagenaar, Murray, & Toomey, 2000) reported encouraging results. The program focused on altering community norms about drinking and on effecting policy changes to reduce the availability of alcohol to youth. Results of a randomized 15-community trial indicated that the intervention reduced the sale of alcohol to minors and reduced alcohol purchases and consumption by 18- to 20-year olds; fewer behavioral changes were observed for younger adolescents (Wagenaar et al., 2000). The intervention was also associated with a decline in alcohol-related arrests and traffic crashes (Wagenaar et al., 2000).

A manual developed by the RAND Corporation to help communities plan and implement substance abuse prevention programs used principles that also can be applied to other troubling youth behaviors such as teen pregnancy and crime. The manual includes 10 steps or "questions" that address needs assessment, goal setting, and program selection, implementation, evaluation, and maintenance (Chinman, Imm, & Wandersman, 2004). While the manual has been used widely, no known outcome evaluations have been undertaken to ascertain the program's effectiveness.

Holder and colleagues (2000) recently reported encouraging results of a multicomponent, community-based intervention to prevent high-risk drinking and related injuries and assaults. The intervention, implemented in three communities in Northern and Southern California and South Carolina, addressed several areas relevant to alcohol consumption and alcohol-related violence and injuries, including media advocacy, the formation of community coalitions, changes in alcohol serving practices, retailer training to reduce alcohol retail sales to young people, increased enforcement of drinking and driving laws, and reductions in the density of alcohol retail outlets. Comparison of intervention communities with matched comparison communities found the intervention to be associated with reduced self-reported binge drinking, alcohol-related car crashes, and alcohol-related injuries and assaults. This promising community-based intervention approach merits further study. Moreover, other research has associated the reduction in alcohol outlet density with reductions in alcohol consumption and in related violence and injuries (C. A. Campbell et al., 2009; Resko et al., 2010; Yu et al., 2008), suggesting that this is an important element for future community-based prevention approaches.

Community-based prevention strategies also have targeted issues such as teen pregnancy prevention (Lesesne et al., 2008), tobacco control (Florin et al., 2006; Merzel, Moon-Howard, Dickerson, Ramjohn, & VanDevanter, 2008), and promoting condom use (Alstead et al., 1999). Although research on these and other community-based prevention initiatives is in its early stages, promising findings with implications for mental health warrant further inquiry.

Prevention at the Level of Society and Policy

Initiatives at the state and federal levels have the potential to shape individuals' behaviors in ways that reduce risks for the onset of mental disorders. Prevention strategies at the societal level generally take a universal approach, such as state-governed excise taxes on harmful substances like tobacco and alcohol. Indicated and selective approaches to prevention include such practices as protecting potential victims of violence by limiting gun access among felons and individuals subject to restraining orders. Some societal-level initiatives focus on children and youth, such as regulations governing school attendance and policies. Others target adults through imposition of such measures as legal limits on blood alcohol concentration and laws governing the purchase of guns. Like community-based prevention strategies, initiatives at the state and federal level are likely to have broad-based effects on the health of groups of different ages (for example, by reducing exposure to crime, violence, or harmful substances). Some researchers argue that despite their considerable potential to create change for the better, federal laws and policies have not been used

productively to that end (Lee, Lee, Lee, & Arch, 2010). Commercial interests with substantial power to oppose the passage of laws and policies (Giesbrecht, 2000) often limit enactment of comprehensive prevention statutes at the federal and state levels. What follows is a brief overview of selected policies with implications for prevention, among them education policies and policies designed to thwart substance use and gun violence.

IMPROVING EDUCATION

Education policy has the potential to exert a significant impact not only on the academic outcomes of children but also on their behavior and social–emotional health. The federal Elementary and Secondary Education Act was enacted in 1965 to provide financial support for public education and was reauthorized as the No Child Left Behind Act of 2001. The No Child Left Behind Act placed greater accountability on school systems to prevent school violence, create safe and orderly school environments, increase student performance, and reduce racial disparities in special education services use, while simultaneously placing a premium on the use of evidence-based practices. Also embedded in the act is an initiative to prevent school dropout.

To assist in the accountability process and to establish evidence-based practices, the Education Sciences Reform Act of 2002 established the Institute of Education Sciences to "provide rigorous evidence on which to ground education practice and policy." Other federal education laws, such as the Individuals with Disabilities Education Act (IDEA) also affect the provision of prevention services (Wright, 2005). For example, IDEA allows school districts to use up to 15% of their special education funds to support preventive interventions for at-risk children. States have the right to set the age for compulsory education, which ranges from 16 to 18 years across the United States. Some researchers have suggested that raising the compulsory education age to 18 nationwide has potential benefits for prevention and health promotion, such as greater economic earnings potential, reduced risks for involvement in deviant and problem behavior, and greater opportunity for exposure to school-based prevention activities and services (Bradshaw, O'Brennan, & McNeely, 2008). While systematic evaluations of these and other educational policies are rare and often yield mixed results (Bradshaw, O'Brennan, & McNeely, 2008), educational policies that focus schools on prevention activities, particularly when coupled with additional funds to support prevention, appear to be a promising means of infusing further mental disorder prevention and health promotion opportunities into the educational setting.

IMPROVING USE OF EVIDENCE-BASED PRACTICES

Federal policy stipulates that schools may only use prevention programs whose effectiveness is supported by solid scientific evidence (Hallfors, Pankratz, & Hartman, 2007; Ringwalt et al., 2008). Several federal agencies, such as the Department of Education, SAMHSA in the Department of Health and Human Services, and the Office of Juvenile Justice and Delinquency Prevention in the Department of Justice have either produced reports or developed guides to facilitate the identification and selection of appropriate evidence-based prevention programs. The web-based National Registry of Evidence-Based Programs and Practices (SAMHSA, 2011), a compilation of over 100 prevention-oriented best practices, is arguably the most comprehensive and influential of those guides. Blueprints for Violence Prevention, developed with the support of the Office of Juvenile Justice and Delinquency Prevention (Center for the Study and Prevention of Violence, 2011), also lists effective prevention programs. These resources have the potential to advance the implementation and dissemination of effective prevention programs.

PREVENTION OF SUBSTANCE ABUSE

Substance abuse prevention initiatives at the societal and policy levels primarily have consisted of the imposition of pricing and tax policies related to substances such as alcohol and tobacco. Recent systematic reviews and meta-analyses of the literature have concluded that increased alcohol excise taxes effectively help reduce both alcohol consumption, including binge drinking, and harmful outcomes such as drunk driving and alcohol-related crash fatalities, even among underage populations (Anderson et al., 2009; Elder et al., 2010; Wagenaar, Salois, & Komro, 2009). A meta-analysis of 112 studies on alcohol tax or price effects (Wagenaar et al., 2009) found, for example, that increased alcohol taxes and prices are associated with decreased sales (aggregate level $r = -0.44$ for total alcohol, $p < 0.001$), with effect sizes exceeding those for many other prevention policies. The magnitudes of the effects were smaller for heavy drinking than for overall drinking. Elder and colleagues (2010) found that the magnitude of an increase in alcohol tax was positively associated with its impact. Other policies and programs also have proven effective in reducing alcohol consumption and alcohol-related harms, among them legislative measures to reduce drunk driving (e.g., reductions in illegal blood alcohol concentration limits for driving) and regulations governing the availability of alcohol (Anderson et al., 2009; Fell & Voas, 2006). Cigarette excise taxes also have been found effective in reducing cigarette use and smoking-related deaths (CDC, 2010).

Mass media campaigns to reduce substance abuse are another society-level prevention strategy. Some campaigns, such as those designed to reduce tobacco and drug use, have sought to reach adolescents and youth through the popular media; to date, however, effects have been mixed (Randolph & Viswanath, 2004). Most public health campaigns have been unable to budget for multimedia strategies of this nature and instead have relied on print materials, graphic media such as billboards, and promotional items like T-shirts and hats.

DECREASING GUN VIOLENCE

Federal gun laws impose certain restrictions on the purchase of guns by individuals at high risk for violent behavior. However, many aspects of gun sales are not federally regulated, including private gun sales by nondealers, the method by which most armed criminals purchase such weapons (Harlow, 2001). To address gaps in federal regulations, a number of states have passed additional laws, such as laws requiring universal background checks, licensing and registration laws, and laws banning gun purchases by individuals with criminal histories. Some states also have enacted statutes increasing oversight and regulation of gun dealers, measures found to lower rates of gun trafficking within states (Webster, Vernick, & Bulzacchelli, 2009). Guns contribute significantly to fatalities and nonfatal wounds among victims of intimate partner violence, the vast majority of whom are female (J. C. Campbell et al., 2003; Saltzman, Mercy, O'Carroll, Rosenberg, & Rhodes, 1992; Wiebe, 2003). Rates of female homicide by partners are 10% lower in states that screen for and prohibit gun purchases by individuals subject to a restraining order (Vigdor & Mercy, 2006). Over one third of states have enacted laws requiring gun owners to store guns in ways that limit access by underage youth; these child access prevention laws have reduced accidental youth gun fatalities (Hepburn, Azrael, Miller, & Hemenway, 2006) and adolescent suicides (Webster, Vernick, Zeoli, & Manganello, 2004).

CURRENT CHALLENGES AND NEXT STEPS

A number of key areas in prevention require attention to promote continued advancement of the field, as highlighted in the 2009 IOM report. We summarize several of these areas below.

Screening

Screening for risk factors is critical to the identification of target populations for prevention efforts. As shown in figure 17-3, screening complements preventive strategies at the universal, selective, and indicated levels by identifying communities, groups or individuals with a risk factor or factors targeted by the preventive intervention. However, screening often poses both funding and logistical challenges. Critically, it also raises ethical issues about the identification of risk factors that may lead to stigma and labeling of individuals, particularly if appropriate, effective preventive interventions are not readily available for individuals who screen positive.

The IOM 2009 report includes a list of 10 suggested criteria for appropriate prevention screening at the individual level, adapted from principles originally developed by the World Health Organization (J. M. G. Wilson & Jungner, 1968). There must be:

1. A disorder to be prevented that poses serious consequences for the individual or those around him or her

2. An empirically supported association of the disorder with the target risk factors

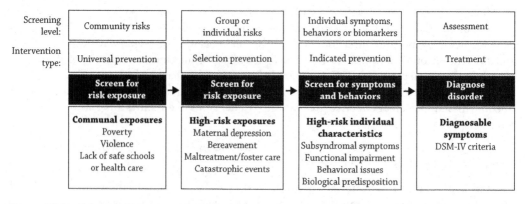

Figure 17-3   **Schema of Opportunities for Screening and Prevention.**

Source: Reprinted with permission from Institute of Medicine, 2009, p. 220.

3. An effective intervention to prevent or reduce target risk factors or early symptoms

4. Appropriate settings for screening and intervention

5. Modifiable risk or protective factors or early symptoms of disorder

6. Validated procedures for identifying risk factors or early symptoms

7. Acceptable, nonstigmatizing screening procedures

8. Consensus regarding whom to refer for further assessment and services

9. Cost-effective screening methods

10. Potential for repeated screenings to identify emerging risks and symptoms over time (IOM, 2009).

For most mental disorders, it is difficult to meet all these criteria at present. However, with increased funding and infrastructure for conducting prevention research, the criteria can provide a solid foundation for the development of effective screening procedures. Strategies to screen and identify high-risk communities, such as the Indices of Multiple Deprivation, have been adopted in the United Kingdom but have yet to be developed in the United States and so warrant further attention (IOM, 2009).

Internet-Based Preventive Interventions

Growing evidence suggests that Internet-based self-help may be an emerging, effective preventive intervention method for highly prevalent disorders such as depression and anxiety (Donker et al., 2009). Large-scale trials are under way to determine the effectiveness of online intervention approaches. For example, Donker and colleagues (2009) are conducting a randomized controlled trial of an Internet-based intervention on 500 subjects ages 18 and up with mild to moderate depression or anxiety. They are interested in discerning whether support by an online coach can improve clinical outcomes, lower dropout rates, and hold down costs and whether the program is equally effective with minimal clinical guidance. In another recent study, van Spijker, van Straten, and Kerkhof (2010) are evaluating the effectiveness of a web-based self-help intervention to reduce suicidal thoughts. These online interventions may both improve accessibility and offer cost-effective alternatives to face-to-face interventions. In a recently completed Australian study, Newton, Teesson, Vogl, and Andrews (2010) found that an Internet-based prevention initiative to reduce alcohol and cannabis use resulted in greater student knowledge about those substances and reduced alcohol use 12 months after program completion.

Replication Studies and Long-Term Follow-up

It is critical that promising prevention programs be subjected to rigorous empirical scrutiny across sites and over time. Most prevention program effects have not been replicated by independent teams of investigators or studied over long follow-up periods to determine if benefits are maintained. Studies to track the developmental course of disorders among participants after the intervention's end are particularly lacking. As noted by Greenberg and colleagues (2001), a number of prevention programs actually show *stronger* effects at later follow-up than immediately following the intervention. Thus it is possible that the magnitudes of near-term intervention effects are underestimates, making the assessment of distal outcomes critical. However, this is not always the case, as noted in the more recent studies of the NFP, which produced significant long-term effects only for girls (Eckenrode et al., 2010), and in the Fast Track studies, which showed relatively few remaining effects by adolescence (Lochman et al., 2010). These findings highlight the need for further long-term studies like those testing the 20-year outcomes of the Good Behavior Game (see Kellam et al., 2008).

Similarly, researchers often are perplexed when seemingly effective programs cannot be replicated either across multiple studies or at different sites within multisite trials (see, e.g., Social and Character Development Research Consortium, 2010). Most recently, questions have arisen about conflicting findings on the effectiveness of prevention programs focused on social and character development and on preventing bullying (e.g., Farrington & Tofi, 2009; Social and Character Development Research Consortium, 2010). Greater emphasis should therefore be placed on the use of meta-analyses, which summarize and contrast findings from multiple trials within a single study (e.g., Durlak et al., 2011).

Cost–Benefit Analyses

The economic and social costs of mental disorders to individuals, families, and societies are very high; the potential of preventive interventions to reduce those costs is great. However, relatively few cost–benefit analyses have been conducted to explore the economic benefits of the prevention of mental and substance abuse disorders (van Gils, Tariq, Verschuuren, & van den Berg, 2011; Zechmeister et al., 2008), particularly with respect to long-term outcomes. Existing analyses do suggest that prevention can yield considerable economic benefits, particularly for interventions among high-risk population subgroups (Aos et al., 2004; van Gils et al., 2011). Better guidelines regarding economic analysis of prevention programs are needed, as are more country- and population-specific economic evaluations (Zechmeister et al., 2008).

Advances in Genetics and Neuroscience

Recent advances in genetics and neuroscience offer the potential to elucidate risk mechanisms for mental disorders with greater clarity and precision. Collaborations among prevention scientists, behavioral geneticists, and neuroscientists can facilitate application of this knowledge to developmental theories of risk and resilience and to prevention strategies (Caspi et al., 2003; Cichetti & Blender, 2006). Moving forward, new statistical methods will be needed to analyze genetic data within a multiple-level framework that incorporates neurobiological, psychological, and environmental–contextual domains. Such methods will enhance the potential of prevention intervention trials to yield further insights into

possible etiologic mechanisms, the degree to which neural plasticity can be enhanced, and interactions between biology and environment in the development of mental disorders and resilience (Cichetti & Blender, 2006).

Implementation and Dissemination

Broad-scale implementation and dissemination of effective preventive interventions in communities and institutions is the long-term goal of prevention research, as shown in figure 17-4. However, the field is currently far more able to develop and evaluate preventive interventions than it is to implement them with fidelity and disseminate them. For example, despite federal requirements to adopt evidence-based curricula when using preventive interventions, the majority of schools have not done so (Domitrovich et al., 2008; Ringwalt et al., 2002). One study reported that only 19% of schools that did use evidence-based prevention programs implemented them with fidelity (Hallfors & Godette, 2002). Other challenges include ensuring that prevention programs are amenable to ready adaptation across disparate populations and settings. The 2009 IOM report highlights the importance of increased emphasis on and funding for implementation and dissemination efforts, including the development of statistical methods to assess the success of such efforts.

Interest also is growing among federal agencies, researchers, and policy makers in moving research findings into real-world settings through what is often referred to as translational research (SPR MAPS II Task Force, 2008). Type I translational research focuses on discovery through clinical trials; type II translational research examines how effective practices, interventions, and treatments can be implemented effectively in real-world settings (Woolf, 2007, 2008). The emerging field of implementation science (Fixsen et al., 2005) focuses on the process of implementing programs with fidelity and sensitivity to organizational, leadership, and other contextual factors at multiple levels (Domitrovich et al., 2008). This area of prevention research will be the subject of growing interest and activity over the next decade and beyond, as it

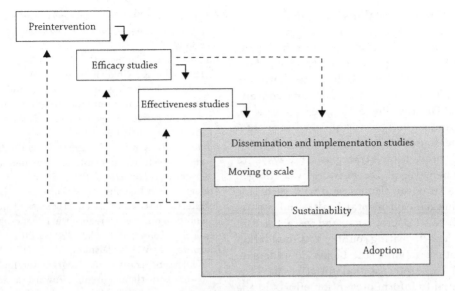

Figure 17-4   **Stages of Research in Prevention Research Cycle.**

Source: Reprinted with permission from Institute of Medicine, 2009, p. 324.

has the potential to optimize the outcomes of prevention programs by ensuring high-quality implementation.

Infrastructure

In 1994, the IOM's first prevention report advocated both the expansion of the infrastructure facilitating government support for prevention research and increased funds to underwrite such research (Muñoz et al., 1996). Since that time, prevention science has achieved substantial gains, yet both the government infrastructure and funding for prevention of mental disorders remain limited. The 2009 IOM report called for a further enhanced prevention infrastructure that includes increased funding for prevention research, development of a coordinated and effective system for delivering preventive interventions, and expansion of a workforce trained in the development, delivery, and evaluation of such interventions. The report noted, however, that there currently were "no targeted funding streams for prevention in the mental health area" (p. 369) and argued for provision of a set-aside within SAMHSA's block grant program for mental health services to fund such activities.

The National Prevention, Health Promotion, and Public Health Council was created in 2010 as a component of the Patient Protection and Affordable Care Act. The council, chaired by the surgeon general with members from across federal agencies and departments, has a mandate to develop a national prevention strategy to guide health promotion and disease prevention. As Beardslee, Chien, and Bell (2011) note, the council has the potential to advance recognition and funding for prevention efforts; advocacy for representation of mental health issues is key to ensuring that mental health is adequately addressed in this prevention agenda.

International Initiatives

A number of exciting international initiatives have been launched in recent years. The World Health Organization, for example, recently collected evidence from a host of countries on the effectiveness of interventions to prevent mental disorders and promote mental health (Herrman, Saxena, & Moodie, 2004; Hosman, Jané-Llopis, & Saxena, 2005). Nations including Australia, the Netherlands, and Scotland have taken significant steps toward the prevention of mental disorders and in most cases are closer to implementing a comprehensive prevention infrastructure than is the United States (e.g., Fudge & Robinson, 2009; Healthier Scotland, 2009). The European Network for Mental Health Promotion and Mental Disorder Prevention, representing 30 European nations, was established as an integrative source of information on evidence-based prevention strategies and ways to implement them. The network was charged by the European Commission with gathering baseline data on mental health and mental health policies, programs, and infrastructure in each participating country as a foundation for future action (Jané-Llopis & Anderson, 2006). These international initiatives have the potential to inform prevention efforts in the United States.

Attention to the areas outlined above will enable prevention science to maintain its momentum and to make progress in achieving population-based reductions in mental disorders. The field has already witnessed dramatic growth, with roughly 400 randomized controlled prevention trials relevant to mental health conducted since the 1994 IOM report (Beardslee et al., 2011). This growing evidence base supports the potential of programs implemented at various ecological levels (individual, family, school, work, community, and society) and targeting a variety of mental disorders at different stages in the life course. These developments suggest that a bright future for prevention is possible. To that end, prevention science merits government funding and policy support; at stake are the reduction of human suffering and promotion of greater well-being among populations in the United States and worldwide.

REFERENCES

Adelman, H. S., & Taylor, L. (2003). On sustainability of project innovations as systemic change. *Journal of Educational and Psychological Consultation, 14*, 1–25.

Albee, G. (1985). The argument for primary prevention. *Journal of Primary Prevention, 5*(4), 213–219.

Albert, M. R. (1999). Fever therapy for general paresis. *International Journal of Dermatology, 38*(8), 633–637.

Alstead, M., Campsmith, M., Halley, C. S., Hartfield, K., Goldbaum, G., & Wood, R. W. (1999). Developing, implementing, and evaluating a condom promotion program targeting sexually active adolescents. *AIDS Education and Prevention, 11*(6), 497–512.

Amato, P. R., & Keith, B. (1991). Parental divorce and the well-being of children: A meta-analysis. *Psychological Bulletin, 110*(1), 26–46.

Anderson, P., Chisholm, D., & Fuhr, D. C. (2009). Effectiveness and cost-effectiveness of policies and programmes to reduce the harm caused by alcohol. *Lancet, 373*(9682), 2234–2246.

Andrews, D. W., & Dishion, T. J. (1995). The Adolescent Transitions Program for high-risk teens and their parents: Toward a school-based intervention. *Education and Treatment of Children, 18*(4), 478–499.

Andrews, G., Issakidis, C., Sanderson, K., Corry, J., & Lapsley, H. (2004). Utilising survey data to inform public policy: Comparison of the cost-effectiveness of treatment of ten mental disorders. *British Journal of Psychiatry, 184*, 526–533.

Andrews, G., & Wilkinson, D. D. (2002). The prevention of mental disorders in young people. *Medical Journal of Australia, 177*(Suppl.), s97–s100.

Aos, S., Lieb, R., Mayfield, J., Miller, M., & Pennucci, A. (2004). *Benefits and costs of prevention and early intervention programs for youth, technical appendix.* Olympia WA: Washington State Institute for Public Policy. Retrieved from http://wsipp. wa.gov/rptfiles/04-07-3901a.pdf

Aronen, E. T., & Arajärvi, T. (2000). Effects of early intervention on psychiatric symptoms of young adults in low-risk and high-risk families. *American Journal of Orthopsychiatry, 70*(2), 223–232.

Aronen, E. T., & Kurkela, S. A. (1996). Long-term effects of an early home-based intervention. *Journal of the American Academy of Child and Adolescent Psychiatry, 35*(12), 1665–1672.

Asparouhov, T., & Muthén, B. O. (2008). Multilevel mixture models. In G. R. Hancock & K. M. Samuelson (Eds.), *Advances in latent variable mixture models* (pp. 27–51). Charlotte, NC: Information Age.

Bair-Merritt, M. H., Jennings, J. M., Chen, R., Burrell, L., McFarlane, E., Fuddy, L., & Duggan, A. K. (2010). Reducing maternal intimate partner violence after the birth of a child: A randomized controlled trial of the Hawaii Healthy

Start Home Visitation Program. *Archives of Pediatric and Adolescent Medicine, 164*(1), 16–23.

Ball, K., Berch, D. B., Helmers, K. F., Jobe, J. B., Leveck, M. D., Marsiske, M.,...Willis, S. L. (2002). Effects of cognitive training interventions with older adults: A randomized controlled trial. *Journal of the American Medical Association, 288*(18), 2271–2281.

Barlow, J., & Coren, E. (2004). Parent-training programmes for improving maternal psychosocial health. *Cochrane Database of Systematic Reviews,* (1), CD002020.

Barlow, J., & Stewart-Brown, S. (2000). Behavior problems and group-based parent education programs. *Journal of Developmental and Behavioral Pediatrics, 21*(5), 356–370.

Barnet, B., Liu, J., DeVoe, M., Alperovitz-Bichell, K., & Duggan, A. K. (2007). Home visiting for adolescent mothers: Effects on parenting, maternal life course, and primary care linkage. *Annals of Family Medicine, 5*(3), 224–232.

Barrera, A. Z., Torres, L. D., & Muñoz, R. F. (2007). Prevention of depression: The state of the science at the beginning of the 21st century. *International Review of Psychiatry, 19*(6), 655–670.

Barrett, S., Bradshaw, C. P., & Lewis-Palmer, T. (2008). Maryland state-wide PBIS initiative: Systems, evaluation and next steps. *Journal of Positive Behavior Interventions, 10,* 105–114.

Barrish, H. H., Saunders, M., & Wolf, M. M. (1969). Good Behavior Game: Effects of individual contingencies for group consequences on disruptive behavior in a classroom. *Journal of Applied Behavior Analysis, 2*(2), 119–124.

Beardslee, W. R., Chien, P. L., & Bell, C. C. (2011). Prevention of mental disorders, substance abuse, and problem behaviors: A developmental perspective. *Psychiatric Services, 62*(3), 247–254.

Bembry, J. X., & Norris, D. F. (2005). An exploratory study of neighborhood choices among Moving to Opportunity participants in Baltimore, Maryland: The influence of housing search assistance. *Journal of Sociology and Social Welfare, 32,* 93–107.

Bennett, J. B., Lehman, W. E., & Reynolds, G. (2000). Team awareness for workplace substance abuse prevention: The empirical and conceptual development of a training program. *Prevention Science, 1*(3), 157–172.

Bennett, J. B., Patterson, C. R., Reynolds, G. S., Wiitala, W. L., & Lehman, W. E. (2004). Team awareness, problem drinking, and drinking climate: Workplace social health promotion in a policy context. *American Journal of Health Promotion, 19*(2), 103–113.

Bharucha, A. J., Pandav, R., Shen, C. Y., Dodge, H. H., & Ganguli, M. (2004). Predictors of nursing facility admission: A 12-year epidemiological study in the United States. *Journal of the American Geriatrics Society, 52*(3), 434–439.

Billings, D. W., Cook, R. F., Hendrickson, A., & Dove, D. C. (2008). A web-based approach to managing stress and mood disorders in the workforce. *Journal of Occupational and Environmental Medicine, 50*(8), 960–968.

Blazer, D. G., Hays, J. C., Fillenbaum, G. G., & Gold, D. T. (1997). Memory complaint as a predictor of cognitive decline—a comparison of African American and White elders. *Journal of Aging and Health, 9*(2), 171–184.

Blitz, C. C., Arthur, M. W., & Hawkins, J. D. (2002). Preventing alcohol, tobacco, and other substance abuse. In L. A. Jason & D. S. Glenwick (Eds.), *Innovative strategies for promoting health and mental health across the life span* (pp. 176–201). New York, NY: Springer.

Botvin, G. J., Griffin, K. W., & Nichols, T. R. (2006). Preventing youth violence and delinquency through a universal school-based prevention approach. *Prevention Science, 7*(4), 403–408.

Botvin, G. J., Mihalic, S. F., & Grotpeter, J. K. (1998). *Life skills training: Blueprints for Violence Prevention, Book 5.* Blueprints for Violence Prevention Series (D.S. Elliott, Series Editor). Boulder, CO: Center for the Study and Prevention of Violence, Institute of Behavioral Science, University of Colorado.

Bowlby, J. (1982). Attachment and loss: Retrospect and prospect. *American Journal of Orthopsychiatry, 52*(4), 664–678.

Bradshaw, C. P., Buckley, J., & Ialongo, N. (2008). School-based service utilization among urban children with early-onset educational and mental health problems: The squeaky wheel phenomenon. *School Psychology Quarterly, 23*(2), 169–186.

Bradshaw, C. P., Koth, C. W., Bevans, K. B., Ialongo, N., & Leaf, P. J. (2008). The impact of school-wide positive behavioral interventions and supports (PBIS) on the organizational health of elementary schools. *School Psychology Quarterly, 23*(4), 462–473.

Bradshaw, C. P., Koth, C. W., Thornton, L. A., & Leaf, P. J. (2009). Altering school climate through school-wide positive behavioral interventions and supports: Findings from a group-randomized effectiveness trial. *Prevention Science, 10*(2), 100–115.

Bradshaw, C. P., Mitchell, M. M., & Leaf, P. J. (2010). Examining the effects of school-wide positive behavioral interventions and supports on student outcomes: Results from a randomized controlled effectiveness trial in elementary schools. *Journal of Positive Behavior Interventions, 12,* 133–148.

Bradshaw, C. P., O'Brennan, L. M., & McNeely, C. A. (2008). Core competencies and the prevention of school failure and early school leaving. *New Directions for Child and Adolescent Development, 122,* 19–32.

Bradshaw, C. P., Zmuda, J. H., Kellam, S. G., & Ialongo, N. S. (2009). Longitudinal impact of two universal preventive interventions in first grade on educational outcomes in high school. *Journal of Educational Psychology, 101*(4), 926–937.

Braga, A. A., Kennedy, D. M., Waring, D. J., & Piehl, A. M. (2001). Problem-oriented policing, deterrence, and youth violence: An evaluation of Boston's Operation Ceasefire. *Journal of Research in Crime and Delinquency, 38,* 195–225.

Breslin, F. C., Sobell, M. B, Sobell, L. C., Cunningham, J. A., Sdao-Jarvie, K., & Borsoi, D. (1999). Problem drinkers: Evaluation of a stepped-care approach. *Journal of Substance Abuse, 10*(3), 217–232.

Bronfenbrenner, U. (1977). Towards an experimental ecology of human development. *American Psychologist, 32,* 513–531.

Bronfenbrenner, U. (1979). *The ecology of human development: Experiments by nature and design.* Cambridge, MA: Harvard University Press.

Bronfenbrenner, U., & Morris, P. A. (1998). The ecology of developmental processes. In W. Damon & R. M. Lerner (Eds.), *Handbook of child psychology: Theoretical models of human development* (5th ed., pp. 993–1028). New York, NY: Wiley.

Brown, C. H., Wang, W., Kellam, S. G., Muthén, B. O., Petras, H., Toyinbo, P.,...Windham, A. (2008). Methods for testing theory and evaluating impact in randomized field trials: Intent-to-treat analyses for integrating perspectives of person, place, and time. *Drug Alcohol Dependence, 95*(Suppl. 1), s74–s104.

Brunwasser, S. M., Gillham, J. E., & Kim, E. S. (2009). A meta-analytic review of the Penn Resiliency Program's effect on depressive symptoms. *Journal of Consulting and Clinical Psychology, 77,* 1042–1054,

Butz, A. M., Lears, M. K., O'Neil, S., & Lukk, P. (1998). Home intervention for in utero drug-exposed infants. *Public Health Nursing, 15*(5), 307–318.

Butz, A. M., Pulsifer, M., Marano, N., Belcher, H., Lears, M. K., & Royall, R. (2001). Effectiveness of a home intervention for perceived child behavioral problems and parenting stress in children with in utero drug exposure. *Archives of Pediatrics and Adolescent Medicine, 155*(9), 1029–1037.

Calear, A. L., & Christensen, H. (2010). Systematic review of school-based prevention and early intervention programs for depression. *Journal of Adolescence, 33,* 429–438.

Campbell, C. A., Hahn, R. A., Elder, R., Brewer, R., Chattopadhyay, S., Fielding, J.,...Middleton, J. C. (2009). The effectiveness of limiting alcohol outlet density as a means of reducing excessive alcohol consumption and alcohol-related harms. *American Journal of Preventive Medicine, 37*(6), 556–569.

Campbell, J. C., Webster, D., Koziol-McLain, J., Block, C., Campbell, D., Curry, M. A.,...Laughon, K. (2003). Risk factors for femicide in abusive relationships: Results from a multisite case control study. *American Journal of Public Health, 93*(7), 1089–1097.

Caplan, G. (1964). *Principles of preventive psychiatry.* New York, NY: Basic Books.

Caplan, R. D., Vinokur, A. D., Price, R. H., & van Ryn, M. (1989). Job seeking, reemployment, and mental health: A randomized field experiment in coping with job loss. *Journal of Applied Psychology, 74*(5), 759–769.

Carlson, M. C., Erickson, K. I., Kramer, A. F., Voss, M. W., Bolea, N., Mielke, M.,...Fried, L. P. (2009). Evidence for neurocognitive plasticity in at-risk older adults: The Experience Corps program. *Journal of Gerontology: Medical Sciences, 64*(12), 1275–1282.

Carlson, M. C., Saczynski, J. S., Rebok, G. W., Seeman, T., Glass, T. A., McGill, S.,...Fried, L. P. (2008). Exploring the effects of an "everyday" activity program on executive function and memory in older adults: Experience Corps. *Gerontologist, 48,* 793–801.

Carpenter, K. J. (1988). *The history of scurvy and vitamin C.* Cambridge, UK: Cambridge University Press.

Caspi, A., Sugden, K., Moffitt, T. E., Taylor, A., Craig, I. W., Harrington, H.,...Poulton, R. (2003). Influence of life stress on depression: Moderation by a polymorphism in the *5-HTT* gene. *Science, 301*(5631), 386–389.

Catalano, R. F., Berglund, M. L., Ryan, J. A. M., Lonczak, H. S., & Hawkins, J. D. (2002). Positive youth development in the United States: Research findings on evaluations of positive youth development programs. *Prevention & Treatment, 5,* Article 15. Retrieved from http://journals.apa.org/prevention/volume5/pre0050015a.html

Caughy, M. O., Nettles, S. M., & O'Campo, P. J. (2008). The effect of residential neighborhood on child behavior problems in first grade. *American Journal of Community Psychology, 42*(1–2), 39–50.

Centers for Disease Control and *Prevention. (2003). Promising practices in chronic disease prevention and control. A public health framework for action.* Atlanta, GA: Department of Health and Human Services.

Centers for Disease Control and Prevention. (2002). *Adolescent and school health: Injury.* Atlanta, GA: Centers for Disease Control and Prevention, US Department of Health and Human Services. Retrieved from http://www.cdc.gov/nccdphp/dash/injury.htm

Centers for Disease Control and Prevention. (2010). State cigarette excise taxes: United States, 2009. *Morbidity and Mortality Weekly Report, 59*(13), 385–388.

Chinman, M., Imm, P., & Wandersman, A. (2004). *Getting to Outcomes 2004: Promoting accountability through methods and tools for planning, implementation, and evaluation* (TR-101-CDC). Santa Monica, CA: RAND Corp.

Cichetti, D., & Blender, J. A. (2006). A multiple-levels-of-analysis perspective on resilience: Implications for the developing brain, neural plasticity and preventive interventions. *Annals of the New York Academy of Sciences, 1094,* 248–258.

Cohen-Katz, J., Wiley, S. D., Capuano, T., Baker, D. M., Kimmel, S., & Shapiro, S. (2005). The effects of mindfulness-based stress reduction on nurse stress and burnout, part II: A quantitative and qualitative study. *Holistic Nursing Practice, 19*(1), 26–35.

Cohen-Katz, J., Wiley, S.D., Capuano, T., Baker, D.M., & Shapiro, S. (2004). The effects of mindfulness-based stress reduction on nurse stress and burnout: A quantitative and qualitative study. *Holistic Nursing Practice, 18*(6), 302–308.

Collins, L. M., Murphy, S. A., & Bierman, K. L. (2004). A conceptual framework for adaptive preventive interventions. *Prevention Science, 5*(3), 185–196.

Collins, L. M., Murphy, S. A., Nair, V., & Strecher, V. (2005). A strategy for optimizing and evaluating behavioral interventions. *Annals of Behavioral Medicine, 30*(1), 65–73.

Collins, W. A., Maccoby, E. E., Steinberg, L., Hetherington, E. M., & Bornstein, M. H. (2000). Contemporary research on parenting: The case for nature and nurture. *American Psychologist, 55*(2), 218–232.

Conduct Problems Prevention Research Group. (2002a). Evaluation of the first 3 years of the Fast Track prevention trial with children at high risk for adolescent conduct problems. *Journal of Abnormal Child Psychology, 30*(1), 19–36.

Conduct Problems Prevention Research Group. (2002b). Using the Fast Track randomized prevention trial to test the early-starter model of the development of serious conduct problems. *Development and Psychopathology, 14*(4), 925–943.

Conduct Problems Prevention Research Group. (2004). The effects of the Fast Track program on serious problem outcomes at the end of elementary school. *Journal of Clinical Child and Adolescent Psychology, 33*(4), 650–661.

Conduct Problems Prevention Research Group. (2007). Fast Track randomized controlled trial to prevent externalizing psychiatric disorders: Findings from grades three to nine. *Journal of the American Academy of Child and Adolescent Psychiatry, 46*(10), 1250–1262.

Conduct Problems Prevention Research Group. (2010). The effects of a multi-year universal social-emotional learning program: The role of student and school characteristics. *Journal of Consulting and Clinical Psychology, 78*(2),156–168.

Connell, A. M., Dishion, T. J., Yasui, M., & Kavanagh, K. (2007). An adaptive approach to family intervention: Linking engagement in family-centered intervention to reductions in adolescent problem behavior. *Journal of Consulting and Clinical Psychology, 75*(4), 568–579.

Cook, R., & Schlenger, W. (2002). Prevention of substance abuse in the workplace: Review of research on the delivery of services. *Journal of Primary Prevention, 23,* 115–142.

Cooper, B., & Morgan, H. G. (1973). *Epidemiological psychiatry.* Springfield, MA: Charles C. Thomas.

Cowen, E. L. (1977). Baby-steps toward primary prevention. *American Journal of Community Psychology, 5*(1), 1–22.

Cowen, E. L. (1980). The wooing of primary prevention. *American Journal of Community Psychology, 8*(3), 258–284.

Craik, F. I. M., Winocur, G., Palmer, H., Binns, M. A., Edwards, M., Bridges, K., … Stuss, D. T. (2007). Cognitive rehabilitation in the elderly: Effects on memory. *Journal of the International Neuropsychological Society, 13*(1), 132–142.

Crockett, K., Zlotnick, C., Davis, M., Payne, N., & Washington, R. (2008). A depression preventive intervention for rural low-income African-American pregnant women at risk for postpartum depression. *Archives of Women's Mental Health, 11*(5–6), 319–325.

Cuijpers, P. (2009). Prevention: An achievable goal in personalized medicine. *Dialogues in Clinical Neuroscience, 11*(4), 447–454.

Cuijpers, P., Muñoz, R. F., Clarke, G. N., & Lewinsohn, P. M. (2009). Psychoeducational treatment and prevention of depression: The Coping with Depression course 30 years later. *Clinical Psychology Review, 29*(5), 449–458.

Cuijpers, P., & Smit, F. (2008). Has time come for broad-scale dissemination for prevention of depressive disorders? *Acta Psychiatrica Scandinavica, 118*(6), 419–420.

Cuijpers, P., van Straten, A., & Smit, F. (2006). Psychological treatment of late-life depression: A meta-analysis of randomized controlled trials. *International Journal of Geriatric Psychiatry, 21*(12), 1139–1149.

Cuijpers, P., van Straten, A., Smit, F., Mihalopoulos, C., & Beekman, A. (2008). Preventing the onset of depressive disorders: A meta-analytic review of psychological interventions. *American Journal of Psychiatry, 165*(10), 1272–1280.

Cunningham, J. A., Humphreys, K., & Koski-Jännes, A. (2000). Providing personalized assessment feedback for problem drinking on the Internet: A pilot project. *Journal of Studies on Alcohol, 61*(6), 794–798.

DeBellis, R., Smith, B. S., Choi, S., & Malloy, M. (2005). Management of delirium tremens. *Journal of Intensive Care Medicine, 20*(3), 164–173.

Dempster, A. P., Laird, N. M., & Rubin, D. B. (1977). Maximum likelihood from incomplete data via the *EM* algorithm. *Journal of the Royal Statistical Society, 39*, 1–38.

Depression Guideline Panel. (1993a). *Depression in primary care: Detection, diagnosis and treatment. Quick reference guide for clinicians.* Rockville, MD: Agency for Health Care Policy and Research, US Department of Health and Human Services.

Depression Guideline Panel. (1993b). *Depression in primary care: Vol. 2. Treatment of major depression.* Rockville, MD: Agency for Health Care Policy and Research, US Department of Health and Human Services.

Devaney, E., O'Brien, M. U., Resnik, H., Keister, S., & Weissberg, R. P. (2006). *Sustainable school-wide social and emotional learning: Implementation guide and toolkit.* Chicago, IL: Collaborative for Academic, Social, and Emotional Learning (CASEL).

Developmental Research and Programs (1997). *Communities That Care: A comprehensive prevention program.* Seattle, WA: Author.

Dishion, T. (1990). The peer context of troublesome child and adolescent behavior. In P. E. Leone (Ed.), *Understanding troubled and troubling youth: Multidisciplinary perspectives.* Newbury Park, CA: Sage.

Dishion, T. J., & Kavanagh, K. (2003). *Intervening in adolescent problem behavior: A family-centered approach.* New York, NY: Guilford.

Dishion, T. J., Kavanagh, K., Schneiger, A., Nelson, S., & Kaufman, N. (2002). Preventing early adolescent substance use: A family-centered strategy for public middle school. *Prevention Science, 3*(3), 191–201.

Dishion, T. J., Kavanagh, K., Veltman, M., McCartney, T., Soberman, L., & Stormshak, E. (2003). *Family management curriculum V. 2. 0: Leader's guide.* Eugene, OR: Child and Family Center.

Dishion, T. J., & Stormshak, E. (2007). *Intervening in children's lives: An ecological, family-centered approach to mental health care.* Washington, DC: APA Books.

Dolan, L. J., Kellam, S. G., Brown, C. H., Werthamer-Larsson, L., Rebok, G. W., Mayer, L. S.,... Wheeler, L. (1993). The short-term impact of two classroom-based preventive interventions on aggressive and shy behaviors and poor achievement. *Journal of Applied Developmental Psychology, 14*, 317–345.

Domitrovich, C. E., Bradshaw, C. P., Greenberg, M. T., Embry, D., Poduska, J., & Ialongo, N. S. (2009). Integrated preventive interventions: The theory and logic. *Psychology in the Schools, 47*, 71–88.

Domitrovich, C. E., Bradshaw, C. P., Poduska, J., Hoagwood, K., Buckley, J., Olin, S.,... Ialongo, N. S. (2008). Maximizing the implementation quality of evidence-based preventive interventions in schools: A conceptual framework. *Advances in School Mental Health Promotion: Training and Practice, Research and Policy, 1,* 6–28.

Donker, T., van Straten, A., Riper, H., Marks, I., Andersson, G., & Cuijpers, P. (2009). Implementation of Internet-based preventive interventions for depression and anxiety: Role of support? The design of a randomized controlled trial. *Trials, 10,* 59.

Doumas, D. M., & Hannah, E. (2008). Preventing high-risk drinking in youth in the workplace: A web-based normative feedback program. *Journal of Substance Abuse Treatment, 34*(3), 263–271.

Dubois, D. L., Holloway, B. E., Valentine, J. C., & Cooper, H. (2002). Effectiveness of mentoring programs for youth: A meta-analytic review.

American Journal of Community Psychology, 30(2), 157–197.

Duggan, A. K., McFarlane, E. C., Windham, A. M., Rohde, C. A., Salkever, D. S., Fuddy, L.,...Sia, C. C. J. (1999). Evaluation of Hawaii's Healthy Start program. *Future Child, 9*, 66–90.

Dupere, V., & Perkins, D. D. (2007). Community types and mental health: A multilevel study of local environmental stress and coping. *American Journal of Community Psychology, 39*(1–2), 107–119.

Durlak, J. A., Weissberg, R. P., Dymnicki, A. B., Taylor, R. D., & Schellinger, K. B. (2011). The impact of enhancing students' social and emotional learning: A meta-analysis of school-based universal interventions. *Child Development, 82*(1), 405–432.

Eaton, W. W., Shao, H., Nestadt, G., Lee, B. H., Bienvenu, O. J., & Zandi, P. (2008). Population-based study of first onset and chronicity in major depressive disorder. *Archives of General Psychiatry, 65*(5), 513–520.

Eckenrode, J., Campa, M., Luckey, D. W., Henderson, C. R., Cole, R., Kitzman, H.,...Olds, D. (2010). Long-term effects of prenatal and infancy nurse home visitation on the life course of youths: 19-year follow-up of a randomized trial. *Archives of Pediatric and Adolescent Medicine, 164*(1), 9–15.

Education Sciences Reform Act, Pub. L. No. 107–279, (2002).

Elder, R. W., Lawrence, B., Ferguson, A., Naimi, T. S., Brewer, R. D., Chattopadhyay, S. K.,...Fielding, J. E. (2010). The effectiveness of tax policy interventions for reducing excessive alcohol consumption and related harms. *American Journal of Preventive Medicine, 38*(2), 217–229.

Elementary and Secondary Education Act, Pub. L. No. 89–10, 79 Stat. 27, 20 U.S.C. 70 (1965).

Erwin, W. E., Williams, D. B., & Speir, W. A. (1998). Delirium tremens. *Southern Medical Journal, 91*(5), 425–432.

Fagan, A. A., Hanson, K., Hawkins, J. D., & Arthur, M. W. (2008). Bridging science to practice: Achieving prevention program implementation fidelity in the Community Youth Development Study. *Journal of Community Psychology, 41*(3–4), 235–249.

Fairchild, A. J., & MacKinnon, D. P. (2009). A general model for testing mediation and moderation effects. *Prevention Science, 10*(2), 87–99.

Farrington, D., & Tofi, M. (2009). School-based programs to reduce bullying and victimization. *Campbell Systematic Reviews*, (6). Retrieved from http://campbellcollaboration.org/reviews_crime_justice/index.php

Feinberg, M. E., Greenberg, M. T., & Osgood, D. W. (2004). Readiness, functioning and perceived effectiveness in community prevention coalitions: A study of Communities That Care. *Journal of Community Psychology, 33*(3–4), 163–176.

Fell, J. C., & Voas, R. B. (2006). The effectiveness of reducing illegal blood alcohol concentration (BAC) limits for driving: Evidence for lowering the limit to .05 BAC. *Journal of Safety Research, 37*(3), 233–243.

Fisher, P. (2005). Gautreaux Assisted Housing Program. In *Electronic encyclopedia of Chicago*. Chicago, IL: Chicago Historical Society. Retrieved from http://www.encyclopedia.chicagohistory.org/pages/507.html

Fixsen, D., Blase, K., Horner, R., & Sugai, G. (2009, March). *Taking evidence-based practices to scale: Building capacity*. Paper presented at the annual meeting of the Association for Positive Behavior Support, Jacksonville, FL.

Fixsen, D. L., Naoom, S. F., Blase, K. A., Friedman, R. M., & Wallace, F. (2005). *Implementation research: A synthesis of the literature*. Tampa, FL: University of South Florida, Louis de la Parte Florida Mental Health Institute, The National Implementation Research Network.

Flay, B. R., Biglan, A., Boruch, R. F., Castro, F. G., Gottfredson, D., Kellam, S.,...Ji, P. (2005). Standards of evidence: Criteria for efficacy, effectiveness and dissemination. *Prevention Science, 6*(3), 151–175.

Flicker, L., Ambrose, T. L., & Kramer, A. F. (2011). Why so negative about preventing cognitive decline and dementia? The jury has already come to the verdict for physical activity and smoking cessation. *British Journal of Sports Medicine, 45*, 465–467.

Florin, P., Celebucki, C., Stevenson, J., Mena, J., Salago, D., White, A.,...Dougal, M. (2006). Cultivating systemic capacity: The Rhode Island Tobacco Control Enhancement Project. *Journal of Community Psychology, 38*(3–4), 213–220.

Forgatch, M. S. (1994). *Parenting Through Change: A training manual*. Eugene, OR: Oregon Social Learning Center.

Forgatch, M. S., and DeGarmo, D. S. (1999). Parenting Through Change: An effective prevention program for single mothers. *Journal of Consulting and Clinical Psychology, 67*(5), 711–724.

Fried, L. P., Carlson, M., Freedman, M., Frick, K. D., Glass, T. A., Hill, J.,...Zeger, S. (2004). A social model for health promotion for an aging population: Initial evidence on the Experience Corps model. *Journal of Urban Health, 81*(1), 64–78.

Fudge, E. A., & Robinson, P. (2009). A public health approach to promoting better mental health outcomes for children of parents with a psychiatric disability. *Psychiatric Rehabilitation Journal, 33*, 83–90.

Gardner, F., Burton, J., & Klimes, I. (2006). Randomized controlled trial of a parenting intervention in the voluntary sector for reducing child conduct problems: Outcomes and mechanisms of change. *Journal of Child Psychology and Psychiatry, 47*(11), 1123–1132.

Giesbrecht, N. (2000). Roles of commercial interests in alcohol policies: Recent developments in North America. *Addiction, 95*(Suppl. 4), 581–595.

Gillham, J. E., Reivich, K. J., & Jaycox, L. H. (2008). *The Penn Resiliency Program.* Unpublished manuscript, University of Pennsylvania.

Goldberger, J. (1914). The etiology of pellagra. *Public Health Reports, 29*(26), 1683–1686.

Gordon, R. S. (1983). An operational classification of disease prevention. *Public Health Reports, 98*(2), 107–109.

Gottfredson, D. C., & Wilson, D. B. (2003). Characteristics of effective school-based substance abuse prevention. *Prevention Science, 4*(1), 27–38.

Gottfredson, G. D., & Gottfredson, D. C. (2001). What schools do to prevent problem behavior and promote safe environments. *Journal of Educational and Psychological Consultation, 12*, 313–344.

Greenberg, M. T. (2004). Current and future challenges in school-based prevention: The researcher perspective. *Prevention Science, 5*(1), 5–13.

Greenberg, M. T., Domitrovich, C., & Bumbarger, B. (2001). The prevention of mental disorders in school-aged children: Current state of the field. *Prevention & Treatment, 4*, 1–62.

Greenberg, M. T., Kusche, C., & Mihalic, S. F. (1998). *Promoting Alternative Thinking Strategies (PATHS): Blueprints for Violence Prevention, Book Ten.* Blueprints for Violence Prevention Series (D.S. Elliott, Series Editor). Boulder, CO: Center for the Study and Prevention of Violence, Institute of Behavioral Science, University of Colorado.

Griffin, K. W., Botvin, G. J., Nichols, T. R., & Doyle, M. M. (2003). Effectiveness of a universal drug abuse prevention approach for youth at high risk for substance use initiation. *Preventive Medicine, 36*(1), 1–7.

Grossman, J. B., & Rhodes, J. E. (2002). The test of time: Predictors and effects of duration in youth mentoring relationships. *Journal of Community Psychology, 30*(2), 199–219.

Hahn, R., Fuqua-Whitley, D., Wethington, H., Lowy, J., Crosby, A., Fullilove, M.,…Dahlberg, L. (2007). Effectiveness of universal school-based programs to prevent violent and aggressive behavior: A systematic review. *American Journal of Preventive Medicine, 33*(Suppl. 2), s114–s129.

Hallfors, D., Cho, H., Livert, D., & Kadushin, C. (2002). Fighting back against substance abuse: Are community coalitions winning? *American Journal of Preventive Medicine, 23*(4), 237–245.

Hallfors, D., & Godette, D. (2002). Will the "Principles of Effectiveness" improve prevention practice? Early findings from a diffusion study. *Health Education Research, 17*(4), 461–470.

Hallfors, D. D., Pankratz, M., & Hartman, S. (2007). Does federal policy support the use of scientific evidence in school-based prevention programs? *Prevention Science, 8*(1), 75–81.

Harlow, C. W. (November 2001, NCJ 189369). *Firearm use by offenders: Survey of inmates in state and federal correctional facilities* (Special Report). The US Department of Justice, Office of Justice Programs, Bureau of Justice Statistics. Retrieved from http://bjs.ojp.usdoj.gov/content/pub/pdf/fuo.pdf

Hawkins, J. D., & Catalano, R. F. (2004). *Communities That Care: Prevention strategies guide.* South Deerfield, MA: Channing Bete.

Hawkins, J. D., Catalano, R. F., & Arthur, M. W. (2002). Promoting science-based prevention in communities. *Addictive Behaviors, 27*(6), 951–976.

Healthier Scotland. (2009). *Towards a mentally flourishing Scotland: Policy and action plan 2009–2011.* Edinburgh, UK: St. Andrew's House.

Heaney, C. A. (1991). Enhancing social support at the workplace: Assessing the effects of the Caregiver Support Program. *Health Education Quarterly, 18*, 477–494.

Heaney, C. A., Price, R. H., & Rafferty, J. (1995). Increasing coping resources at work: A field experiment to increase social support, improve work team functioning, and enhance employee mental health. *Journal of Organizational Behavior, 16*, 335–352.

Hegyi, J., Schwartz, R. A., & Hegyi, V. (2004). Pellagra: Dermatitis, dementia and diarrhea. *International Journal of Epidemiology, 43*(1), 1–5.

Heirich, M., & Sieck, C. J. (2000). Worksite cardiovascular wellness programs as a route to substance abuse prevention. *Journal of Occupational and Environmental Medicine, 42*(1), 47–56.

Hepburn, L., Azrael, D., Miller, M., & Hemenway, D. (2006). The effect of child access prevention laws on unintentional child firearm fatalities, 1979–2000. *Journal of Trauma, 61*(2), 423–428.

Herrman, H., Saxena, S., & Moodie, R. (2004). *Promoting mental health: Concepts, emerging evidence, practice.* Geneva, Switzerland: World Health Organization.

Hertzog, C., Kramer, A. F., Wilson, R. S., & Lindenberger, U. (2009). Enrichment effects on adult cognitive development: Can the functional capacity of older adults be preserved and enhanced? *Psychological Science in the Public Interest, 9,* 1–65.

Hetheringon, E. M., & Stanley-Hagan, M. (1999). The adjustment of children with divorced parents: A risk and resiliency perspective. *Journal of Child Psychology and Psychiatry, 40*(1), 129–140.

Hoagwood, K. E., Olin, S. S., Kerker, B. D., Kratochwill, T. R., Crowe, M., & Saka, N. (2007). Empirically based school interventions targeted at academic and mental health functioning. *Journal of Emotional and Behavioral Disorders, 15,* 66–92.

Holder, H. D., Gruenewald, P. J., Ponicki, W. R., Treno, A. J., Grube, J. W., Saltz, R. F., ... Roeper, P. (2000). Effect of community-based interventions on high-risk drinking and alcohol-related injuries. *Journal of the American Medical Association, 284*(18), 2341–2347.

Horner, R. H., Sugai, G., Smolkowski, K., Eber, L., Nakasato, J., Todd, A. W., & Esperanza, J. (2009). A randomized, wait-list controlled effectiveness trial assessing school-wide positive behavior support in elementary schools. *Journal of Positive Behavior Interventions, 11,* 133–144.

Horowitz, J. L., & Garber, J. (2006). The prevention of depressive symptoms in childhood: A meta-analytic review. *Journal of Clinical and Community Psychology, 74*(3), 401–415.

Hosman, C., Jané-Llopis, E., & Saxena, S. (Eds.). (2005). *Prevention of mental disorders: Effective interventions and policy options.* Oxford, UK: Oxford University Press.

Hughes, T. F., & Ganguli, M. (2009). Modifiable risk factors for late-life cognitive impairment and dementia. *Current Psychiatry Review, 5*(2), 73–92.

Ialongo, N. S., Kellam, S. G., & Poduska, J. (2000). A developmental framework for clinical child and pediatric psychology research. In D. Drotar (Ed.), *Handbook of research in pediatric and clinical child psychiatry: Practical strategies and methods* (pp. 3–19). New York, NY: Kluwer Academic/Plenum.

Ialongo, N., Poduska, J., Werthamer, L., & Kellam, S. (2001). The distal impact of two first grade preventive interventions on conduct problems and disorder and mental health service need

and utilization in early adolescence. *Journal of Emotional and Behavioral Disorders, 9,* 146–160.

Ialongo, N. S., Werthamer, L., Kellam, S. G., Brown, C. H., Wang, S., & Lin, Y. (1999). Proximal impact of two first-grade preventive interventions on the early risk behaviors for later substance abuse, depression, and antisocial behavior. *American Journal of Community Psychology, 27,* 599–641.

Individuals with Disabilities Education Act, Pub. L. No. 101–476 (1990).

Individuals with Disabilities Education Improvement Act of 2004, Pub. L. No. 108–446 (2004).

Institute of Medicine. (2009). *Preventing mental, emotional, and behavioral disorders among young people: Progress and possibilities.* Washington, DC: National Academies Press.

Ireland, J. L., Sanders, M. R., & Markie-Dadds, C. (2003). The impact of parent training on marital functioning: A comparison of two group versions of the Triple P–Positive Parenting Program for parents of children with early-onset conduct problems. *Behavioural and Cognitive Psychotherapy, 31,* 127–142.

Irvine, A. B., Biglan, A., Smolkowski, K., Metzler, C. W., and Ary, D. V. (1999). The effectiveness of a parenting skills program for parents of middle school students in small communities. *Journal of Consulting and Clinical Psychology, 67*(6), 811–825.

Jané-Llopis, E., & Anderson, P. (Eds). (2006). *Mental health promotion and mental disorder prevention across European member states: A collection of country stories.* Luxembourg: European Communities.

Jané-Llopis, E., Hosman, C., Jenkins, R., & Anderson, P. (2003). Predictors of efficacy in depression prevention programmes: Meta-analysis. *British Journal of Psychiatry, 183,* 384–397.

Jones, D. E., Godwin, J., Dodge, K. A., Bierman, K. L., Coie, J. D., Greenberg, M. T., ... Pinderhughes, E. E. (2010). Impact of the Fast Track prevention program on health services use by conduct-problem youth. *Pediatrics, 125*(1), e130–e136.

Judd, L. L. (1997). The clinical course of unipolar major depressive disorders. *Archives of General Psychiatry, 54*(11), 989–991.

Jukes, T. H. (1989). The prevention and conquest of scurvy, beri-beri, and pellagra. *Preventive Medicine, 18*(6), 877–883.

Kam, C., Greenberg, M. T., & Kusche, C. A. (2004). Sustained effects of the PATHS curriculum on the social and psychological adjustment of children in special education. *Journal of Emotional and Behavioral Disorders, 12*, 66–78.

Kaplan, H. I., Sadock, B. J., & Grebb, J. A. (1994). *Kaplan and Sadock's synopsis of psychiatry.* Baltimore, MD: Williams & Wilkins.

Kaufman, J. E., & Rosenbaum, J. (1992). The education and employment of low-income black youth in white suburbs. *Educational Evaluation & Policy Analysis, 14*, 229–240.

Keels, M. (2008). Neighborhood effects examined through the lens of residential mobility programs. *American Journal of Community Psychology, 42*(3–4), 235–250.

Kellam, S. G., Branch, J. D., Agrawal, K. C., & Ensminger, M. E. (1975). *Mental health and going to school: The Woodlawn program of assessment, early intervention and evaluation.* Chicago, IL: University of Chicago Press.

Kellam, S. G., Brown, C. H., Poduska, J. M., Ialongo, N. S., Wang, W., Toyinbo, P.,...Wilcox, H. C. (2008). Effects of a universal classroom behavior management program in first and second grades on young adult behavioral, psychiatric, and social outcomes. *Drug and Alcohol Dependence, 95*(Suppl. 1), 1–28.

Kellam, S. G., Koretz, D., & Mościcki, E. K. (1999). Core elements of developmental epidemiologically based prevention research. *American Journal of Community Psychology, 27*(4), 463–482.

Kellam, S. G., Ling, X., Merisca, R., Brown, C. H., & Ialongo, N. (1998). The effect of the level of aggression in the first grade classroom on the course and malleability of aggressive behavior into middle school. *Development and Psychopathology, 10*(2), 165–185.

Kellam, S. G., & Rebok, G. W. (1992). Building etiological theory through developmental epidemiologically-based preventive intervention trials. In J. McCord & R. E. Tremblay (Eds.), *Preventing antisocial behavior: Interventions from birth through adolescence* (pp. 162–195). New York, NY: Guilford.

Kellam, S. G., Rebok, G. W., Ialongo, N., & Mayer, L. S. (1994). The course and malleability of aggressive behavior from early first grade into middle school: Results of a developmental epidemiologically-based preventive trial. *Journal of Child Psychology, Psychiatry and Allied Disciplines, 35*(2), 259–281.

Kelly, J. G., Ryan, A. M., Altman, B. E., & Stelzner, S. P. (2000). Understanding and changing social systems: An ecological view. In J. Rappaport & E. Seidman (Eds.), *Handbook of community psychology* (pp. 133–159). New York, NY: Kluwer Academic/Plenum.

Kessler, R. C., Anthony, J. C., Blazer, D. G., Bromet, E., Eaton, W. W., & Kendler, K. (1997). The U.S. National Comorbidity Survey: Overview and future directions. *Epidemiologia e Psichiatria Sociale, 6*(1), 4–16.

Kessler, R. C., Chiu, W. T., Demler, O., & Walters, E. E. (2005). Prevalence, severity and comorbidity of 12-month DSM-IV disorders in the National Comorbidity Survey replication. *Archives of General Psychiatry, 62*(6), 617–627.

Kessler, R. C., & Frank, R. G. (1997). The impact of psychiatric disorders on work loss days. *Psychological Medicine, 27*(4), 861–873.

Kitzman, H. J., Olds, D. L., Cole, R. E., Hanks, C. A., Anson, E. A., Arcoleo, K. J.,...Holmberg, J. R. (2010). Enduring effects of prenatal and infancy home visiting by nurses on children: Follow-up of a randomized trial among children at age 12 years. *Archives of Pediatrics and Adolescent Medicine, 164*(5), 412–418.

Kitzman, H., Olds, D. L., Sidora, K., Henderson, C. R., Hanks, C., Cole, R.,...Glazner, J. (2000). Enduring effects of nurse home visitation on maternal life course: A 3-year follow-up of a randomized trial. *Journal of the American Medical Association, 283*(15), 1983–1989.

Klosterkötter, J., Schultze-Lutter, F., & Ruhrmann, S. (2008). Kraepelin and psychotic prodromal conditions. *European Archives of Psychiatry and Clinical Neuroscience, 258*(Suppl. 2), 74–84.

Koniak-Griffin, D., Anderson, N. L., Brecht, M. L., Verzemnieks, I., Lesser, J., & Kim, S. (2002). Public health nursing care for adolescent mothers: Impact on infant health and selected maternal outcomes at 1 year post-birth. *Journal of Adolescent Health, 30*(1), 44–54.

Koniak-Griffin, D., Anderson, N. L., Verzemnieks, I., & Brecht, M. L. (2000). A public health nursing early intervention program for adolescent mothers: Outcomes from pregnancy through 6 weeks postpartum. *Nursing Research, 49*(3), 130–138.

Koniak-Griffin, D., Verzemnieks, I. L., Anderson, N. L., Brecht, M. L., Lesser, J., Kim, S., & Turner-Pluta, C. (2003). Nurse visitation for adolescent mothers: Two-year infant health and maternal outcomes. *Nursing Research, 52*(2), 127–136.

Koretz, D. S., & Mościcki, E. K. (1997). An ounce of prevention research: What is it worth? *American Journal of Community Psychology, 25*(2), 189–195.

Kuh, D., & Ben-Shlomo, Y. (1997). *A life course approach to chronic disease epidemiology.* New York, NY: Oxford University Press.

Last, J. M. (2001). *A dictionary of epidemiology.* New York, NY: Oxford University Press.

Launer, L. J. (2005). The epidemiologic study of dementia: A life-long quest? *Neurobiology of Aging, 26*(3), 335–340.

Lavery, L. L., Dodge, H. H., Snitz, B., & Ganguli, M. (2009). Cognitive decline and mortality in a community-based cohort: The Monongahela Valley Independent Elders Survey. *Journal of the American Geriatrics Society, 57*(1), 94–100.

Lee, P. R., Lee, D. R., Lee, P., & Arch, M. (2010). 2010: U.S. drug and alcohol policy, looking back and moving forward. *Journal of Psychoactive Drugs, 42*(2), 99–114.

Lesesne, C. A., Lewis, K. M., White, C. P., Green, D. C., Duffy, J. L., & Wandersman, A. (2008). Promoting science-based approaches to teen pregnancy prevention: Proactively engaging the three systems of the interactive systems framework. *American Journal of Community Psychology, 41*(3–4), 379–392.

Leventhal, T., & Brooks-Gunn, J. (2000). The neighborhoods they live in: The effects of neighborhood residence on child and adolescent outcomes. *Psychological Bulletin, 126*(2), 309–337.

Leventhal, T., & Brooks-Gunn, J. (2004). A randomized study of neighborhood effects on low-income children's educational outcomes. *Developmental Psychology, 40*(4), 488–507.

Leventhal, T., Fauth, R. C., & Brooks-Gunn, J. (2005). Neighborhood poverty and public policy: A 5-year follow-up of children's educational outcomes in the New York City Moving to Opportunity demonstration. *Developmental Psychology, 41*(6), 933–952.

Lewinsohn, P. M., Antonuccio, D. O., Steinmetz, J. L., & Teri, L. (1984). *The Coping with Depression course: A psychoeducational intervention for unipolar depression.* Eugene, OR: Castalia.

Lilienfeld, A. M., & Lilienfeld, D. E. (1980). *Foundations of epidemiology* (2nd ed.). New York, NY: Oxford University Press.

Lochman, J. E., Bierman, K. L., Coie, J. D., Dodge, K. A., Greenberg, M. T., McMahon, R. J., & Pinderhughes, E. E. (2010). The difficulty of maintaining positive intervention effects: A look at disruptive behavior, deviant peer relations, and social skills during the middle school years. *Journal of Early Adolescence, 30,* 593–624.

Lochman, J. E., & van den Steenhoven, A. (2002). Family-based approaches to substance abuse prevention. *Journal of Primary Prevention, 23,* 49–114.

Lochman, J. E., & Wells, K. C. (1996). A social-cognitive intervention with aggressive children: Prevention effects and contextual implementation issues. In R. D. Peters & R. J. McMahon (Eds.), *Prevention and early intervention: Childhood disorders, substance use, and delinquency* (pp. 111–143). Newbury Park, CA: Sage.

Lochman, J. E., & Wells, K. C. (2002). The Coping Power program at the middle school transition: Universal and indicated prevention effects. *Psychology of Addictive Behaviors, 16*(Suppl. 4), s40–s54.

Lochman, J. E., & Wells, K. C. (2004). The Coping Power program for preadolescent aggressive boys and their parents: Outcome effects at the one-year follow-up. *Journal of Consulting and Clinical Psychology, 72*(4), 571–578.

Mair, J. S., & Mair, M. (2003). Violence prevention and control through environmental measures. *Annual Review of Public Health, 24,* 209–225.

Manger, T. H., Hawkins, J. D., Haggerty, K. P., & Catalano, R. F. (1992). Mobilizing communities to reduce risks for drug abuse: Lessons on using research to guide prevention practice. *Journal of Primary Prevention, 13,* 3–22.

Marcenko, M. O., & Spence, M. (1994). Home visitation services for at-risk pregnant and postpartum women: A randomized trial. *American Journal of Orthopsychiatry, 64*(3), 468–478.

Marcenko, M. O., Spence, M., & Samost, L. (1996). Outcomes of a home visitation trial for pregnant and postpartum women at-risk for child placement. *Children and Youth Services Review, 18,* 243–259.

Martinez, C. R., Jr., & Forgatch, M. S. (2001). Preventing problems with boy's noncompliance: Effects of a parent training intervention for divorcing mothers. *Journal of Consulting and Clinical Psychology, 69*(3), 416–428.

Mayer, G. R. (1995). Preventing antisocial behavior in the schools. *Journal of Applied Behavior Analysis, 28*(4), 467–478.

McFarlane, W. R. (2007). *Prevention of schizophrenia.* Washington, DC: National Academies Press.

Merzel, C., Moon-Howard, J., Dickerson, D., Ramjohn, D., & VanDevanter, N. (2008). Making the connections: Community capacity for tobacco control in an urban African American community. *American Journal of Community Psychology, 41*(1–2), 74–88.

Mrazek, P. J., & Haggerty, R. J. (1994). *Reducing risks for mental disorders: Frontiers for preventive intervention research.* Washington, DC: National Academies Press.

Muñoz, R. F. (2001). On the road to a world without depression. *Journal of Primary Prevention, 21,* 325–338.

Muñoz, R. F., Le, H., Clarke, G., & Jaycox, L. (2002). Preventing the onset of major depression. In

I. H. Gotlib & C. L. Hammen (Eds.), *Handbook of depression* (pp. 343–359). New York, NY: Guilford.

Muñoz, R. F., Le, H., Ippen, C. G., Diaz, M. A., Urizar, G. G., Soto, J., . . . Lieberman, A. F. (2007). Prevention of postpartum depression in low-income women: Development of the *Mamás y Bebés*/Mothers and Babies course. *Cognitive and Behavioral Practice, 14,* 70–83.

Muñoz, R. F., Mrazek, P. J., & Haggerty, R. J. (1996). Institute of Medicine report on prevention of mental disorders: Summary and commentary. *American Psychologist, 51*(11), 1116–1122.

Murray, C. J., Lopez, A. D., Mathers, C. D., & Stein, C. (2001). *The Global Burden of Disease 2000 project: Aims, methods and data sources.* (Global Programme on Evidence for Health Policy Discussion paper No. 36—revised). World Health Organization, Geneva.

Muthén, B. (2004). Latent variable analysis: Growth mixture modeling and related techniques for longitudinal data. In D. Kaplan (Ed.), *The Sage handbook of quantitative methodology for the social sciences* (pp. 345–368). Thousand Oaks, CA: Sage.

Muthén, B., & Asparouhov, T. (2006). Growth mixture analysis: Models with non-Gaussian random effects. In G. Fitzmaurice, M. Davidian, G. Verbeke, & G. Molengerghs (Eds.), *Advances in longitudinal data analysis.* London, UK: Chapman and Hall/CRC.

Muthén, B., Brown, C. H., Masyn, K., Jo, B., Khoo, S. T., Yang, C. C., . . . Liao, J. (2002). General growth mixture modeling for randomized preventive interventions. *Biostatistics, 3*(4), 459–475.

Muthén, B. O., & Curran, P. J. (1997). General longitudinal modeling of individual differences in experimental designs: A latent variable framework for analysis and power estimation. *Psychological Methods, 2,* 371–402.

Nagin, D. S. (2005). *Group-based modeling of development over the life course.* Cambridge, MA: Harvard University Press.

National Institute of Mental Health Prevention Research Steering Committee. (1994). *The prevention of mental disorders: A national research agenda.* Bethesda, MD: National Institute of Mental Health.

National Institutes of Health (2010). *Preventing Alzheimer's disease and cognitive decline. NIH State-of-the-Science Consensus Conference. Final panel statement.* Bethesda, MD: Author. Retrieved from http://consensus.nih.gov/2010/alzstatement.htm

Newton, N. C., Teesson, M., Vogl, L. E., & Andrews, G. (2010). Internet-based prevention for alcohol and cannabis use: Final results of the Climate Schools course. *Addiction, 105*(4), 749–759.

No Child Left Behind Act of 2001, Pub. L. No. 107–110, 115 Stat. 1425 (2002).

Olds, D. L. (2006). The Nurse–Family Partnership: An evidence-based preventive intervention. *Infant Mental Health Journal, 27,* 5–25.

Olds, D., Henderson, C. R., Jr., Cole, R., Eckenrode, J., Kitzman, H., Luckey, D., . . . Powers, J. (1998). Long-term effects of nurse home visitation on children's criminal and antisocial behavior: 15-year follow-up of a randomized controlled trial. *Journal of the American Medical Association, 280*(14), 1238–1244.

Olds, D. L., Henderson, C. R., Jr., Kitzman, H. J., Eckenrode, J. J., Cole, R. E., & Tatelbaum, R. C. (1999). Prenatal and infancy home visitation by nurses: Recent findings. *Future Child, 9*(1), 44–65, 190–191.

Olds, D. L., Kitzman, H. J., Cole, R. E., Hanks, C. A., Arcoleo, K. J., Anson, E. A., . . . Stevenson, A. J. (2010). Enduring effects of prenatal and infancy home visiting by nurses on maternal life course and government spending: Follow-up of a randomized trial among children at age 12 years. *Archives of Pediatrics and Adolescent Medicine, 164*(5), 419–424.

Olds, D. L., Kitzman, H., Cole, R., Robinson, J., Sidora, K., Luckey, D. W., . . . Holmberg, J. (2004). Effects of nurse home-visiting on maternal life course and child development: Age 6 follow-up results of a randomized trial. *Pediatrics, 114*(6), 1550–1559.

Olds, D. L., Kitzman, H., Hanks, C., Cole, R., Anson, E., Sidora-Arcoleo, K., . . . Bondy, J. (2007). Effects of nurse home visiting on maternal and child functioning: Age-9 follow-up of a randomized trial. *Pediatrics, 120*(4), e832–e845.

Olds, D. L., Robinson, J., O'Brien, R., Luckey, D. W., Pettitt, L. M., Henderson, C. R., Jr., . . . Talmi, A. (2002). Home visiting by paraprofessionals and by nurses: A randomized, controlled trial. *Pediatrics, 110*(3), 486–496.

Olds, D. L., Robinson, J., Pettitt, L., Luckey, D. W., Holmberg, J., Ng, R. K., . . . Henderson, C. R., Jr. (2004). Effects of home visits by paraprofessionals and by nurses: Age 4 follow-up results of a randomized trial. *Pediatrics, 114*(6), 1560–1568.

Orr, L., Feins, J. D., Jacob, R., Beecroft, E., Sanbonmatsu, L., Katz, L. F., . . . Kling, J. (2003). *Moving to Opportunity for Fair Housing demonstration program.* Washington, DC: US Department of Housing and Urban Development.

Osborn, M. W. (2006). Diseased imaginations: Constructing delirium tremens in Philadelphia,

1813–1832. *Social History of Medicine, 19*, 191–208.

Papp, K. V., Walsh, S. J., & Snyder, P. J. (2009). Immediate and delayed effects of cognitive interventions in healthy elderly. *Alzheimer's & Dementia, 5*(1), 50–60.

Park-Higgerson, H. K., Perumean-Chaney, S. E., Bartolucci, A. A., Grimley, D. M., & Singh, K. P. (2008). The evaluation of school-based violence prevention programs: A meta-analysis. *Journal of School Health, 78*(9), 465–479.

Patient Protection and Affordable Care Act, Pub. L. No. 111–148 (2010).

Patterson, G. R., DeBaryshe, B. D., & Ramsey, E. (1989). A developmental perspective on antisocial behavior. *American Psychologist, 44*(2), 329–335.

Patterson, G. R., DeGarmo, D. S., and Forgatch, M. S. (2004). Systematic changes in families following prevention trials. *Journal of Abnormal Child Psychology, 32*(6), 621–633.

Patterson, G. R., Reid, J. B., & Dishion, T. J. (1992). *A social interactional approach: Vol. 4. Antisocial boys.* Eugene, OR: Castalia.

Petras, H., Kellam, S. G., Brown, C. H., Muthén, B. O., Ialongo, N. S., & Poduska, J. M. (2008). Developmental epidemiological courses leading to antisocial personality disorder and violent and criminal behavior: Effects by young adulthood of a universal preventive intervention in first- and second-grade classrooms. *Drug and Alcohol Dependence, 95*(Suppl. 1), 45–59.

Poduska, J. M., Kellam, S. G., Wang, W., Brown, C. H., Ialongo, N. S., & Toyinbo, P. (2008). Impact of the Good Behavior Game, a universal classroom-based behavior intervention, on young adult service use for problems with emotions, behavior, or drugs or alcohol. *Drug and Alcohol Dependence, 95*(Suppl. 1), 29–44.

Price, R. H., van Ryn, M., & Vinokur, A. D. (1992). Impact of a preventive job search intervention on the likelihood of depression among the unemployed. *Journal of Health and Social Behavior, 33*(2), 158–167.

Prinz, R. J., Sanders, M. R., Shapiro, C. J., Whitaker, D. J., & Lutzker, J. R. (2009). Population-based prevention of child maltreatment: The U.S. Triple P system population trial. *Prevention Science, 10*(1), 1–12.

Prochaska, J. O., Velicer, W. F., Fava, J. L., Rossi, J. S., & Tsoh, J. Y. (2001). Evaluating a population-based recruitment approach and a stage-based expert system intervention for smoking cessation. *Addictive Behaviors, 26*(4), 583–602.

Rajakumar, K. (2000). Pellagra in the United States: A historical perspective. *Southern Medical Journal, 93*(3), 272–277.

Randolph, W., & Viswanath, K. (2004). Lessons learned from public health mass media campaigns: Marketing health in a crowded media world. *Annual Review of Public Health, 25*, 419–438.

Rapp-Paglisi, L. A., & Dulmas, C. N. (2005). Prevention across the adult life span. In C. N. Dulmas and L. A. Rapp-Paglisi (Eds.), *Handbook of preventive interventions for adults* (pp. 3–13). New York, NY: Wiley.

Raudenbush, S. W., & Bryk, A. S. (2002). *Hierarchical linear models: Applications and data analysis* (2nd ed). Newbury Park, CA: Sage.

Rebok, G. W. (2008). *Cognitive training: Influence on neuropsychological and brain function in later life. State-of-science review.* London, UK: Government Foresight Mental Capital and Mental Wellbeing Project, Government Office for Science.

Rebok, G. W., Carlson, M. C., Glass, T. A., McGill, S., Hill, J., Wasik, B. A.,...Rasmussen, M. D. (2004). Short-term impact of Experience Corps participation on children and schools: Results from a pilot randomized trial. *Journal of Urban Health, 81*(1), 79–93.

Reid, J. B., Eddy, J. M., Fetrow, R. A., & Stoolmiller, M. (1999). Description and immediate impacts of a preventive intervention for conduct problems. *American Journal of Community Psychology, 27*(4), 483–517.

Reid, M. J., Webster-Stratton, C., & Hammond, M. (2003). Follow-up of children who received the Incredible Years intervention for oppositional-defiant disorder: Maintenance and prediction of 2-year outcome. *Behavior Therapy, 34*, 471–491.

Resko, S. M., Walton, M. A., Bingham, C. R., Shope, J. T., Zimmerman, M., Chermack, S. T.,... Cunningham, R. M. (2010). Alcohol availability and violence among inner-city adolescents: A multi-level analysis of the role of alcohol outlet density. *American Journal of Community Psychology, 46*(3–4), 253–262.

Riggs, N. R., Greenberg, M. T., Kusche, C. A., & Pentz, M. A. (2006). The mediational role of neurocognition in the behavioral outcomes of a social–emotional prevention program in elementary school students: Effects of the PATHS curriculum. *Prevention Science, 7*(1), 91–102.

Ringwalt, C. L., Ennett, S., Vincus, A., Thorne, J., Rohrbach, L. A., & Simons-Rudolph, A. (2002). The prevalence of effective substance use prevention curricula in U.S. middle schools. *Prevention Science, 3*(4), 257–265.

Ringwalt, C., Hanley, S., Vincus, A. A., Ennett, S. T., Rohrbach, L. A., & Bowling, J. M. (2008). The prevalence of effective substance use prevention curricula in the nation's high schools. *Journal of Primary Prevention, 29*(6), 479–488.

Roenker, D. L., Cissell, G. M., Ball, K. K., Wadley, V. G., & Edwards, J. D. (2003). Speed-of-processing and driving simulator training result in improved driving performance. *Human Factors, 45*(2), 218–233.

Rose, G. (1992). *The strategy of preventive medicine.* Oxford, UK: Oxford University Press.

Saltzman, L. F., Mercy, J. A., O'Carroll, P. W., Rosenberg, M. L., & Rhodes, P. H. (1992). Weapon involvement and injury outcomes in family and intimate assaults. *Journal of the American Medical Association, 267*(22), 3043–3047.

Sampson, R. J., Morenoff, J. D., & Earls, F. (1999). Beyond social capital: Spatial dynamics of collective efficacy for children. *American Sociological Review, 64,* 633–660.

Sampson, R. J., Raudenbush, S. W., & Earls, F. (1997). Neighborhoods and violent crime: A multilevel study of collective efficacy. *Science, 277*(5328), 918–924.

Sanders, M. R., Markie-Dadds, C., Tully, L. A., & Bor, W. (2000). The Triple P–Positive Parenting Program: A comparison of enhanced, standard, and self-directed behavioral family intervention for parents of children with early onset conduct problems. *Journal of Consulting and Clinical Psychology, 68,* 624–640.

Sanders, M. R., Pidgeon, A. M., Gravestock, F., Connors, M. D., Brown, S., & Young, R. W. (2004). Does parental attributional retraining and anger management enhance the effects of the Triple P–Positive Parenting Program with parents at risk of child maltreatment? *Behavior Therapy, 35,* 513–535.

Sandler, I. N., Ayers, T. S., Wolchik, S. A., Tein, J.-Y., Kwok, O. M., Lin, K.,…Griffin, W. A. (2003). Family Bereavement Program: Efficacy of a theory-based preventive intervention for parentally bereaved children and adolescents. *Journal of Consulting and Clinical Psychology, 71*(3), 587–600.

Sandler, I. N., Ma, Y., Tein, J., Ayers, T. S., Wolchik, S., Kennedy, C., & Millsap, R. (2010). Long-term effects of the Family Bereavement Program on multiple indicators of grief in parentally bereaved children and adolescents. *Journal of Consulting and Clinical Psychology, 78*(2), 131–143.

Sandler, I., Ostrom, A., Bitner, M. J., Ayers, T. S., Wolchik, S., & Daniels, V.-S. (2005). Developing effective prevention services for the real world: A prevention service development model. *American Journal of Community Psychology, 35*(3–4), 127–142.

Sandler, I. N., Wolchik, S. A., Ayers, T. S., Tein, J.-Y., Coxe, S., & Chow, W. (2008). Linking theory and intervention to promote resilience of children following parental bereavement. In M. Stroebe, M. Hanson, W. Stroebe, & H. Schut (Eds.), *Handbook of bereavement research: Consequences, coping, and care* (pp. 531–550). Washington, DC: American Psychological Association.

Schmiege, S. J., Khoo, S. T., Sandler, I. N., Ayers, T. S., & Wolchik, S. A. (2006). Symptoms of internalizing and externalizing problems: Modeling recovery curves after the death of a parent. *American Journal of Preventive Medicine, 31*(6 Suppl. 1), 152–160.

Shadish, W. R., Cook, D. T., & Campbell, D. T. (2002). *Experimental and quasi-experimental designs for generalized causal inference.* Boston, MA: Houghton Mifflin.

Skogan, W. G., Hartnett, S. M., Bump, N., & Dubois, J. (2008). *Evaluation of CeaseFire-Chicago.* Washington, D.C.: US Department of Justice, Office of Justice Programs, National Institute of Justice. Retrieved from http://www.northwestern.edu/ipr/publications/ceasefire.html

Sobell, M. B., & Sobell, L. C. (2000). Stepped care as a heuristic approach to the treatment of alcohol problems. *Journal of Consulting and Clinical Psychology, 68*(4), 573–579.

Social and Character Development Research Consortium (2010). *Efficacy of school-wide programs to promote social and character development and reduce problem behavior in elementary school children* (NCER 2011–2001). Washington, DC: US Department of Education.

Spoth, R. L., & Greenberg, M. T. (2005). Toward a comprehensive strategy for effective practitioner–scientist partnerships and large-scale community health and well-being. *American Journal of Community Psychology, 35*(3–4), 107–126.

Spoth, R., Redmond, C., & Lepper, H. (1999). Alcohol initiation outcomes of universal family-focused preventive interventions: One- and 2-year follow-ups of a controlled study. *Journal of Studies on Alcohol and Drugs, 13*(Suppl.), 103–111.

Spoth, R., Redmond, C., & Shin, C. (2000). Modeling factors influencing enrollment in family-focused preventive intervention research. *Prevention Science, 1*(4), 213–225.

Spoth, R., Shin, C., Guyll, M., Redmond, C., & Azevedo, K. (2006). Universality of effects: An examination of the comparability of long-term family intervention effects on substance use across risk-related subgroups. *Prevention Science, 7*(2), 209–224.

SPR MAPS II Task Force (2008). *Type 2 translational research: Overview and definitions.* Retrieved from http://preventionscience.org/SPR_Type%20 2%20Translation%20Research_Overview%20 and%20Definition.pdf

Strein, W., Hoagwood, K., & Cohn, A. (2003). School psychology: A public health perspective I. Prevention, populations, and systems change. *Journal of School Psychology, 41,* 23–38.

Studenski, S., Carlson, M. C., Fillit, H., Greenough, W. T., Kramer, A., & Rebok, G. W. (2006). From bedside to bench: Does mental and physical activity promote cognitive vitality in late life? *Science of Aging Knowledge Environment, 2006*(10), 21.

Substance Abuse and Mental Health Services Administration. (2011). *National registry of evidence-based programs and practices.* Rockville, MD: Substance Abuse and Mental Health Services Administration, US Department of Health and Human Services. Retrieved from http://www.nrepp.samhsa.gov/

Substance Abuse and Mental Health Services Administration. (2010). *Results from the 2009 National Survey on Drug Use and Health: Mental health findings.* Rockville, MD: Substance Abuse and Mental Health Services Administration, US Department of Health and Human Services.

Sugai, G., & Horner, R. (2006). A promising approach for expanding and sustaining school-wide positive behavior support. *School Psychology Review, 35,* 245–259.

Sugai, G., Horner, R., & Gresham, F. (2002). Behaviorally effective school environments. In M. R. E. Shinn, H. M. E. Walker, & G. E. Stoner (Eds.), *Interventions for academic and behavior problems II* (pp. 315–350). Bethesda, MD: NASP Publications.

Tandon, S. D., Perry, D. F., Mendelson, T., Kemp, K., & Leis, J. A. (2011). Preventing perinatal depression in low-income home visiting clients: A randomized controlled trial. *Journal of Consulting and Clinical Psychology, 79,* 707–712.

Tobin, T., Sugai, G., & Colvin, G. (1996). Patterns in middle school discipline records. *Journal of Emotional and Behavioral Disorders, 4,* 82–94.

Tremblay, G. C., & Israel, A. C. (1998). Children's adjustment to parental death. *Clinical Psychology: Science and Practice, 5,* 424–438.

Trudeau, L., Spoth, R., Randall, G. K., & Azevedo, K. (2007). Longitudinal effects of a universal family-focused intervention on growth patterns of adolescent internalizing symptoms and polysubstance use: Gender comparisons. *Journal of Youth and Adolescence, 6,* 725–740.

van Gils, P. F., Tariq, L., Verschuuren, M., & van den Berg, M. (2011). Cost-effectiveness research on preventive interventions: A survey of the publications in 2008. *European Journal of Public Health, 21*(2), 260–264.

van Lier, P. A. C., Verhulst, F. C., & Crijnen, A. A. M. (2003). Screening for disruptive behavior syndromes in children: The application of latent class analyses and implications for prevention programs. *Journal of Consulting and Clinical Psychology, 71*(2), 353–363.

van Spijker, B. A., van Straten, A., & Kerkhof, A. J. (2010). The effectiveness of a web-based self-help intervention to reduce suicidal thoughts: A randomized controlled trial. *Trials, 11,* 25.

Vigdor, E. R, & Mercy, J. A. (2006). Do laws restricting access to firearms by domestic violence offenders prevent intimate partner homicide? *Evaluation Review, 30*(3), 313–346.

Vinokur, A. D., Price, R. H., & Schul, Y. (1995). Impact of the JOBS intervention on unemployed workers varying in risk for depression. *American Journal of Community Psychology, 23*(1), 39–74.

Vinokur, A. D., Schul, Y., Vuori, J., & Price, R. H. (2000). Two years after a job loss: Long-term impact of the JOBS program on reemployment and mental health. *Journal of Occupational Health Psychology, 5*(1), 32–47.

Vinokur, A. D., van Ryn, M., Gramlich, E. M., & Price, R. H. (1991). Long-term follow-up and benefit–cost analysis of the Jobs Program: A preventive intervention for the unemployed. *Journal of Applied Psychology, 76*(2), 213–219.

Vuori, J., Silvonen, J., Vinokur, A. D., & Price, R. H. (2002). The Tyohon job search program in Finland: Benefits for the unemployed with risk of depression or discouragement. *Journal of Occupational Health Psychology, 7*(1), 5–19.

Waasdorp, T. E., Bradshaw, C. P., & Leaf, P. J. (2012). The impact of School-wide Positive Behavioral Interventions and Supports (SWPBIS) on bullying and peer rejection: A randomized controlled effectiveness trial. *Archives of Pediatrics and Adolescent Medicine, 116*(2), 149–156.

Wagenaar, A. C., Murray, D. M., & Toomey, T. L. (2000). Communities Mobilizing for Change on Alcohol (CMCA): Effects of a randomized trial on arrests and traffic crashes. *Addiction, 95*(2), 209–217.

Wagenaar, A. C., Salois, M. J., & Komro, K. A. (2009). Effects of beverage alcohol price and tax levels on drinking: A meta-analysis of 1003 estimates from 112 studies. *Addiction, 104*(2), 179–190.

Wagner, A. K., Soumerai, S. B., Zhang, F., & Ross-Degnan, D. (2002). Segmented regression analysis of interrupted time series studies in medication use research. *Journal of Clinical Pharmacy and Therapeutics, 27*(4), 299–309.

Walker, H. M., Horner, R. H., Sugai, G., Bullis, M., Sprague, J. R., Bricker, D., & Kaufman, M. J. (1996). Integrated approaches to preventing antisocial behavior patterns among school-age children and youth. *Journal of Emotional and Behavioral Disorders, 4*, 194–209.

Wang, C., Brown, C. H., & Bandeen-Roche, K. (2005). Residual diagnostics for growth mixture models. *Journal of the American Statistical Association, 100*, 1054–1076.

Wang, P. S., Patrick, A., Avorn, J., Azocar, F., Ludman, E., McCulloch, J., . . . Kessler, R. (2006). The costs and benefits of enhanced depression care to employers. *Archives of General Psychiatry, 63*(12), 1345–1353.

Wang, P. S., Simon, G. E., Avorn, J., Azocar, F., Ludman, E. J., McCulloch, J., . . . Kessler, R. C. (2007). Telephone screening, outreach, and care management for depressed workers and impact on clinical and work productivity outcomes: A randomized controlled trial. *Journal of the American Medical Association, 298*(12), 1401–1411.

Wang, P. S., Simon, G. E., & Kessler, R. C. (2008). Making the business case for enhanced depression care: The National Institute of Mental Health–Harvard Work Outcomes Research and Cost-effectiveness Study. *Journal of Occupational and Environmental Medicine, 50*, 468–475.

Watson-Thompson, J., Fawcett, S. B., & Schultz, J. A. (2008). Differential effects of strategic planning on community change on two urban neighborhood coalitions. *American Journal of Community Psychology, 42*(1–2), 25–38.

Webster, D. W., Vernick, J. S., & Bulzacchelli, M. T. (2009). Effects of state-level firearm seller accountability policies on firearm trafficking. *Journal of Urban Health, 86*(4), 525–537.

Webster, D. W., Vernick, J. S., & Mendel, J. (2009). *Interim evaluation of Baltimore's Safe Streets program.* Baltimore, MD: Center for the Prevention of Youth Violence, Johns Hopkins Bloomberg School of Public Health. Retrieved from http://www.baltimorehealth.org/info/2009_01_13.SafeStreetsEval.pdf

Webster, D. W., Vernick, J. S., Zeoli, A. M., & Manganello, J. A. (2004). Association between youth-focused firearm laws and youth suicides. *Journal of the American Medical Association, 292*(5), 594–601.

Webster-Stratton, C. (1990). *The Incredible Years parent training program manual: Effective communication, anger management and problem-solving (ADVANCE).* Seattle, WA: Incredible Years.

Webster-Stratton, C. & Hammond, M. (1997). Treating children with early-onset conduct problems: A comparison of child and parent training interventions. *Journal of Consulting and Clinical Psychology, 65*(1), 93–109.

Webster-Stratton, C., & Herman, K. C. (2008). The impact of parent behavior-management training on child depressive symptoms. *Journal of Counseling Psychology, 55*, 473–484.

Weist, M. (2001). Toward a public mental health promotion and intervention system for youth. *Journal of School Health, 71*(3), 101–104.

Weisz, J. R., Sandler, I. N., Durlak, J. A., & Anton, B. S. (2005). Promoting and protecting youth mental health through evidence-based prevention and treatment. *American Psychologist, 60*(6), 628–648.

Whalley, L. J., Dick, F. D., & McNeill, G. (2006). A life-course approach to the aetiology of late-onset dementias. *Lancet Neurology, 5*(1), 87–96.

Wiebe, D. J. (2003). Sex differences in the perpetrator–victim relationship among emergency department patients presenting with nonfatal firearm-related injuries. *Annals of Emergency Medicine, 42*(3), 405–412.

Williams, J. W., Plassman, B. L., Burke, J., Holsinger, T., & Benjamin, S. (2010). *Preventing Alzheimer's disease and cognitive decline.* Rockville, MD: Agency for Healthcare Research and Quality, US Department of Health and Human Services. Retrieved from http://www.ahrq.gov/clinic/tp/alzcogtp.htm

Willis, S. L., Tennstedt, S. L., Marsiske, M., Ball, K., Elias, J., Koepke, K. M., . . . Wright, E. (2006). Long-term effects of cognitive training on everyday functional outcomes in older adults. *Journal of the American Medical Association, 296*(23), 2852–2854.

Wills, E. F. (1930). Delirium tremens: Its causation, prevention, and treatment. *British Journal of Inebriety, 28*, 43–49.

Wilson, J. M., Chermack, S., & McGarrell, E. F. (2010). *Community-based violence prevention: An assessment of Pittsburgh's One Vision One Life program.* Santa Monica, CA: RAND Corporation.

Wilson, J. M. G., & Jungner, G. (1968). *Principles and practice of screening for disease.* Geneva, Switzerland: World Health Organization.

Wilson, S. J., & Lipsey, M. W. (2007). School-based interventions for aggressive and disruptive behavior: Update of a meta-analysis. *American*

Journal of Preventive Medicine, 33(2 Suppl.), s130–s143.

Wilson, S. J., Lipsey, M. W., & Derzon, J. H. (2003). The effects of school-based intervention programs on aggressive behavior: A meta-analysis. *Journal of Counseling and Clinical Psychology, 71*(1), 136–149.

Wittchen, H. U., Beesdo, K., Bittner, A., & Goodwin, R. D. (2003). Depressive episodes—evidence for a causal role of primary anxiety disorders? *European Psychiatry, 18*(8), 384–393.

Wolchik, S. A., Sandler, I. N., Millsap, R. E., Plummer, B. A., Greene, S. M., Anderson, E. R., . . . Haine, R. A. (2002). Six-year follow-up of a randomized, controlled trial of preventive interventions for children of divorce. *Journal of the American Medical Association, 288*(15), 1874–1881.

Wolchik, S. A., West, S. G., Sandler, I., Tein, J., Coatsworth, D., Lengua, L., . . . Griffin, W. A. (2000). An experimental evaluation of theory-based mother and mother–child programs for children of divorce. *Journal of Consulting and Clinical Psychology, 68*(5), 843–856.

Wolinsky, F., Unverzagt, F., Smith, D., Jones, R., Stoddard, A., & Tennstedt, S. (2006). The ACTIVE cognitive training trial and health-related quality of life: Protection that lasts for 5 years. *Journal of Gerontology: Medical Sciences, 61*(12), 1324–1329.

Woolf, S. H. (2007). Potential health and economic consequences of misplaced priorities. *Journal of the American Medical Association, 297*(5), 523–526.

Woolf, S. H. (2008). The meaning of translational research and why it matters. *Journal of the American Medical Association, 299*(2), 211–213.

Wright, P. W. (2005). *IDEA 2004: Proposed changes to the code of federal regulations.* Washington, DC: US Department of Education. Retrieved from http://www.wrightslaw.com/idea/law/idea.regs.propose.pdf

Yu, Q., Scribner, R., Carlin, B., Theall, K., Simonsen, N., Ghosh-Dastidar, B., . . . Mason, K. (2008). Multilevel spatio-temporal dual changepoint models for relating alcohol outlet destruction and changes in neighborhood rates of assaultive violence. *Geospatial Health, 2*(2), 161–172.

Yung, A. R., Killackey, E., Hetrick, S. E., Parker, A. G., Schultze-Lutter, F., Klosterkoetter, J., . . . McGorry, P. D. (2007). The prevention of schizophrenia. *International Review of Psychiatry, 19*(6), 633–646.

Yung, A. R., Phillips, L. J., Yuen, H. P., Francey, S. M., McFarlane, C. A., Hallgren, M., & McGorry, P. D. (2003). Psychosis prediction: 12-month follow up of a high-risk ("prodromal") group. *Schizophrenia Research, 60*(1), 21–32.

Zandi, P. P., & Rebok, G. W. (2007). Introduction to the special issue on psychiatric prevention. *International Review of Psychiatry, 19*(6), 593–595.

Zechmeister, I., Kilian, R., & McDaid, D. (2008). Is it worth investing in mental health promotion and prevention of mental illness? A systematic review of the evidence from economic evaluations. *BMC Public Health, 8*, 20.

Zins, J. E., Weissberg, R. P., Wang, M. C., & Walberg, H. J. (Eds.) (2004). *Building academic success on social and emotional learning: What does the research say?* New York, NY: Teachers College Press.

Zlotnick, C., Miller, I. W., Pearlstein, T., Howard, M., & Sweeney, P. (2006). A preventive intervention for pregnant women on public assistance at risk for postpartum depression. *American Journal of Psychiatry, 163*(8), 1443–1445.

18

Progress Made, but Much More to Be Done

PHILIP J. LEAF

LAYSHA OSTROW

RONALD W. MANDERSCHEID

DAVID L. SHERN

WILLIAM W. EATON

Key Points

- The recent surge of understanding about the etiology of mental and behavioral disorders and the disability, distress, and dollars associated with them has not been sufficiently translated into public health efforts

- The public health approach to mental health will not prevail without changes in the way we conduct research, train and collaborate with professionals and consumers, and advocate for public health practices and health-promoting policies

- Understanding resilience—the capacity for health despite exposure to risk—is important in public health efforts

- The concept of recovery as defined by consumers rather than symptom mitigation has become an important principle in both mental health policy making and research

- Now is an opportune time to integrate mental health care (such as psychiatry and psychotherapy) with formal support services (such as vocational rehabilitation) and natural supports (family, friends, peers, and the community)

- Now is an opportune time to integrate mental and physical health services, from prevention through recovery, into community health services available to everyone

- Consumer involvement in both individual care and policy making improves outcomes and recovery potential for individuals with serious mental illness

- Consumer-operated or self-help services have been found to improve outcomes

- The Patient Protection and Affordable Care Act will significantly change the financing and organization of health services and prevention efforts in the United States and provides an opportunity for important advances in public mental health

OVERVIEW

In his 1926 presidential address before the American Public Health Association, "Public Health at the Crossroads," Charles-Edward A. Winslow (1926) highlighted the need for increased attention to the prevention, treatment, and remediation of mental illnesses. He forecast a future in which mental health would play a far more significant role in efforts to promote, maintain, and restore health and to reduce the consequences of ill health, observing:

> It is impossible to consider, even in the briefest summary, the future program of the public health movement without at least some reference to the vast and fertile fields of mental hygiene. Today, the attention devoted to this problem by municipal health departments is so slight that it has not even been included in our Appraisal Form for city health work; but in the not-distant future I am inclined to believe that the care of mental health will occupy a share of our energies perhaps as large as that devoted to the whole range of disorders affecting other organs of the body. (p. 1078)

Over 75 years later, some progress has been made in the prevention and treatment of mental disorders and in the reduction of disabilities associated with them. Despite this progress, however, the mental health field has yet to achieve the role in public health policy, programs, and services envisioned by Winslow. This is not because mental disorders and their consequences have become less important to our individual and collective

health and well-being. Quite the opposite is the case. Indeed, earlier chapters in this volume have spoken eloquently to the progress made in our understanding of mental disorders, their etiology and course, their prevalence and incidence, and their prevention and treatment. Further, the impact of mental disorders on individual health and the public health has been highlighted in policy reports at national and international levels, accompanied by data that underscore the significant human and economic impact of mental disorders on people and on economies (an issue discussed below).

Earlier chapters summarized our current knowledge and areas where our understanding of mental disorders is likely to increase. The current chapter has a different goal. It posits that it is time to move from paper to practice and to change the landscape of that practice. We aim to provide a glimpse of what could and should occur in the future. Rather than describe a world in which our impact on the incidences, courses, and consequences of mental disorders continues to be minimal, we prefer to envision a world in which existing knowledge is used and outcomes for real people change.

To achieve that aim, the field of public mental health must move beyond a narrow focus on clinical interventions to embrace the impact of community and population dynamics in promoting mental health, preventing mental illnesses, and fostering recovery. Thus, this chapter begins with an overview of what has come before, examining progress and pitfalls. This is followed by a section that discusses the evolution needed to bring about Winslow's vision of mental health care as an integral part of the public health. That forward-looking section examines the growing role of such factors as the social determinants of health, attention to the full spectrum of mental health and illness from prevention through recovery across the life span, the importance of resilience in preventing behavioral problems, the still evolving key role of consumers in treatment and recovery, and the policy changes needed to embrace mental health as an intrinsic part of the public health.

PAST AS PROLOGUE: THE NEED FOR A PUBLIC HEALTH MODEL

Data and Policy Documents Don't Always Inform Progress

As articulated in chapter 1, mental disorders have been recognized as among the most common disabling and often chronic disorders. The World Health Organization (WHO) has found that globally, mental illnesses including depression, schizophrenia, bipolar disorder, and alcohol use are ranked among the 10 leading causes of disability (Murray & Lopez, 1996; WHO, 2008a). For women ages 15–44 years, depression constitutes the leading cause of disability in the entire range of low-, middle-, and high-income countries (WHO, 2008a). Among older adults, both depression and dementias (including Alzheimer's disease) are a significant source of disability (WHO, 2008a). Critically, compared with other chronic disorders such as hypertension, heart disease, and diabetes, most mental and behavioral disorders tend to arise far earlier in the life span—in childhood, adolescence and young adulthood (Carter et al., 2010; Kessler et al., 2007; Kessler, Berglund, Demler, Jin, & Walters, 2005; Merikangas et al., 2010; Patel, Flisher, Hetrick, & McGorry, 2007). This fact has significant implications for services and supports, education, and employment. (See also chapter 6.)

Moreover, as discussed in chapter 13, awareness has been growing about the significant impact mental disorders have on health, on quality of life, and also, in this era of cost containment and health reform, on the costs of health care. As the director of the National Institute of Mental Health (NIMH) recently observed (Insel, 2011):

> The annual economic costs of mental illness in the United States are enormous. The direct costs of mental health care represent around 6% of overall health care costs. Among all Americans, 36.2 million people paid for mental health services totaling $57.5 billion in 2006—the most recent year we have this type of data available. This places mental health care expenditures as this nation's third costliest medical conditions, behind heart conditions and trauma, and tied with cancer. Of course, the costs of mental health care are only a fraction of the costs of mental illness, which can result in substantial costs for co-morbid medical conditions as well as social costs due to disability, unemployment, and incarceration.

Unfortunately, the knowledge that mental disorders constitute significant health and economic challenges for the United States and other countries around the world has not been adequately translated into the sorely needed public health effort commensurate with the individual and collective disability, distress, and dollars associated with these disorders. Thus, as discussed in detail in chapter 15 and elsewhere in this volume, despite significant changes in public understanding of the causes of mental illnesses (Pescosolido et al., 2010) and a history of successes in reducing barriers to care around the world, the vast majority of individuals with mental disorders never receive care (Kessler, Demler, et al., 2005; Merikangas et al., 2010; Substance Abuse and Mental Health Services Administration [SAMHSA], 2010). Stigma remains a deterrent to care (Link & Phelan, 2006; Pescosolido et al., 2010), and recognition that treatment can improve the course of these chronic disorders varies broadly by ethnic and racial background, economic status, and geographic region (Anglin, Alberti, Link, & Phelan, 2008). Thus even when specialized mental health care is available, many people are unwilling or unable to surmount existing barriers to using those services.

In part, that is why when mental health services are sought, they frequently are received from providers outside the mental health specialty sector, such as primary care clinicians, schools, child welfare agencies, and correctional facilities (Atkins, Hoagwood, Kutash, & Seidman, 2010; Manderscheid, 2010; Redlich & Cusack, 2010). These providers and settings are the first door to health care as a whole for most people around the world. However, these providers may not have the same state-of-the-science knowledge and skills to diagnose and provide care for people with serious mental disorders that are available through the specialty mental health sector. Moreover, treatment received from these practitioners may not be grounded in existing best practices, and consumers and caregivers may not be engaged as partners in that care (Institute of Medicine [IOM], 2006, 2009).

Even if the data alone have provided insufficient impetus to change, over the past three decades high-level reports also have advanced the cause of mental health in eloquent ways, urging change in policy and programs. In the United States, the President's Commission on Mental Health (1978) and the surgeon general's report on mental health (Surgeon General of the United States, 1999) both urged major changes in how the country addresses the needs of persons with mental disorders. However, their impetus for action was not long-lived. It remains to be seen whether the recommendations of the New Freedom Commission on Mental Health (2003), with its emphasis on recovery as a benchmark for success, will meet the same fate. Even more recently, as a component of national health care reform, SAMHSA (2011) announced a plan using a public health approach to promote positive social and emotional competencies as well as mental health and wellness. It will be interesting to see whether this becomes simply another report that barely makes a ripple or whether it results in fundamental changes in the strategies communities, service providers, and funders use in efforts to promote wellness and to prevent and remediate mental disorders.

Worldwide, the United Nations and the WHO have highlighted place-based interventions along with inequalities and disadvantages in global mental health and mental illnesses (United Nations Economic and Social Council, 2008; WHO, 2002, 2003, 2004, 2008b, 2009a, 2009b, 2010). Through its reports and other activities, each agency has encouraged efforts to ensure that persons with mental disorders are included globally as candidates not only for clinical services but also for other priority initiatives aimed at reducing mortality, morbidity, and improving quality of life (WHO, 2010). Sadly, the United Nations General Assembly did not include mental disorders among the illnesses for discussion at the agency's September 2011 high-level meeting on preventing noncommunicable diseases. Paper is far less expensive than policy implementation on a global scale.

New Knowledge May Not Always Inform Change in Programs and Policy

As described in previous chapters, some advances in the descriptive epidemiology of mental disorders have been made over the past half century. In 1950, toward the conclusion of the first generation of psychiatric epidemiology (Dohrenwend and Dohrenwend, 1982), knowledge of the burden of mental disorders was limited to estimates of those in treatment (Hollingshead & Redlich, 1958; Kramer, 1969). When second-generation studies concluded that more than 50% of the US population suffered from emotional problems, as in the Midtown Manhattan study (Srole, 1975), the estimate was ignored, because it was based on a model of mental functioning that did not refer to specific diagnoses. The third generation of studies, beginning with the Epidemiologic Catchment Area Program (ECA) (Robins & Regier, 1991), based estimates of prevalence on improved measurement of specific disorders (as described in chapter 4) and was harder to ignore. The ECA was followed by several national and international studies reinforcing its credibility and establishing the considerable burden of mental disorders, as described in the 1996 study of the global burden of disease (Murray & Lopez, 1996) reviewed in chapter 1. Even with acceptance of the burden of mental disorders and the growing body of prevalence data, however, further advances are needed in the assessment of specific disorders, as shown in chapter 4. Similarly, although prevalence studies have established social and demographic correlates of specific psychiatric disorders, as described in chapter 7, relatively few prospective studies have established how these same social and demographic correlates may be associated with increased risk for specific disorders; even fewer studies consider more than one or two risk factors simultaneously.

The exponential growth in basic science, including genetics, over the past 50 years has yielded dramatic advances in our understanding of the role genes play in human behavior (see chapter 8). For the most part, however, we have yet to experience practical results of these advances; there are very few examples comparable to the discovery of the genetic and environmental basis of phenylketonuria (as described in chapter 17) that have led to screening or treatment preventing a disorder from occurring in the first place. Knowledge about the brain, its functions, and its dysfunctions has grown markedly, in large measure because of advances in measurement techniques. Indeed, the pace of new findings about brain development, structure, and actions was so remarkable in the closing decade of the 20th century that it led the US Congress and the president to proclaim the 1990s "the decade of the brain" (www.loc.gov/loc/brain/proclaim.html). Much of this understanding has revealed the developmental sequences of both the growth and plasticity of the brain, as described in chapter 9. Again, however, this advance has not yet been well translated into improvements in the mental health of the public or in the diagnosis, treatment, and recovery of people with mental illnesses.

These advances in the knowledge of brain development have been paralleled by recent advances in our understanding both of the development of disorders (chapter 6) and of responses and adaptations to stress over the life span (chapter 10) and to crises and traumas (chapter 11). These advances have suggested how effective preventive interventions might be developed and implemented when both structured and well timed to the developmental stage of the individual, as described in chapter 17.

Over the last century, findings from epidemiologic studies, primarily associated with physical health and illnesses, have been translated into clinical practice and subsequently into community-based public health interventions at the national and international levels (McKinlay & McKinlay, 1977; Wynder, 1994). When it comes to mental disorders, it will be critical to look past efficacy research to emphasize translating our understanding of the factors affecting onset, recovery, and relapse that can help reduce the incidence, prevalence, and impact of mental disorders on populations (Insel, 2009).

Services, Improving Slowly

More than research needs to change, however, to bring mental health to the fore in public health. The content of this volume shows that while progress has been made, more substantial change is needed when it comes to the mental health care system and how mental health care is practiced. Change is needed in naming mental and behavioral disorders, bringing science to scale in mental health service systems, and treating and preventing these disorders.

NAMING MENTAL ILLNESSES

In chapter 2, McHugh notes that our great advances in understanding mental illnesses has not been translated into a commensurate reduction of the burdens to those experiencing these illnesses. He further questions the extent to which future nosologic efforts will prove useful for prevention or reduction of impairment. There is a need for a nosology that facilitates the targeting of efforts at prevention, treatment, and recovery, one that is more closely linked with the interventions to be used. The current nosology provides little help in understanding why some individuals respond to pharmacologic treatments, psychosocial treatments, or both while others do not.

BRINGING SCIENCE TO SCALE

Too few individuals with the most severe forms of mental illness receive treatments consistent with existing scientific evidence (Wang, Demler, & Kessler, 2002). (See also chapter 15.) New practices born of scientific knowledge simply have not been translated into community-based mental health care, much less into more global public health. Although earlier chapters have highlighted many opportunities for reducing the incidence, prevalence, and consequences of mental disorders, current prevention efforts and interventions do not reflect a cohesive strategy, whether at the national level or more globally. Rather, they arise as idiosyncratic applications of interventions in particular contexts that have rarely if ever been brought to scale in large metropolitan areas. As a result, the benchmarks for successful treatment have continued to be access to care and symptom reduction rather than the more important and possible benchmark of recovery.

In the United States and elsewhere, little connection, much less collaboration, exists between those individuals and groups who are knowledgeable of risk and protective factors and those creating fiscal and other public policies. Although this may be particularly true for countries and contexts with fewer resources (See chapters 3 and 16), there is only limited evidence that efforts anywhere to promote mental health and treat mental disorders incorporate findings from the latest research advances on effectiveness and dissemination. What limited efforts have been undertaken to reduce risk, increase access, and facilitate use of state-of-the-science preventive and treatment interventions and recovery supports have been underfunded and often limited to a single agency or program. Moreover, current monitoring efforts have not proven fruitful in planning for and monitoring changes in the prevalence of mental disorders.

Current strategic plans for the NIMH (2008) and the SAMHSA (2011) hold some hope for change. They focus on reducing the occurrence and consequences of mental disorders in the United States. Attention appears to be shifting from a disease model to one that emphasizes the many facets of full and productive lives because in most communities, our knowledge of prevention, treatment, and recovery from mental disorders has had little impact on individuals experiencing the disorders or those charged with creating more effective policies and practices to treat and prevent them.

TREATING AND PREVENTING MENTAL ILLNESSES

Efforts to prevent and treat mental disorders are lagging behind efforts for other illnesses. Ward and colleagues (2004), for example, concluded that between 1970 and 2006 there was a significant reduction in the mortality rates of most cancers in the United States. They attributed those declines to improved screening and to the general population's knowledge about risks for cancer, both of which resulted in earlier detection of cancers and improvements in the treatments available. Data described elsewhere in this book do not suggest similar reductions in the prevalences or consequences of mental disorders.

For more than a century, public health has focused on preventing disease, prolonging life, and promoting health by stimulating and reinforcing educational and organizational efforts of federal, state, and local governments; communities; and community-based organizations. Efforts were directed at individuals with predominantly acute diseases or at high risk for such diseases (Winslow, 1926). Unfortunately, mental and behavioral disorders—which are chronic, remitting illnesses—often were excluded in these efforts or marginalized and not seen as critical to the broader community-wide health effort.

While we are not suggesting that there has been a wholesale lack of attention to mental health issues despite the magnitude of the worldwide need, we do contend that action has not kept pace with this growing recognition. The public health implications of mental and behavioral disorders do not rank high on the list of criteria considered in crafting public policy or new directions in public health. Simply put, until recently, knowledge that mental disorders constitute significant health challenges for the United States and other countries has not been translated into a public health effort commensurate with the disabilities, distress, and human and economic costs associated with these disorders.

What Is Needed?

It is unlikely that outcomes from mental disorders will change significantly without a fundamental change in the way we study, organize services for, and educate about mental illnesses. To that end, we are tempted to paraphrase Winslow's statement from early in the past century: It is impossible to consider a world where future efforts at improving health and well-being will not focus greater attention and resources on preventing mental disorders and reducing the consequences for those that do occur. Unless we marshal new approaches and engage policy makers, service providers, consumers, academic researchers, and community activists in creating, implementing, and sustaining solutions to these problems, we will experience another century in which we fail to ensure that mental health is embraced as essential to overall public health and well-being.

It is not likely that a multifaceted public health approach will prevail as the new mental health paradigm without changes in the way we conduct research, train professionals and consumers, and advocate for effective public health practices and policies. We need to move beyond periodic "thought pieces" to ensuring that these components of the strategy are as important as efforts to increase research funding, if not more so. Thus what is called for is a wholesale change in the approach to mental health and mental illnesses. That change requires looking through a different prism as well as using different tools to change the focus of mental health culture from pathology to wellness, from clinical to community, and from individual care to public health. It needs to include not just families and practitioners but consumers and communities. It needs to focus on individuals, not just disorders; on social determinants of mental health and illness, not just pathology; and on recovery, not just remission. That is why in the rest of this chapter we frame a picture of where the field of public mental health needs to be headed to become an integral part of public health. We explain why an understanding of social determinants of health is needed, the important protective role of the community in promoting both positive mental health and resilience in the face of adversity, the changing role of consumers and self-determination, and the nature of recovery and recovery supports.

THE ROAD TO TOMORROW

The public health mission here—to prevent the distress and disruption that too often accompany mental disorders—includes the need to focus beyond services, looking toward policies and practices that both promote mental health and allow individuals with mental disorders to achieve and sustain recovery, thereby experiencing the least possible disruption in their lives at all phases of the illness. We need to move beyond a focus only on changing the pathology within an individual; rather, we must attend to the structural, economic, policy, and ecological factors that contribute to the onset and persistence of behavioral disorders. Below, we suggest key areas to which attention must be directed to achieve those ends.

Social Determinants of Health

COMMUNITY

As national health reform (in the form of the Patient Protection and Affordable Care Act of 2010) moves forward, we will need to increase attention to community contexts, which often involve the social determinants of health for the population overall as well as for persons with mental and behavioral disorders. As documented in the final report of the WHO's Commission on Social Determinants of Health (2008), recognition is growing that the community in which one resides has important effects in such areas as child development, self-concept, sociality, social networks, marriage, sense of well-being, criminal behavior, and even physical and emotional health. We readily acknowledge considerable differences in the health and well-being of communities and that some communities that provide personal, social, economic, and cultural opportunities for residents also convey a positive sense of well-being and good quality of life. At the same time, we know of communities with more limited fiscal and personal resources in which individuals are likely to feel isolated from others and perceive few positive opportunities to be available. As the United States moves toward implementation of the national Healthy People 2020 project of the US Department of Health and Human Services (see http://www.healthypeople.gov/2020/default.aspx), those of us concerned with the mental health of populations—with public mental health—must focus our efforts on activities to strengthen communities and the ability of all to participate in their communities, much in the way we sought to create and make effective treatments available for those with mental disorders.

The role of community context is no more powerfully represented than in the social determinants of health. These are the environmental variables that interact with genetic vulnerabilities to produce either well-being or illness. Social determinants are the conditions in which children and families are born and mature. Toxins, noise, crowding, poor housing conditions, and low-quality, unsafe schools and workplaces all affect health and quality of life (Evans & Kantrowitz, 2002). Perhaps the best known social determinant is socioeconomic status, shown to have a consistent, graded effect on health status (Braverman, Egerter, Woolf, & Marks, 2011). Socioeconomic status helps determine health status through several mechanisms, including both the direct acquisition of needed material resources and the cognitive and emotional skills needed to participate successfully in community life (Braverman et al., 2011). Not only is the absolute level of income an important determinant of health, but, as Wilkinson and Pickett (2010) demonstrate, the degree of disparity between the richest and the poorest is a powerful predictor of variety of health and well-being indicators. The United States is particularly notable with regard to health and income inequalities that predict reduced life expectancy, increased infant mortality, increased obesity, and higher rates of homicide and imprisonment as well as other indicators of decrements in both individual and community health.

State-level differences in inequality are correlated with prevalence of depression in the individual states (Messias, Eaton, & Grooms, 2011). Racial differences in health and mental health status reflect the effects of discrimination, its attendant social-psychological effects on self-image, and material effects on access to equal opportunity (Williams, Neighbors, & Jackson, 2008).

The impact of these and other social determinants is likely mediated through both psychological and physiological mechanisms. Toxins can be either material (e.g., lead exposure) or psychological (e.g., discrimination); they can produce physical and emotional ill health through multiple pathways. Of particular relevance are the toxic health effects of chronic stress and trauma. We have known for some time that chronic stress is associated with neurobiological changes in the brain that are mediated by cortisol and other stress hormones and that are predictive of poorer mental and general health status (McEwen, 2007). (See also chapters 10 and 11.) These hormonal assaults on the brain result in structural and functional changes that place individuals at increased risk for the development of a broad range of illnesses. The Adverse Childhood Experiences study documents the long-term effects of childhood trauma on the expression of mental and general health disorders (Felitti & Anda, 2010).

DISPARITIES AND INEQUITIES

Most efforts to improve health have focused on increasing the overall level of health in a community. While this is an important objective, it does not reflect the knowledge that within a community, health is not necessarily distributed either equally or uniformly. Some groups may experience greater exposure to risks, coupled with lower resilience and less access to resources. In the United States, significant differences in health have been found to be based on income, age, gender, and race. These differences are not simply health disparities; rather, they represent inequities with important implications for later success for individuals, families, and communities. One of the most consistent epidemiologic findings is the relationship between poverty and mental disorders. It is clear that access to social and economic resources frequently results in increased protective factors and services (Costello, Compton, Keeler, & Angold, 2003; Costello, Erkanli, Copeland, & Angold, 2010).

Recent work toward the goals of the Healthy People 2020 program (http://www.healthypeople.gov/2020/default.aspx) recognized the importance of this linkage and implemented a model to address health and health care disparities, including disparities in mental illness and its care. This work emphasizes that health-related disparities can be addressed only through approaches that promote social equity, since those disparities are based on social disadvantage (Braverman et al., 2011). A major emphasis of the Patient Protection and Affordable Care Act is on eliminating current disparities in health and health care by changing insurance coverage, paying for prevention and promotion interventions, and directly addressing mental illness and health care without distinction from other illnesses or treatments.

RESILIENCE

While the risk factors associated with social determinants create an increased likelihood that illnesses and disability will develop, the effects of such risk factors are mediated by one's resilience, a function of both personal and environmental variables. Resilience refers to the capacity for health despite exposure to risk (Bonanno, 2004). It involves rapid, effective recovery after stress by using both personal skills and other capacities as well as by relying on social and other external, environmental supports. Resilience can be a characteristic of individuals as well as communities (F. H. Norris, Stevens, Pfefferbaum, Wyche, & Pfefferbaum, 2008). For individuals, resilience is associated with temperamental variables and environments that promote the development of problem-solving and social skills as well as with a social environment that helps buffer stress. Similarly, in families, supportive, secure, and caring parents foster resilience in children and in the family as a whole. At both the community and school levels, a sense of

cohesion and belonging, supported by prosocial peer relations and an environment that provides opportunities to develop competencies, is associated with the development of resilience.

PROMOTION OF MENTAL HEALTH AND PREVENTION OF MENTAL ILLNESS

Many of the variables that underlie the development of resilience have been operationalized in interventions that seek to promote positive mental health as well as to reduce the incidence of mental illnesses, including substance use and abuse. As discussed in chapter 17, a wide range of evidence-based interventions have been found effective in achieving those ends. At the individual, family, school, and community levels, interventions have promoted healthful behaviors and reduced the occurrence of problem behaviors and diagnosable mental illnesses. As noted by the IOM (2009), however, the challenge in realizing the benefits of these known-effective preventive interventions is bringing them to scale, with fidelity, in a broad, global way. With testing and implementation of preventive efforts widely dispersed across government entities, no one is providing sufficient strategic leadership in the prevention and promotion sphere to realize the extraordinary potential of these interventions. Building both the political will to develop the next generation of prevention and promotion efforts and accountability structures to gauge our success will be critical to the success of those efforts.

Improving the System of Mental Health Care

INTEGRATING CARE

In many ways, until recently, modern-day efforts to bring mental health into public health have paralleled efforts of more than 100 years ago to include mental health as part of the public hygiene movement, which, sadly, proved largely unsuccessful (Grob, 1991). Throughout much of the last century, mental disorders and, to an even greater extent, addictions were considered the province of a separate system of care and not susceptible to the same sorts of interventions and preventive strategies that were effective in strengthening overall public health.

The situation has changed today for a number of reasons, among them the burgeoning cost of health care as a whole and the trend to focus the majority of health care dollars—as much as 75%—on chronic, rather than acute, disorders. These developments have been accompanied by the marked strength of the behavioral health science base and the compelling evidence of both the extreme disease burden attributable to mental disorders and their coexistence with other chronic and acute illnesses. With the increased appreciation that mental disorders represent more than half of the world's most disabling conditions, coupled with the growing armamentarium of effective prevention and promotion technologies as well as treatments, now is the time to fully integrate mental health services, from prevention through recovery, into community health available to everyone. Now is also the time to integrate mental health care (such as psychiatry and psychotherapy) with formal support services (such as vocational rehabilitation) and natural supports (family, friends, peers, and the community), all similarly essential components of both a person-centered, not disease-centered, system and a system that uses a public health approach.

COORDINATING CARE

In the United States, many individuals with a mental disorder will also experience a substance use disorder, particularly since undiagnosed individuals frequently self-medicate chronic mental disorders such as depression with alcohol or drugs of abuse. Moreover, people with serious mental illnesses today run a high risk of co-occurring chronic physical conditions that have been found to reduce their life expectancy by an average of 25 years (Colton & Manderscheid, 2006). (See chapter 6.) Finally, people with mental disorders also can get sick with acute illnesses that require treatment, as is the case for people with other chronic health problems such as heart disease, diabetes and asthma.

In each case, more than one provider is likely to be involved in the provision of services. To be most effective—and to best serve their patients—they need not only to share information (medications prescribed, diagnoses made, etc.) but also to work together toward their patients' overall health. That is what coordinated care is about. It is essential to a public health approach that patients are viewed from a holistic perspective, as people with behavioral *and* physical health care needs, and are treated as people, not as disease entities. Thus it is essential for mental health care providers to collaborate with physical health care providers. Opportunities may be presented with the ongoing health care reforms in the United States that emphasize the importance of coordination among physical, mental, and substance abuse care providers. However, the historical division between physical and mental health in training, service provision, and advocacy means that groups who need to work together have little history of success in doing so. Successful models of integration and positive outcomes need to be identified, disseminated, and supported by mentoring and coaching. This presents a particular challenge, because the different treatment disciplines possess divergent views about the concept of, even the possibility of, recovery from mental and substance use disorders.. More training for providers, purchasers, and consumers is needed to help the workforce move from "parallel play" to collaborative care.

Further, whether in health and mental health prevention or treatment, collaboration can significantly benefit systematic efforts to measure community health status, which in turn can help target increasingly limited resources to meet emerging threats and to evaluate the overall effectiveness of interventions. Just as we monitor the rates of infectious and noncommunicable diseases and systematically assess the safety of food and water, we should assess the quality of our lived and psychological environments. Just as we require children to be vaccinated against a range of infectious illnesses as a condition of attending school, we should expect that children's social and emotional health will be monitored and effective techniques implemented to boost their resilience to toxic stress and trauma. This new focus on an approach that fully integrates and coordinates prevention and promotion technologies is essential for the future of individuals and communities alike.

BUILDING A STRUCTURE FOR A SUSTAINED EFFORT

If we continue simply to do what we've been doing, there is little likelihood of substantial changes in the mental health of our communities. As recognized by the health care reforms described earlier in this chapter and elsewhere in this volume, health and well-being must be promoted and the consequences of illnesses when they do occur must be reduced by moving toward solutions aimed toward positive outcomes in populations. This must be achieved not simply by conducting clinical trials, which often exclude many individuals who have comorbid conditions or who are unable or unwilling to participate in the research requirements that accompany the treatment. Implementing and sustaining the necessary initiatives will require greater attention to fiscal sustainability as well as to both organizational and structural impediments. Necessary initiatives include but are not limited to health benefits, medical homes, accountable care organizations, patient- and consumer-focused tools, and clear peer and community leadership. We need to increase and support population-based structures that foster mental health (among other things) along with efforts to provide more effective treatments with an increased emphasis on implementation at scale and on sustainability (Fixsen, Naoom, Blase, Friedman, & Wallace, 2005). We also must recognize there is much to be learned about ways to improve the mental health of populations by building on the research and practices of other sectors, such as criminal justice (Fox & Berman, 2002) and education (Domitrovich et al., 2008; Fixsen, Blase, Horner, & Sugai, 2009).

Putting People First in Public Mental Health

Just as mental health care must be fully integrated with general health care, individuals with mental disorders must be integrated fully into the primary care system and be empowered to participate meaningfully in their treatment. Just as mental health services traditionally have been segregated from general health services, persons with severe mental and substance use disorders have been segregated from their communities. Full inclusion in the community with equitable opportunities to participate in all aspects of community life is a goal for all people in our communities. Assistive technologies and skill sets to promote this integration involve health literacy and rehabilitative supports (discussed below). As Carl Bell (2011) has asserted, health promotion and disease prevention are essential tools to eliminate community health disparities.

Consumer involvement in both individual care and policy making improves both outcomes and recovery potential for individuals with serious mental illness (Fisher & Spiro, 2010; IOM, 2006; New Freedom Commission on Mental Health, 2003). Participation in the health and social service delivery systems also improves a sense of citizenship in the population with serious mental illnesses (Chamberlin, 1998). Consumer involvement, person-centered care, and recovery have emerged as priorities for mental health system policy and programming in numerous recent policy documents, among them *Mental Health: A Report of the Surgeon General* (Surgeon General of the United States, 1999), the Institute of Medicine's *Improving the Quality of Health Care for Mental and Substance-Use Conditions* (2006), and the New Freedom Commission report (2003).

IS MENTAL HEALTH LAGGING BEHIND IN CONSUMER INVOLVEMENT?

Both the practice of and evidence base for patient-centeredness, self-management, and peer support appear less developed in the mental health field than in other areas of health care, including treatment for addictions and substance use. Overall, when it comes to mental health, patient-centeredness, self-management, and peer support (discussed below) have yet to be recognized as important elements of quality care, resulting in far fewer documented improved outcomes than in other fields. For example, evidence for improved outcomes due to patient-centeredness in primary care and other specialties has developed markedly over the past decade (Battersby et al., 2010).

In 2007, the National Cancer Institute issued *Patient-Centered Communication in Cancer Care: Promoting Healing and Reducing Suffering* (Epstein & Street, 2007), a report documenting the importance of patient-centeredness for achieving desired outcomes of cancer care. Enough research has been conducted to allow for meta-analyses on studies of patient-centeredness and cancer care (Venetis, Robinson, Turkiewicz, & Allen, 2009). Research on self-management of other chronic conditions, such as limb loss and type 2 diabetes, has shown these types of patient-centered interventions to be effective (S. L. Norris, Engelgau, & Venkat Narayan, 2001; Wegener, Mackenzie, Ephraim, Ehde, & Williams, 2009). The US Department of Veterans Affairs, one of the largest providers of services to persons who have lost limbs, recently announced the creation of its Office of Patient-Centered Care and Cultural Transformation, which focuses on demonstrating new models of care, such as the patient-aligned care team, and analyzing their outcomes.

Peer support has been an essential part of substance abuse treatment since Alcoholics Anonymous (AA) was created in 1935. Courts often mandate AA as part of substance use rehabilitation, sometimes as a condition of jail diversion. Peers also have worked as addiction support specialists in traditional settings since the mid-20th century (White, 2004). Certainly in mental health, an evidence base is rapidly developing for shared decision making, self-management interventions, and peer support (all described below). Yet, despite this trend, stigma remains a barrier to consumer involvement in care—even in person-centered intervention—in clinical practice (IOM, 2006). Complicating the situation still further, research into the evidence base for promising practices in mental health care is fraught with diverse and complex outcomes and variations in study design (Drake et al., 2001). The result is that research evidence is difficult to synthesize and disseminate. Other chronic disease research may not face these challenges and is therefore more accepted and advanced.

CENTRALITY OF RECOVERY

Recovery has been defined as "a journey of healing and transformation enabling a person with a mental health problem to live a meaningful life in a community of his or her choice while striving to achieve his or her full potential" (SAMHSA, 2004). The concept of recovery, rather than symptom mitigation, as a goal has become an important principle in both mental health policy making (SAMHSA, 2004) and research (Surgeon General of the United States, 1999). The public health relevance of this definition of recovery lies in the idea of individuals' ability to lead lives as fully participating members of society, with a right to community integration. It completes the overall public health vision of illness prevention, wellness promotion, patient-focused treatment interventions, and reclaiming psychosocial functioning (Miles, Espiritu, Horen, Sebian, & Waetzig, 2009).

Despite the all too common misconception that consumers of mental health services have impaired decision-making ability, the evidence shows that such incapacity is no more common in this population than in the general population (IOM, 2006). Therefore, in our vision for the future of the public mental health system, we include opportunities for consumers to make decisions at the individual and population levels about prevention, promotion, treatment, and reclaiming life roles (Miles et al., 2009). The next discussions consider specific but not exhaustive strategies for consumer-guided services.

PERSON-CENTERED SERVICES

Patient-centered services are receiving increased attention across a wide array of health issues. The IOM has defined patient-centered care as "care that is respectful of and responsive to individual patient preferences, needs, and values and ensuring that patient values guide all clinical decisions" (IOM, 2006, p. 78) and has used patient-centeredness as an indicator of a high-quality health care system (IOM, 2001).

Since publication of the 2006 IOM report, three maxims of patient-centeredness have been proposed (Berwick, 2009):

- "The needs of the patient come first" asserts that patients know their own interests better than physicians do.
- "Nothing about me without me," a classic slogan from the disability rights movement, speaks to both transparency and participation in care.
- "Every patient is the only patient" emphasizes customized care at the level of the individual and that providers are "guests" in a patient's life rather than "hosts" in the health care system.

For patient-centered care to exist, patients must have access to information that facilitates well-informed health care decisions. "Patient activation"—the skills, knowledge, beliefs, and behaviors necessary for an individual to manage a chronic illness—is an important part of patient-centered care (IOM, 2006). Because the potential for maximal wellness is defined by a person's abilities and resources to improve health behavior (Bruhn, Cordova, Williams, & Fuentes, 1977), person-centeredness must be a part of any public health approach to prevention and health promotion.

HEALTH LITERACY

Health literacy is a key element of the just-mentioned "patient activation," since information about mental health, medical conditions, recovery, and self-direction is an essential consumer empowerment tool. Health literacy can help consumers better independently understand their health and wellness as they engage with providers in planning their care. It also can help healthy individuals stay healthy. According to the IOM (2006), an individual's decision-making capacity rests on three factors: (1) the ability at a point in time to understand, appreciate, reason, and communicate preferences, (2) knowledge of the risks and benefits in specific decisions to be made; and (3) the knowledge and biases of the person making decisions about the individual's capacity.

Evidence suggests that health disparities are related both to an individual's health knowledge and to the perceptions and biases brought to the table by persons advising or making health decisions for the individual. Increased opportunities for improving health literacy can benefit these areas by preparing consumers to make risk–benefit decisions and reasonably assess preferences and by helping providers feel more comfortable with patient-centered decision making. Moreover, health literacy addresses the public need for a better overall understanding of wellness and illness, which in turn can promote healthy and empowered communities (Nielsen-Bohlman, Panzer, & Kindig, 2004). As information-based interventions and systems (e.g., personal health records that the consumer maintains and controls) are developed and implemented as part of health care reform, health literacy will become increasingly important. It will be critical that mental health issues are attended to along with efforts focusing on the broader health care system.

SHARED DECISION MAKING

Shared decision making is "the collaboration between patients and caregivers to come to an agreement about a healthcare decision" (Dartmouth Center for Shared Decision-Making, 2010, http://cancer.dartmouth.edu/pf/cancer_care/shared_decision.html). Most often, it involves the introduction and use of decision aids and patient education. From a practical perspective, shared decision making requires creation of a collaborative process between client and practitioner, both of whom recognize one another as experts and work together to exchange information and clarify values to arrive at health care decisions (Deegan, Rapp, Holter, & Riefer, 2008).

Shared decision making has been shown to be effective in helping patients experiencing any of a variety of physical conditions (e.g., cancer and multiple sclerosis) to make more informed decisions (Frosch & Kaplan, 1999; Heesen et al., 2007; Volk, Cass, & Spann, 1999). The consumer is encouraged to take as much responsibility as possible in making decisions about treatment and in carrying out treatment objectives.

In some cases, evidence-based medicine assumes that informed consumer preferences and choices outweigh objective scientific evidence (Adams & Drake, 2006). For that reason, greater attention should be paid to the content of decision aids—"information interventions" to help consumers understand the pros and cons of a decision (Adams & Drake, 2006). At the same time, research is needed to develop even more effective mental health care decision aids and to integrate those efforts with broader health efforts while still working to improve outcomes for persons with mental illnesses (Adams & Drake, 2006; Joosten et al., 2008).

The importance of shared decision making has been codified in the Patient Protection and Affordable Care Act, which directs the US Department of Health and Human Services to produce decision aids that are meaningful for patients across the life span and disease conditions. Some stakeholders see shared decision making as a vehicle for cost containment (Braddock, 2010), but it also promotes a partnership of providers and patients that allows both to view health care in the context of individual needs and community resources.

SELF-MANAGEMENT AND WELLNESS

Efforts to improve self-management for persons with mental illness should approach wellness promotion, treatment, and recovery from a holistic perspective—one that values the mental, physical, and social aspects of a person's life. Self-management has many dimensions, including empowerment, self-efficacy, personal responsibility, and interdependence with other persons in the community. As such, the use of self-management and wellness tools is an important part of sustaining long-term recovery. Self-management interventions, such as Illness Management and

Recovery (a SAMHSA evidence-based practice [EBP]) and the Wellness Recovery Action Plan have been shown to improve both recovery and symptom-related outcomes (Cook, 2009; Mueser et al., 2002). Self-management interventions can be used to promote both mental health recovery and more holistic definitions of wellness. For instance, self-management interventions are seen frequently for control of diseases such as diabetes (Funnell et al., 2009).

With the recent enactment of the Patient Protection and Affordable Care Act, an emerging emphasis on the integration of mental and physical wellness has prompted the development of new consumer-focused treatment and recovery interventions for persons with mental illness. A skeletal prototype that emerged from the recent ACMHA Summit in New Orleans (an annual meeting of leaders in the behavioral health field) is a peer-led, accountable community wellness organization. These organizations would be "peer-led healthy communities that promote wellness and are accountable for the whole health of members" (Manderscheid, 2011, p. 1) that would be similar in role and structure to accountable care organizations. Self-help centers already provide peer support for wellness promotion among persons recovering from mental disorders (Swarbrick & Ellis, 2009) and are training peer wellness coaches to join the mental health workforce to help others with or in recovery from mental illnesses to identify health-related goals and maintain a healthy lifestyle (Swarbrick, Murphy, Zechner, Spagnolo, & Gill, 2011).

PEER SUPPORT

Peer support, a system of giving and receiving help, is founded on the core principles of respect, shared responsibility, and mutual agreement on what is helpful. Peer support programs, which are available for people experiencing or recovering from any number of illnesses (e.g., cancer, amputation, and addictions), recognize peers as more likely than other people to understand the situation of others with the similar experiences of illness and service use empathically through common experience and shared emotional and psychological pain (Mead & MacNeil, 2006).

In mental health, peer support is the outgrowth of a political movement: the mental health consumer movement, which has changed the shape and structure of mental health services in ways that inform a public health approach. Behavioral health peer support services are provided by individuals who self-identify as having mental illnesses, who are receiving or have received mental health services, and who in turn deliver services to help others with mental disorders bring about desired social or personal change (Temple University Collaborative on Community Inclusion of Individuals with Psychiatric Disabilities, 2011). Peer-run services include but are not limited to drop-in centers, crisis services, and employment services that are planned, operated, and managed by people with mental disorders.

As adjuncts to traditional mental health services, consumer-operated or self-help services have been found to improve outcomes compared to traditional services alone (Campbell, 2009; Segal, Silverman, & Temkin, 2010). The SAMHSA and its Center for Mental Health Services have designated both support delivered by peer specialists in traditional settings and consumer-operated services as evidence-based practices (Campbell et al., 2006; Mann, 2010; Van Tosh & del Vecchio, 2000). Peer support offers positive role models for persons with severe mental illnesses, benefiting both the giver and the receiver. Thus peer support can assist persons with serious mental illnesses in combating negative self-images or self-stigma. With more positive self-images, such individuals are more likely to engage in productive roles as a part of the larger community.

Although numerous programs engage peers in service provision, the value of peer intervention has been less noticeable in the emerging work on communities and the social and physical determinants of health. Peer support in that area needs to be explored in greater depth, since the tools developed by the modern consumer movement in the United States can facilitate implementation of the public health model in mental health and implementation of the Patient Protection and Affordable Care Act. Peer support is a vehicle to enable community participation in health promotion and disease prevention; through it, persons with mental illnesses can provide consumer leadership to promote a holistic approach to both wellness and prevention (Manderscheid, 2011).

SELF-DIRECTED CARE

Whether well or ill, people want to be in charge of their lives. Self-directed care is a direct response to that issue for people with mental illnesses. Instead of insurers paying providers for care, self-directed care enables consumers to select and pay for the goods and services available in the health care marketplace that will best promote their individual recovery. Self-directed care also allows a person to purchase community-based wellness services, such as those that provide opportunities for physical fitness or provide supports for community participation.

In self-directed care, consumers will create a budget with the help of a "recovery coach" to purchase services tailored to their individualized recovery and rehabilitation needs. It will be possible to purchase both traditional and nontraditional services (Barczyk & Lincove, 2010). Self-directed care programs have a five-part basic framework (Doty, Mahoney, & Simon-Rusinowitz, 2007):

- Develop a "recovery plan," including services to be purchased and supports to be used, potential barriers to goals, and coping strategies.
- Create a budget allocating dollars to the goods and services included in the recovery plan.
- Receive assistance from a life coach trained in self-directed planning and recovery-oriented care.
- Work with a financial intermediary on managing one's funds, such as paying providers, tracking the budget, and documenting purchases. Financial intermediaries usually work either directly for or on contract to the self-directed care program.
- Monitor and implement the self-directed care plan and budget with the support of the life coach.

Self-directed care programs are offered through Medicaid in some states and counties; programs vary significantly. The Patient Protection and Affordable Care Act offers an opportunity to expand this model through its provisions to expand Medicaid state waivers. While only limited data are available, it appears that self-directed care programs reduce use of crisis services and improve consumer satisfaction (Alakeson, 2010; Cook, Russell, Grey, & Jonikas, 2008).

Consumer Self-Direction and the Public Health

Achieving or maintaining health is a complex process that requires advocates, including consumers (who, accustomed to being disempowered, frequently need to be taught, coached, and mentored), to take on roles as effective change makers (Fisher & Spiro, 2010). Preferences for involvement may depend on an individual's level of insight and recovery status. As consumers progress in recovery, they may become more empowered. Because persons who take a more active role in decision making and managing their illnesses are healthier over time, engaging consumers in motivational techniques can promote health (Torrey & Drake, 2009). This kind of responsibility for one's own health is an essential component of the public health approach, as it empowers people as members of a community to promote both mental and physical wellness. Consumer involvement presents both opportunities to promote population mental health and challenges to a mental health care system that is changing under newly enacted health care reform policies.

Unfortunately, insufficient research has been undertaken on person-centered care, peer support, and the outcomes of consumer involvement. As health coverage policies become more focused on evidence-based interventions, it is critical that research be conducted on all aspects of the public health model: community effects, prevention, promotion, treatment, and recovery. The resulting evidence should allow identification of the strategies that work when outcomes are measured at the level of the population as well

as those that are effective when implemented state-wide and in urban and suburban communities with large populations.

CONCLUSION

Although we are hesitant to predict the future, it is likely that the adverse consequences of mental and behavioral disorders for overall health and well-being will continue until those problems become more salient to policy makers, planners, and the general public. As this chapter suggests, a public health orientation, while no panacea, offers a promising mix of models, intervention approaches, and methodological techniques to address the challenges being confronted by multiple health and human service systems (Kolko, Hoagwood, & Springgate, 2010; Miles et al., 2009). An important aspect of a public health perspective is expanding attention beyond access to and effectiveness of treatments to include reducing the incidence of mental and behavioral problems and maximizing health and well-being even after the occurrence of a mental disorder.

As the current director of NIMH has acknowledged:

> None of the progress we are seeing in clinical research will have the necessary impact on public health unless we can close the gap between what we know and what we apply in practice. This translational gap exists throughout medicine, but the problem is more acute in psychiatry because so much of mental health care takes place outside the health care system. (Insel, 2009, p. 131)

It is hardly likely that continuing the same strategy will result in the improvements in outcomes seen with other disorders and in other countries. If we are to aim to improve the health of the population by increasing overall health and by reducing disparities and inequities, we will need a theory of change that focuses on those outcomes. Efforts to improve individual services and to create a better understanding of risk will, in and of themselves, not likely translate into effects observed in the population.

As we move through the 21st century, we will need to begin with a clear focus on the outcomes we seek to achieve in collaboration with consumers, family members, community-based organizations, government organizations, and health care providers. We must implement with high fidelity those policies and practices most certain to promote positive mental health and functioning for those with mental disorders. We need to include consumers, health care providers, and other service providers in the development, implementation, and monitoring of strategies to reduce the prevalence and consequences of mental disorders in the population. Any other strategy is likely to perpetuate the unacceptably slow developments that have occurred since Winslow's 1926 presidential address and that continue to lag behind progress in other fields of health and illness.

The public health approach envisioned here for the future of the mental health field will coalesce work on communities and on the social and physical determinants of health not only with developments in self-direction and peer supports but also with the new programs and incentives of the Patient Protection and Affordable Care Act. This is all very exciting. We should be optimistic about the potential of these new linkages for addressing many of the problems identified in this text.

REFERENCES

Adams, J., & Drake, R. (2006). Shared decision-making and evidence-based practice. *Community Mental Health Journal, 42*(1), 87–105.

Alakeson, V. (2010). International development in self-directed care. *Commonwealth Fund Issue Brief, 78*, 1–12.

Anglin, D. M., Alberti, P. M., Link, B. G., & Phelan, J. C. (2008). Racial differences in beliefs about the effectiveness and necessity of mental health treatment. *American Journal of Community Psychology, 41*(1–2), 17–24.

Atkins, M. S., Hoagwood, K. E., Kutash, K., & Seidman, E. (2010). Toward the integration of education and mental health in schools. *Administration and Policy in Mental Health and Mental Health Services Research, 37*(1), 40–47.

Barczyk, A. N., & Lincove, J. A. (2010). Cash and Counseling: A model for self-directed care programs to empower individuals with serious mental illnesses. *Social Work in Mental Health, 8*(3), 209–224.

Battersby, M., Von Korff, M., Schaefer, J., Davis, C., Ludman, E., Greene, S.,…Wagner, E. (2010). Twelve evidence-based principles for implementing self-management support in primary care. *Joint Commission Journal on Quality and Patient Safety, 36*(12), 561–570.

Bell, C. C. (2011). NIMH needs stronger prevention focus. *Clinical Psychiatry News, 39*, 19.

Berwick, D. M. (2009). What "patient-centered" should mean: Confessions of an extremist. *Health Affairs, 28*(4), 555–565.

Bonanno, G. A. (2004). Loss, trauma, and human resilience: Have we underestimated the human capacity to thrive after extremely adversive events? *American Psychologist, 59*(1), 20–28.

Braddock, C. H. (2010). The emerging importance and relevance of shared decision making to clinical practice. *Medical Decision Making, 30* (5 Suppl.), 5s–7s.

Braverman, P. A., Egerter, S. A., Woolf, S. H., & Marks, J. S. (2011). When do we know enough to recommend action on the social determinants of health? *American Journal of Preventive Medicine, 40*(1 Suppl.), s58–s66.

Bruhn, J. G., Cordova, F. D., Williams, J. A., & Fuentes, R. G. (1977). The wellness process. *Journal of Community Health, 2*(3), 209–221.

Campbell, J. (2009). *Federal multi-site study finds consumer-operated service programs are evidence-based practices.* St. Louis, MO: Missouri Institute of Mental Health.

Campbell, J., Lichtenstein, C., Teague, G., Johnsen, M., Yates, B., & Sonnefeld, J. (2006). *The Consumer Operated Service Programs (COSP) multi-site research initiative: Final report.* St. Louis, MO: Coordinating Center at the Missouri Institute of Mental Health.

Carter, A. S., Wagmiller, R. J., Gray, S. A. O., McCarthy, K. J., Horwitz, S. M., & Briggs-Gowan, M. J. (2010). Prevalence of DSM-IV disorder in a representative, healthy birth cohort at school entry: Sociodemographic risks and social adaptation. *Journal of the American Academy of Child and Adolescent Psychiatry, 49*(7), 686–698.

Chamberlin, J. (1998). Citizenship rights and psychiatric disability. *Psychiatric Rehabilitation, 21*, 405–408.

Colton, C., & Manderscheid, R. (2006). Congruencies in increased mortality rates, years of potential life lost, and causes of death among public mental health clients in eight states. *Preventing Chronic Disease, 3*(2), 1–14.

Commission on Social Determinants of Health of the World Health Organization. (2008). *Closing the gap in a generation: Health equity through action on the social determinants of health.* Geneva, Switzerland: World Health Organization. Retrieved from http://www.who.int/social_determinants/thecommission/finalreport/en/index.html

Cook, J. A. (2009). *Mental illness self-management through wellness recovery action planning: WRAP evidence base.* West Dummerston, VT: Copeland Center.

Cook, J. A., Russell, C., Grey, D. D., & Jonikas, J. A. (2008). Economic grand rounds: A self-directed care model for mental health recovery. *Psychiatric Services, 59*(6), 600–602.

Costello, E. J., Compton, S. N., Keeler, G., & Angold, A. (2003). Relationships between poverty and psychopathology: A natural experiment. *Journal of the American Medical Association, 290*(15), 2023–2029.

Costello, E. J., Erkanli, A., Copeland, W., & Angold, A. (2010). Association of family income supplements in adolescence with development of psychiatric and substance use disorders in adulthood. *Journal of the American Medical Association, 303*(19), 1954–1960.

Dartmouth Center for Shared Decision-Making. (2010). *Mission, vision, and goals.* Retrieved from http://www.dhmc.org/shared_decision_making.cfm

Deegan, P., Rapp, C., Holter, M., & Riefer, M. (2008). Best practices: A program to support shared decision making in an outpatient psychiatric medication clinic. *Psychiatric Services, 59*(6), 603–605.

Dohrenwend, B. S., & Dohrenwend, B. P. (1982). Perspectives on the past and future of psychiatric epidemiology: The 1981 Rema Lapouse Lecture. *American Journal of Public Health, 72,* 1271–1279.

Domitrovich, C. E., Bradshaw, C. P., Poduska, J., Hoagwood, K., Buckley, J., Olin, S., . . . Ialongo, N. S. (2008). Maximizing the implementation quality of evidence-based preventive interventions in schools: A conceptual framework. *Advances in School Mental Health Promotion: Training and Practice, Research and Policy, 1*(3), 6–28.

Doty, P., Mahoney, K. J., & Simon-Rusinowitz, L. (2007). Designing the Cash and Counseling demonstration and evaluation. *Health Services Research, 42*(1 Pt. 2), 378–396.

Drake, R. E., Goldman, H. H., Leff, H. S., Lehman, A. F., Dixon, L., Mueser, K. T., & Torrey, W. C. (2001). Implementing evidence-based practices in routine mental health service settings. *Psychiatric Services, 52*(2), 179–182.

Epstein, R., & Street, R., Jr. (2007). *Patient-centered communication in cancer care: Promoting healing and reducing suffering.* Bethesda, MD: National Cancer Institute, National Institutes of Health, US Department of Health and Human Services.

Evans, G. W., & Kantrowitz, E. (2002). Socioeconomic status and health: The potential role of environmental risk exposure. *Annual Review of Public Health, 23*(1), 303–331.

Felitti, V. J., & Anda, R. F. (2010). The relationship of adverse childhood experiences to adult medical disease, psychiatric disorders, and sexual behavior: Implications for healthcare. In R. Lanius & E. Vermetten (Eds.), *The impact of early life trauma on health and disease: The hidden epidemic.* London, UK: Cambridge University Press.

Fisher, D., & Spiro, L. (2010). Finding and using our voice: How consumer/survivor advocacy is transforming mental health care. In L. D. Brown & S. Wituk (Eds.), *Mental health self-help* (pp. 213–233). New York, NY: Springer.

Fixsen, D. L., Blase, K. A., Horner, R., & Sugai, G. (2009). *Concept paper: Developing the capacity for scaling up the effective use of evidence-based programs in state departments of education.* Retrieved from University of Connecticut web site: http://www.uconnucedd.org/lend/readings/2011/pdfs/Session%2025%20-%20Mar%2025,%202011/Concept_Paper_SISEP_0409_WEB.

Fixsen, D. L., Naoom, S. F., Blase, K. A., Friedman, R. M., & Wallace, F. (2005). *Implementation research: A synthesis of the literature.* Tampa, FL: Louis de la Parte Florida Mental Health Institute, University of South Florida.

Fox, A., & Berman, G. (2002). Going to Scale: A Conversation About the Future of Drug Courts. *Court Review, 39*(3), 4–13.

Frosch, D. L., & Kaplan, R. M. (1999). Shared decision making in clinical medicine: Past research and future directions. *American Journal of Preventive Medicine, 17*(4), 285–294.

Funnell, M. M., Brown, T. L., Childs, B. P., Haas, L. B., Hosey, G. M., Jensen, B., . . . Weiss, M. A. (2009). National standards for diabetes self-management education. *Diabetes Care, 32*(Suppl. 1), S87–S94.

Grob, G. (1991). *From asylum to community: Mental health policy in modern America.* Princeton, NJ: Princeton University Press.

Heesen, C., Kasper, J., Köpke, S., Richter, T., Segal, J., & Mühlhauser, I. (2007). Informed shared decision making in multiple sclerosis—inevitable or impossible? *Journal of Neurological Sciences, 259*(1–2), 109–117.

Hollingshead, A. B., & Redlich, F. C. (1958). *Social class and mental illness: Community study.* New York, NY: Wiley.

Insel, T. R. (2009). Translating scientific opportunity into public health impact: A strategic plan for research on mental illness. *Archives of General Psychiatry, 66*(2), 128–133.

Insel, T. R. (2011, January 26). *Director's blog: The economics of health care reform.* Retrieved from National Institute of Mental Health web site at www.nimh.nih.gov/about/director/2011/the-economics-of-health-care-reform.shtml

Institute of Medicine. (2001). *Crossing the quality chasm: A new health system for the 21st century.* Washington, DC: National Academies Press.

Institute of Medicine. (2006). *Improving the quality of health care for mental and substance-use conditions.* Washington, DC: National Academies Press.

Institute of Medicine. (2009). *Preventing mental, emotional, and behavioral disorders among young people: Progress and possibilities.* Washington, DC: National Academies Press.

Joosten, E., DeFuentes-Merillas, L., De Weert, G., Sensky, T., Van der Staak, C., & De Jong, C. (2008). Systematic review of the effects of shared decision-making on patient satisfaction, treatment adherence and health status. *Psychotherapy and Psychosomatics, 77*(4), 219–226.

Kessler, R. C., Amminger, G. P., Aguilar-Gaxiola, S., Alonso, J., Lee, S., & Ustun, T. B. (2007). Age of onset of mental disorders: A review of recent literature. *Current Opinion in Psychiatry, 20*(4), 359–364.

Kessler, R. C., Berglund, P., Demler, O., Jin, R., & Walters, E. E. (2005). Lifetime prevalence and age-of-onset distributions of DSM-IV disorders in the National Comorbidity Survey Replication. *Archives of General Psychiatry, 62*(6), 593–602.

Kessler, R. C., Demler, O., Frank, R. G., Olfson, M., Pincus, H. A., Walters, E. E.,...Zaslavsky, A. M. (2005). Prevalence and treatment of mental disorders: 1990–2003. *New England Journal of Medicine, 352*(24), 2515–2523.

Kolko, D. J., Hoagwood, K. E., & Springgate, B. (2010). Treatment research for children and youth exposed to traumatic events: Moving beyond efficacy to amp up public health impact. *General Hospital Psychiatry, 32*(5), 465–476.

Kramer, M. (1969) Applications of mental health statistics: Uses in mental health programmes of statistics derived from psychiatric services and selected vital and morbidity records. Geneva, Switzerland: World Health Organization.

Link, B. G., & Phelan, J. C. (2006). Stigma and its public health implications. *Lancet, 367*(9509), 528–529.

Manderscheid, R. W. (2010). Evolution and integration of primary care services with specialty services. In B. Lubotsky Levin, K. Hennessy, & J. Petrila (Eds.), *Mental health services: A public health perspective* (pp. 389–400). New York, NY: Oxford University Press.

Manderscheid, R. (2011, March 23). Are peer-led wellness communities in our future? *Behavioral Healthcare.* Retrieved from http://www.behavioral.net/article/are-peer-led-wellness-communities-our-future

Mann, C. (2010, May). *Communication to state Medicaid directors on Community Living Initiative.* Baltimore, MD: Center for Medicaid, CHIP, and Survey and Certification, Center for Medicare and Medicaid Services, US Department of Health and Human Services. Retrieved from https://www.cms.gov/smdl/downloads/smd10008.pdf

McEwen, B. S. (2007). Physiology and neurobiology of stress and adaptation: Central role of the brain. *Physiological Reviews, 87*(3), 873–904.

McKinlay, J. B., & McKinlay, S. M. (1977). The questionable contribution of medical measures to the decline of mortality in the United States in the twentieth century. *Milbank Memorial Fund Quarterly. Health and Society, 55*(3), 405–428.

Mead, S., & MacNeil, C. (2006). Peer support: What makes it unique? *International Journal of Psychosocial Rehabilitation, 10*(2), 29–37.

Merikangas, K. R., He, J., Burstein, M., Swendsen, J., Avenevoli, S., Case, B.,...Olfson, M. (2010). Service utilization for lifetime mental disorders in US adolescents: Results of the National Comorbidity Survey–Adolescent Supplement (NCS-A). *Journal of the American Academy of Child and Adolescent Psychiatry, 50*(1), 32–45.

Messias, E., Eaton, W. W., & Grooms, A. N. (2011). Economic grand rounds: Income inequality and depression prevalence across the United States: An ecological study. *Psychiatric Services, 62*(7), 710–712.

Miles, J., Espiritu, R., Horen, N., Sebian, J., & Waetzig, E. (2009). *A public health approach to children's mental health: A conceptual framework.* Washington, DC: Georgetown University Center for Child and Human Development.

Mueser, K. T., Corrigan, P. W., Hilton, D. W., Tanzman, B., Schaub, A., Gingerich, S.,...Herz, M. I. (2002). Illness management and recovery: A review of the research. *Psychiatric Services, 53*(10), 1272–1284.

Murray, C. J. L., & Lopez, A. D. (1996). *The global burden of disease: A comprehensive assessment of mortality and disability from diseases, injuries, and risk factors in 1990 and projected to 2020.* Cambridge, MA: Harvard University Press.

National Institute of Mental Health. (2008). *National Institute of Mental Health strategic plan.* Rockville, MD: National Institute of Mental Health, National Institutes of Health, US Department of Health and Human Services

New Freedom Commission on Mental Health. (2003). *Achieving the promise: Transforming mental health care in America.* Rockville, MD: Substance Abuse and Mental Health Services Administration, US Department of Health and Human Services.

Nielsen-Bohlman, L., Panzer, A., & Kindig, D. (2004). *Health literacy: A prescription to end confusion.* Washington, DC: National Academies Press.

Norris, F. H., Stevens, S. P., Pfefferbaum, B., Wyche, K. F., & Pfefferbaum, R. L. (2008). Community resilience as a metaphor, theory, set of capacities, and strategy for disaster readiness. *American Journal of Community Psychology, 41*(1), 127–150.

Norris, S. L., Engelgau, M. M., & Venkat Narayan, K. M. (2001). Effectiveness of self-management training in type 2 diabetes. *Diabetes Care, 24*(3), 561–587.

Patel, V., Flisher, A. J., Hetrick, S., & McGorry, P. (2007). Mental health of young people: A global public-health challenge. *Lancet, 369*(9569), 1302–1303.

Patient Protection and Affordable Care Act, Pub. L. No. 111–148, 124 Stat. 119 *through* 124 Stat. 1025 (2010).

Pescosolido, B. A., Martin, J. K., Long, J. S., Medina, T. R., Phelan, J. C., & Link, B. G. (2010). A disease like any other? A decade of change in public reactions to schizophrenia, depression, and alcohol dependence. *American Journal of Psychiatry, 167*(11), 1321–1330.

President's Commission on Mental Health. (1978). *Report to the president from the President's Commission on Mental Health.* Washington, DC: US Government Printing Office.

Redlich, A. D., & Cusack, K. J. (2010). Mental health treatment in criminal justice settings. In B. Lubotsky Levin, K. Hennessey, & J. Petrila (Eds.), *Mental health services: A public health perspective* (pp. 421–440). New York, NY: Oxford University Press.

Robins, L. N., & Regier, D. A. (1991). *Psychiatric disorders in America: The Epidemiologic Catchment Area study.* New York, NY: Free Press.

Segal, S. P., Silverman, C. J., & Temkin, T. L. (2010). Self-help and community mental health agency outcomes: A recovery-focused randomized controlled trial. *Psychiatric Services, 61*(9), 905–910.

Srole, L. (1975). Measurement and classification in socio-psychiatric epidemiology: Midtown Manhattan study (1954) and Midtown Manhattan restudy (1974). *Journal of Health and Social Behavior, 16*(4), 347–364.

Substance Abuse and Mental Health Services Administration. (2004). *National consensus statement on mental health recovery.* Rockville, MD: Substance Abuse and Mental Health Services Administration, US Department of Health and Human Services.

Substance Abuse and Mental Health Services Administration. (2010). *Results from the 2009 National Survey on Drug Use and Health: Summary of national findings.* Rockville, MD: Substance Abuse and Mental Health Services Administration, US Department of Health and Human Services

Substance Abuse and Mental Health Services Administration. (2011). *Leading change: A plan for SAMHSA's role and actions 2011–2014.* Rockville, MD: Substance Abuse and Mental Health Services Administration, US Department of Health and Human Services.

Surgeon General of the United States. (1999). *Mental health: A report of the surgeon general.* Rockville, MD: Office of the Surgeon General, US Department of Health and Human Services.

Swarbrick, M., & Ellis, J. (2009). Peer-operated self-help centers. *Occupational Therapy in Mental Health, 25*(3), 239–251.

Swarbrick, M., Murphy, A. A., Zechner, M., Spagnolo, A. B., & Gill, K. J. (2011). Wellness coaching: A new role for peers. *Psychiatric Rehabilitation Journal, 34*(4), 328–331.

Temple University Collaborative on Community Inclusion of Individuals with Psychiatric Disabilities. (2011). *Fact sheet on peer support.* Retrieved from http://tucollaborative.org/comm_inclusion/peer_support.html

Torrey, W., & Drake, R. (2009). Practicing shared decision making in the outpatient psychiatric care of adults with severe mental illnesses: Redesigning care for the future. *Community Mental Health Journal, 46*(5), 433–440.

United Nations Economic and Social Council. (2008, December). *Realizing the Millennium Development Goals for persons with disabilities through the implementation of the World Programme of Action concerning Disabled Persons* and the Convention on the Rights of Persons with Disabilities (Resolution A/RES/63/160). Retrieved from http:www.un.org/disabilities/default.asp?id=1463

Van Tosh, L., & del Vecchio, P. (2000). *Consumer-operated self-help programs: A technical report.* Rockville, MD: Substance Abuse and Mental Health Services Administration, US Department of Health and Human Services.

Venetis, M., Robinson, J., Turkiewicz, K., & Allen, M. (2009). An evidence base for patient-centered cancer care: A meta-analysis of studies of observed communication between cancer specialists and their patients. *Patient Education and Counseling, 77*(3), 379–383.

Volk, R. J., Cass, A. R., & Spann, S. J. (1999). A randomized controlled trial of shared decision making for prostate cancer screening. *Archives of Family Medicine, 8*(4), 333–340.

Wang, P. S., Demler, O., & Kessler, R. C. (2002). Adequacy of treatment for serious mental illness in the United States. *American Journal of Public Health, 92*(1), 92–98.

Ward, E., Jemal, A., Cokkinides, V., Singh, G. K., Cardinez, C., Ghafoor, A., & Thun, M. (2004). Cancer disparities by race/ethnicity and socioeconomic status. *CA: A Cancer Journal for Clinicians, 54*(2), 78–93.

Wegener, S. T., Mackenzie, E. J., Ephraim, P., Ehde, D., & Williams, R. (2009). Self-management improves outcomes in persons with limb loss. *Archives of Physical Medicine and Rehabilitation, 90*(3), 373–380.

White, W. (2004, March). *The history and future of peer-based addiction recovery support services.* Paper presented at the SAMHSA Consumer and Family Direction Initiative Summit, Washington, DC. Retrieved from http://www.facesandvoicesofrecovery.org/pdf/peer-based_recovery.pdf

Wilkinson, R., & Pickett, K. (2010). *The spirit level: Why equality is better for everyone* (2nd ed.). London, UK: Penguin.

Williams, D. R., Neighbors, H. W., & Jackson, J. S. (2008). Racial/ethnic discrimination and health: Findings from community studies. *American Journal of Public Health, 93*(2), 200–208.

Winslow, C.-E. A. (1926). Public health at the crossroads. *American Journal of Public Health, 16*(11), 1075–1085.

World Health Organization. (2002). *Prevention and promotion in mental health.* Geneva, Switzerland: Author.

World Health Organization. (2003). *Caring for children and adolescents with mental disorders: Setting WHO directions.* Geneva, Switzerland: Author.

World Health Organization. (2004). *Prevention of mental disorders: Effective interventions and policy options.* Geneva, Switzerland: Author.

World Health Organization. (2008a). *The global burden of disease: 2004 update.* Geneva, Switzerland: Author.

World Health Organization. (2008b). *Mental health: Integrating mental health into primary care: A global perspective.* Geneva, Switzerland: Author.

World Health Organization. (2009a). *Improving health systems and services for mental health.* Geneva, Switzerland: Author.

World Health Organization. (2009b). *Mental health, resilience and inequalities.* Geneva, Switzerland: WHO Regional Office for Europe, World Health Organization.

World Health Organization. (2010). *Mental health and development: Targeting people with mental health conditions as a vulnerable group.* Geneva, Switzerland: Author.

Wynder, E. L. (1994). Revealing the causes of chronic disease epidemics: From research to prevention. *Annals of Medicine, 26*(1), 57–59.

Index

bipolar disorder (*Cont.*)
  socioeconomic status and, 161
  universal prevalence rates, 156
  urban living and, 183, 183
Bowlby, John, 282
brain development, executive functions and, 246–248
  declines in, 248
  IADL and, 248
brain fag, 44
Brandeis, Louis D., 355
Breuer, Josef, 270
bulimia nervosa
  diagnostic criteria for, 13
  symptoms of, 12
Burger, Warren, 365
Burlingham, Dorothy, 273
Bush, George H. W., 428

Cache County Study of Memory in Aging, 110
CAGE scale, 76
Canadian Community Health Survey (CCHS), 9, 10
Cannon, Walter, 271
career. *See* work, stress and
case-control studies, 92
case management, in CBHOs, 407–408
  care models for, 408
  development of, 407
  goals of, 407
  integrative structure for, 407–408
CBHOs. *See* community behavioral health organizations
CBM. *See* Christian Blind Mission
CBT. *See* cognitive-behavioral therapy
CCHS. *See* Canadian Community Health Survey
CeaseFire program, 485–486
Center for Epidemiologic Studies Depression Scale-Revision
  (CESD-R), 76
CESD-R. *See* Center for Epidemiologic Studies Depression
  Scale-Revision
child development
  cultural influences on, 51
  stress and
    acute exposure, 273
    attachment theory and, 286
    life-course perspective on, 285
    maltreatment as influence on, 282, 286–287
    peer relationships and, 287–288
    school relationships and, 287–288
    youth mentoring for, 487–488
Child Health Insurance Plan (CHIP), 433
child sexual abuse
  as trauma, 307
  and PTSD, 307
  and suicide, 310
children's rights. *See also* juvenile justice system
  juvenile justice as, 369–371
    In re Gault, 354–355, 370–371
  mental health and, 368–371
    informed consent, 368–369
    right to refuse treatment, 368–369
    right to treatment, 369
children's services, in U.S., 383
Chile, mental illness in, treatment therapies for, cultural
  influences on, 53
China, neurasthenia in, 44
CHIP. *See* Child Health Insurance Plan
Christian Blind Mission (CBM), 454
Christoffel, Ernst Jakob, 454
chromosomes, 202–203
  DNA in, 203

histones in, 203
Churchill, Winston, 355
CIDI. *See* Composite International Diagnostic Interview
Civil Rights of Institutionalized Persons Act (U.S.), 366
Clinical Descriptions and Diagnostic Guidelines (WHO), 32
clozapine, 403
clubhouse model, for CBHOs, 409–411
  Fountain House, 410
  goals of, 410
  humanistic model of rehabilitation in, 411
  ICCD surveys for, 410
  limitations of, 411
  We Are Not Alone program and, 409–410
CMHC Act. *See* Mental Retardation Facilities and
  Community Mental Health Centers Construction Act
CNCG studies. *See* Cross-National Collaborative
  Group studies
cognitive-behavioral therapy (CBT), 404
  socio-cultural influences on, 53
  TF-CBT, 331–332
cognitive disorders
  dementia. *See also* Alzheimer's disease
    age of onset for, 137
    costs for treatment, in U.S., 392
    in GBD, 19
    pellagra and, 463
  in GBD, 17–19
  schizophrenia
    in Africa, local community response to, 50
    age of onset for, 136–137, 250
    chronic medical conditions and, 142
    classifications of, 18
    costs for treatment, in U.S., 391
    diagnostic criteria for, 18
    diathesis-stress models for, 280
    ethnicity and, 169–171
    etiology of, 250
    executive functions with, 250–251, 251
    in GBD, 17–19
    genetic studies for, 215–217
    IPSS, 45–46, 50
    marital status and, 178, 179
    outcome analysis for, 142–144
    prevention strategies for, 471–472
    race and, 169–171
    socioeconomic status and, 160–162, 162
    universal prevalence rates, 156
    urban living and, 183–184, 184
cohort studies, 92. *See also* Epidemiologic Catchment Area
  program
Collaborative Psychiatric Epidemiology Surveys (CPES), 9,
  10. *See also* ethnicity, mental disorders and; marital
  status, mental disorders and; race, mental disorders
  and; socioeconomic status, mental disorders and;
  urbanicity, mental disorders and
  methodology, 153–155
  SDS in, 10
college students, mental health and, 376–378
  confidentiality, 376–378
  liability issues, 376–378
Collins, Francis, 202
communities, prevention strategies for, 483–489. *See also*
  specific community programs
  advantages of, 483
  as broad-based, 484–485
  institutional interventions for, 486–487
  as social determinants of health, 517–518
  for substance abuse, 488–489
  for underserved populations, 486–487

for violence prevention, 485–486
through youth mentoring, 487–488
Communities That Care (CTC) program, 484–485
community behavioral health organizations (CBHOs), 397–399
ACT in, 408–409
clinical effectiveness of, 409
development of, 408–409
function of, 409
case management in, 407–408
care models for, 408
development of, 407
goals of, 407
integrative structure for, 407–408
as change agent, during community tools era, 405–406
clubhouse model for, 409–411
Fountain House, 410
goals of, 410
humanistic model of rehabilitation in, 411
ICCD surveys for, 410
limitations of, 411
We Are Not Alone program and, 409–410
functions of, 397–398
management structure for, 397
for mental disorder treatment, 398
professional staffing in, 398–399
rehabilitation services under, 404–405
services in, 397, 407–412
continuum of, 398
supported employment services in, 411–412
community health services, in U.S.
under CMHC Act, 402–405
community support tools under, 404–405
psychoactive drug development under, 403–404
psychotherapy under, 404
during community tools era, 402–406
change agents during, 405–406
rehabilitation services during, 404–405
during institutional era, 401–402
asylums, 399–400, 400, 402
expansion of facilities, 401
treatment goals, 401–402
under Medicaid, 405–406
under Medicare, 405
during recovery era, 406
conceptual goals during, 406
under Mental Health Parity and Addiction Equity Act, 406, 417, 433
under Patient Protection and Affordable Care Act, 393, 406, 433
under Social Security Act, 405
SSDI program in, 405
SSI program in, 405
Community Mental Health Centers and Mental Retardation Act of 1963 (U.S.), 383
Community Support Program, 383
community tools era, for U.S. health services, 402–406
change agents during, 405–406
rehabilitation services during, 404–405
competency for consent, 360–361
APA guidelines for, 361
competency to stand trial, 374
complicated grief, 308
composite estimators, 109
Composite International Diagnostic Interview (CIDI), 47
for assessment of mental disorders, 73
in U.S., 386
concentration camp survivors, PTSD in, 318–321

conduct disorder
characteristics of, 12
cost of treatment, in U.S., 391, 392
genetic studies for, 225
confidentiality, 358–359
for college students, 376–378
consciousness. *See also* the mind
in behavior perspective of psychiatry, 37
definition of, 33
in dimensional perspective of psychiatry, 36–37
in disease perspective of psychiatry, 34–36
experiential modalities of, 37–38
extrinsic modalities of, 37–38
in life-story perspective of psychiatry, 37–38
self-differentiating modalities of, 36–37
structure of, 33
teleological modalities of, 37
Constitution, U.S., 354–358
due process under, 354–355, 354–355
hypothetical case for, 358
equal protection clause under, 355–356
ADA under, 356, 366, 367
law of supremacy and, 353
reserved powers under, 357–358
parens patriae, 358
police powers, 357–358
right to liberty under, 356
right to privacy under, 356–357
as source of laws, 353
construct validity, 67
consumers, for mental health care systems
consumer-directed care, 521
in global mental health systems, 521
content validity, 67
coping
resilience and, 283, 283–284
Coping Power program, 479
Coping with Depression (CWD) course, 471
cortisol
release of, after acute crisis response, 304
salivary, stress measurement with, 276
CPES. *See* Collaborative Psychiatric Epidemiology Surveys
crime, exposure to, as traumatic event, 314–317
criminal law. *See also* juvenile justice system
basic concepts in, 371
competency to stand trial, 374
mental health and, 371–375
duty to protect and, 374–375
GBMI, 372, 373–374
insanity defense, 372, 371–373
special courts for, 375
transinstitutionalization, 375
criterion validity, 66–67
Cross-National Collaborative Group (CNCG) studies, 46–47
cross-sectional studies, 92
CTC program. *See* Communities That Care program
culture, psychopathology and, 38–39. *See also* emic approach, to mental health; etic approach, to mental health
by age, 51
for alcohol abuse, 51
with CBT, 53
child development influenced by, 51
combined approaches in, 47–48
definitions for, 42
for eating disorders, 51–52
economic development as influence on, 42, 52

with prescription opioids, 174–175
race and, 171–175, 172
  among African Americans, 174
socioeconomic status and, 162–165, 164
universal prevalence rates, 156–157
urban living and, 184–185, 184
DSM-IV. *See* Diagnostic and Statistical Manual, Fourth
  Edition
DTC advertising. *See* direct-to-consumer advertising
DUD. *See* drug use disorder
due process, under U.S. Constitution, 354–355, 354–355
  hypothetical case for, 358
duty to protect, 374–375
eating disorders, 12–13
anorexia nervosa
  diagnostic criteria for, 13
  symptoms of, 12
bulimia nervosa
  diagnostic criteria for, 13
  symptoms of, 12
cultural influences on, 51–52
in GBD study, 13

EB estimation. *See* empirical Bayes estimation
EBLUP. *See* empirical best linear unbiased predictor
ECA program. *See* Epidemiologic Catchment Area program
ecological systems theory, for stress, 278–279
in life-course perspective, 285
in prevention strategies, 468–469
economic development
global mental health system and, financing for, 448–449
mental health influenced by, 42, 52
Edinburgh Postpartum Depression Scale, 49
emic approach, to mental health, 42–43
for culture-bound syndromes, 45
etic approach combined with, 47–48
knowledge of mental disorders in, 43–45
for MDD, 44
for panic attack, 44–45
symptom classification with, 43–44
syndrome description in, 44
emotions, during/after acute crisis, 304–305, 305, 311
empirical Bayes (EB) estimation, 108–109
empirical best linear unbiased predictor (EBLUP), 108–109
employment. *See also* work, stress and
through CBHOs, for people with disabilities, 411–412
ENCODE Project, 202
epidemics, as traumatic event, 325–328
Epidemiologic Catchment Area (ECA) program, 22
in Baltimore, 127, 139
  MDD assessment, 141
as cohort study, 92
needs assessment guidelines, 81
respondent categorization in, 93
socioeconomic status as variable, for mental disorder
  prevalence, 157–157
during third generation of psychiatric epidemiology, 65
epidemiology. *See* psychiatric epidemiology
epigenetics, 233–234
equal protection clause, in U.S. Constitution, 355–356
ADA under, 356, 366
  right to community treatment under, 367
ethics, in prevention strategies for mental disorders, 462
ethnicity, mental disorders and, 165–175
alcohol abuse and, 171–175, 172
  among Latino Americans, 171
  among Native Americans, 171

anxiety disorders, 165–168, 167
  panic disorder, 166–168
bipolar disorder, 169, 170
data review methods, 152–154
DUD and, 171–175, 172
  among Latino Americans, 173
  among Native Americans, 173–174
  with prescription opioids, 174–175
for Latino Americans
  alcohol abuse, 171
  DUD among, 173
  MDD, 168–169
  in NLAAS, 10, 154
MDD, 168–169
for Mexican-Americans, 165
  agoraphobia, 165–166
for Native Americans
  alcohol abuse, 171
  DUD, 173–174
schizophrenia, 169–171
simple phobia and, 167
social phobia and, 167
traumatic events and, risk factors for, 329
etic approach, to mental health, 42–43, 45–47
in CNCG studies, 46–47
emic approach combined with, 47–48
in ICPE surveys, 47
in IPSS, 45–46, 50
executive functions
with AD, 253
with ADHD, 249–250
biological windows of vulnerability for, 248–249
biomarkers for, with mental disorders, 254–256
  in animal models, 255
  in clinical practice, 255
  diagnostic accuracy and, 254–255
  for pathophysiological research, 255
  for therapeutic development, 255–256
brain development and, 246–248
  declines in, 248
  IADL and, 248
components of, 247
with HD, 253–254
interventions for, 256–257
  Experience Corps, 256–257
with MDD, 251–252
with neurodegenerative disorders, 253–254
with PD, 253–254
PFC and, 246
  with ADHD, 249–250
  functions of, 247
  maturation of, 247–248
  with MDD, 251–252
  with schizophrenia, 250–251
  HPA axis and, 251
Experience Corps, 256–257
experimental study design, 91–92
external validity for, 97
generalizability in, 96–98
limitations of, 91–92
exposure therapy, 332–333

family interventions, for mental disorders, 473–477. *See also*
  specific family programs
advantages of, 473
after death of parent, 476–477
after divorce, 476–477

active, environmental stressors and, 281
passive, environmental stressors and, 280–281
reactive, environmental stressors and, 281
Global Burden of Disease (GBD) study, 4
  ADHD in, 12
  affective disorders in, 16–17
  alcoholism in, 21
  anxiety disorders in, 13–16
  autistic disorder in, 11–12
  bipolar disorder in, 16–17
  cognitive disorders in, 17–19
  DALYs in, 4, 21–22
  dementia in, 19
  drug abuse in, 21
  eating disorders in, 13
  MDD in, 16
  measures of disability in, 9, 9–10
  OCD in, 14
  panic disorder in, 13–14
  PTSD in, 14–16
  schizophrenia in, 17–19
  simple phobias in, 14
  social phobia in, 14
  substance use disorders in, 19–21
global mental health systems, 521–522
  action areas for, 446
  BasicNeeds and, 454
  CBM and, 454
  design for, 446
  financing for, 448–449
  human resources in, 447–448
  improvement strategies for, 519–525
    consumer involvement in, 521, 525
    through health literacy, 522
    infrastructural reform, 521
    integration/coordination of care, 519–521
    with patient-centered care, 521–522
    through peer support, 523–524
    as people-centered, 521–525
    recovery in, 521
    with self-directed care, 524–525
    with self-management, 523
    with shared decision-making, 522–523
    through wellness programs, 523
  indicators in, 442–443
  infrastructure for, 445–446
  international data sources for, 443–445
    European baseline surveys, 445
    Mental Health Atlas, 443–444
    in published literature, 445
    WHO-AIMS, 444–445
  International Union of Psychological Sciences and, 454–455
  legislation for, 445–447
    against discrimination, 446–447
  within primary health care, 449–452
    access for, 449
    advocacy for, 450–451
    collaborative organizations for, 452
    coordinators in, 451–452
    as cost-effective, 450
    financial support for, 452
    health care providers in, 451
    health outcome improvements from, 450
    as human rights issue, 449–450
    institutional support for, 451
    medication access in, 451

as process, 451
  public policy for, 450
  training requirements for, 451
public policy for, 445–447
  in primary health care, integration within, 450
research infrastructure for, 452
  economic gaps in, by nation, 452
UNHCR and, 453–454
UNICEF and, 453
WHO and, 453
  WHO-AIMS, 444–445
WPA and, 454
Goethe, Johann Wolfgang von, 44
Goldberger, Joseph, 463
Good Behavior Game, 100, 478–479
Gould, Stephen Jay, 33
grief
  complicated, 308
  traumatic, 308
Griswold v. Connecticut, 356–357
guilty but mentally ill (GBMI), 372, 373–374
GWAS. *See* genome-wide association studies

handicap, definition of, 9
HapMap Project, 202
Hargave v. Vermont, 376
Harlow, Harry, 282
HB estimation. *See* hierarchical Bayes estimation
HD. *See* Huntington's disease
Head Start program
  long-term effects of, 101–102
  regression discontinuity and, 99
health. *See* public mental health
Health and Retirement Survey, 292
health care systems. *See also* global mental health systems
  financing for, 442
  governance structure in, 442
  information systems within, 441–442
  leadership in, 442
  medical technologies in, 442
  service delivery for, 441
  WHO guidelines for, 441
  workforce resources for, 441
health insurance, in U.S., prevalence of, 387–389
health literacy, 522
health-related burden, of mental disorders, 4. *See also* Global Burden of Disease study
  GBD study, 4, 9, 9–10
heterotypic continuity, 285
hierarchical Bayes (HB) estimation, 108–109
Hinckley, John, 372
Hispanic. *See* Latino Americans
histones, 203
HIV. *See* human immunodeficiency virus
homeostasis, stress as influence on, 270
homotypic continuity, 285
Hopi tribe, culture-bound syndromes among, 45
household interview surveys, 64
  in study design, 95
HPA axis. *See* hypothalamic-pituitary-adrenal axis
5-HTT gene, 232
  in stress response, 281
Human Genome Project, 202
human immunodeficiency virus (HIV), 52
human rights. *See also specific rights*
  integration of mental health care in primary care as, 449–450

mental disorders (*Cont.*)
  cultural knowledge of, 43–48
  data analysis of, as latent constructs, 104–107
  disabilities with, 8
  within disease perspective of psychiatry, 35
  in DSM-IV, 4
  emic approach to, 43–45
  epidemiology of, historical challenges with, 4
  executive function and, biomarkers for, 254–256
    in animal models, 255
    in clinical practice, 255
    diagnostic accuracy and, 254–255
    for pathophysiological research, 255
    for therapeutic development, 255–256
  explicit diagnostic criteria for, development of, 4
  family interventions for, 473–477. *See also specific family programs*
    advantages of, 473
    after death of parent, 476–477
    after divorce, 476–477
    with home visiting, 474–475
    limitations of, 473–474
    through parental training, 475–476
  during first generation of psychiatric epidemiology, definitions of, 63
  GBD study, 4, 9, 9–10
  genetic factors for, 206–232. *See also* adoption studies, for mental disorders; family studies, for mental disorders; twin studies, for mental disorders
    for ADHD, 220, 221–224
    for Alzheimer's disease, 231, 218, 219
    association studies for, 230, 231
    for autism spectrum disorder, 226
    for bipolar disorder, 213–214
    challenges with, 232–234
    for conduct disorder, 225
    DNA sequencing for, 233
    environmental factors a influence on, 232
    epigenetics for, 233–234
    family studies for, 207–208, 209, 210, 211–212
    generational transmission of, 228–229
    heritability and, 227, 227–228
    5-HTT gene and, 232
    linkage studies for, 229–230, 230–231
    new approaches to, 233–234
    for OCD, 207–208
    for panic disorder, 209
    for schizophrenia, 215–217
    segregation studies for, 229
    susceptibility genes and, 229–232
    twin studies for, 227, 207–208, 209
  health-related burden of, 4
  among Latino Americans
    alcohol abuse, 171
    DUD, 173
    MDD, 168–169
    in NLAAS, 10, 154
  law and, involuntary commitment, 362–363, 363
  marital status and, 175–181
    alcohol abuse and, 178–181, 180
    anxiety disorders, 175–177
    bipolar disorder, 178, 178
    data review methods, 152–154
    DUD and, 178–181, 180
    MDD and, 177–178, 176
    schizophrenia and, 178, 179

  among Mexican-Americans, 165
    agoraphobia, 165–166
  mortality and, 144, 143
  among Native Americans
    alcohol abuse, 171
    DUD, 173–174
  phenotypes for, definition of, 206
  population disparities for, 153, 186
  prevalence rates for, 6–7
  prevention strategies, research methodologies for, 467–468, 468
  screening programs for, 491–492
  as social stigma, in dark ages of public mental health, 399
  social stigma for
    during adolescence, 424
    among African Americans, 424
    changes in public attitudes, 427–428
    in dark ages of public mental health, 399
    in non-Western societies, 424
    public campaigns for prevention of, 424–426
    for treatment seeking, 423–424
  urbanicity and, 181–185
    alcohol abuse and, 184–185, 184
    anxiety disorders, 181, 182
    bipolar disorder, 183, 182
    data review methods, 152–154
    DUD and, 184–185, 184
    MDD, 181–183, 182
    schizophrenia, 183–184, 184
  in U.S., prevalence rates for, 386, 386–390
mental health. *See also* assessment, of mental disorders; emic approach, to mental health; etic approach, to mental health; global mental health systems; health care systems; needs, assessment of; study design, for mental health
  competency to stand trial, 374
  criminal law and, 371–375
    competency to stand trial, 374
    duty to protect and, 374–375
    GBMI, 372, 373–374
    insanity defense, 372, 371–373
    special courts for, 375
    transinstitutionalization, 375
  cultural impacts on, 42–43, 49–50
  economic development as influence on, 42, 52
  gender and, cultural influences on, 50–51
  law and, 358–371. *See also* children's rights; right to refuse treatment; right to treatment in safe/humane environment
    for college students, 376–378
    competency for consent, 360–361
    for confidentiality, 358–359, 376–378
    during disasters, 379
    for informed consent, 359–360, 361
    public policy and, 352
    right to community treatment, 367–368
    in treatment seeking interventions, 432–433
  public health model for, 513–517
    improved data sources for, 513–514
    prevention goals in, 516
    requirements for, 517
    scientific knowledge in, adjusted weight of, 514–515, 515–516
    service improvements in, 515–516
    treatment goals in, 516
  social determinants of, 517–519
    communities as, 517–518

economic disparity as, 518–519
promotion and prevention strategies as, 519
resilience as, 519
trauma and, 313–314
treatment seeking for, pathways to, 422–433
barriers to, 423, 430–432
through DTC advertising, 429, 429–430, 428–430
financial barriers to, 430–432
increased public knowledge of, 428
through institutions, 422
legislative interventions for, 432–433
medication trends in, 428–430
social stigma and, 423–424, 424–426, 427–428
in U.S., 382–385, 384. *See also* community health services, in U.S.
ambulatory admission rates in, 385
bed turnover rates for, 385
children's services in, 383
with CIDI, 386
Community Support Program, 383
costs of, 390–393, 392. *See also specific disorders*
general health care, 383
hospital system in, expansion of, 383–385
human service sector, 383
insurance prevalence in, 387–389
in juvenile justice system, 390
multi-service organizations in, 386
in NCS-R, 386, 386–390
patterns of care in, 385, 389–390
prevalence of mental disorders, 386, 386–390
prevalence of substance abuse disorders, 386–390
professional human resources in, 385
residential treatment services in, 383
revenues from, 392–393
under SAMHSA, 389–390
self-help sector, 383
specialty sector, 383–384
treatment prevalence in, 387–389
workforce resources for, 441
Mental Health Atlas, 443–444
Mental Health Parity and Addiction Equity Act (U.S.), 406, 417, 433
Mental Retardation Facilities and Community Mental Health Centers Construction (CMHC) Act, 402–405
community support tools under, 404–405
psychoactive drug development under, 403–404
psychotherapy under, 404
mentoring. *See* youth mentoring, as intervention strategy
Methods for the Epidemiology of Child and Adolescent Mental Disorders (MECA) study, 110
Mexican-Americans, mental disorders among, 165
agoraphobia, 165–166
military personnel. *See also* posttraumatic stress disorder
war as traumatic event for, 318
Mills v. Rogers, 364
the mind
attributes of, 33
features of, 33
mitosis, 203–204
M'Naghten, Daniel, 372
monoamine oxidase A (MAOA), 281
mood disorders. *See* affective disorders; major depressive disorder
mortality, mental disorders and, 144, 143
multi-service organizations, in U.S., 386

National Anxiety Disorders Screening Day, 425
National Comorbidity Survey (NCS), 127, 131, 139
National Comorbidity Survey-Replication (NCS-R), 10, 76, 154
MDD in, 77
for mental disorder prevalence in U.S., 386, 386–390
for substance abuse disorder prevalence in U.S., 386–390
National Epidemiologic Study on Alcohol and Related Conditions (NESARC) survey, 140, 140. *See also* ethnicity, mental disorders and; marital status, mental disorders and; race, mental disorders and; socioeconomic status, mental disorders and; urbanicity, mental disorders and
alcohol abuse in, urbanicity as variable for, 184
anxiety disorders in, urbanicity as variable for, 182
bipolar disorders in, urbanicity as variable for, 183
DUD in, urbanicity as variable for, 184
MDD in, urbanicity as variable for, 182
schizophrenia in, urbanicity as variable for, 184
National Latino and Asian American Survey (NLAAS), 10
National Longitudinal Alcohol Epidemiology Study (NLAES), 162
National Survey of American Life (NSAL), 10, 154
National Survey on Drug Use and Health (NSDUH), 110
Native Americans, mental disorders among
alcohol abuse, 171
DUD, 173–174
natural disasters, as traumatic events, 321–325, 327–328
natural killer cell cytotoxicity (NKCC) levels, 290
nature *versus* nurture, 202
NCS. *See* National Comorbidity Survey
NCS-R. *See* National Comorbidity Survey-Replication
needs, assessment of, 79–83
definitions in, 80
demand for care compare to, 80–81
direct clinical, 82–83
ECA program guidelines, 81
for mental disability, 80
for mental impairment, 80
for populations, 81
negligence doctrine, 359–360
NESARC survey. *See* National Epidemiologic Study on Alcohol and Related Conditions survey
neurasthenia, in China, 44
neurodegenerative disorders, executive functions and, 253–254. *See also* Alzheimer's disease; Huntington's disease; Parkinson's disease
New Beginnings program, 476–477
NFP. *See* Nurse Family Partnership
NGOs. *See* nongovernmental organizations
Nigeria, 44
NKCC levels. *See* natural killer cell cytotoxicity levels
NLAAS. *See* National Latino and Asian American Survey
NLAES. *See* National Longitudinal Alcohol Epidemiology Study
No Child Left Behind Act (U.S.), 478
non-experimental study design, 92
Berkson bias in, 94–95
case-control, 92
cohort, 92
cross-sectional, 92
external validity in, 98
generalizability in, 94–96
instrumental variables methods, 99
interrupted time series in, 99
long-term follow-up strategies in, 101–102
propensity score matching in, 99–100

prevalence studies, for mental disorders
  data analysis for, estimation methods, 107–109
  gender separation in, 9
  lifetime prevalence, 7
  methodology for, 7–10
  one-year prevalence, 7
  population-based, 8–9
  sample sizes for, 8
prevention strategies, for mental disorders
  advancements in neuroscience, 493
  Alzheimer's disease, 472–473
  at community level, 483–489. *See also specific community programs*
    advantages of, 483
    as broad-based, 484–485
    institutional interventions for, 486–487
    for substance abuse, 488–489
    for underserved populations, 486–487
    for violence prevention, 485–486
    through youth mentoring, 487–488
  cost-benefit analyses for, 493
  current status of, 468
  definitions for, 463–465
  for delirium tremens, 462–463
  disease burden in, 461–462
  dissemination of, 493–494
  ecological systems theory in, 468–469
  epidemiology in, 466–467
  ethics of, 462
  through family intervention, 473–477. *See also specific family programs*
    advantages of, 473
    after death of parent, 476–477
    after divorce, 476–477
    with home visiting, 474–475
    limitations of, 473–474
    through parental training, 475–476
    programs for, 476, 476–477
  for general paresis, 463
  goal-setting in, 463–466
  historical perspective on, 462–463
  implementation of, 493–494
  institutional infrastructure development for, 494
  integrated framework for, 466–468
  international initiatives for, 494
  Internet-based, 492
  intervention trials research for, 467
  IOM guidelines, 463–465
  life-course development in, 467
  life-course perspective on, 470
  MDD, 470–471
    CWD course, 471
  for pellagra, 463
  primary, 463
  in public health model, 516
  through public policy, 489–491
    through education improvements, 489–490
    with evidence-based practices, 490
    through firearms legislation, 490–491
    for substance abuse, 490
  rationale for, 461–462
  through replication studies, 492–493
  research methodologies for, 467–468
    growth modeling techniques, 468
  schizophrenia, 471–472
  in schools, 477–481. *See also specific school programs*
    for college students, 376–378

  development of, 477–478
    indicated models for, 479–480
    integrated models for, 480–481
    universal models for, 478–480
  through screening programs, 491–492
  for scurvy, 462
  secondary, 465
  as social determinant for mental health, 519
  successful approaches in, 464
  tertiary, 465
  timing of, age and, 469–470
  in workplace, 481–483
primary health care systems, global mental health systems integrated within, 449–452
  access for, 449
  advocacy for, 450–451
  collaborative organizations for, 452
  coordinators in, 451–452
  as cost-effective, 450
  financial support for, 452
  health care providers in, 451
  health outcome improvements from, 450
  as human rights issue, 449–450
  institutional support for, 451
  medication access in, 451
  as process, 451
  public policy for, 450
  training requirements for, 451
Primary Health Questionnaire-9, 76
primary prevention strategies, for mental disorders, 463
private law, 353
probability sampling, 95
prodrome period, 128–129
Project Atlas, 432
propensity score matching, 99–100
Prozac. *See* fluoxetine
psychiatric epidemiology
  first generation of, 62, 63, 62–64
    assessment methods for, 62–63
    classic studies in, 62
    mental illness during, definition of, 63
  historical background of, 62–65
  historical challenges with, 4
  second generation of, 64
    household interview surveys during, 64
  third generation of, 4, 64–65
    ECA during, 65
psychiatric examinations, 67–69
  with SCAN, 68–69, 73–74, 74
  with SCID, 69
psychiatrists, 33
  increases in, 416
psychiatry, perspectives of, 34–39
  behavior perspective, 37
    consciousness in, 37
    public health applications of, 37
    substance abuse disorders and, 37
  combinations of, 38–39
  dimensional perspective, 36, 36–37
    affective disorders within, 36
    consciousness in, 36–37
    public health applications of, 36–37
  disease perspective, 34–35, 35–36, 35
    consciousness and, 34–36
    mental disorders within, 35
    neuropathology in, 34–35
    public health applications, 35–36

external validity in, 98
generalizability in, 94–96
instrumental variables methods, 99
interrupted time series in, 99, 99
long-term follow-up strategies in, 101–102
propensity score matching in, 99–100
with rare outcomes, 102
regression analysis for, 98
regression discontinuity in, 99, 99
population specificity in, 92–98
Berkson bias in, 94–95
in experimental studies, 96–98
external validity for, 97
generalizability in, 94–98
household surveys for, 95
internal validity for, 97–98
in non-experimental studies, 94–96
prevalence data and, 93–94
probability sampling for, 95
in randomized trials, 96
random sampling for, 95
Substance Abuse and Mental Health Services
　Administration (SAMHSA), 389–390
substance abuse disorders
age of onset for, 136
alcohol abuse
after acute crisis, 309
CAGE scale for, 76
costs for treatment, in U.S., 392
cultural distinctions for, 51
delirium tremens and, 462–463
ethnicity, 171, 171–175, 172
in GBD, 21
among Latino Americans, 171
literature studies for, 21
marital status and, 178–181, 180
among Native Americans, 171
race and, 174, 171–175, 172
socioeconomic status and, 162–165, 164
universal prevalence rates, 156–157
urban living and, 184–185, 184
in behavior perspective of psychiatry, 37
cost of treatment, in U.S., 391
DUD, 20–21
after acute crisis, 309
among African Americans, 174
costs for treatment, in U.S., 392
diagnostic criteria for, 156–157
educational level and, 163
ethnicity, 171–175, 172
in GBD study, 21
among Latino Americans, 173
marital status and, 178–181, 180
among Native Americans, 173–174
race, 171–175, 172
socioeconomic status and, 162–165, 164
universal prevalence rates, 156–157
urban living and, 184–185, 184
in GBD study, 19–21
with marijuana, 174
with prescription opioids, 174–175
prevention strategies for
at community level, 488–489
through public policy, 490
substance dependence compared to, 19
in U.S., prevalence rates, 386–390
substance dependence, 19

diagnostic criteria for, 20
suicide
after acute crises, 310
signs of ideation, 322–323
Sundram, Clarence, 365
Supplemental Security Disability Income (SSDI)
　program, 405
Supplemental Security Income (SSI) program, 405
Supreme Court, U.S., 353
survey contractors, 79
susceptibility genes, 229–232
for stress, 280–281
Sutton, Thomas, 463
syndromes. *See* culture-bound syndromes
synthetic estimation methods, 107–108
Tarasoff v. the Regents of the University of California, 374–375
10th Amendment. *See* reserved powers, under U.S.
　Constitution
terrorism, as traumatic event, 323–324
tertiary prevention strategies, for mental disorders, 465
test-retest reliability, 65
TF-CBT. *See* trauma-focused cognitive-behavioral therapy
theory of cumulative risk. *See* cumulative risk, theory of
theory of reasoned action. *See* reasoned action, theory of
third generation, of psychiatric epidemiology, 4, 64–65
ECA during, 65
tobacco use, after acute crisis, 309
PTSD and, 309
tolerable stress, 272
total institution, 402
toxic stress, 272
transcultural approach, to mental health. *See* etic approach,
　to mental health
transinstitutionalization, 375
trauma-focused cognitive-behavioral therapy (TF-CBT),
　331–332
traumatic events
definition of, 313–314
disasters as, 321–328
mental health access after, as law, 379
natural, 321–325, 327–328
individual, 314–321
accidents as, 317
acute physical injury as, 317
child sexual abuse as, 307
crime as, exposure to, 314–317
illness as, 317–318
for military personnel, 318
for refugees, 318–321
violence as, 314–317
intervention strategies for, 330–334
exposure therapy, 332–333
IPT, 333–334
mixed, 333
non trauma-focused, 333
PFA, 330–331
resources for, 332
TF-CBT, 331–332
mass, 321–328
bioterrorism as, 325–328
emerging epidemics as, 325–328
industrial accidents as, 321, 325
terrorism as, 323–324
violence, 321
mental health and, 313–314
methodological measurements for, 314
prevalence of exposure to, 314, 326–327

Venter, Craig, 202
violence
  prevention strategies for
    at community level, 485–486
    through firearms legislation, 490–491
  as traumatic event
    for individuals, 314–317
    for large populations, 321

war, as traumatic event, 320–321
  for citizens, as refugees, 318–321
  for military personnel, 318
We Are Not Alone program, 409–410
wellness programs, in global mental health systems, 523
Wellness Recovery Action Plan (WRAP), 523
WHO. See World Health Organization
WHO Assessment Instrument for Mental Health Systems
    (WHO-AIMS), 444–445
Wilson, William Julius, 282
Winslow, Charles-Edward A., 512
WMH surveys. See World Mental Health surveys
women
  cultural influences on mental health for, 50–51
  Edinburgh Postpartum Depression Scale for, 49
  exposure to traumatic events, 328
  postpartum depression in, cultural influences on
    treatment, 51

in romantic relationships, stress from, 289
in work environment, stress from, 290–291
Women's Health Initiative, 96
work
  prevention strategies at, for mental disorders,
    481–483
  stress and, 290–291
    gender differences and, 290–291
    NKCC levels, 290
World Health Organization (WHO)
  Clinical Descriptions and Diagnostic Guidelines, 32
  global health care system guidelines, 441
  global mental health systems and, 453
  ICPE surveys, 47
  IPSS, 45–46, 50
  Mental Health Atlas, 443–444
  WHO-AIMS, 444–445
World Mental Health (WMH) surveys, 47
World Psychiatric Association (WPA), 454
worry, GAD and, 252–253
WPA. See World Psychiatric Association
WRAP. See Wellness Recovery Action Plan
Wyatt standards, for safe/humane treatment, 365
Wyatt v. Stickney, 365

Youngberg v. Romeo, 364, 365
youth mentoring, as intervention strategy, 487–488

CPSIA information can be obtained at www.ICGtesting.com
Printed in the USA
LVOW03s0559120915

453639LV00017B/18/P